Teaching Atlas of Musculoskeletal Imaging

Thieme

Teaching Atlas of Musculoskeletal Imaging

Peter L. Munk, M.D., C.M., F.R.C.P.C.
Professor
Departments of Radiology and Orthopaedics
University of British Columbia
Head
Section of Musculoskeletal Radiology
Vancouver General Hospital and Health Science Center
Vancouver, British Columbia, Canada

Anthony G. Ryan, M.B., B.C.H., B.A.O., F.R.C.S.I., M.Sc. (Engineering and Physical Sciences in Medicine), D.I.C., F.R.C.R., F.F.R.R.C.S.I.
Consultant Musculoskeletal and Interventional Radiologist
Waterford Regional Teaching Hospital
Ardkeen, Waterford City, Republic of Ireland
Radiologic Tutor and Clinical Instructor in Radiology
The Royal College of Surgeons in Ireland
Dublin, Republic of Ireland

Thieme
New York • Stuttgart

Thieme Medical Publishers, Inc.
333 Seventh Ave.
New York, NY 10001

Editor: Birgitta Brandenburg
Assistant Editor: Ivy Ip
Vice President, Production and Electronic Publishing: Anne T. Vinnicombe
Production Editor: Print Matters, Inc.
Vice President, International Marketing: Cornelia Schulze
Sales Director: Ross Lumpkin
Chief Financial Officer: Peter van Woerden
President: Brian D. Scanlan
Compositor: Compset, Inc.
Printer: The Maple-Vail Book Manufacturing Group

Library of Congress Cataloging-in-Publication Data

Munk, Peter L.
Teaching atlas of musculoskeletal imaging / Peter L. Munk, Anthony G. Ryan.
p. ; cm.
Includes bibliographical references and index.
ISBN-13: 978-1-58890-372-3 (alk. paper)
ISBN-10: 1-58890-372-9 (alk. paper)
ISBN-13: 978-3-13-141981-1 (alk. paper)
ISBN-10: 3-13-141981-4 (alk. paper)
1. Musculoskeletal system—Diseases—Imaging—Atlases. 2. Musculoskeletal system—Diseases—Case studies. I. Ryan, Anthony G. II. Title.
[DNLM: 1. Musculoskeletal Diseases—diagnosis—Atlases. 2. Musculoskeletal Diseases—diagnosis—Case Reports. 3. Diagnostic Imaging—Atlases. 4. Diagnostic Imaging—Case Reports. 5. Musculoskeletal System—injuries—Atlases. 6. Musculoskeletal System—injuries—Case Reports. WE 17 M966t 2007]
RC925.5.M86 2007
616.7'0754—dc22

2006102651

Printed in the United States
5 4 3 2 1

The Americas ISBN 978-1-58890-372-3

Rest of World ISBN 978-3-13-141981-1

DEDICATIONS

To my wife, Alice Maria Chung, who has loved me and stuck by me through difficult and easy times; to my daughters, Charlotte Gisele Munk, Eleanor Ruth Munk, and Sophie Alexis Munk, who have taught me the meaning of true affection; and to our Lord, Jesus Christ.

—Peter L. Munk

For those to whom I owe the greatest debt of gratitude: my parents, Margaret and Jeremiah Ryan (Ní bheidh a leithéidí ann arís); and for those for whom I am continually grateful—my wife, Caitríona, and son, Michael.

—Anthony G. Ryan

CONTENTS

PREFACE

If *Teaching Atlas of Musculoskeletal Imaging* had been written 30 or 40 years ago, it no doubt would have looked much different from the current volume and in some ways would have been much simpler to put together. At that time, the book would have consisted almost exclusively of radiographs, with the occasional tomogram and arthrogram or other infrequent imaging technique. The current volume, although, of course, using radiography throughout, includes a great deal of cross-sectional imaging; particularly computed tomography and magnetic resonance imaging, which have come to revolutionize the way musculoskeletal imaging has been performed.

Trying to cover all of musculoskeletal radiology in one book is, of course, nearly impossible, and the task to me sounded like having an examination question posed that reads "explain the universe and give three examples." This volume is not meant to be an exhaustive compilation of the imaging features of every clinical entity that occurs in the musculoskeletal system—if it were, this mammoth task would have taken many more authors, many more years, and many more volumes to complete. What we have sought to do is show a broad range of representative clinical conditions with some of the more classical imaging findings. Certainly not all common conditions will be found in this book, and a few infrequently encountered ones have been included for the sake of variety and scope. The atlas is organized into eight broad sections totaling 130 cases. For each case a selection of representative images is provided, as is a discussion centered on clinical and imaging features. Differential diagnosis and a few representative references are also typically included. The emphasis varies depending on the individual case.

This text was particularly designed for trainees in radiology and those practicing general radiology who have an interest in musculoskeletal disease. We hope it will also be useful to other practitioners of musculoskeletal medicine, including those in orthopedics.

ACKNOWLEDGMENTS

As with most projects like this, the amount of effort required and complexity always seem to be more than originally anticipated. The encouragement of my wife and three daughters has been critical to my completion of this project. In addition, several friends and colleagues made a genuine difference. Among these are Rev. David Demchuk of Vancouver, Rev. Michael J. Voll of Edmonton, and Dr. Mark J. Lee of Calgary, whose unflagging friendship and encouragement were critical. I cannot fail to mention as well two of my colleagues at the Vancouver General Hospital, Mr. Laurel O. Marchinkow and Dr. Gerald M. Legiehn. I also would be remiss if I did not acknowledge the good sense of humor and help of my secretary, Ms. Jenny Silver, and the technical wizardry of my research associate, Mr. Michael Mudri. The encouragement of Dr. Tommy Pope of Charleston was also appreciated.

—Peter L. Munk

I thank Pete Munk for giving me the opportunity to coauthor this book (an honor and a privilege), for an awesome year's fellowship at Vancouver General Hospital, and for his ongoing friendship. I cannot really give thanks for the grey hairs, my constant pained expression, and the encephalomalacia resulting from the actual authoring.

I thank all the other authors for their invaluable contributions.

I thank Jenny Silver and Lorie Marchinkow of Vancouver General Hospital for their tireless work in drafting the manuscript and the fantastic line diagrams respectively. I also thank Judith Tomat and Birgitta Brandenburg of Thieme, and Richard Rothschild of Print Matters for their unstinting efforts in producing a finished volume from the rough-hewn manuscript with which they were presented.

Most of all, I thank my wife Caitríona, without whose patience and forbearance my contribution to this volume could never have happened.

Last but not least, I thank my son Michael for his patience while waiting for Dad to play. The back of my head is now more recognizable to him from watching me returning to the office to "just do some work on another chapter." Now that the book is on the shelf, it's time to play ball!

—Anthony G. Ryan

CONTRIBUTORS

Editors

Peter L. Munk, M.D., C.M., F.R.C.P.C.
Professor
Departments of Radiology and Orthopaedics
University of British Columbia
Head
Section of Musculoskeletal Radiology
Vancouver General Hospital and Health Science Center
Vancouver, British Columbia, Canada

Anthony G. Ryan, M.B., B.C.H., B.A.O., F.R.C.S.I., M.Sc. (Engineering and Physical Sciences in Medicine), D.I.C., F.R.C.R., F.F.R.R.C.S.I.
Consultant Musculoskeletal and Interventional Radiologist
Waterford Regional Teaching Hospital
Ardkeen, Waterford City, Republic of Ireland
Radiologic Tutor and Clinical Instructor in Radiology
The Royal College of Surgeons in Ireland
Dublin, Republic of Ireland

Contributors

Hema N. Choudur, M.B.B.S., D.N.B.
Assistant Professor
Wentworth/Halton X-Ray and Ultrasound, Inc.
Central Business Office
Hamilton, Ontario, Canada

Sam Y. Chun, M.D., F.R.C.P.C.
Valley Radiologists
Federal Way, Washington

Bruce B. Forster, M.Sc., M.D., F.R.C.P.C.
Associate Professor and Vice Chair, Research
Department of Radiology
University of British Columbia
Vancouver General Hospital and Health Science Center
Vancouver, British Columbia, Canada

Ali Islam, M.D., F.R.C.D.
Associate Professor
Department of Radiology
Schulich School of Medicine and Dentistry
Director of Cardiac CT and MRI
St. Joseph's Health Care
London, Ontario, Canada

Laurel O. Marchinkow, R.T.R.
Department of Radiology
Vancouver General Hospital and Health Science Center
Vancouver, British Columbia, Canada

Mark Murphey, M.D.
Chief
Department of Radiologic Pathology
Armed Forces Institute of Pathology
Washington, District of Columbia

Nizar Al-Nakshabandi, M.D., F.R.C.P.C.
Assistant Professor
Department of Radiology
College of Medicine
King Saud University
King Khalid University Hospital
Riyadh, Saudi Arabia

George Nomikos, M.D.
Assistant Professor
Department of Radiology
New York University Medical Center
Hospital for Joint Diseases Orthopaedic Institute
New York, New York

Thomas Pope, M.D., F.A.C.R.
Professor
Departments of Radiology and Orthopaedics
Medical University of South Carolina
Charleston, South Carolina
Consulting Radiologist
Frankin and Seidelmann Subspecialty Radiology
Beachwood, Ohio

Brian Edward Reeves, D.O.
The Woman's Place
Florida Hospital
Orange City, Florida

Kevin Rowan, M.D., F.R.P.C.
Clinical Instructor
Department of Radiology
University of British Columbia
Vancouver, British Columbia, Canada

Alison Spouge, M.D., F.R.C.P.C.
Associate Professor
Department of Radiology
University of Western Ontario
Department of Diagnostic Imaging
University Hospital
London Health Sciences Centre
London, Ontario Canada

CASE 1

Anthony G. Ryan and Peter L. Munk

Clinical Presentation

A 23-year-old man presented after a skiing injury with a painful knee that had swollen gradually over a period of hours since the injury. Clinical examination revealed an obvious effusion but no excessive motion (i.e., a negative drawer sign).

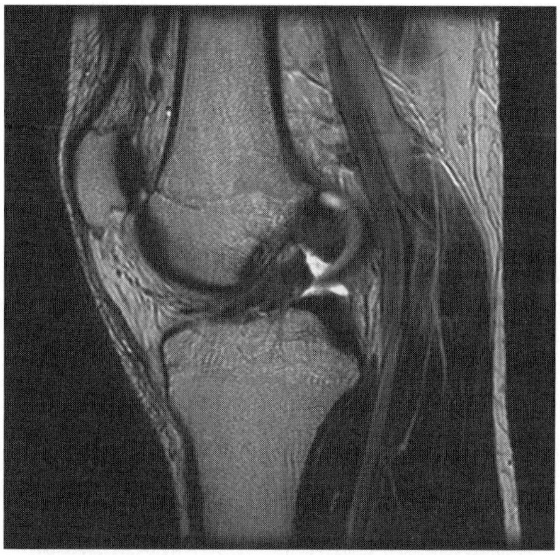

Figure 1A

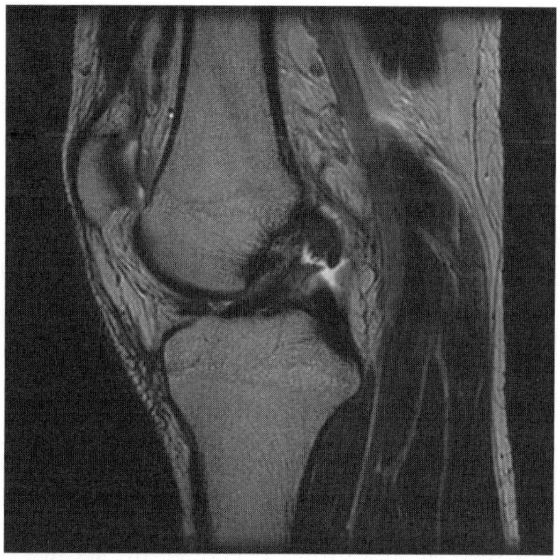

Figure 1B

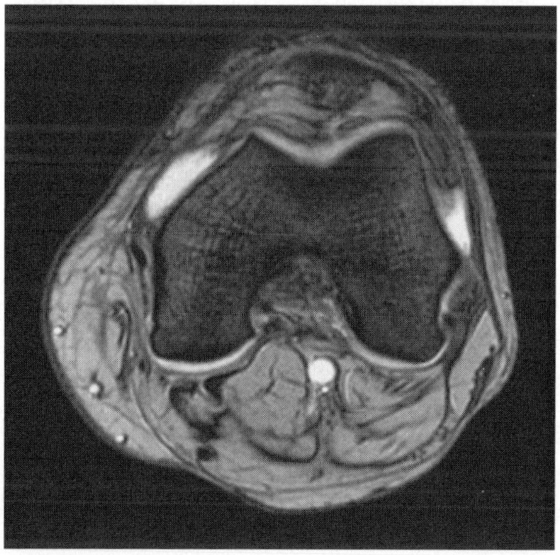

Figure 1C

Radiologic Findings

MRI (**Figs. 1A–1C**) revealed a focal discontinuity of the cranial third of the anterior cruciate ligament (ACL).

Diagnosis

Complete tear of the cranial third of the ACL.

Discussion

Background

The typical pattern of injury (see below) is partially explained by the internal structure of the ligament. The distal attachment of the ligament is stronger than the proximal, having a broader base and an attachment to the anterior horn of the lateral meniscus in addition to the tibia. The ligament consists of two distinct components: anterior and posterior bands. The anterior band is stronger, containing more tightly packed fibers and thus conferring greater stability to the knee joint and resisting anterior tibial displacement. Although the fibers of the posterior band are packed less tightly, they remain taut in extension, thus resisting hyperextension.

Etiology

The classic mode of ACL injury is forced valgus strain on a fixed leg. It occurs in sports such as American football, soccer, and, less commonly, rugby. An almost equal and increasing incidence of ACL tears is seen in skiers, however, when the femur is forced into external rotation on a fixed tibia. In football players, the tear tends to occur in the midportion of the ligament, as a result of the direct impact and resultant "snapping"; in skiers, the ligament tends to tear proximally, as a result of the forced longitudinal strain.

Clinical Findings

The typical pattern of ACL injury is that of an acute event, resulting in severe pain, an accompanying "snap," and immediate disability. Delayed knee swelling is usual, with an immediate effusion more frequently seen in association with an intra-articular fracture. A hemarthrosis frequently accompanies complete ACL tears, but is seen less commonly with partial tears.

Clinical examination is especially limited acutely, secondary to the associated pain and muscular spasm, with the anterior drawer and Lachman's tests having sensitivities in the region of 78 to 89%, respectively.

Arthroscopy, although clearly more accurate than physical exam, is invasive and expensive. False-negative arthroscopy may occur secondary to an obscuring infrapatellar plica, a partially healed torn ligament, or an intact synovial envelope (the ACL being intracapsular but extrasynovial).

Complications

Knees with deficient ACLs are particularly susceptible to developing arthritis secondary to the increased translation of the femur on the tibia. In athletes, the resultant loss of strength and stability may be career-ending if the ligament is not repaired; even then, some professionals never return to their previous level of performance.

Imaging Findings

RADIOGRAPHY

If an associated fracture of the lateral tibial plateau is present (Segond fracture, **Figs. 1D,1E**), a "lateral capsular" sign may be present, whereby the bony fragment is seen projected adjacent to the lateral tibial plateau, which may be oriented in any direction, depending on the degree of hemarthrosis and so on that is present.

The "deep lateral notch" sign (**Figs. 1F,1G**) is a notch produced in the lateral femoral condyle as a result of impaction of the condyle against the posterolateral tibial plateau. There may be an associated fracture of the tibial plateau.

The tibial attachment may be avulsed without an accompanying tear of the ACL (**Fig. 1H**); this latter pattern is seen more commonly in male children.

MAGNETIC RESONANCE IMAGING

MRI is the investigation of choice for a complete tear, with sensitivities reported between 92 and 100%. A standard internal derangement protocol (oblique sagittal fast spin-echo [FSE] T2, coronal fast-recovery fast spin-echo (FRFSE) T2 with fat-saturation, sagittal T1, sagittal MPGR [multiplaner gradient

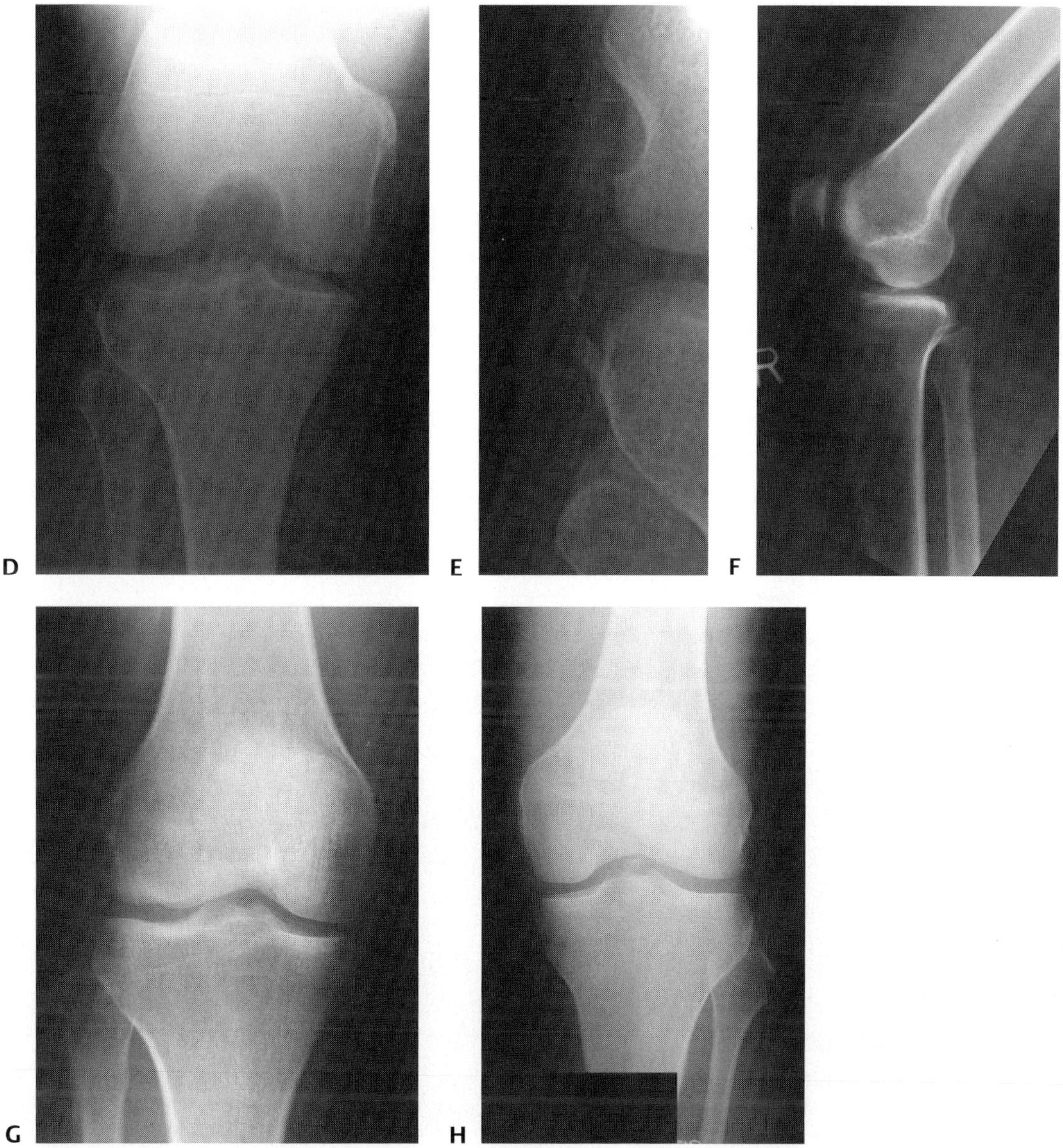

Figures 1D "Tunnel" view of the knee in a patient with a previously ruptured anterior cruciate ligament (ACL) shows the previous fracture and subsequent capsular calcification. **1E** Magnified view of the injury shown in **Figs. 1D**. **1F** and **1G** The "deep lateral notch" is produced as a result of impaction of the lateral femoral condyle against the posterolateral tibial plateau when the ACL snaps. **1H** Avulsion of the tibial attachment, which in this case was not associated with an ACL tear.

recall], and axial MPGR) will show the majority of acute injuries, with the sagittal oblique T2 and sagittal MPGR most likely to demonstrate the disruption to best effect. The axial sequences are thought by some authors to increase the sensitivity for partial tears.

The normal ACL appears as a dark, 3- to 4-mm band extending from the anterior tibia to the medial aspect of the lateral femoral condyle, with the stronger anterior band noticeably darker than the posterior component. If an effusion is present, fluid may track between the anterior and posterior bands of an intact ACL, producing apparent intrasubstance high signal intensity suggestive of a tear.

If an acute complete tear is present, this will be evident by ligamentous discontinuity and associated high signal intensity on fluid-sensitive sequences. The ligament, or portions of it, may be indistinct and surrounded by ill-defined, heterogeneous signal intensity secondary to hemorrhage (**Figs. 1I,1J**).

A delay of several weeks after the initial injury may be advantageous, as in the interim, hemorrhage and edema will subside, making the ACL findings more conspicuous. The remaining intact fibers typically assume a wavy pattern and may sometimes be seen lying flat along the floor of the tibial intercondylar region. This latter finding may be appreciated by first noting the loss of parallelism of the ligament with the intercondylar roof. The ligament may begin to retract secondary to ischemia.

If imaging is delayed over 2 months, the appearances may become less easy to interpret. If a remotely torn ligament has had an opportunity to heal by scar formation, the ligament may appear intact but clinically will be much weaker and the joint will be unstable. If the tear is of the cranial portion, the femoral attachment may be seen to be avulsed and in some cases, it may actually reattach by granulation tissue to the adjacent posterior cruciate ligament (PCL).

Partial tears

Although axial images are said to provide a high sensitivity for partial tears, the diagnosis remains challenging. Sagittal and coronal images may show focal areas of increased signal, or the ligament may be diffusely thickened and demonstrate patchy increased high signal. It is generally considered,

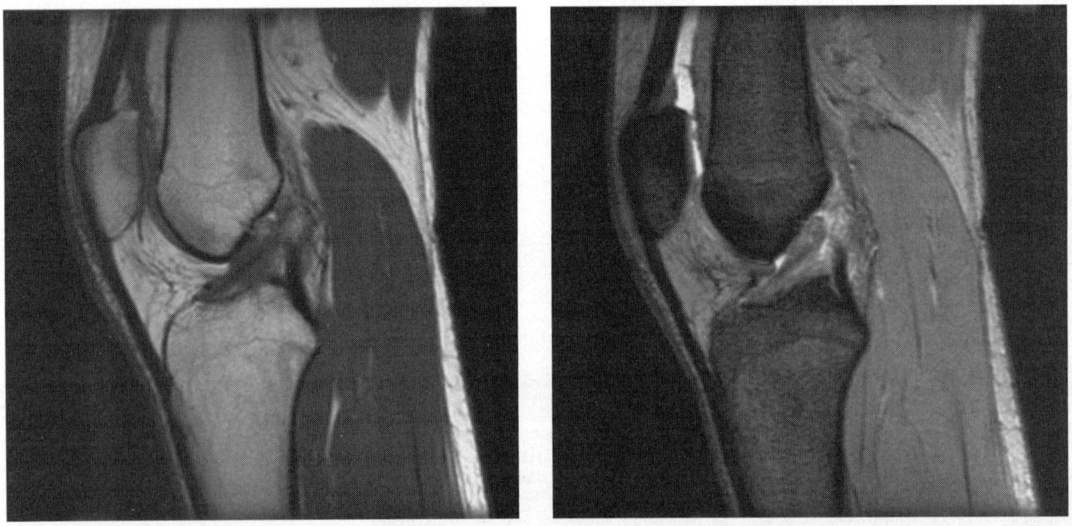

I J

Figures 1I and **1J** T1- and T2-weighted images, respectively, of an undisplaced complete tear of the cranial anterior cruciate ligament. The ligament is indistinct, returns heterogeneous signal intensity, and is surrounded by ill-defined, heterogeneous signal intensity secondary to hemorrhage. Discontinuity is evident at the cranial extent of the visualized ligament.

however, that if a partial tear is evident, it is likely to be clinically significant, as even small, so-called stable tears can progress over time to become complete with subsequent disability. Conversely, it is thought that if a tear is not visible, it is not likely to be clinically relevant.

Ancillary evidence of ACL tears

Anterior subluxation greater than 7 mm of the tibia with respect to the femur is 100% specific for ACL tear. Translation to this extent is also likely to cause obvious PCL buckling.

Bone bruises

Given the nature of the forces involved in rupturing the ACL, it is not surprising that there are expected patterns of "kissing" bone contusion, which will be evident on fluid-sensitive sequences such as short tau inversion recovery (STIR) or T2 fat-saturated. Poorly defined areas of low signal intensity on T1-weighted images are suggestive but typically less conspicuous than on the aforementioned sequences (**Figs. 1K,1L**).

The edema is typically seen in the lateral femoral condyle adjacent to the anterior horn of the lateral meniscus and in the posterolateral tibial plateau. Impaction forces may produce osteochondral fractures of the lateral femoral condyle, which may be seen on radiographs as the deep lateral notch sign.

Avulsion fractures

Segond fractures are clearly identified by MRI performed acutely. Less commonly, avulsions may be seen at the insertions of the semimembranosus and arcuate ligament insertions. Avulsion of the tibial attachment without an accompanying tear of the ACL is seen most frequently in boys.

Treatment

In the nonprofessional athlete, a conservative approach is more likely, with physical therapy given to strengthen the quadriceps muscles to restore knee joint stability.

K

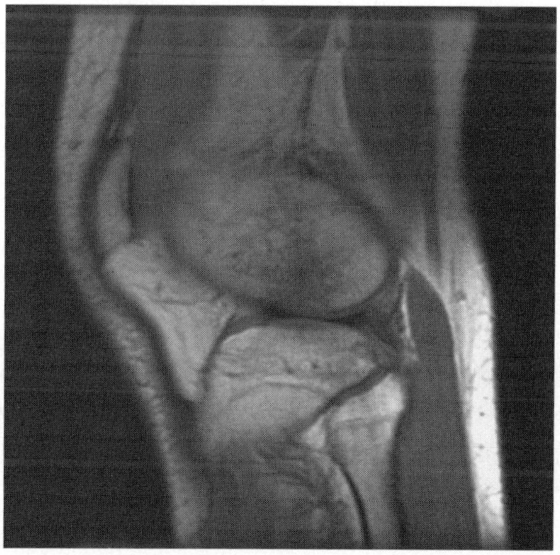

L

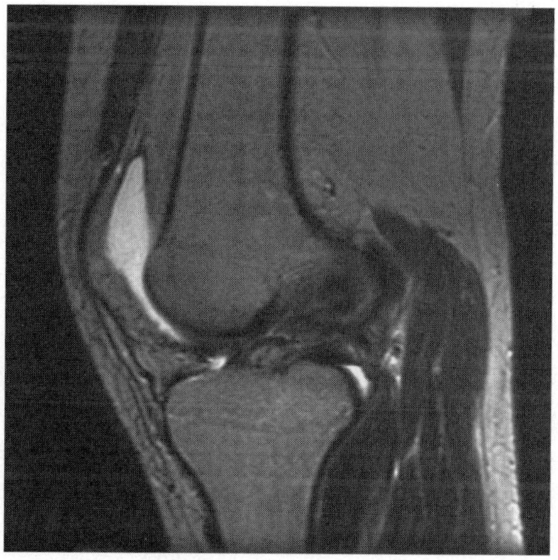

Figures 1K and **1L** Bone contusion of the lateral femoral condyle is evident on the sagittal T1-weighted image (**1K**) as a poorly marginated triangular area of low signal intensity in this patient with a midsubstance tear. The T2-weighted image (**1L**) shows focal discontinuity and surrounding high signal intensity.

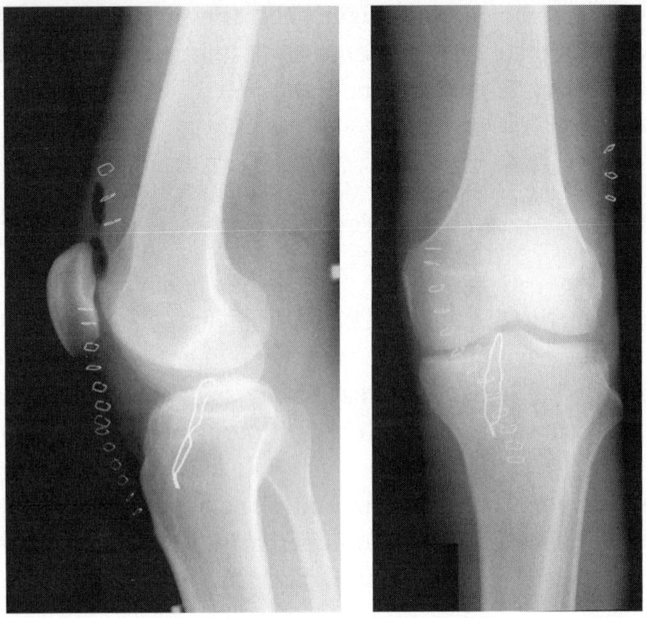

Figures 1M and **1N** Previously avulsed tibial insertion has been surgically reattached, and continuity has been restored by use of a length of orthopedic wire.

In a professional athlete, repair is typically undertaken. If an avulsion is present, the fragment will be "tacked" back in place with subsequent restoration of continuity (**Figs. 1M,1N**).

"Stout" sutures may be employed to repair a midsubstance tear.

In the chronically torn ligament, or where initial attempts at treatment have failed, ligament reconstruction by use of a "neoligament," for example, transposed patellar tendon, may be employed.

Prognosis

In the hands of an expert, a repaired ligament should restore normal function, even to the professional athlete.

A conservatively treated knee or a knee that has failed treatment measures is at risk for chronic instability, frequently "giving way," and consequently osteoarthrosis.

PEARLS

- The ACL is intracapsular but extrasynovial.
- Although reference is frequently made to the concurrence of medial meniscal and ACL tears (which, with an associated medial collateral ligament tear, make up O'Donoghue's "unhappy triad"), lateral meniscal tears are in fact more frequent than medial meniscal tears in association with ACL tears.
- A line drawn through the distal posterior edge of the PCL on a sagittal view should intersect the medullary cavity of the femur. If it does not, significant buckling is present and is highly suggestive of an ACL tear.

PITFALLS

- A pseudomass in the region of the proximal ACL, mimicking a proximal tear, may be seen secondary to partial voluming with the femoral condyle.
- A ganglion cyst of the ACL, thought possibly to represent a result of remote trauma, will cause intrasubstance high signal and mass effect and thus mimic a tear. The focal nature of the high signal and the lack of other evidence should lead to a diagnosis of the former.
- If an effusion is present, fluid may track between the anterior and posterior bands of an intact ACL, producing apparent intrasubstance high signal intensity suggestive of a tear.

Suggested Readings

Lee JK, Yao L, Phelps CT, et al. Anterior cruciate ligament tears: MR imaging compared with arthroscopy and clinical tests. Radiology 1988;166:861–864

Roychowdhury S, Fitzgerald SW, Sonin AH, Peduto AJ, Miller FH, Hoff FL. Using MR imaging to diagnose partial tears of the anterior cruciate ligament: value of axial images. Am J Roentgenol 1997;168:1487–1491

Vellet AD, Lee DH, Munk PL, et al. Anterior cruciate ligament tear: prospective evaluation of diagnostic accuracy of middle- and high-field-strength MR imaging at 1.5 and 0.5 T. Radiology 1995;197:826–830

CASE 2

Anthony G. Ryan and Peter L. Munk

Clinical Presentation

A 28-year-old man presented with knee pain and swelling after a high-speed skiing injury.

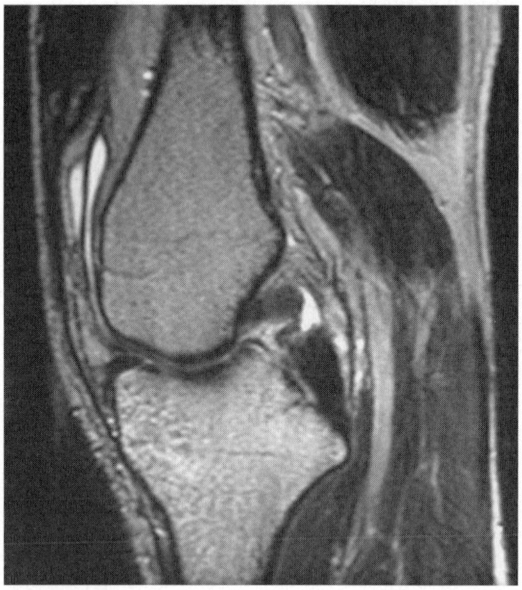

Figure 2A

Radiologic Findings

A sagittal T2-weighted image of the knee (**Fig. 2A**) revealed a focal discontinuity of the posterior cruciate ligament (PCL) and a small joint effusion.

Diagnosis

Acute tear of the PCL.

Differential Diagnosis

None.

Discussion

Background

The PCL stabilizes the knee by preventing anterior translation of the femur on the tibia. It takes its origin from the posterolateral aspect of the medial femoral condyle and attaches on the posterior tibia ~1 cm distal to the articular surface. It is intracapsular but extrasynovial, lying in the same synovial compartment as the anterior cruciate ligament (ACL).

Similar to the ACL, there is a larger anterolateral band and a smaller posteromedial band; the former tightens in flexion, the latter in extension. The PCL is relatively stronger than the ACL and is thus less frequently injured (by a factor of 9).

The ligament tears most frequently in its midsubstance (50 to 75%). PCL tears occur in isolation in only ~30% of injuries, with 30 to 35% associated with a femoral avulsion and 20 to 30% associated with a tibial avulsion.

The most frequent complex of injuries is that of a torn PCL, an associated ACL tear, and a posterolateral corner disruption (including the posterolateral capsule and the popliteus tendon).

Etiology

The usual mechanism of action is that of a direct force on the tibia in a flexed leg, for example, against a dashboard in a sudden-deceleration motor vehicle accident. The ligament is less commonly injured at the extremes of flexion and extension (as is the mechanism in skiing injuries).

If a motor vehicle accident is the cause, typically the leg strikes the dashboard, driving the proximal tibia backward, stretching and tearing the PCL. In this setting, bone contusions will be evident at the anterior tibial plateau and the posterior femoral condyles.

If there is a hyperextension injury, there is likely to be a tibial attachment avulsion with preservation of the PCL itself (**Figs. 2B,2C**).

The PCL is at particular risk in a posterior dislocation of the knee.

Rarely, the PCL may tear in association with closed fractures of the femoral shaft (found in one study to occur in 21% of such fractures), although in this setting, the medial collateral ligament is the most frequent accompanying ligamentous injury (38%).

Clinical Findings

If a direct force on the anterior tibia has been the mechanism, a pretibial hematoma may be present, and there may be an associated fracture of the hip or patella, secondary to the same impact.

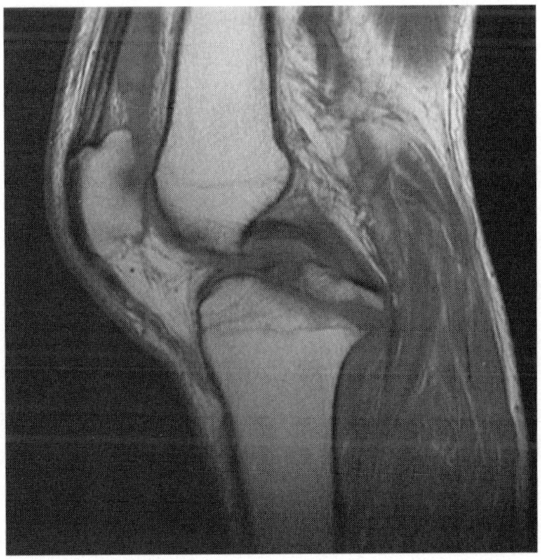

B

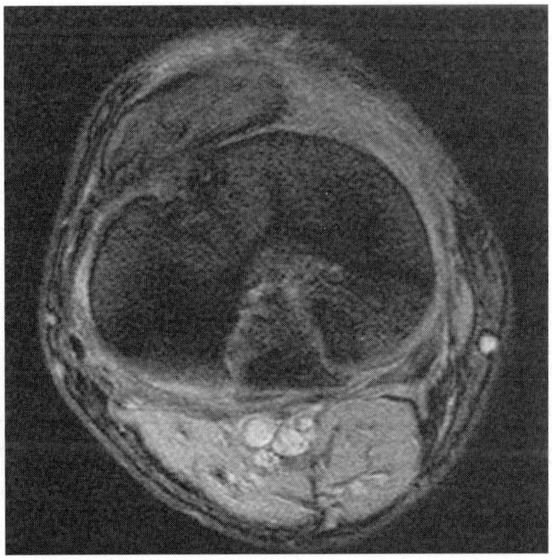

C

Figures 2B Midline sagittal T1-weighted image shows a continuous posterior cruciate ligament with an attached avulsed fragment from the tibial insertion. **2C** Axial MPGR from the same patient shows the bony fragment at the tibial insertion site.

Clinical examination may be significantly limited by the attendant soft tissue injuries, for example, hamstring spasm and hemarthrosis. If the posterolateral structures are otherwise intact, the posterior drawer may be falsely negative, reducing this test's accuracy to between 50 and 60%.

Arthroscopy

The PCL can be difficult to visualize at arthroscopy and requires two ports, posteromedial and posterolateral. It may be necessary to open the synovial envelope, as a tear may be missed and the arthroscopy called falsely negative if the envelope has not actually been ruptured secondary to the injury. The difficulty in assessing the PCL arthroscopically is reduced if there is a corresponding tear of the ACL.

The meniscofemoral ligaments may be mistaken for an intact PCL, again leading to a false-negative investigation.

Complications

Premature patellofemoral osteoarthrosis.

Imaging Findings

RADIOGRAPHY

A bony avulsion of the posterior tibial insertion occurs in less than 10% of cases, best seen on the lateral plain film.

A cortical avulsion off the medial tibial plateau may be evident, associated with tears of the PCL and medial meniscus. This pattern of injury is described as a "reverse" Segond fracture.

ULTRASOUND

The PCL is scanned in the longitudinal plane with a curvilinear transducer. A normal PCL should be homogeneously hypoechoic with a well-defined posterior border.

A torn PCL is characterized by the following:

- Heterogeneously hypoechoic with an indistinct posterior margin
- Significantly thicker: 12.0 to 20.0 mm compared with 3.8 to 5.8 mm for normal PCL
- Focal discontinuity may be demonstrable.

MAGNETIC RESONANCE IMAGING

MRI is the current imaging modality of choice for visualizing the PCL, which is well seen on a single image (sagittal midline) in up to 95% of studies. The PCL is typically seen as a uniformly dark band convex posteriorly. The adjacent meniscofemoral ligaments (anterior = Humphrey, posterior = Wrisberg) may produce apparent thickening of the ligament in its midportion. On coronal images, the PCL is seen on the medial aspect of the intracondylar notch.

Acute tear

A complete tear is evident by failure to identify the ligament. There may be amorphous areas of high signal intensity on both T1- and T2-weighted images with loss of fiber definition. Focal disruptions are unusual, and the more common pattern is that of a midsubstance interstitial tear.

When a midsubstance tear is present, it will typically cause diffuse widening of the ligament with increased signal on both T1- and T2-weighted images. A PCL of higher signal intensity than the ACL on any pulse sequence is abnormal.

Should a complete tear be present, the gap will be evident, and the torn edges may be clearly visible (**Fig. 2A**). If an avulsion injury is associated, hemorrhage and edema will be evident on fluid-sensitive sequences. Redundancy of an avulsed ligament may be evident.

Given the significant energy required to rupture the PCL, other associated injuries are common, including the ACL, the collateral ligaments, meniscal tears, and osteochondral injury.

In the event of a dashboard injury, bone contusions will be evident at the anterior tibial plateau and the posterior femoral condyles. In the presence of an associated ACL rupture, bone contusions may be evident on the anterior tibial plateau and the anterior aspect of the femoral condyle.

Partial tear

Abnormal signal intensity within the substance of the ligament is usual, with some intact and some discontinuous fibers (**Fig. 2D**).

Chronic tear

Because most torn PCLs are interstitial rather than focally disrupted, a chronically torn PCL will usually be seen as a continuous structure (**Fig. 2E**). There may be some thickening with associated irregularity of the surface of the ligament.

When imaging the knee, PCL ganglia are seen relatively frequently as well-defined multilocular lesions, hypo- or slightly hyperintense to muscle on T1 images with homogeneously high signal intensity on T2-weighted images. Their significance is uncertain, and the theory that they represent a post-traumatic phenomenon remains unproven. Whatever their etiology, ganglion cysts may cause symptoms by virtue of local mass effect, resulting in limited range of motion and osseous erosion.

Treatment

The torn PCL is rarely surgically repaired, as it is not thought to be a significant cause of instability, particularly if the anterior compartment muscles are well developed.

If an avulsed tibial fragment is present, it is replaced by open reduction and fixation with subsequent restoration of PCL function.

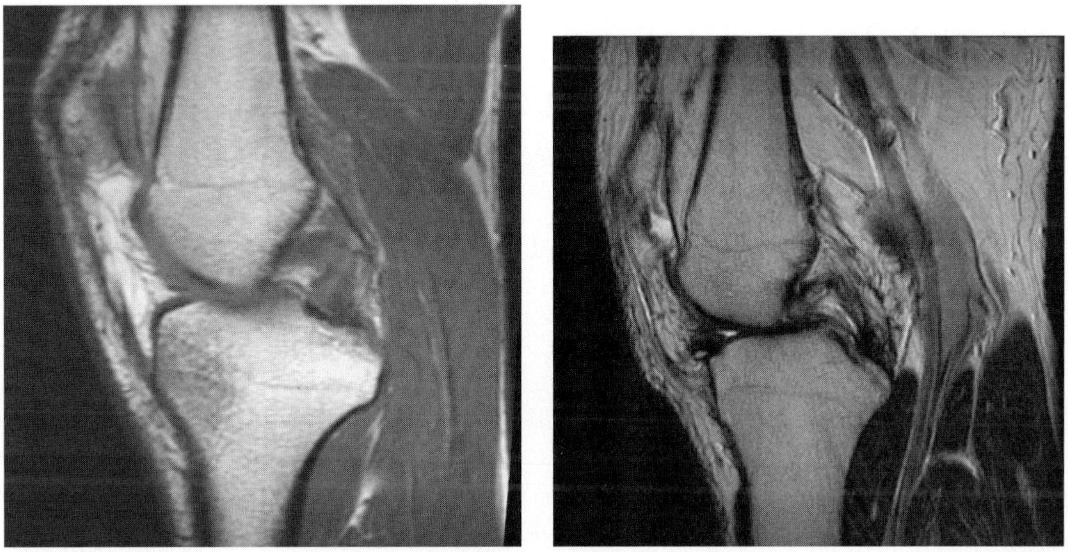

D E

Figures 2D Sagittal T2-weighted image shows heterogeneous high signal within a continuous ligament consistent with an acute intrasubstance tear. **2E** Sagittal T2-weighted image shows a thinned, heterogeneous posterior cruciate ligament with surface irregularity consistent with a chronic tear.

Prognosis

If a PCL injury goes undetected, increased femorotibial translation places abnormal increased stress on the patellofemoral joint, leading to premature osteoarthrosis.

PEARLS

- A PCL of higher signal intensity than the ACL on any pulse sequence is abnormal.
- If, on preoperative imaging, the ACL is shown to be torn, the likelihood of arthroscopy being falsely negative in the assessment of the PCL is decreased.

PITFALLS

- At arthroscopy, the meniscofemoral ligaments may be mistaken for an intact PCL, leading to a false-negative investigation.
- With T1 weighting, the magic angle phenomenon may produce artefactual increased signal along the convex portion of the ligament, which should not be present on the other longer TE sequences performed.

Suggested Readings

Cohen AP, King D, Gibbon AJ. Impingement fracture of the andromeda tibial margin: a radiographic sign of combined posterolateral complex and posterior cruciate ligament disruption. Skeletal Radiol 2001;30:114–116

Miller TT. Sonography of injury of the posterior cruciate ligament of the knee. Skeletal Radiol 2002;31:149–154

Sonin AH, Fitzgerald SW, Friedman H, Hoff FL, Hendrix RW, Rogers LF. Posterior cruciate ligament injury: MR imaging diagnosis and patterns of injury. Radiology 1994;190:455–458

CASE 3

Hema N. Choudur, Anthony G. Ryan, and Peter L. Munk

Clinical Presentation

Five different patients presented with joint line pain. A history of trauma to the knee accompanied by an audible "pop" was given by the three younger patients. Limitation in knee flexion with no history of trauma was given by the two older patients.

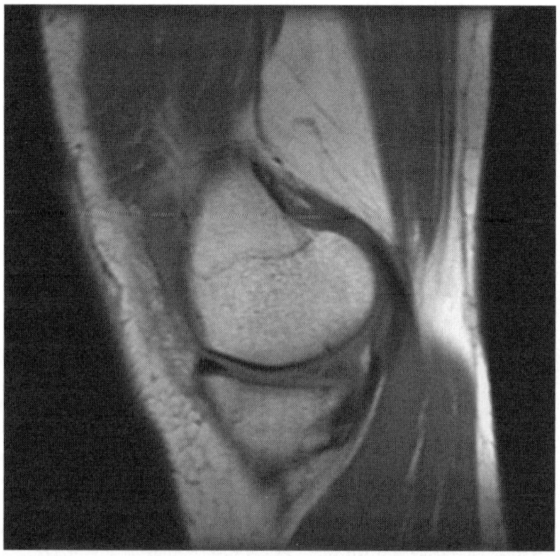

Figure 3A

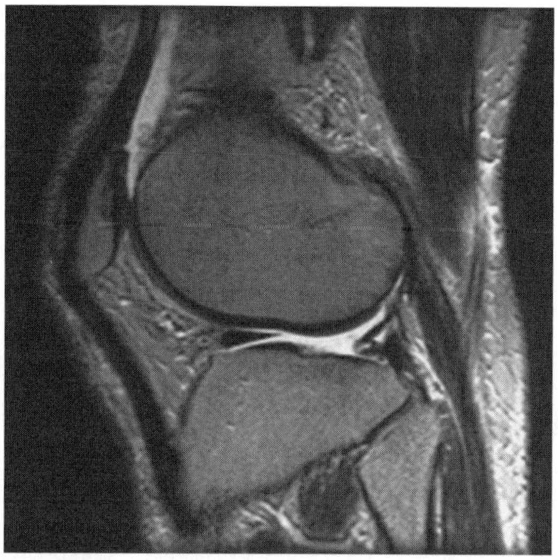

Figure 3B

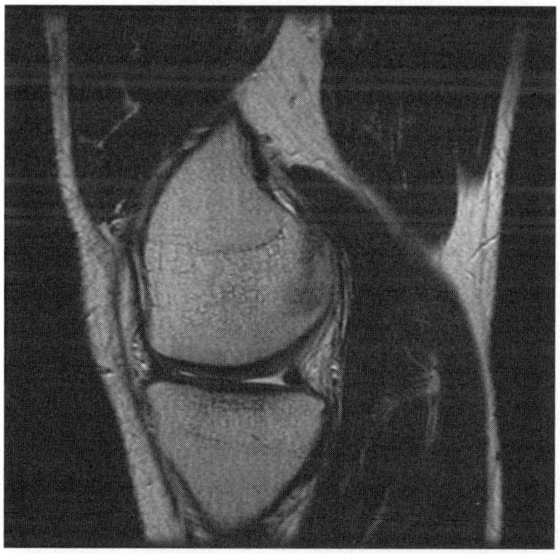

Figure 3C

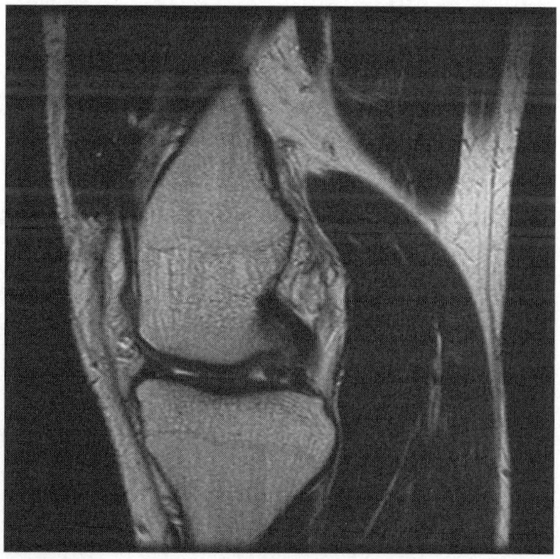

Figure 3D

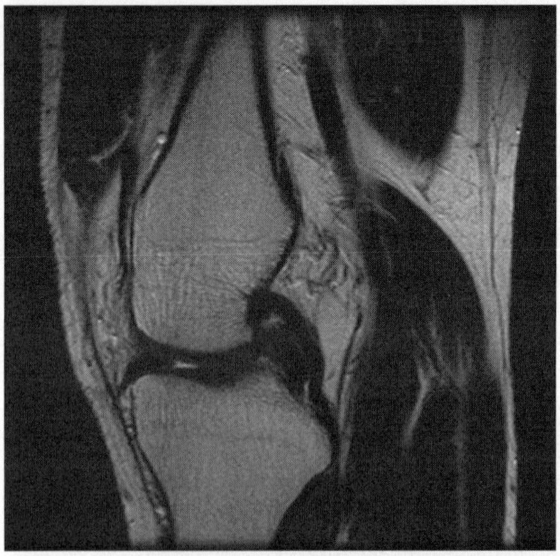

Figure 3E

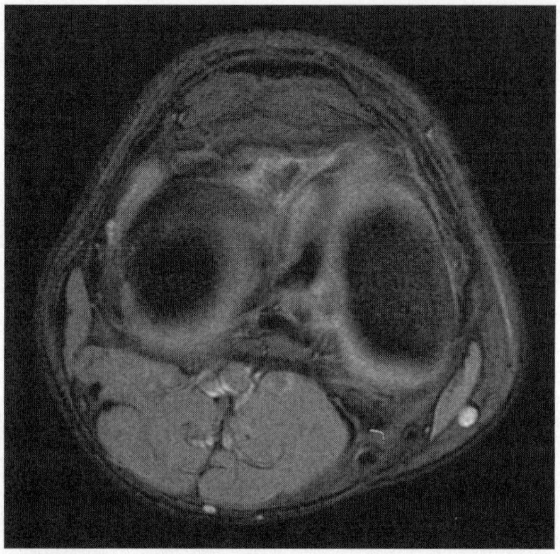

Figure 3F

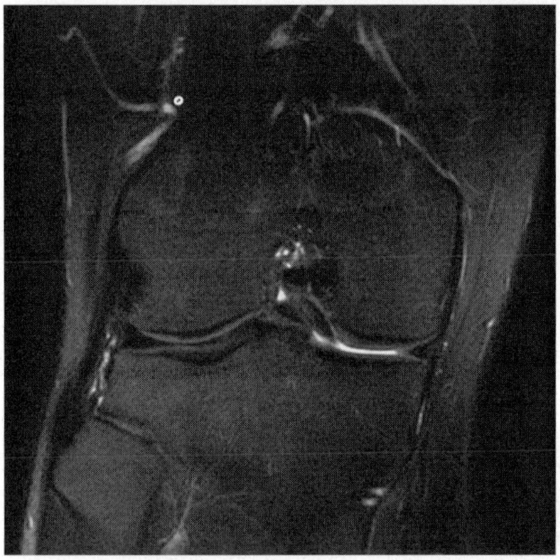

Figure 3G

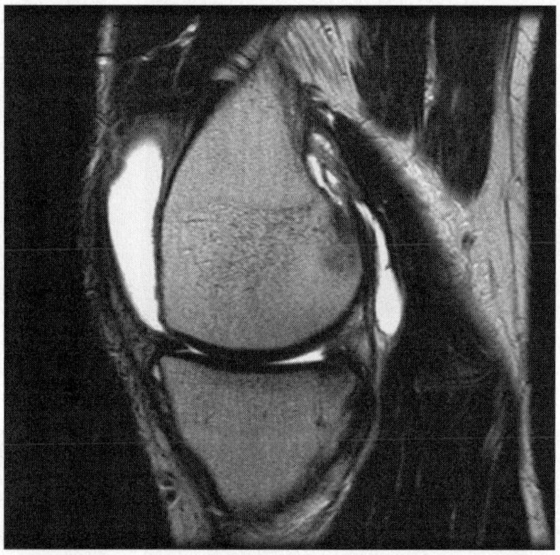

Figure 3H

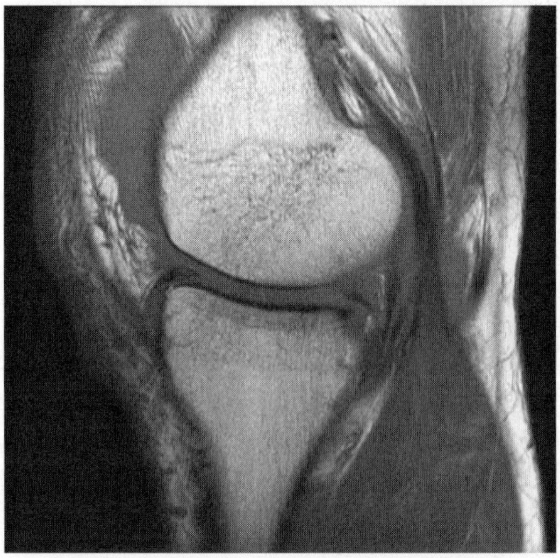

Figure 3I

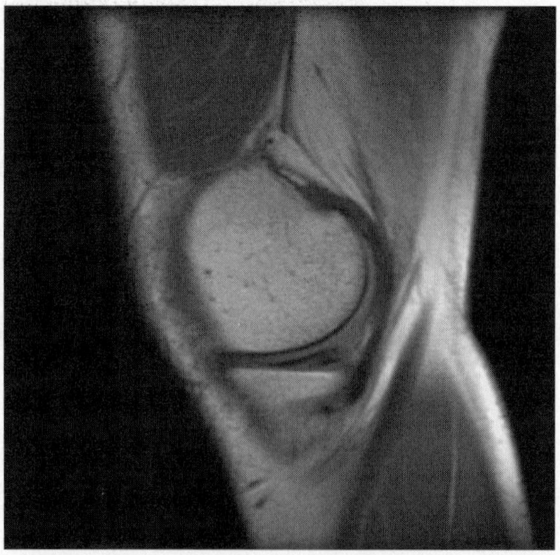

Figure 3J

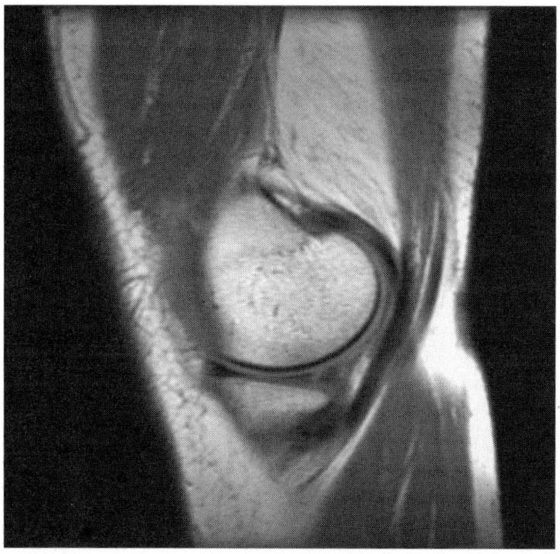

Figure 3K

Radiologic Findings

A T1-weighted sagittal image (**Fig. 3A**) shows a complex tear in the posterior horn of the medial meniscus. A T2-weighted sagittal image shows a complex tear in the posterior horn of the lateral meniscus (**Fig. 3B**).

Figures 3C–3G show a flipped fragment of the posterior horn of the medial meniscus with the characteristic double posterior cruciate ligament sign.

Sagittal T2-weighted (**Fig. 3H**) and sagittal T1-weighted (**Fig. 3I**) images show a missing segment of the posterior horn of the medial meniscus. A sagittal T1-weighted image (**Fig. 3J**) shows a linear oblique tear surfacing inferiorly in the posterior horn of the medial meniscus. Another sagittal T1-weighted image (**Fig. 3K**) shows a linear vertical tear in the posterior horn of the medial meniscus.

Diagnosis

Meniscal tears.

Differential Diagnosis

None.

Discussion

Background

The menisci are semilunar cartilages that serve to increase the congruency between the femoral condylar articular surfaces and the tibial plateau. The menisci serve various functions, including load transmission, stability, joint proprioception, shock absorption, and articular cartilage nutrition.

The medial meniscus is thicker than the lateral, with the anterior horn about one third the thickness of the posterior, covering ~50% of the tibial plateau. The lateral meniscus is of uniform thickness anteroposteriorly and covers ~75% of the tibial plateau. When viewed from above, the meniscus has a crescent shape (*meniscus* means "little moon" in Greek). The meniscal ring is thickest at the periphery and tapers off centrally, creating a shallow cup to hold the rounded condyles of the femur. In cross section, the meniscus has a triangular wedge shape.

The lateral meniscus is more mobile than the medial, as the latter is tightly adherent to the capsule. The meniscocapsular attachment on the lateral aspect is interrupted by the popliteal tendon.

The menisci become progressively avascular from the periphery to the center. By about the ninth month of life, the central portion loses its vascularity, with only 10 to 30% of the meniscus retaining its vascularity. At birth, the menisci are also very cellular, composed mostly of circumferentially oriented collagen fibers, in addition to a few radially, vertically, and obliquely oriented fibers. Following the above vascular pattern, the periphery of the menisci is innervated, but the central portions are not.

Etiology

Although there are different mechanisms of injury, sudden deceleration or change of direction while running and direct blunt trauma are the most frequent. Shearing and compressive forces affect the central menisci, and blunt injuries have the greatest impact peripherally. The usual mechanism of injury resulting in a meniscal tear is a rotational force applied when the knee is partly or completely flexed. Football and tennis are the most frequent inciting sports.

There is a 60% incidence of degenerative meniscal tears after age 60 years. The medial meniscus is most commonly injured in the stable knee or in the chronic anterior cruciate ligament- (ACL-) deficient knee. The lateral meniscus is most commonly injured with an acute ACL tear. The majority of meniscal tears have a posterior horn flap pattern.

Pathophysiology

Certain meniscal tears occur gradually over a long period of time. In older patients, these may represent so-called degenerative meniscal tears and may not be symptomatic. These tears are more frequent in the medial meniscus.

Clinical Findings

The patient usually complains of joint line pain, recurrent swelling, and occasional "giving way." An acute meniscal tear may be heard as a "pop" and felt as a tear or rip in the knee. Within a few minutes to hours, there is often swelling of the knee as a result of joint effusion. Patients with meniscal tears often describe a "catch" in their knees. In the most dramatic situations, the knee will actually lock, preventing the patient from fully extending or straightening the knee. Tears are typically quite painful initially, but over time, most of the pain disappears except with certain activities. In some patients, the tear becomes asymptomatic, especially if their activity level decreases significantly.

Tenderness is elicited by deep palpation along the joint line. Twisting the knee while flexing it will occasionally cause or reproduce the patient's symptoms. McMurray's and Apley's compressions are specific tests for detecting meniscal injury. Hemarthrosis within 3 hours of injury is unlikely to be due to a meniscal tear and usually indicates an ACL tear or a fracture.

Stages of Disease

In older people, chronic myxoid degeneration may progress to a tear without a history of injury.

Complications

Osteoarthritis is the most significant complication of an untreated meniscal tear. Altered biomechanical stress results in varying degrees of bone marrow edema in the tibial and femoral condyles, which may present as focal knee pain. In an ACL-deficient knee, the progress of osteoarthritis is faster.

Pathology

GROSS

At arthroscopy, the peripheral vascular zone tears are seen as reddish breaks, whereas those in the central menisci are whitish due to their avascularity.

Imaging Findings

RADIOGRAPHY

Conventional radiographs are useful in ruling out associated avulsion fractures (Segond) and other injury-related osteochondral defects. Loose bodies and/or chondral calcifications may be identified.

MAGNETIC RESONANCE IMAGING

MRI is the imaging procedure of choice. Its negative predictive value is most helpful in deciding appropriate management. If the MRI is normal, there is more than 90% certainty that no abnormality exists in the joint. A necessary criterion is the visualization of an abnormal signal contacting the articular meniscal surface in at least two slices or in two planes. Having met the MRI criteria for a tear, it is important to characterize it to facilitate management.

O'Conner's classification of tears consists of the following:

- *Longitudinal tear* Oriented parallel to the edge of the meniscus; may be complete or partial. When complete, the displaceable fragment may represent a bucket handle tear.
- *Horizontal tear* Separates the superior from the inferior meniscus and can predispose the patient to complex or flap tears. It is most common in older patients secondary to degeneration.
- *Oblique full-thickness tear* Located within the anterior or posterior meniscus, the tear cuts obliquely through the entire meniscus.
- *Radial tear* Vertically oriented, extending from the inner edge of the meniscus to the periphery; can be complete or incomplete.
- *Flap tear* Similar to an oblique tear but has a horizontal cleavage element separating the superior from the inferior meniscus.
- *Complex tear* Most common in chronic meniscal lesions; has all other types of tears in its configuration. It occurs most often in older individuals.

If surgery is contemplated, the surgeon must know the type of tear, location, extent, and associated ligamentous injury/cartilage involvement. The tear should be imaged in at least two planes.

Longitudinal tears occur in young people following acute trauma, and horizontal tears occur in older individuals with degenerative changes in the knee. The bucket handle, flap, and oblique tears require a greater degree of rotatory stress.

In various studies,

- The accuracy of MRI ranged from 64 to 95% in detecting medial meniscus lesions and from 83 to 94% in detecting lateral meniscus lesions.

- Seventeen percent of the grade II lesions (intrameniscal high signal) were found to be torn on arthroscopy.
- The highest accuracy was in detecting grade III (abnormal signal extending to the articular surface) lesions.
- With MRI, false-positive results were much more common than false-negative results.

A more challenging area is the postoperative knee with a retear. An MR arthrogram has a high degree of accuracy if gadolinium is seen to enter a fresh tear, which can thus be differentiated from high signal granulation tissue in relation to an old tear or repair.

Treatment

Appropriate treatment depends on the accurate localization of the tear.

- If the tear is located in the vascular peripheral 3 mm, called the "red" zone, it is amenable to arthroscopic repair, as it has the greatest potential to heal.
- If located in the avascular white zone (5 mm from the periphery), it is less amenable to repair.
- Other factors are the stability and length of the tear. If less than 1 cm in length, tears are considered stable and amenable to repair, and if more than 1 cm, they are considered unstable and require partial meniscectomy.
- In deciding between repair and excision, the length of the tear is an important factor. If the tear is less than 4 mm, it heals well; therefore, repair may be considered. If it is more than 4 mm, an excision is the line of treatment offered.
- This factor is especially important in concomitant ACL reconstruction. Partial meniscectomy is indicated for all isolated complex tears and flap tears, radial tears more than 5 mm in length, and irreparable tears.
- Fibrin clots are routinely deposited within the tear at the time of arthroscopic repair.

Prognosis

Vertical tears in the peripheral zone in young individuals heal very well, as do stable tears. Partial meniscectomy of complex tears provides temporary relief of symptoms but does not halt the progression to osteoarthritis. Research is ongoing in the use of allografts following meniscectomy to promote better healing and function.

PEARLS

- To meet the MRI criteria of a tear, the intrameniscal high signal should surface in at least two slices or in two planes. Not all meniscal tears are symptomatic unless associated with bone marrow edema.
- An MR arthrogram is imperative to assess retears following arthroscopic repair. Contrast imbibing into the tear is the characteristic feature of a retear.

PITFALL

- Radial tears are the most difficult to diagnose and should be looked for carefully in sagittal and coronal planes.

Suggested Readings

Jee WH, McCauley TR, Kim JM, et al. Meniscal tear configurations: categorization with MR imaging. Am J Roentgenol 2003;180:93–97

Magee T, Shapiro M, Rodriguez J, Williams D. MR arthrography of postoperative knee: for which patients is it useful? Radiology 2003;229:159–163

Magee T, Shapiro M, Williams D. MR accuracy and arthroscopic incidence of meniscal radial tears. Skeletal Radiol 2002;31:686–689

CASE 4

Hema N. Choudur, Anthony G. Ryan, and Peter L. Munk

Clinical Presentation

Two patients presented with focal knee pain, anterolateral in the first and posteromedial in the second, with a palpable mass in the latter.

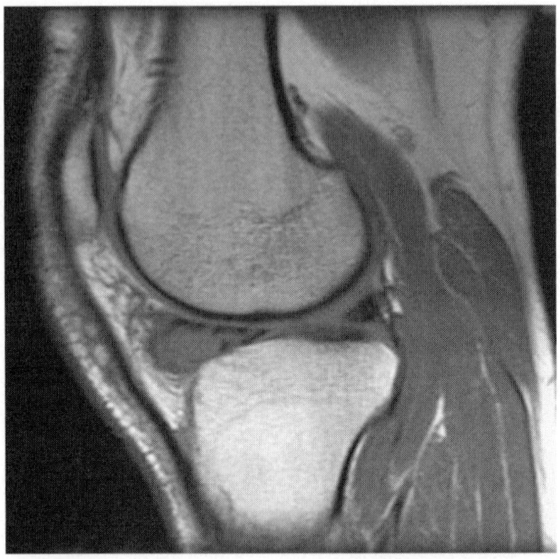

Figure 4A

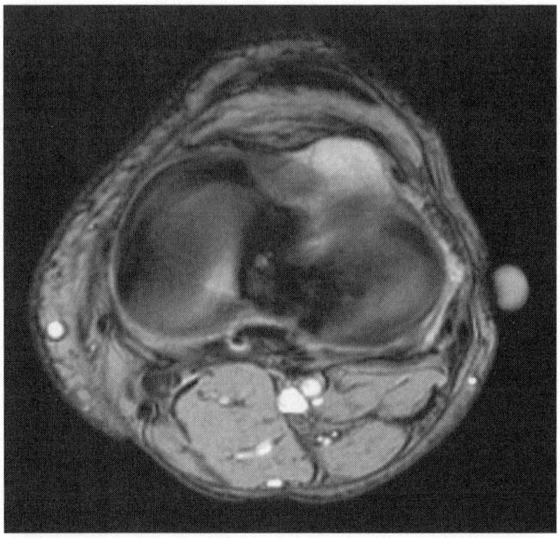

Figure 4B

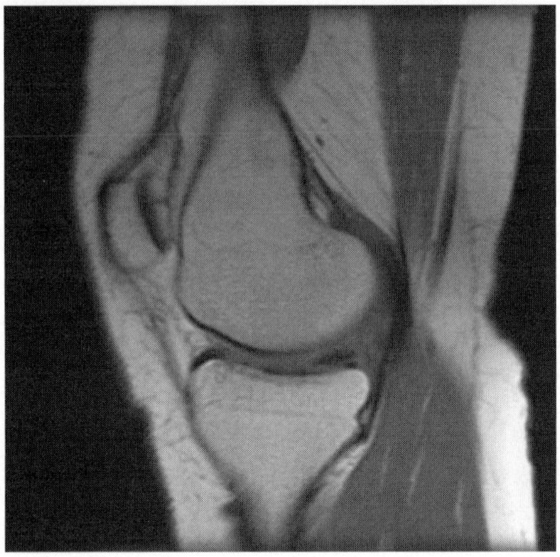

Figure 4C

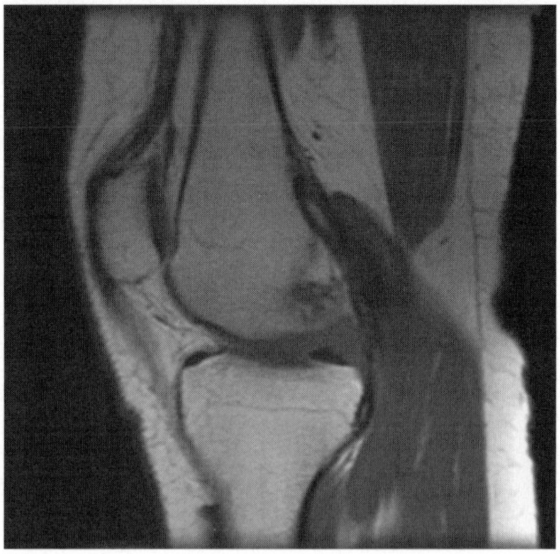

Figure 4D

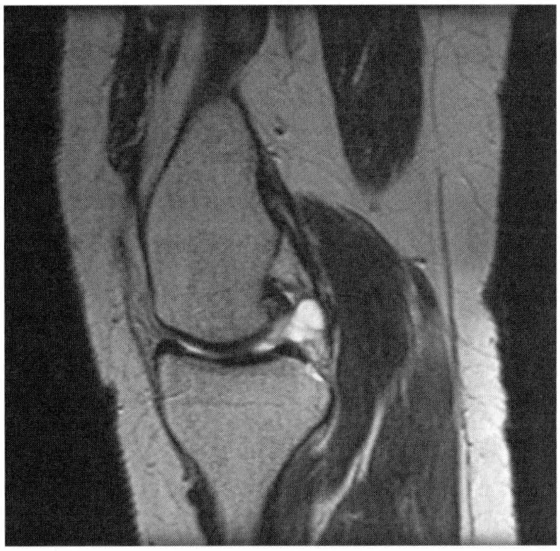

Figure 4E

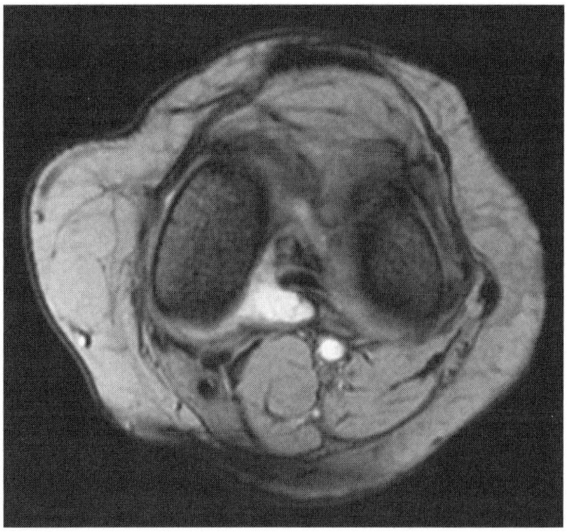

Figure 4F

Radiologic Findings

T1-weighted sagittal (**Fig. 4A**) and T2-weighted axial (**Fig. 4B**) images reveal a meniscal cyst arising from the anterior horn of the lateral meniscus.

T1-weighted sagittal (**Figs. 4C,4D**), T2-weighted sagittal (**Fig. 4E**), and T2-weighted axial (**Fig. 4F**) images reveal a parameniscal cyst arising from the posterior horn of the medial meniscus.

In the first case, the T2-weighted images show a well-defined cystic lesion within the anterior horn of the lateral meniscus. A similar lesion was noted extending from the posterior horn of the medial meniscus in the second. An associated meniscal tear was evident in both.

Diagnosis

Meniscal cyst.

Differential Diagnosis

- Ganglion
- Synovial cyst
- Proximal tibiofibular cyst
- Traumatic bursitis
- Masses (including pigmented villonodular synovitis, hemangioma, lipoma, and synovial sarcoma)

The clue to the diagnosis lies in demonstrating the fluid nature of the cyst and the associated horizontal tear in the meniscus with which it communicates.

Discussion

Background

Meniscal cysts were first described by Ebner in 1904. In 1923, the first series of meniscal cysts were reported as seen in 1% of meniscectomies. Magnetic resonance imaging (MRI) has revolutionized the detection and imaging of meniscal cysts.

Meniscal cysts occur twice as often in men as in women—at an average age of 30 years. Lateral meniscal cysts are more common than medial by a ratio of 3:1.

In the illustrative cases, the meniscal cysts were seen adjacent to the lateral and medial meniscus, respectively.

Etiology and Pathophysiology

The most common theory is that the knee joint, acting as a pump, pushes fluid into a preexisting micro- or macroscopic horizontal tear. The horizontal tears typically arise as a result of a combination of degeneration and trauma. The cystic tract balloons out along the line of least resistance, that is, parameniscally. The loose peripheral attachment of the lateral meniscus to the joint capsule renders enough freedom for growth, unlike the medial meniscus, which is tightly adherent to the capsule, limiting its expansion.

Clinical Findings

The usual presentation is a dull, aching pain in the medial or lateral compartment adjacent to the knee joint. On physical examination, fullness and tenderness are noted along the joint line on the affected side. Occasionally, a mass can be palpated adjacent to the joint line. The size of the lesions may decrease in flexion and increase in extension.

Stages of Disease

Small meniscal cysts are difficult to differentiate from horizontal cleavage tears. The key to diagnosis lies in the appreciation of a mass effect and/or a bulky meniscus. As the cysts grow, they extend parameniscally, often maintaining a communication with the meniscal tear.

Medial meniscal cysts, which tend to grow to a larger size than their lateral counterparts, can be seen extending from the posterior horn and dissecting peripherally. They are usually found deep to the medial collateral ligament or in the posteromedial corner deep to the posterior oblique ligament.

Lateral meniscal cysts are usually located anterior to the lateral collateral ligament or between the lateral collateral ligament and popliteus tendon.

Complications

Large medial meniscal cysts rarely cause compression of the saphenous nerve.

Pathology

GROSS

Meniscal cysts are typically multilocular and are lined with synovial endothelial tissue.

MICROSCOPIC

Barrie performed histopathologic studies and postulated that meniscal cyst formation originated by an influx of synovial fluid through microscopic and gross tears in the substance of the meniscus. In 112 cysts, he demonstrated a meniscal tear with a horizontal component, as well as a tract that provided an exchange of fluid between the joint and the cyst. In the absence of a meniscal tear, it has been proposed that a parameniscal cyst may develop from a compression injury to the periphery of a meniscus that has central degeneration. A meniscal cyst may then develop more peripherally, leaving the body of the meniscus abnormal but not torn.

Imaging Findings

RADIOGRAPHY

Plain radiographs of the knee may show pressure erosions of the adjacent tibial plateau.

ULTRASOUND

Sonography is excellent for detecting the fluid within the cyst but has a limited role in evaluating the relationship of the cyst to intra-articular structures.

COMPUTED TOMOGRAPHY

CT shows the cyst and intra-articular structures, but with its limited soft tissue resolution, it cannot demonstrate a meniscal tear.

CT arthrography can detect the communication between the cyst and the joint space but gives little information about noncommunicating cysts.

MAGNETIC RESONANCE IMAGING

MRI is an excellent modality to diagnose meniscal cysts as a result of its multiplanar acquisition, excellent soft tissue contrast, and lack of invasivity. Sagittal, coronal, and axial planes are usually acquired.

- On T1-weighted images, meniscal cysts appear iso-/hypointense to surrounding muscle.
- On proton density images, they are isointense or slightly hyperintense to skeletal muscle.
- They show an increased signal intensity on T2-weighted fast spin-echo, short tau inversion recovery (STIR), and T2* gradient echo images.
- They are well circumscribed with smooth walls and are not infrequently septated. Because cysts may also contain bloody or gelatinous fluid with an increased protein content, there may be some variation in their signal intensities on T1- and T2-weighted images.

Treatment

- Arthroscopic or open cyst decompression

In the presence of a small meniscal tear, an arthroscopic partial meniscectomy may be performed, followed by arthroscopic cyst decompression, consisting of deroofing and débridement.

If no tear is present, open-cyst decompression with peripheral meniscal repair, leaving the central meniscus untouched, is said to be the treatment of choice. The cyst is removed, the residual wall is débrided, and the resultant space is packed with fibrin to preserve the stability of the meniscus.

Prognosis

Good or excellent results can be expected from either open or arthroscopic treatment of meniscal cysts.

PEARL

- The clue to the diagnosis lies in demonstrating the fluid nature of the cyst and the associated horizontal tear in the meniscus with which it communicates.

PITFALL

- Noncommunicating meniscal cysts will frequently be missed at arthroscopy.

Suggested Readings

Barrie HJ. The pathogenesis and significance of meniscal cysts. J Bone Joint Surg Br 1979;61-B:184–189

Blair TR, Schweitzer M, Resnick D. Meniscal cysts causing bone erosion: retrospective analysis of seven cases. Clin Imaging 1999;23:134–138

Campbell SE, Sanders TG, Morrison WB. MR imaging of meniscal cysts: incidence, location, and clinical significance. Am J Roentgenol 2001;177:409–413

Mills CA, Henderson IJ. Cysts of the medial meniscus: arthroscopic diagnosis and management. J Bone Joint Surg Br 1993;75:293–298

Passariello R, Trecco F, de Paulis F, et al. Meniscal lesions of the knee joint: CT diagnosis. Radiology 1985;157:29–34

Seymour R, Lloyd DC. Sonographic appearances of meniscal cysts. J Clin Ultrasound 1998;26:15–20

CASE 5

Anthony G. Ryan and Peter L. Munk

Clinical Presentation

A 26-year-old man presented with focal medial joint line pain, having received a heavy tackle to the outside of the leg while playing ice hockey.

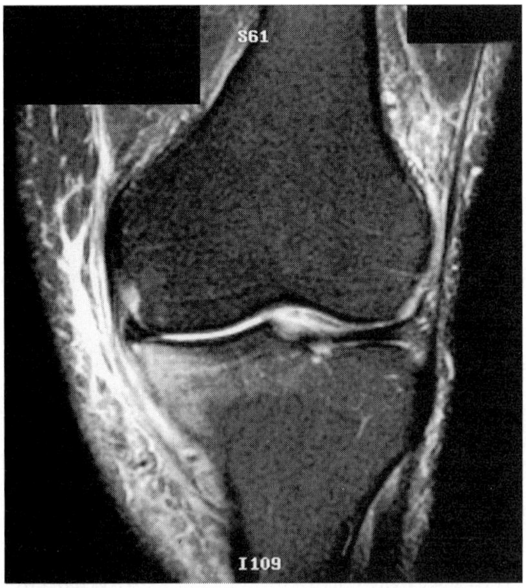

Figure 5A

Radiologic Findings

A coronal T2-weighted image (**Fig. 5A**) shows diffuse high signal and splitting of the medial collateral ligament (MCL). The intact proximal portion of the ligament is clearly seen. The distal half is poorly seen, attenuated, and discontinuous, and high signal fluid is shown internal and external to the ligament.

Diagnosis

MCL tear (grade III).

Differential Diagnosis

None.

Discussion

Background

Anatomically, the MCL consists of superficial and deep parts. The deep portion is inseparable from the true capsule of the joint, which in turn is adherent to the medial meniscus via meniscofemoral and meniscotibial ligaments.

Between the deep and superficial parts of the MCL lies a bursa surrounded by a variable amount of fat.

The superficial part of the MCL may be further divided into vertical and posterior oblique components. The vertical portion arises from the medial femoral epicondyle 5 cm above the joint line and inserts distally onto the medial tibial metaphysis 7 cm below the joint. The posterior oblique component extends from the femoral epicondyle to the posteromedial tibia and adjacent semimembranosus tendon.

Functionally, the ligament resists valgus forces at the knee and prevents excessive external rotation and anterior tibial translation. The vertical component remains constant in length throughout flexion, whereas the posterior oblique component becomes lax in flexion.

Etiology

Isolated MCL injury typically occurs with pure valgus stress without a rotatory component such as occurs in ice hockey injuries.

MCL disruption is said to occur in up to 60% of skiing injuries, usually occurring when valgus stress is applied to the flexed knee.

The MCL is the most frequent site of ligamentous injury (38%) found in association with closed fractures of the distal femoral shaft.

Pathophysiology

The MCL is strong and when injured is frequently associated with internal derangements of the knee, particularly anterior cruciate ligament (ACL) and meniscal tears. When rotation is combined with valgus, the posterior oblique portion tends to be injured first, followed by the ACL, and then the remainder of the MCL.

Clinical Findings

Patients frequently present with pain, swelling, and tenderness directly over the ligament. If an effusion develops immediately after the inciting injury, there is a high probability of an associated internal derangement, as the MCL is extra-articular. As a corollary, isolated tears should not produce an effusion.

MCL integrity is assessed by valgus strain on the knee; however, the associated tenderness and muscle spasm limit the sensitivity of the examination, which is thus associated with a high false-negative rate. Valgus strain is applied at different angles of flexion: laxity at 30% implies isolated disruption of the MCL, whereas laxity in extension signifies a more extensive injury, as, for example, to the cruciate ligaments.

O'Donoghue's "unhappy" triad, consisting of an ACL tear, an MCL tear, and a medial meniscal tear with an associated lateral compartment bone bruise, occurs secondary to valgus with rotation.

Stages of Disease

MCL injuries are graded on a three-point scale:

Grade 1 Strain Microtears and irreversible stretching of the collagenous fibers of the MCL. This injury is associated with no loss of function.

Grade 2 Partial tear that may be associated with some mild to moderate loss of function and laxity
Grade 3 Complete tear and consequent loss of function

Complications

Loss of joint stability.

Imaging Findings

RADIOGRAPHY

Although uncommon, fractures of the lateral femoral condyle and lateral tibial plateau may be present.

ULTRASOUND

Despite the superficial location of the structure, ultrasound is infrequently utilized in the assessment of acute MCL injuries.

COMPUTED TOMOGRAPHY

CT will define associated bony injuries elegantly but has no role in the assessment of the acutely injured MCL.

MAGNETIC RESONANCE IMAGING

The deep and superficial MCL may be identified on MR as parallel dark bands on both axial and coronal sequences. The bands may be seen to be clearly separated by fatty tissue on coronal MRI (T1).

The superficial MCL is seen to best advantage on the coronal sequences at the level of the intracondylar notch parallel with the distal ACL insertion. The ligament should be seen as a dark, thin stripe paralleling the cortices of the femoral condyle and proximal tibia.

Between the superficial and deep MCL is the bursa, surrounded by fibrofatty tissue, which will appear bright on T1 and T2 if no fluid is present within the bursa but will appear low signal on T1 and high on T2 in the presence of bursitis.

Fluid within the bursa may be mistaken for an acute tear of the ligament.

Grade 1 Strain: intact low-signal MCL with surrounding fluid secondary to perifascicular edema. Abnormal signal will be seen in the adjacent subcutaneous fat.

Grade 2 Partial tear: thickening of the ligament with diffuse intrasubstance signal heterogeneity, perifascicular edema, and elevation of the fibers from the bony attachment by accompanying edema and/or hemorrhage (**Fig. 5B**)

Grade 3 Complete tear: loss of continuity of the ligament, disruption of the capsular ligaments, and subcutaneous fat edema (**Figs. 5A, 5C,** and **5D**). Complete avulsions are usually secondary to high-energy trauma, such as a motor vehicle accident.

Associated injuries

The MCL attaches anteriorly to the patellar retinaculum. Injuries to the MCL may well be associated with retinacular tears. These latter injuries are best seen on the axial sequences.

Two typical patterns of bone contusions occur with MCL injuries:

1. Lateral contusion secondary to valgus impaction (**Fig. 5E**)
2. Medial avulsion injuries in either femur or tibia

Injuries to the deep MCL are almost always associated with disruption of the meniscofemoral or meniscotibial ligaments, which will appear as disruption of the normally dark, thin bands on T1 and T2 in the presence of a displaced medial meniscus.

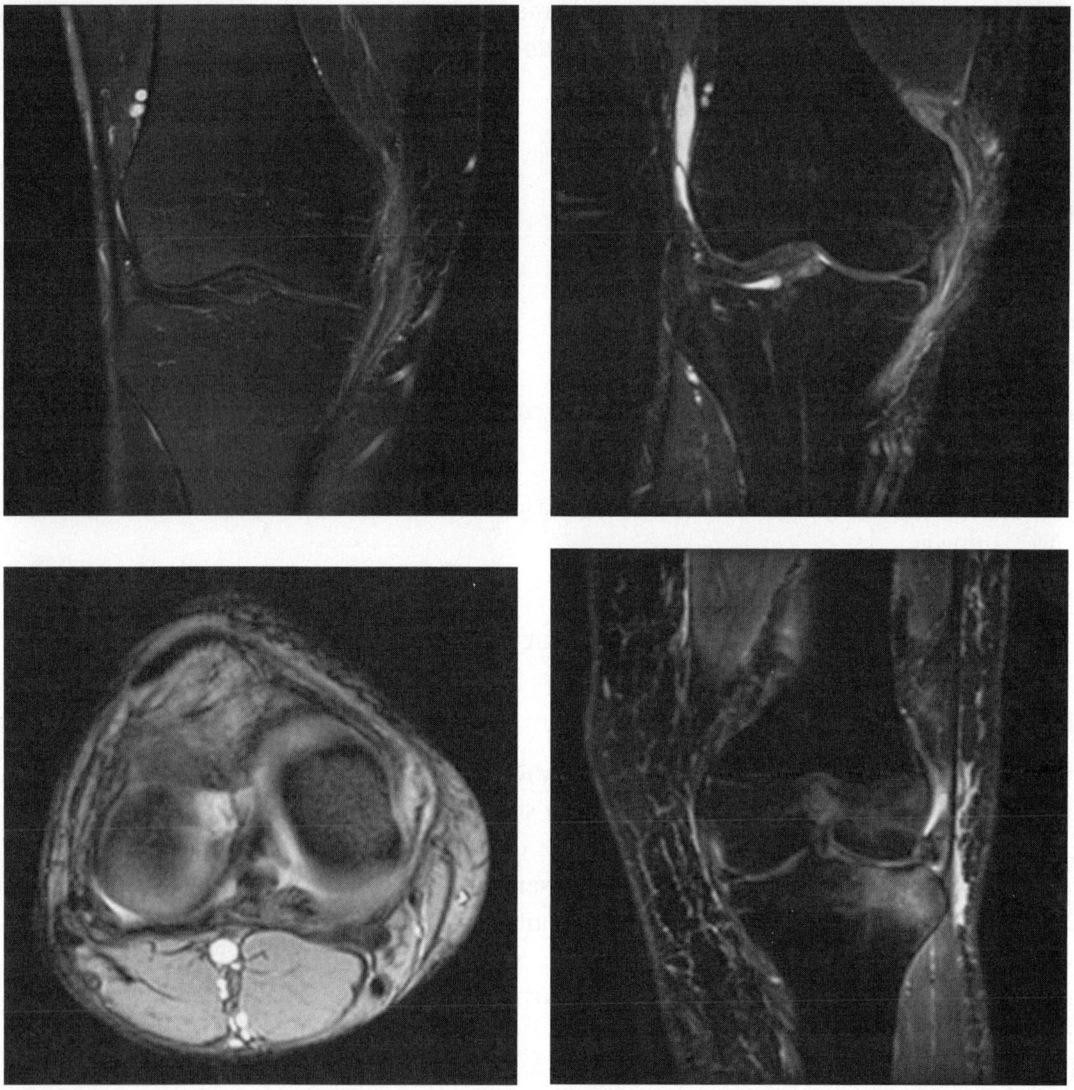

B C D E

Figures 5B–5E **5B** Coronal T2-weighted fat-saturated image shows a high-grade partial tear (grade II) of the proximal half of the medial collateral ligament (MCL). Thickening and diffuse intrasubstance signal heterogeneity is evident proximally. Although more than 50% of the MCL thickness is torn, fiber continuity persists. **5C** Coronal T2-weighted fat-saturated image shows a grade III/complete tear of the distal half of the MCL with fluid evident between the deep and superficial components of the ligament, fluid interposed between the distal ligament and the subjacent tibia, and abundant subcutaneous edema. Note that the meniscocapsular complex remains intact; that is, no fluid is seen interposed between the meniscus and the capsule/deep ligament. **5D** Axial T2-weighted image shows discontinuity of fibers medially at the level of the distal medial femoral condyle. Fluid is evident on either side of the torn ligament. **5E** Coronal T2-weighted fat-saturated image shows a torn medial collateral ligament with meniscocapsular separation and contusions of the lateral tibial plateau and lateral femoral condyle secondary to impaction. The lateral meniscus is torn and extruded laterally.

Meniscocapsular separation frequently occurs in association with an MCL injury and is demonstrated by visualizing joint fluid extending between the medial meniscus and the capsule. Coronal T2 or gradient images are required for this, as T1 images will most likely miss the fluid, particularly if only a small amount is present. Because the injury to the meniscus affects the vascular portion, this is an area that responds to surgical repair and is thus important to recognize.

Chronic injuries

The chronically torn MCL is usually seen as a thick, dark band on all sequences secondary to the presence of dense scar. Very low signal intensity may be demonstrated if the proximal ligament becomes calcified, as, for example, in the Pellegrini-Stieda pattern.

In the absence of calcifications, a chronic MCL tear is often best appreciated by the loss of distinction of the MCL from adjacent fat on T1-weighted images.

Treatment and Prognosis

Grades 1 and 2 Conservative nonsurgical management is the treatment of choice, aimed at preventing extension of the existing injury.

Grade 3 If immobilized in a long-leg cast for a minimum of 6 weeks, the ligament eventually heals by granulation tissue and subsequent scar formation but with loss of original strength. This is usually inconsequential to the amateur, but it may limit the activities of a professional athlete. In this cohort, surgeons may consider attempting repair by reinforcement with tensor fasciae latae or semitendinosis or adductor tendons.

PEARLS

- Most MCL injuries will heal spontaneously, and the crucial aspect of imaging is to identify the other associated injuries.
- As the MCL is extra-articular, isolated tears should not produce an effusion.
- Meniscocapsular separation frequently occurs in association with an MCL injury and is demonstrated by visualizing joint fluid extending between the medial meniscus and the capsule.
- Between the superficial and deep MCL, the bursa is surrounded by fibrofatty tissue, which will appear bright on T1 and T2 if no fluid is present within the bursa, but which will appear low signal on T1 and high on T2 in the presence of bursitis.

PITFALLS

- A thickened MCL is a frequent attendant in osteoarthrosis and thus may be mistaken for a chronic tear. There will usually be a varus deformity at the knee, which causes buckling of the MCL and thickening of the tissues around the ligament.
- In the above circumstances, a chronic MCL tear is often best appreciated by the loss of distinction of the MCL from adjacent fat on T1-weighted imaging.
- Fluid within the bursa may be mistaken for an acute tear of the ligament.

Suggested Readings

Garvin GJ, Munk PL, Vellet AD. Tears of the medial collateral ligament: magnetic resonance imaging findings and associated injuries. Can Assoc Radiol J 1993;44:199–204

Rasenberg EI, Lemmens JA, Van Kampen A, et al. Grading medial collateral ligament injury: comparison of MR imaging and instrumented valgus varus laxity test device. A prospective double blind study. Eur J Radiol 1995;21:18–24

Schweitzer ME, Tran D, Dely DM, Hume EL. Medial collateral ligament injuries: evaluation of multiple signs, prevalence and location of associated bone bruises, and assessment with MR imaging. Radiology 1995;194:825–829

Staron RB, Haramati N, Feldman F, et al. O'Donoghue's triad: magnetic resonance imaging evidence. Skeletal Radiol 1994;23(8):633–666

CASE 6

Anthony G. Ryan and Peter L. Munk

Clinical Presentation

Our patient presented with recurrent pain and locking after a remote trauma.

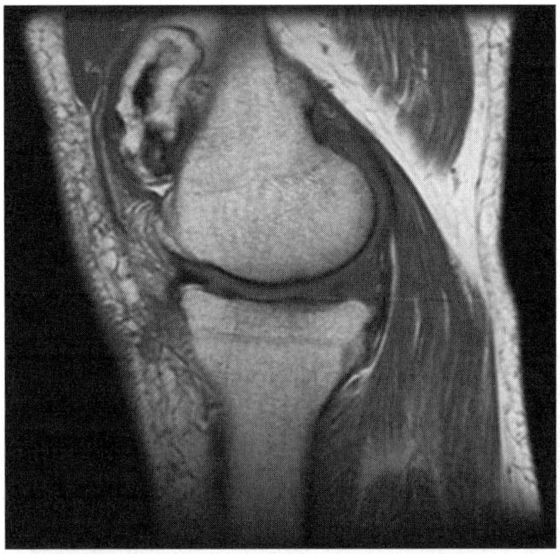

Figure 6A

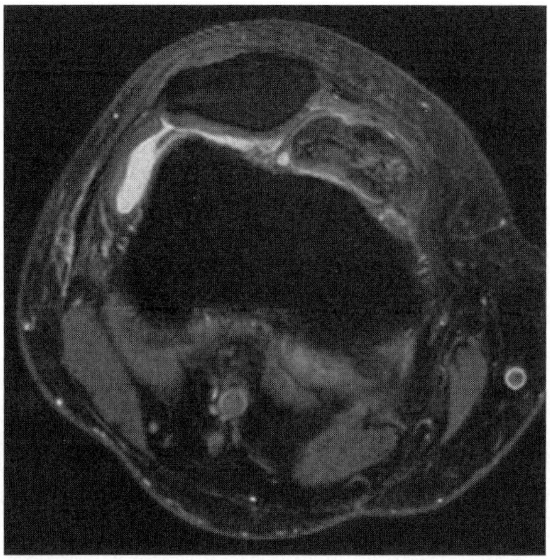

Figure 6B

Radiologic Findings

A sagittal T1-weighted image (**Fig. 6A**) and an axial proton density (PD) fat-saturated image (**Fig. 6B**) show a very large irregular intra-articular loose body in the superomedial patellar recess secondary to degenerative osteoarthritis. Speckled low density scattered throughout the lesion is evident, consistent with calcifications. Chondromalacia patella is evident on the axial image. Articular surface irregularity and subchondral sclerosis are evident on the sagittal image.

Diagnosis

Intra-articular loose body.

Differential Diagnosis

Solitary loose body:

1. Chip fracture from trauma (**Figs. 6C–6F**)
2. Osteochondral fracture
3. Usually affecting the knee (**Fig. 6G**), talus, and elbow. A donor site may be visible.
4. Severe degenerative joint disease (**Figs. 6A,6B**)
5. Detached osteophyte; usually other signs of degenerative arthritis. The fragments are typically larger and more variable than those found in synovial osteochondromatosis.

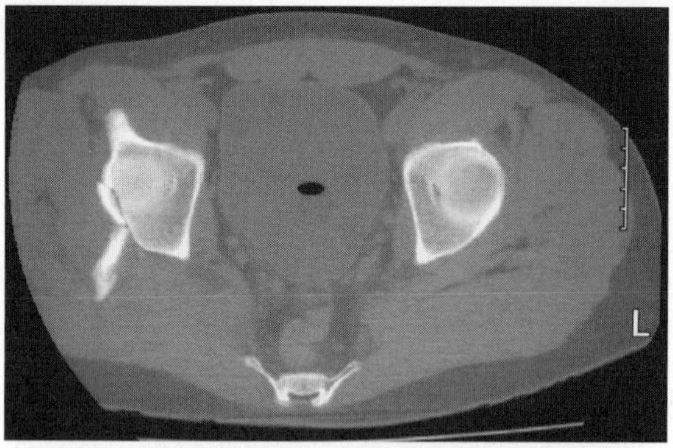

C

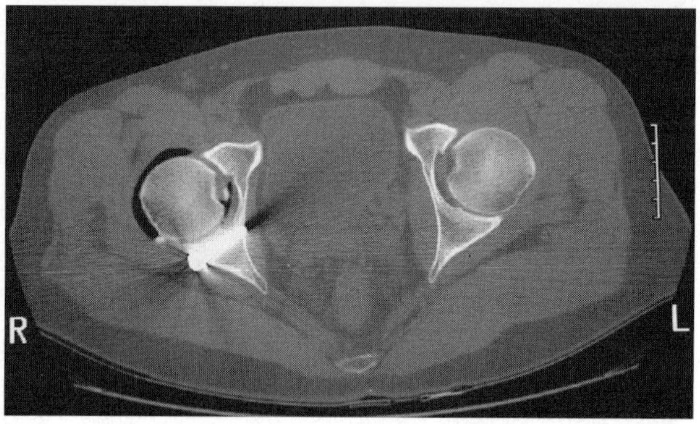

D

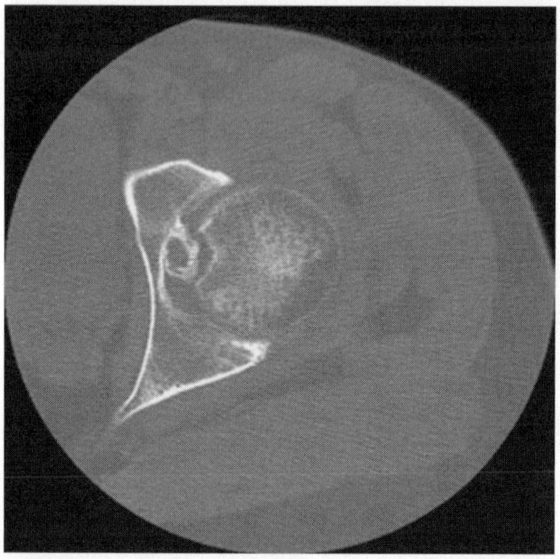

E

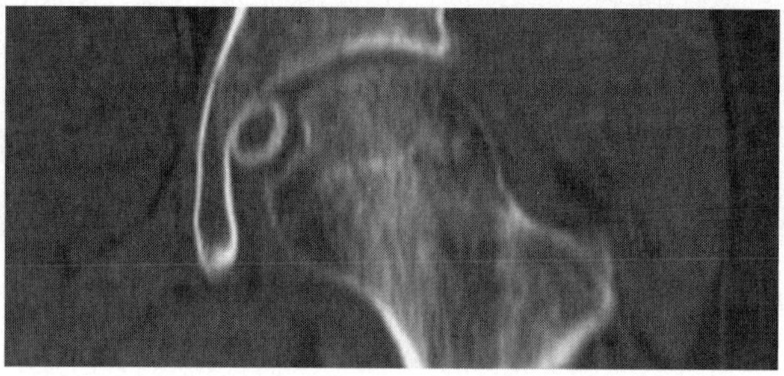

F

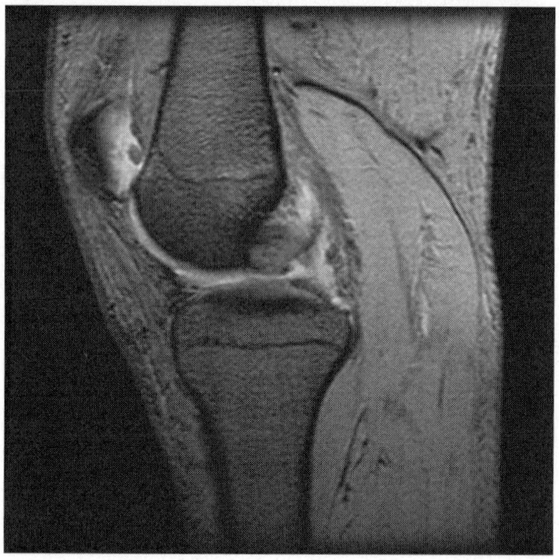

G

Figures 6C Transaxial CT pelvis posttrauma shows a comminuted fracture of the posterosuperior acetabular margin. **6D** Same patient as in **6C**. Postreduction CT shows two small intra-articular fragments, one medially at the level of the fovea capitis and a second lying posteriorly at the level of the posterior acetabular margin. **6E** and **6F** Axial and coronal reformat, respectively, of the left hip shows an untreated posttraumatic loose body medial to the femoral head. Erosion and irregularity of the femoral head is evident, as are secondary degenerative changes (articular surface irregularity, superior joint space narrowing, and subchondral sclerosis). **6G** Sagittal T2-weighted image of the knee shows a small loose body posterior to the patella. The donor site secondary to an osteochondral defect on the posterior aspect of the patella is not shown.

Multiple loose bodies:

1. Neuropathic arthropathy (the debris of the six Ds)
2. Rice bodies (rheumatoid arthritis, seronegative inflammatory arthritis, juvenile rheumatoid arthritis, and tuberculous joints)
3. Synovial osteochondromatosis (**Fig. 6H**)

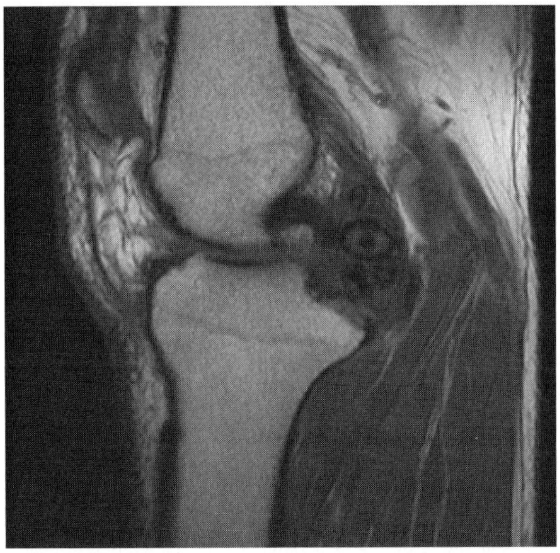

Figure 6H Sagittal T1-weighted image of the knee shows multiple well-defined loose bodies secondary to synovial osteochondromatosis posterior to the posterior cruciate ligament.

Discussion

Background

Emphasis will be placed on those conditions causing multiple small loose bodies, as the other conditions are dealt with at length elsewhere in the atlas.

Etiology

The etiology of large, solitary loose bodies is self-evident from the differential above.

The so-called rice bodies associated with juvenile rheumatoid arthritis are composed of fragments of sloughed infarcted hypertrophied synovium, which are not typically calcified.

The etiology of synovial osteochondromatosis is unknown, although neoplastic and infectious mechanisms have been proposed.

Pathophysiology

Regardless of origin, the presence of loose bodies interferes with the mechanical function of the joint, disrupting congruency and preventing normal articulation. In addition, they act as potent cartilaginous irritants, causing cartilaginous destruction and eventual osteoarthritis if left untreated.

RICE BODIES

Rice bodies arise as a nonspecific response to synovial inflammation, most frequently occurring in association with inflammatory arthritides, especially rheumatoid and its juvenile variant. It is thought they represent sloughed infarcted synovium. Multiple rice body formation is a recognized complication of chronic bursitis.

SYNOVIAL OSTEOCHONDROMATOSIS

Multiple small nodules of synovial origin are broken off with joint motion and are shed into the joint. After a period of mobility, during which time they are referred to as "joint mice," they tend to reattach to the synovium. The nodules tend to be of similar size and are scattered uniformly throughout the joint. These may be only faintly calcified initially but over time may progress to frank ossification, although up to 30% of them do not calcify at all.

These fragments eventually cause secondary erosion of the intracapsular bone; joint space narrowing and osteophyte formation may occur later in the disease.

Clinical Findings

Joint locking, clicking, and crunching occur.

A patient may relate a several-year history of joint pain and limited range of motion. The knee, hip, elbow, shoulder, and temporomandibular joints (TMJs) are most commonly involved.

Complications

The presence of intra-articular loose bodies, regardless of etiology, predisposes to accelerated osteoarthritis secondary to erosion of the cartilage and subchondral bone.

Incomplete reduction of an intra-articular fracture has been reported as a result of an osteochondral body becoming entrapped between the fracture fragments, necessitating open treatment.

Imaging Findings

RADIOGRAPHY

- Uncalcified lesions, such as hypertrophied synovium, rice bodies, osteochondromatosis, and intra-articular fibrinous debris, are not visible on conventional radiographs.
- The nodules of synovial osteochondromatosis may be only faintly calcified initially but over time progress to frank ossification, affecting the knee, hip (**Figs. 6I, 6J**), ankle, wrist, shoulder, and TMJs, in descending order.
- Secondary erosions, joint space narrowing, and osteophyte formation may be evident.

ULTRASOUND

- Reported sensitivity and specificity of ultrasound were 100 and 95%, respectively, in the identification of intra-articular bodies.

COMPUTED TOMOGRAPHY

- Calcifications and small ossific fragments not seen on conventional radiographs will be demonstrated with ease on CT (**Figs. 6D,6K**).

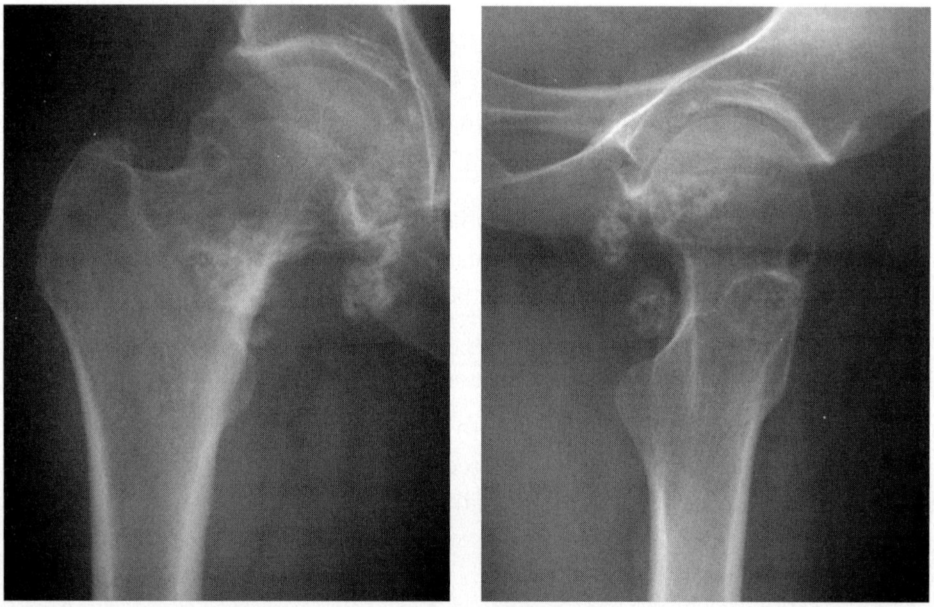

I J

Figures 6I and **6J** Anteroposterior and lateral radiographs, respectively, of the right hip show multiple round calcified densities of similar size, characteristic of synovial osteochondromatosis.

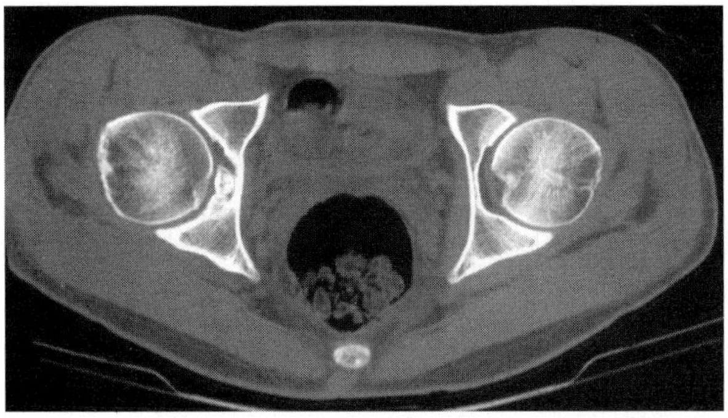

Figure 6K Transaxial CT of the pelvis at the level of the femoral heads shows an ossified loose body between the femoral head and the acetabulum medially on the right, not seen on conventional radiography, in a patient with synovial osteochondromatosis.

- Joint manipulation preceding CT increases the sensitivity of the examination in establishing a definitive diagnosis.
- CT arthrography also increases the accuracy of the examination (80%).
- CT has been used to identify the lesions of synovial osteochondromatosis in the TMJ joints, demonstrating increased soft-tissue density within the joints in addition to multiple small peripherally calcified densities.
- CT demonstrates associated bony changes elegantly, as, for example, erosions of the condylar process and fossa and, if present, thinning of the walls of the external auditory and carotid canals.

MAGNETIC RESONANCE IMAGING

- The presence of intra-articular fluid and performance of saline-enhanced MR arthrography improve detectability of intra-articular bodies.
- MR arthrography is the most accurate (92%) technique for detection of individual osseous and cartilaginous intra-articular bodies, best demonstrated by spoiled GRASS and T2-weighted SE sequences.
- MRI without arthrography has an accuracy of between 57 and 70%.
- Bony loose bodies may be seen to contain high-signal fatty marrow surrounded by a low signal intensity rim.
- Rice bodies are seen as conspicuous, innumerable, well-defined nodules within the joint demonstrating intermediate signal intensity on T1 and relatively lower signal intensity on T2, reflecting their fibrous structure. After intravenous gadolinium, synovium enhances brightly, but rice bodies do not.
- The cartilaginous bodies of synovial osteochondromatosis are of high signal intensity on T2 with respect to skeletal muscle (unless calcified, in which case they will be of low signal intensity on all sequences) (**Figs. 6L,6M**).

Treatment

Arthroscopic retrieval of smaller loose bodies may be possible, although arthrotomy may be necessary. Synovectomy is the treatment for synovial osteochondromatosis.

Prognosis

The prognosis depends on the underlying condition.

Early detection and removal help to prevent secondary degeneration and loss of function.

PEARLS

- After intravenous gadolinium, synovium enhances brightly; however, rice bodies do not.
- Calcifications and small ossific fragments not seen on conventional radiographs will be demonstrated with ease on CT.

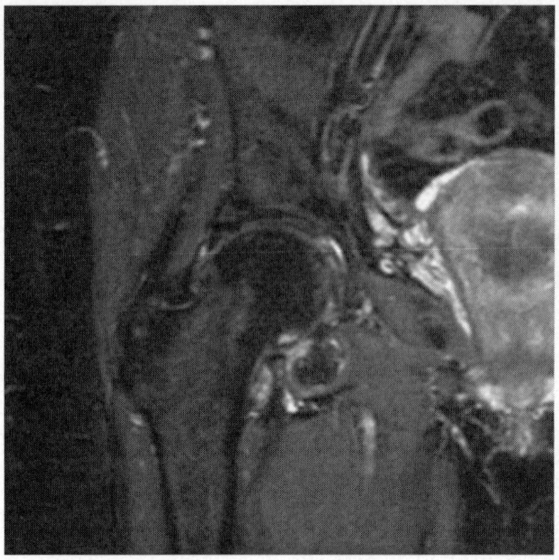

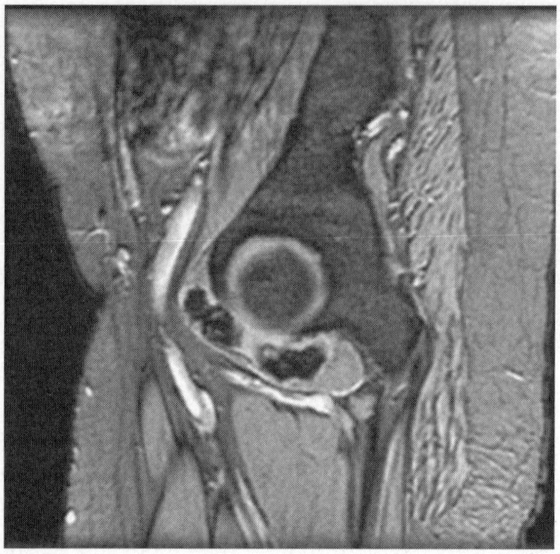

Figures 6L and **6M** MRI of the same patient as in **Figs. 6I** and **6J**. The calcified bodies are clearly seen within the joint space on both T2 fat-saturated (**6L**) and gradient sequences (**6M**). The dense low signal intensity reflects the calcified nature of these lesions. Speckled high signal intensity remains in keeping with persistent cartilage content.

- Rice bodies are not typically calcified, whereas 70% of the nodules of synovial osteochondromatosis will calcify eventually.

PITFALLS

- MRI without arthrography has an accuracy of between 57 and 70%, compared with 92% for saline MR arthrography in the detection of loose intra-articular bodies.
- The lack of calcifications does not exclude the diagnosis of synovial osteochondromatosis, as the lesions may be only faintly calcified initially.
- Incomplete reduction of an intra-articular fracture has been reported as a result of osteochondral body entrapment between the fracture fragments, necessitating open treatment.

Suggested Readings

Chen A, Wong LY, Sheu CY, Chen BF. Distinguishing multiple rice body formation in chronic subacromial-subdeltoid bursitis from synovial chondromatosis. Skeletal Radiol 2002;31:119–121

Connell DG, Parikh JR, Forster BB, Munk PL. Post-manipulation CT of the knee joint: an aid in diagnosis of intraarticular loose bodies. J Comput Assist Tomogr 1991;15:511–512

Munk PL, Helms CA. Temporomandibular joint synovial osteochondromatosis: CT manifestations. Can Assoc Radiol J 1989;40:274–276

CASE 7

Anthony G. Ryan and Peter L. Munk

Clinical Presentation

A 26-year-old insulin-dependent patient with diabetes sustained a combined extension against resistance and direct impact injury as a result of a heavy tackle while playing amateur soccer. He complained of immediate excruciating pain in his distal thigh and had almost complete loss of active knee extension on examination.

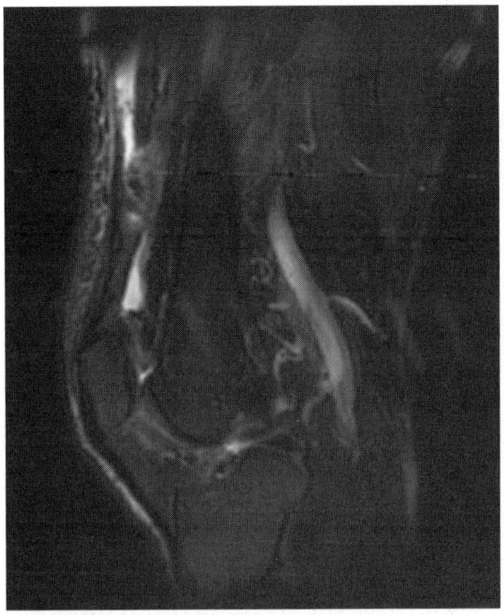

Figure 7A

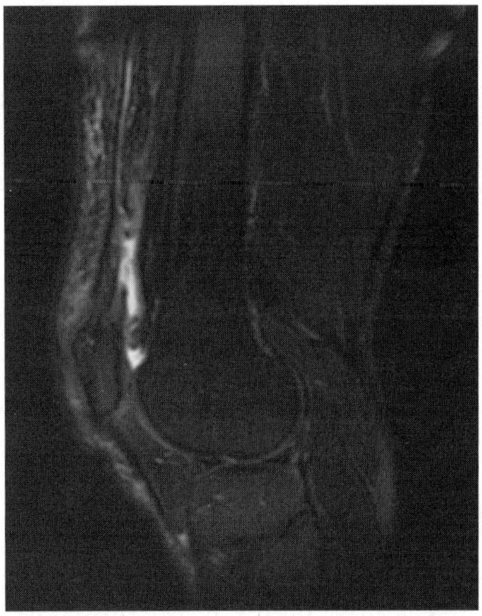

Figure 7B

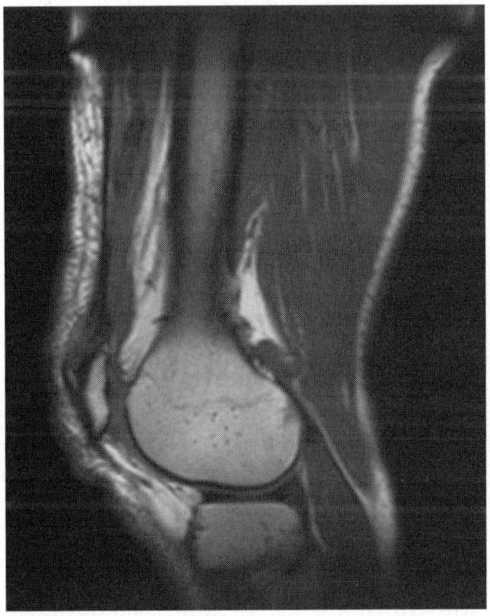

Figure 7C

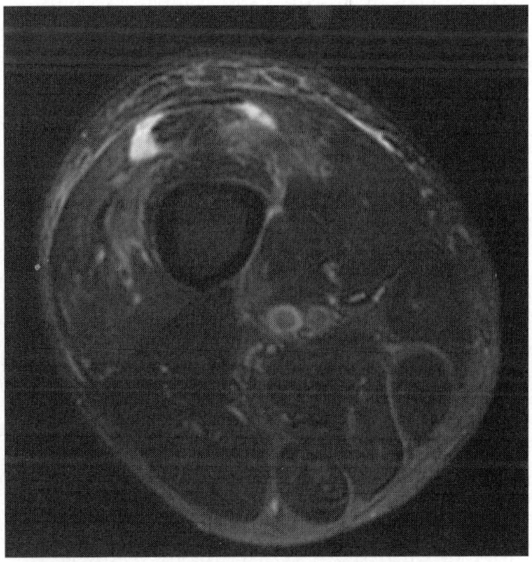

Figure 7D

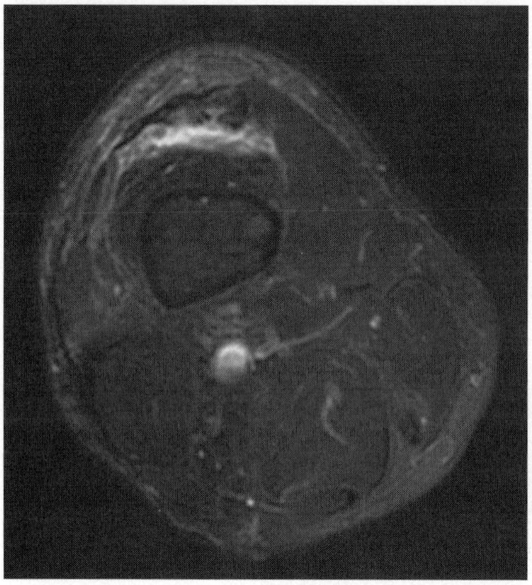

Figure 7E

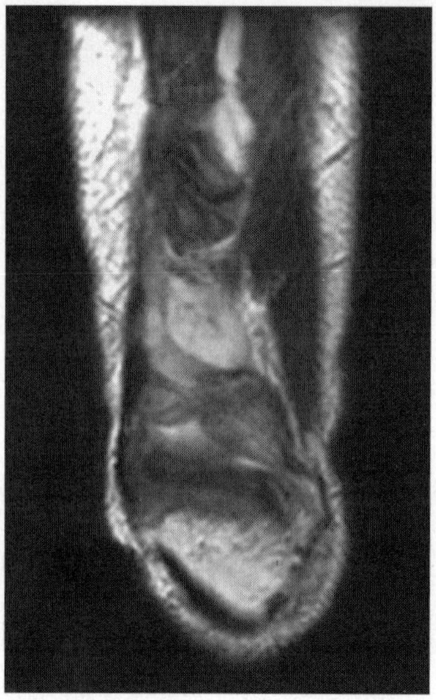

Figure 7F

Radiologic Findings

Sagittal T2 (**Figs. 7A,7B**), sagittal T1 (**Fig. 7C**), axial proton density fat-saturated (**Figs. 7D,7E**), and coronal T2 (**Fig. 7F**) images show focal discontinuity, thickening, and signal heterogeneity within the proximal quadriceps tendon at the level of the musculotendinous condensation. Fluid signal intensity is evident on the T2 images anterior and posterior to the tendon. High signal intensity is also evident within the substance of the adjacent muscles of the anterior compartment: rectus femoris, vastus intermedius, vastus medialis, and vastus lateralis.

Diagnosis

Quadriceps tendon tear.

Differential Diagnosis

None.

Discussion

Background

The extensor mechanism of the knee joint consists of the quadriceps muscle and tendon, patella, patellar tendon, and patellar retinacula.

The quadriceps tendon itself is a conjoint tendon of the four muscles of the anterior compartment of the thigh—the rectus femoris, vastus lateralis, vastus medialis, and vastus intermedius—which are the major extensors, and consequently stabilizers, of the knee joint.

Injuries of these structures may be classified as acute or chronic contusions or partial or complete tears.

Etiology

Rupture of the quadriceps tendon is uncommon in the absence of conditions predisposing to tendinopathy.

The tendon may be weakened because of chronic degeneration or inflammation, which may then produce an exercise-related rupture secondary to less forceful contraction.

Endogenous disorders giving rise to tendon weakness include diabetes mellitus, rheumatoid arthritis, and seronegative spondyloarthropathy.

Primary and secondary hyperparathyroidism: End-stage renal disease is frequently associated with distal quadriceps rupture, secondary to a combination of the secondary hyperparathyroidism and subtendinous bone resorption.

Exogenous factors predisposing to tendinopathy include mechanical impingement, repetitive overuse, systemic steroid use or abuse, and repeated intra-articular or bursal injection of steroids.

As many as 50% of patients with closed femoral shaft fractures have accompanying injuries of the extensor mechanism (**Fig. 7G**). Contusions to the muscle belly are usually sustained by direct trauma secondary to contact sport activities or motor vehicle collisions.

Strain of the complex is most likely to happen at the musculotendinous junction.

Pathophysiology

Rupture of the distal quadriceps secondary to end-stage renal disease occurs as a result of the combination of secondary hyperparathyroidism and subtendinous bone resorption.

Acute injuries are associated with edema, hemorrhage, and fluid collections.

Complete disruption of the extensor mechanism may be associated with osseous avulsion of the superior pole of the patella (**Figs. 7H,7I**).

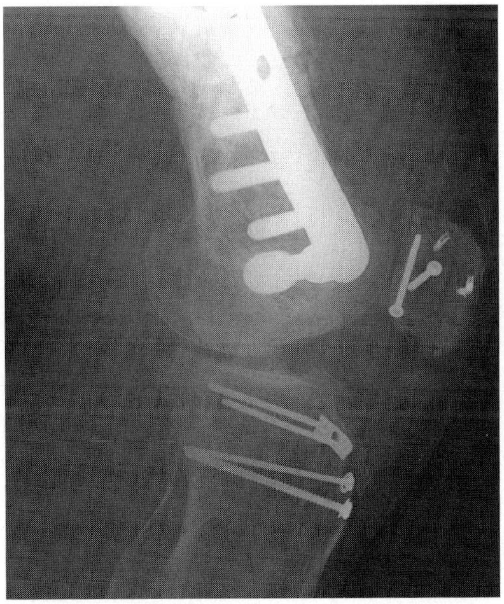

Figure 7G Lateral radiograph of the knee after fixation of distal femoral and proximal tibial fractures. Calcifications are evident in both quadriceps and patellar tendons, indicative of the combined injury sustained at the time of the initial insult.

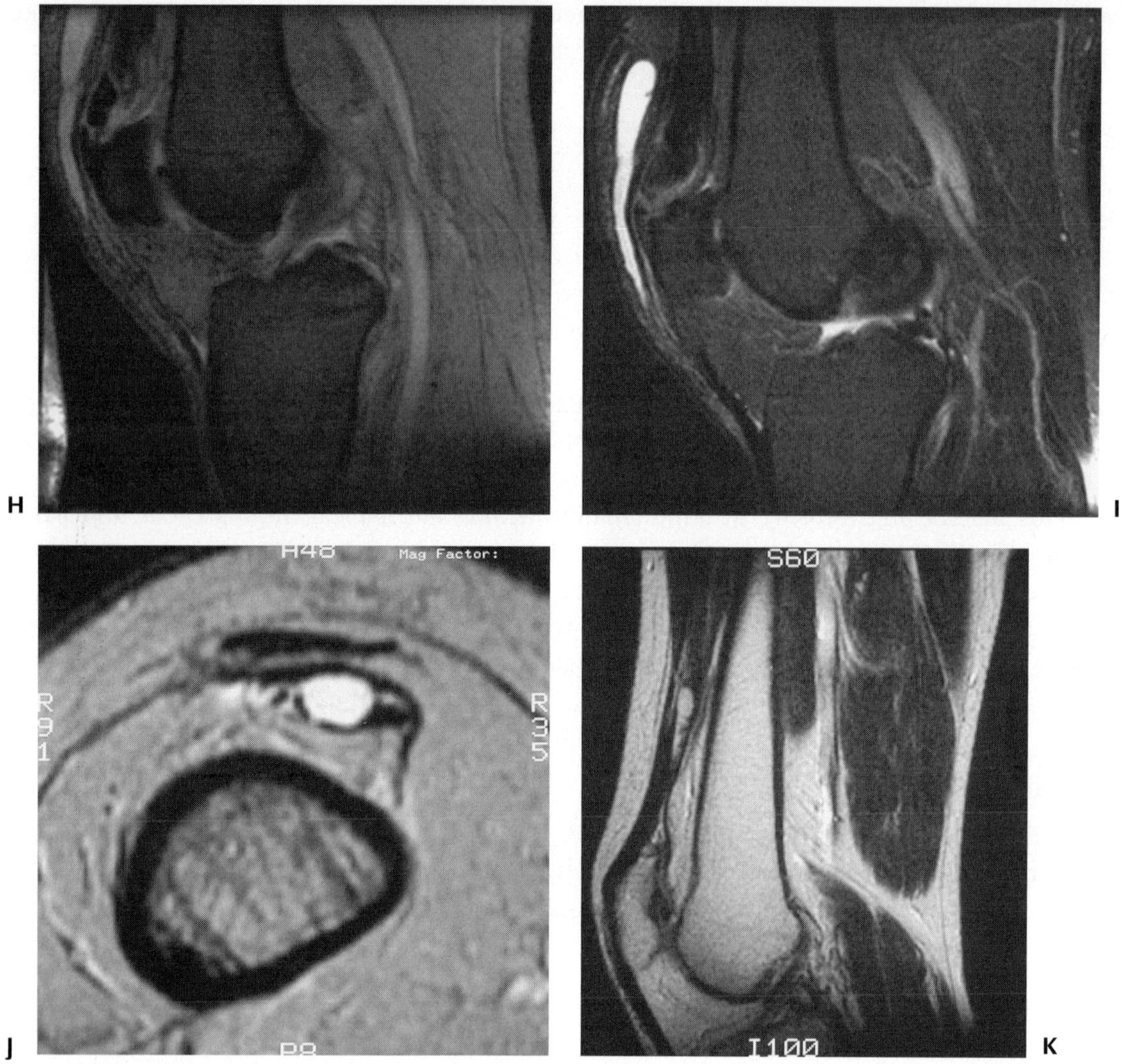

Figures 7H and **7I** Sagittal MPGR (**7H**) and sagittal T2 (**7I**) images demonstrate focal discontinuity of the distal quadriceps tendon with avulsion of the superior pole of the patella. Note also the slightly wavy or corrugated appearance of the patellar tendon, secondary evidence of the more cephalad injury. **7J** and **7K** Axial (**7J**) and sagittal (**7K**) T2 images from a follow-up study performed in a 47-year-old man with a post-partial quadriceps tendon tear. Note that the cyst is located at the musculotendinous condensation of the vastus intermedius.

Chronic injuries often demonstrate redundancy, atrophy, and retraction of the affected structures. Cyst formation may be evident as a late sequel of quadriceps injury (**Figs. 7J,7K**).

In the chronic state, the tendon itself and its bony attachment tend to be affected to a greater extent. This will generally cause progressive tendon weakening, at which point the tendon then becomes the weakest link in the myotendinous unit.

The tendon may be weakened because of chronic degeneration or inflammation, which may then produce an exercise-related rupture secondary to less forceful contraction.

Clinical Findings

Traumatic rupture of the quadriceps tendon is an uncommon knee injury that occurs in the elderly and/or the obese and in those with underlying systemic disease.

Clinically, the patient has anterior knee pain and cannot actively extend the knee. In a partial tear, extension is maintained but is likely to be weak and painful. The clinical evidence of the tear may be concealed by hematoma or hemarthrosis.

Undiagnosed rupture predisposes to chronic loss of function.

Stages of Disease

Acute tears may extend and/or become chronic, and partial tears may progress to complete tears if undiagnosed.

Complications

- Chronic discontinuity, loss of function, muscle atrophy, weakness
- Muscle fibrosis after an injury; for example, in the vastus lateralis, this may give rise to a contracture, leading to recurrent patellar dislocation.
- In the presence of a chronic quadriceps tendon tear, the muscle belly may undergo atrophy, which may begin within 10 days after immobilization. After 20 days of continuous bed rest, 10% of the muscle mass of a healthy man is lost. If established for 4 months, the atrophy becomes partially irreversible.

Imaging Findings

RADIOGRAPHY

- On the lateral view of the knee, there may be loss of normal quadriceps outline and a soft-tissue mass representing the retracted quadriceps tendon.
- In a chronic tear, the retracted tendon may be calcified.
- Most patients have a hemarthrosis, which may be evident as a dense effusion.
- Lateral radiographs of the knee may show a corrugated patellar tendon.

ULTRASOUND

- Longitudinal and transverse sonograms, including dynamic scanning, may be critical to diagnosing a partial quadriceps tendon tear.
- Sonography may aid in differentiation of partial-thickness tears from complete quadriceps tendon tears, particularly in the acute setting.
- Partial rupture demonstrated as a focal hypoechoic defect in the tendon
- Complete rupture demonstrated as a complete disruption of the tendon fibers
- Ultrasound appears to have a high sensitivity and specificity for complete tears but may have difficulty detecting partial or chronic partial tears, the latter sensitivity is further reduced by the presence of scar tissue.

MAGNETIC RESONANCE IMAGING

Normal

- The quadriceps tendon is typically seen as a uniformly low signal intensity band on all sequences, extending superiorly from the superior margin of the patella, and is best visualized on the sagittal T1 sequence.
- On higher field scanners (1.5 T and up), the quadriceps tendon may be visualized as a multilayered structure, with separate layers arising from different muscles, the superficial layer originating from the posterior fascia of the rectus femoris muscle and the deep layer originating from

the anterior fascia of the midline vastus intermedius muscle. The middle layer(s) arise(s) from the deep fascia separating the vastus medialis and the vastus lateralis muscles from the vastus intermedius muscle.

- The typical quadriceps tendon measures 5 cm in length and is 7 to 8 mm thick.

Tears

- Complete
  - A complete tear will obviously result in a focal discontinuity, the gap being filled by hemorrhagic fluid.
  - Sagittal MRI may show a corrugated appearance of the patellar tendon.
  - Unsuspected nondisplaced patellar fractures may be disclosed by MRI.
  - Transient dislocation of the patella is an often clinically unsuspected entity for which MRI can serve an important diagnostic role.
- Partial
  - A partial tear will typically be evident on MRI by abnormal size and increased internal signal.
  - The laminated configuration of the quadriceps tendon allows distinction between partial and complete tears. Both may be accompanied by edema and hemorrhage, manifest as fluid/high signal intensity on T2-weighted images.
  - Incomplete ruptures may be seen as focal discontinuities of individual layers, with the other layers remaining (**Figs. 7L,7M**).
- Chronic
  - In the presence of a chronic quadriceps tendon tear, the muscle belly may undergo atrophy, which, on MRI, would be seen as fatty degeneration ± loss of muscle bulk.
  - Cyst formation is an uncommon finding in the presence of a chronic tear.
  - Muscle fibrosis after an injury, for example, vastus lateralis with recurrent patella dislocation, may occur, and fibrosis may give rise to a contracture that may be amenable to surgical treatment.

L

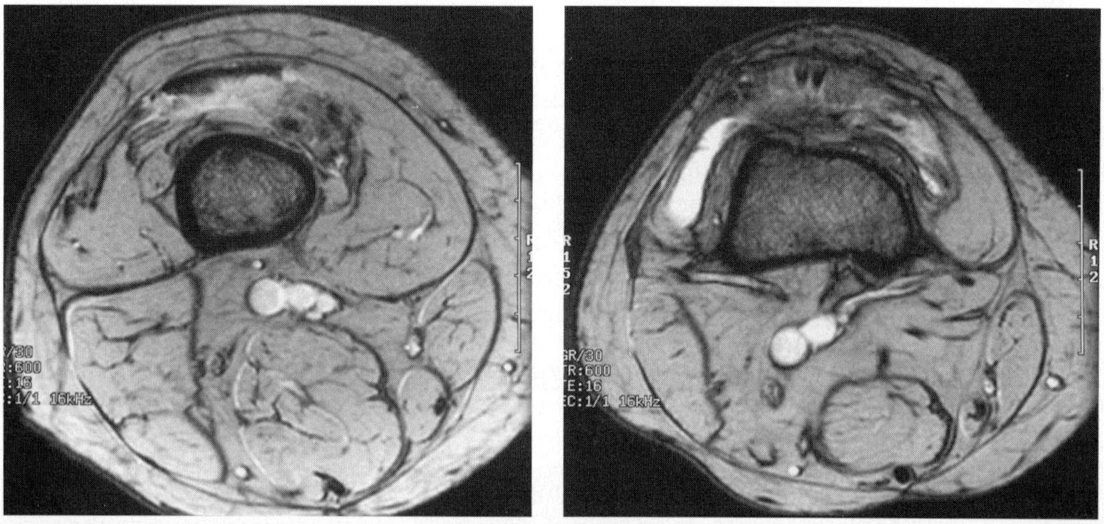

M

Figures 7L and **7M** Axial T2 images (**7L** more cephalad than **7M**) show thickening, discontinuity, and signal heterogeneity at the level of the proximal musculotendinous condensation, similar to the case in **Figs. 7A–7F**. The distortion is most evident on the medial aspect of the condensation, affecting the vastus intermedius and vastus medialis to a greater degree, reflecting a greater degree of injury and retraction. Fluid signal intensity is seen posterior to the tendon on **7L**.

Strain

- Acute strain on the myotendinous unit can give rise to characteristic findings on MRI with high signal intensity centered on the tendinous condensation.
- Fat-suppressed T2 and inversion recovery sequences will demonstrate high signal intensity with a geographic or diffuse appearance with feathery margins. High T1 signal intensity is usually indicative of subacute blood. No fibrous discontinuity or laxity should be observed, differentiating these injuries from high-grade strain injury.

Hematoma

- The majority of intramuscular hematomas resolve spontaneously after a period of 6 to 8 weeks.
- Methemoglobin gives rise to characteristically high signal intensity on T1 sequences.
- Chronic hematomas will usually show a low signal intensity rim, reflecting the presence of hemosiderin and fibrosis.

Treatment

Partial tendon tears may be treated conservatively by immobilization and supervised physiotherapy until the return to full function.

Complete tears require reapposition of the discontinuous margins to restore full function.

Contractures secondary to fibrosis may be amenable to surgical treatment. If the injury is chronic, and the tendon has retracted significantly, a pin may be placed through the distal tendon and traction applied with a view to lengthening it to reappose the tendon margins.

If sufficient length is still unavailable, repair may be achieved by use of a transposed distal iliotibial band.

Prognosis

- Partial tears tend to do well with conservative management.
- Complete tears do well if the ends are reapposed acutely.
- The longer the delay between injury and repair, the poorer the likelihood of a return to full function.

PEARLS

- The clinical diagnosis is often overlooked, and the radiologist could be the first to suggest the diagnosis.
- A corrugated appearance of the patellar tendon on sagittal images indicates a reduction in the normal tensile force applied to it and the need for careful evaluation of the patella and quadriceps tendon mechanism.
- After intravenous gadolinium, hematomas will not be expected to show any enhancement, whereas a neoplasm may demonstrate some nodular enhancement, particularly peripherally.

PITFALLS

- The presence of scar tissue in the setting of chronic injury may represent a potential pitfall in the sonographic assessment of partial versus complete quadriceps tears.
- Fat-suppressed T2 and inversion recovery sequences may demonstrate high signal intensity within a geographic area or diffuse appearance with feathery margins. High T1 signal intensity

is usually indicative of subacute blood. No fibrous discontinuity or laxity should be observed, differentiating these injuries from high-grade strain injury.

- Operative repair is, by definition, open joint surgery and should not be undertaken in the presence of infection, particularly in chronic cases. Thus, if there is such a suspicion, preoperative aspiration may be indicated. Alternatively, post-gadolinium MRI will aid in confirming the diagnosis.

Suggested Readings

Berlin RC, Levinsohn EM, Chrisman H. The wrinkled patellar tendon: an indication of abnormality in the extensor mechanism of the knee. Skeletal Radiol 1991;20:181–185

La S, Fessell DP, Femino JE, Jacobson JA, Jamadar D, Hayes C. Sonography of partial-thickness quadriceps tendon tears with surgical correlation. J Ultrasound Med 2003;22:1323–1331

Zeiss J, Saddemi SR, Ebraheim NA. MR imaging of the quadriceps tendon: normal layered configuration and its importance in cases of tendon rupture. Am J Roentgenol 1992;159:1031–1034

CASE 8

Anthony G. Ryan and Peter L. Munk

Clinical Presentation

A 54-year-old man presented with a painful mass posterior to the knee.

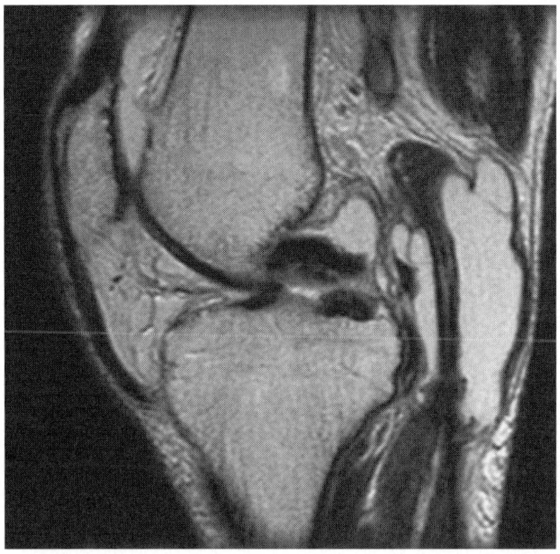

Figure 8A

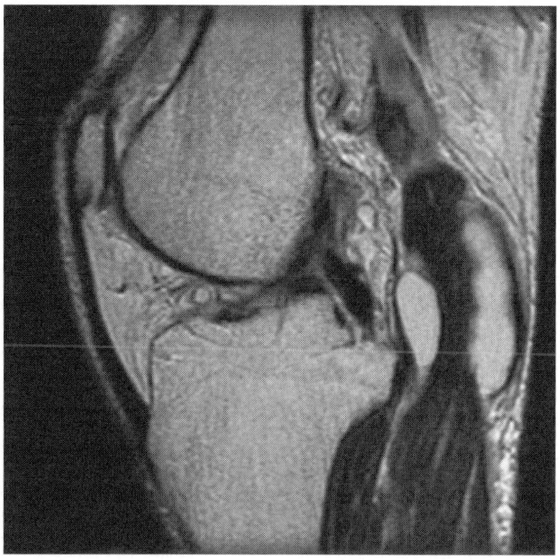

Figure 8B

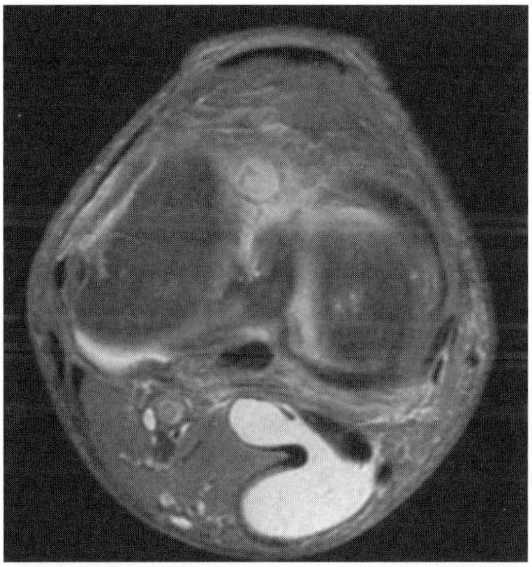

Figure 8C

Radiologic Findings

Sagittal T2 MRI (**Figs. 8A,8B**) and axial proton density fat-saturated images (**Fig. 8C**) show a lobulated high-signal intensity lesion communicating with a knee joint effusion via the interval between the tendons of the medial head of gastrocnemius and semimembranosus muscles.

Diagnosis

Popliteal (Baker's) cyst.

Differential Diagnosis

Although the appearances are typical of a popliteal cyst, in the appropriate circumstances, a popliteal artery aneurysm should be excluded.

When a cyst is seen around the knee, the primary differential is between a meniscal cyst, tibiofibular cyst, cruciate cyst ganglion, and synovial cyst. A meniscal tear is typically found in the presence of a meniscal cyst.

The proximal tibiofibular joint communicates with the knee joint in up to 10% of cases.

If the mass is a cruciate cyst, its typical relationship to the anterior or posterior cruciate ligament should be clearly evident.

Discussion

Background

Commonly found in patients with rheumatoid arthritis (60%) and less frequently found in non-rheumatoid patients, popliteal cysts are synovial cysts that communicate with the knee joint, unless the intervening channel is blocked secondary to recurrent inflammation.

Popliteal cysts occur most frequently in the gastrocnemius-semimembranosus bursa, found, as its name suggests, between the tendons of the medial head of the gastrocnemius and the distal semimembranosus tendon. The larger the cyst, the more likely it will extend into unusual locations. Inferior and medial extension is relatively common, whereas lateral or cephalad extension is rare.

The supralateral bursa may fill between the lateral head of the gastrocnemius and the distal end of the biceps, although this is uncommon, as is filling of the popliteal bursa, found beneath the lateral meniscus and anterior to the popliteus, where it may be confused for a meniscal cyst.

If arthrography is performed, communication with the bursa is expected unless the channel is blocked, as above.

The cysts may form different morphologies. For example, if intact, a cyst will be expected to have a smooth, well-defined contour. Most cysts are unilocular, although multiloculated cysts are not uncommon (**Figs. 8D–8F**).

As the cyst enlarges, it may dissect along fascial planes (usually between the gastrocnemius and the soleus).

If the cyst has ruptured, then a defined structure will not be seen; however, increased edema within the tissues of the calf will be demonstrated.

Etiology

The cyst is most commonly found secondary to rheumatoid arthritis, as in the reference case. However, cysts may occur secondary to degenerative arthritis, internal derangement (joint effusion, meniscal tear), and least frequently in pigmented villonodular synovitis (PVNS).

Studies have shown no association between anterior cruciate ligament tear or medial collateral ligament injury and the presence of a Baker's cyst.

Pathophysiology

The cyst is formed by the escape of an effusion into one of the bursae adjacent to the knee joint. As the volume within the bursa increases, it compresses the communicating channel, preventing further

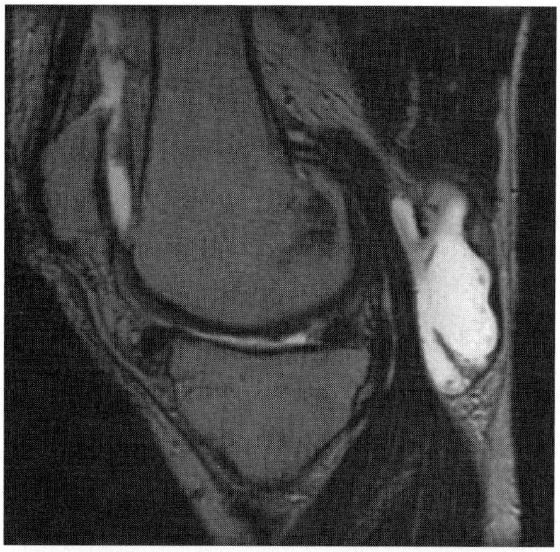

D

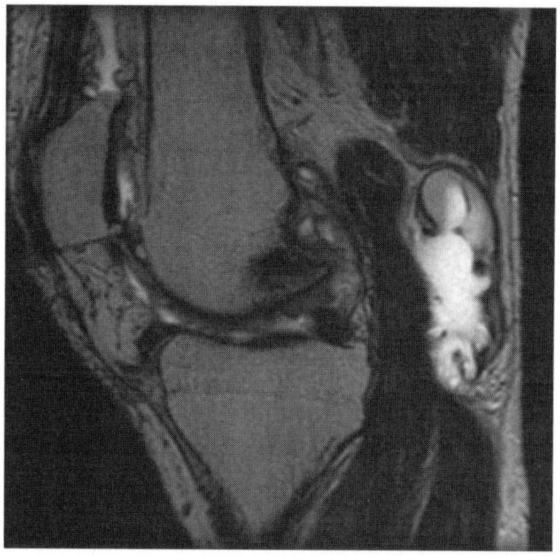

E

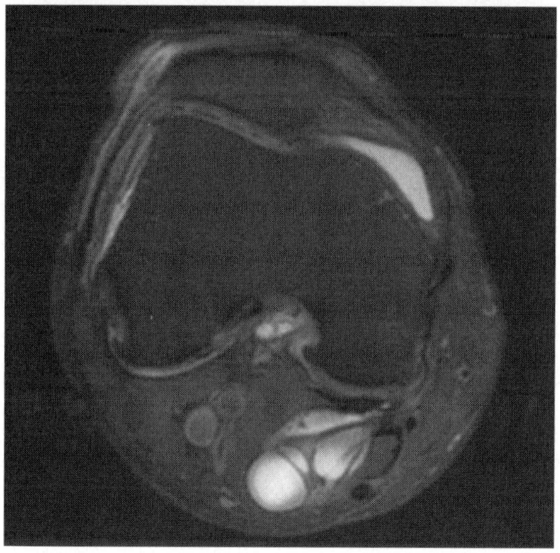

F

Figures 8D–8F Sagittal T2 (**8D,8E**) and axial proton density fat-saturated (**8F**) images show a single large cyst with multiple septations of varying thicknesses. A small joint effusion is also evident, as are findings of degenerative arthritis (thinned irregular cartilage, subchondral sclerosis, patellofemoral and central osteophytosis) secondary to underlying rheumatoid arthritis. Note also the diffusely hypertrophied and irregular synovium in **8D** and **8E**. The cyst is otherwise uncomplicated.

filling or drainage. The channel may also be obstructed by debris from the effusion or subsequently from the cyst so formed.

If the cyst ruptures, fluid tracking subcutaneously can provoke a chemical cellulitis, which may be mistaken for deep venous thrombosis (DVT).

Clinical Findings

Baker's cysts are said to become symptomatic when their total volume measures ~10 cc. The patient typically presents with pain and swelling in the calf, which may raise suspicion of a DVT. Occasionally, both conditions may coexist, as the cyst may compress the popliteal vein, predisposing to thrombophlebitis ± DVT.

Complications

Cysts will cause symptoms by virtue of being palpable, compression on adjacent structures, or rupture.

If the cyst is large enough, it may interfere with flexion of the knee. Compression on adjacent nerves may simulate a nerve entrapment syndrome.

If a DVT is incorrectly diagnosed and consequently anticoagulated on clinical grounds, development of a calf hematoma and secondary compartment syndrome may result. Similarly, patients on anticoagulants will be at risk for developing spontaneous hemorrhage into the cysts.

Baker's cysts contain a synovial lining and may thus share disease processes found in the adjacent knee joint. Calcified bodies secondary to trauma, arthropathy, or synovial osteochondromatosis may be found. Chondrometaplasia may give rise to de novo calcified loose bodies within the cyst. If PVNS is present, then the presence of hemosiderin on MRI would identify the condition.

Cysts are liable to develop chronic inflammation and may be seeded hematogenously by infection, thus resulting in abscess formation. Repeated hemorrhage may give rise to blood degradation products on MRI and a fluid-fluid level on axial imaging.

When a bursitis is chronic, there may be a hypertrophied synovium with heterogeneous contained fluid. In severe cases, erosion of adjacent bone may occur.

Pathology

GROSS

Synovium-lined sac in continuity with the knee joint.

MICROSCOPIC

Synovial lining with many inflammatory cells, especially when there has been repeated infection.

Imaging Findings

RADIOGRAPHY

Conventional radiographs may aid in reaching a diagnosis by identifying underlying osteoarthritis or rheumatoid arthritis, and occasionally calcified debris. A soft-tissue mass may be demonstrable on lateral films.

Direct arthrography with double contrast combined with joint mobilization was at one time the gold standard for demonstrating the bursa and its communications.

Lack of communication, however, does not exclude the diagnosis, as the channel may be obstructed by inflammatory debris.

ULTRASOUND

- Anechoic (fluid-filled) well-defined lesions
- Debris will frequently be seen, as will multiple thin septae.
- Ultrasound will easily differentiate between other causes of clinically evident popliteal swelling (e.g., popliteal aneurysms and ganglion cysts).
- Ultrasound is sufficiently sensitive to identify cysts as small as 3 mm in diameter. They will be well defined and echoic, and may contain thin septae.
- Occasionally, the cephalic portion of a cyst may be identified with a poorly defined inferior portion and accompanying soft-tissue edema, suggesting cyst rupture.
- Complete decompression may result in a false-negative diagnosis.

COMPUTED TOMOGRAPHY

- Although not used routinely in the diagnosis of popliteal cysts, CT arthrography will elegantly demonstrate communication with the joint when contrast is introduced prior to CT.

MAGNETIC RESONANCE IMAGING

- Popliteal cysts demonstrate typical fluid signal: hypointense on T1 and hyperintense on T2.
- If inflammation is present, changes may be apparent in the surrounding muscle and subcutaneous tissues, best appreciated on T2-weighted and fat-suppressed inversion recovery images.

- Repeated hemorrhage may give rise to blood degradation products on MRI and a fluid-fluid level on axial imaging.
- If PVNS is present, then the presence of hemosiderin on MRI would identify the condition.

Treatment

- Conservative, including rest, elevation, cold packs, anti-inflammatories ± aspiration and steroid injection
- Treatment of underlying degenerative disorders may aid in the cyst's resolution.
- Surgical excision may be necessary if local symptoms are excessive.
- Cysts in the pediatric population are usually self-limited and require no intervention.

Prognosis

The majority requires no, or minimal, treatment. If treated, particularly by surgery, recurrence is uncommon, unless the underlying intra-articular condition remains untreated.

PEARL

- The key differentiating point is that, despite the degree of lobulation, the epicenter of the cyst will remain at the location of the gastrocnemius-semimembranosus bursa.

PITFALL

- It is important to ensure prior to diagnosing a Baker's cyst, that no definite solid component exists that could represent the presence of a synovial tumor. This is best established by the absence of enhancing material within the lesion. The walls of the cyst may enhance, however, especially if the cyst has been inflamed.

Suggested Readings

Miller TT, Staron RB, Koenigsberg T, Levin TL, Feldman F. MR imaging of Baker cysts: association with internal derangement, effusion, and degenerative arthropathy. Radiology 1996;201:247–250

Munk PL, Vellet AD, Levin MF. Leaking Baker's cyst detected by magnetic resonance imaging. Can Assoc Radiol J 1993;44:125–128

Torreggiani WC, Al-Ismail K, Munk PL, et al. The imaging spectrum of Baker's (popliteal) cysts. Clin Radiol 2002;57:681–691

CASE 9

Anthony G. Ryan and Peter L. Munk

Clinical Presentation

A 13-year-old boy presented to his family doctor with a history of anterior knee pain. Direct questioning revealed he had recently taken part in a track and field competition. Physical exam revealed focal tenderness over the tibial tuberosity. He had full range of passive motion but a somewhat limited knee extension secondary to the pain. The practitioner sent the boy for a radiograph, which revealed no significant abnormality, but because the boy had ongoing pain, he was referred to an orthopedic surgeon, who requested an MRI.

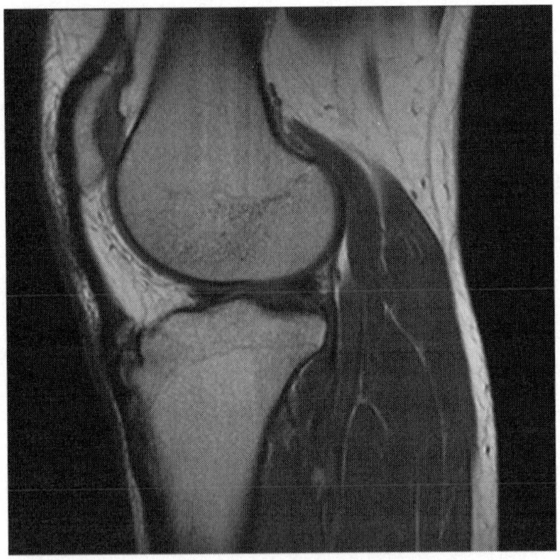

Figure 9A

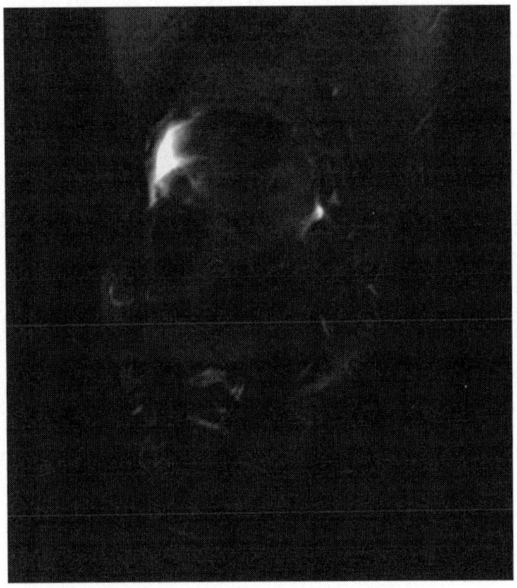

Figure 9B

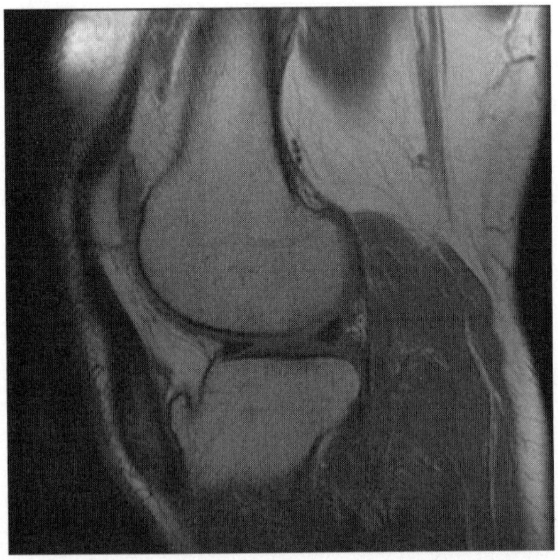

Figure 9C

Radiologic Findings

A sagittal T1 (**Fig. 9A**) image shows minimal fragmentation of the proximal aspect of the tibial tuberosity apophysis and fiber discontinuity in the adjacent patellar tendon insertion. A coronal short tau inversion recovery (STIR) sequence (**Fig. 9B**) through the tibial tuberosity reveals focal high signal intensity surrounding the cephalad fragment. Sagittal T2 (**Fig. 9C**) shows a markedly thickened patellar tendon at the level of its insertion with demonstrated high signal intensity within the tendon.

Diagnosis

Osgood-Schlatter disease.

Differential Diagnosis

- *Normal Variant* The normal ossification pattern between 8 and 14 years may simulate a fragmented tuberosity. The patient will not be symptomatic, however.
- *Osteitis* In the appropriate setting, tuberculous osteitis may be considered.

Discussion

Background

The etiology of Osgood-Schlatter disease remains unclear, although there is consensus that trauma is the underlying cause.

The debate arises in how one describes the actual injury; that is, all the following may be described in the complex of injuries described as Osgood-Schlatter disease: a cartilaginous avulsion fracture of the tibial tuberosity, a tear of the patellar tendon at its tibial insertion, or chronic tendinitis of the patellar tendon with secondary ossification. The features common to all the above involve a tendon abnormality, with or without an attendant osseus component, as evinced by the characteristic findings of persistent ossific fragments within a thickened patellar tendon in the later stages of the disease. This begs the question regarding the existence of an actual fracture at the time of injury or whether it is ossification within a chronic tendinitis.

The normal tibial tuberosity ossifies from distal to proximal between the ages of 7 and 9 years, while at the same time, the main tibial ossification center expands down to meet the tuberosity ossification center. Sandwiched between the two ossification centers is a layer of apophyseal cartilage, present until closure of the physis. This chondro-osseous region at the patellar tendon insertion is thus mechanically susceptible, and it is postulated that acute or chronic trauma may give rise to an Osgood-Schlatter lesion.

The condition most commonly affects males (males:females, 5:1) between the ages of 10 and 15 years. It is bilateral in 25% of cases.

Etiology

Two theories pertain to the development of this condition: the avulsion fracture theory and the tendinitis theory. In the avulsion fracture theory, the tibial tuberosity fragmentation is ascribed to a recent traumatic event, whereas in the tendinitis theory, it is thought the fragmentation arises secondary to repeated microtrauma to the deep fibers of the patellar tendon with resultant ossification.

Pathophysiology

According to the avulsion fracture theory, fracture follows sudden acute or repeated trauma/strain on the patellar tendon.

According to the tendinitis theory, tendinitis is secondary to repeated trauma to the deep fibers of the patellar tendon, which, during the reparative phase, demonstrates ossification.

Clinical Findings

There is usually a history of recent athletic activity, including kicking, jumping, or squatting. A recent growth spurt may be evident on direct questioning. The patient complains of local pain and, on examination, will have focal tenderness over the tibial tuberosity. Swelling of the overlying soft tissue may be visible.

Stages of Disease

There are five stages of Osgood-Schlatter disease, based on MRI appearances:

- Normal
- Early
- Progressive
- Terminal
- Healing

Complications

- Nonunion of the avulsed fragment
- The patellar tendon may be completely avulsed at its insertion.
- Secondary to the subsequent weakness induced in the tendon, the patella may become prone to subluxation and chondromalacia patellae.
- Genu recurvatum may be evident in severe cases.

Imaging Findings

RADIOGRAPHY

- Lateral radiographs may reveal pretibial soft-tissue swelling, reflecting the presence of edema within the skin and subcutaneous tissues overlying the tuberosity.
- Thickening of the distal portion of the patellar tendon with an indistinct posterior margin
- There may be increased radiodensity of the infrapatellar fat pad, in severe cases leading to obliteration of the fat pad.
- Ossific fragments secondary to avulsion of small ossicles from the tibial tuberosity ossification center

- Irregularity of the tibial tuberosity, which is most likely to be bilateral, is quite common in this age group.
- Radiographs at the early stage may appear completely normal.
- Even in the later stages, radiographs may not show the avulsed fragments.

ULTRASOUND

- Cartilaginous swelling and edema
- Fragmentation of the ossification center
- Thickening of the patellar tendon
- Infrapatellar bursitis
- If the above findings are clearly evident, then ultrasound may suffice as a means of follow-up.

COMPUTED TOMOGRAPHY

- Enlarged patellar tendon
- Decreased attenuation, suggestive of tendinitis
- Distended deep infrapatellar bursa
- Ossific fragments may be seen (in up to 32% of cases).
- On follow-up studies, these fragments may remain nonunited despite the disappearance of pain.

MAGNETIC RESONANCE IMAGING

- Increased signal intensity on T1- and T2-weighted images at the tibial insertion site of the patellar tendon, reflecting the presence of blood products and edema
- Distention of the deep infrapatellar bursa may be visible.
- Marrow edema may be evident occasionally within the tibial tuberosity and the tibial apophysis, manifested as low signal intensity on T1 and high on T2 and inversion recovery sequences.
- A tear may be evident within the secondary ossification center, widening to an "opened shell"-like shape (**Fig. 9D**).
- This may be seen on follow-up studies to fragment and separate, leading to partial avulsion and proximal retraction of a portion of the secondary ossification center (**Fig. 9E**).
- Terminal: complete separation of the avulsed fragments of the secondary ossification center (**Fig. 9F**)

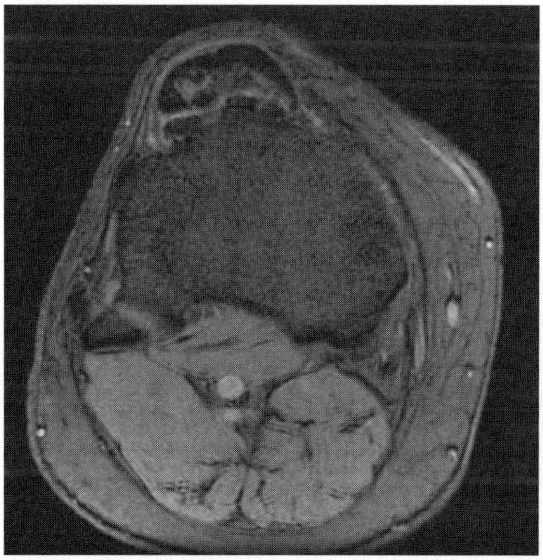

D

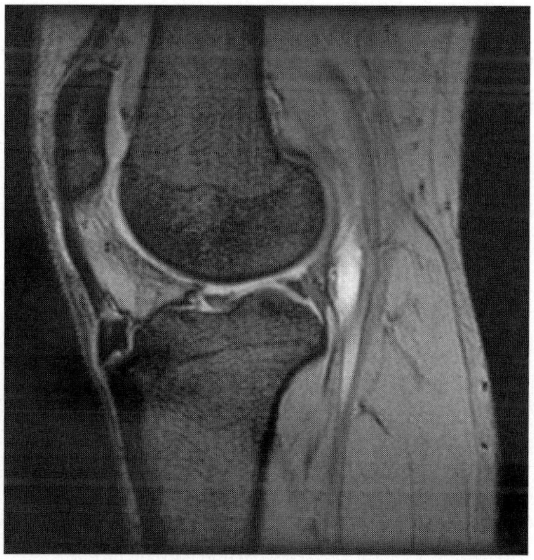

E

Figures 9D Axial inversion recovery at the level of the tibial tuberosity shows central high signal in the so-called open shell configuration. **9E** Sagittal T2-weighted image shows a combined avulsion of the patellar tendon insertion and an intratendon tear at the tendon-osseous interface. Pretibial high signal is also evident.

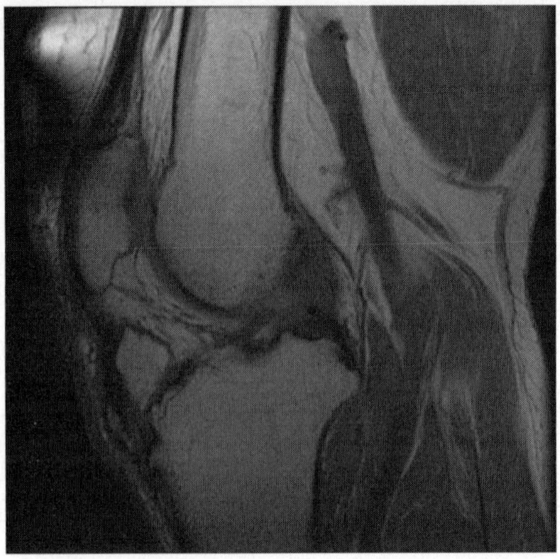

F

Figure 9F Sagittal T1-weighted image shows chronic nonunion of a large avulsed fragment, with a further smaller intratendinous ossicle also evident.

Treatment

Immobilization ± steroid injection.

Prognosis

Typically, full recovery, depending on stage.

PEARLS

- Presence of clinical symptoms is paramount.
- Soft-tissue swelling/MRI findings should be present for the diagnosis to be clinched, with the caveat that, rarely, MRI may be negative in the early stages of the disease.
- Concentrating on subtle abnormalities of the patellar tendon is more likely to yield results than hunting for an avulsed fragment that may not be present.
- High signal on T2-weighted/STIR will differentiate an avulsed, fractured fragment from a physiologically nonunited secondary ossification center.

PITFALLS

- Resist the desire to image the contralateral limb unless symptoms are present. If it is a normal variant, it is quite likely to be bilateral, so you will be none the wiser.
- Fragmentation of the tibial tuberosity is common.
- Radiographs are frequently normal and may miss the presence of an avulsed fragment, which may be evident on contemporaneous MRI.
- Occasionally MRI may be normal in the initial phase of the disease.
- The normal patellar tendon may demonstrate foci of increased signal intensity at its distal end on 3D gradient sequences.

Suggested Readings

De Flaviis L, Nessi R, Scaglione P, Balconi G, Albisetti W, Derchi LE. Ultrasonic diagnosis of Osgood-Schlatter and Sinding-Larsen-Johansson diseases of the knee. Skeletal Radiol 1989;18:193–197

Hirano A, Fukubayashi T, Ishii T, Ochiai N. Magnetic resonance imaging of Osgood-Schlatter disease: the course of the disease. Skeletal Radiol 2002;31:334–342

Rosenberg ZS, Kawelblum M, Cheung YY, Beltran J, Lehman WB, Grant AD. Osgood-Schlatter lesion: fracture or tendinitis? Scintigraphic, CT, and MR imaging features. Radiology 1992;185:853–858

CASE 10

Anthony G. Ryan and Peter L. Munk

Clinical Presentation

A 20-year-old man presented with anterior knee pain, localized to the lower pole of the patella, focal tenderness at this site on examination, and moderate limitation of active knee extension secondary to pain.

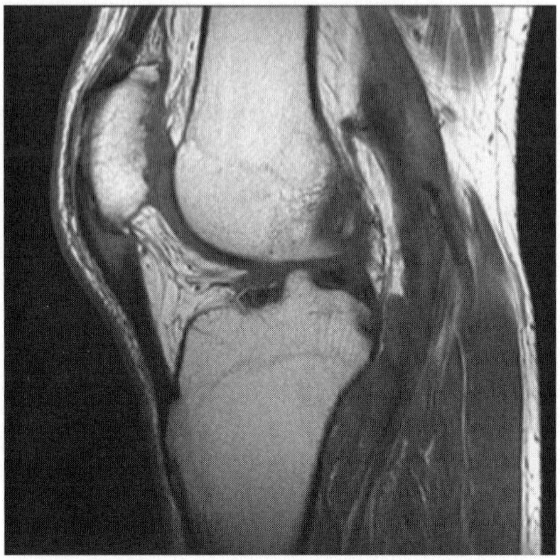

Figure 10A

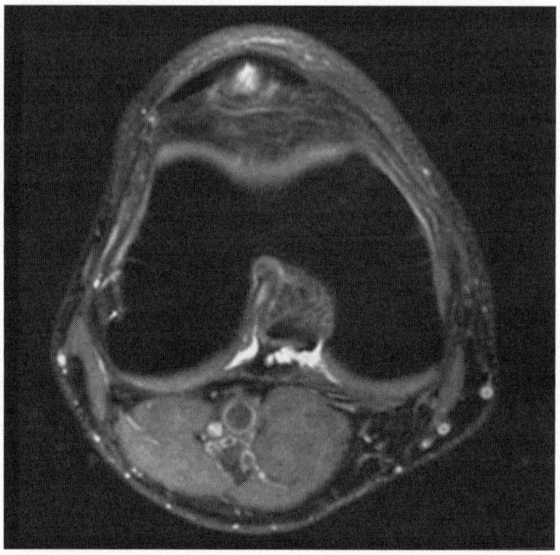

Figure 10B

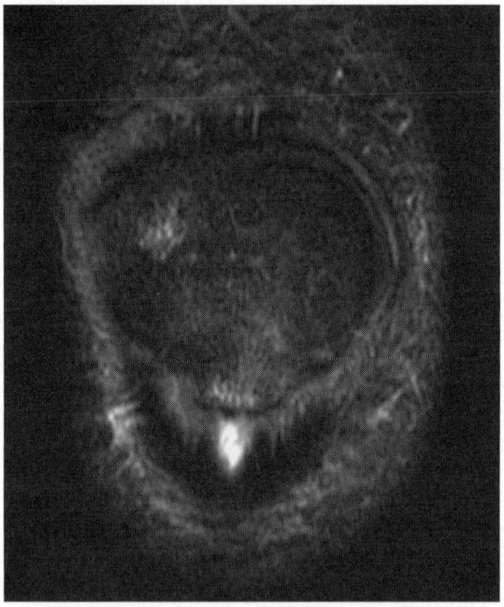

Figure 10C

Radiologic Findings

A sagittal T1-weighted image (**Fig. 10A**) shows focal tendon thickening of the proximal patellar tendon and intratendinous intermediate signal intensity. Focal low signal intensity is shown at the inferior pole of the patella. An axial proton density fat-saturated image (**Fig. 10B**) shows a focal "cone-shaped" focus of high signal intensity in the proximal patellar tendon. STIR sequence (**Fig. 10C**) shows a similar "cone-shaped" focus of high signal intensity at the same location. Ill-defined high signal is also demonstrated in the adjacent inferior pole of the patella.

Diagnosis

Jumper's knee.

Differential Diagnosis

- *Sinding-Larsen-Johansson (SLJ) disease* Although frequently used synonymously with jumper's knee, this term should be reserved for osteochondrosis affecting young adolescents (10 to 14 years). Cerebral spastic children are particularly predisposed. SLJ is caused by persistent traction at the cartilaginous junction of the patella and the patellar ligament, usually at the inferior patellar pole, and usually seen in an active preteen boy who complains of activity-related pain.
- *Infrapatellar bursitis* is based on the clinical presentation (easily differentiated from jumper's knee on ultrasound).
- *Inferior pole sleeve avulsion fracture* This entity should be considered in a younger patient.

Discussion

Background

In adults, the weakest link in the muscle-tendon-bone chain is the musculotendinous insertion. In adolescents, prior to epiphyseal fusion, the weakest point is at the tendon-epiphyseal or tendon-apophyseal junction.

Jumper's knee is the common name given to a partial tear of the patellar insertion of the patellar tendon, most commonly seen in younger athletes, including football players and track and field participants.

Etiology

Patellar tendinosis is thought to be caused by repetitive trauma resulting in microtears at the patellar tendon enthesis, on which background a partial or complete tear may more easily occur. Repetitive violent contractions of the quadriceps occur in "jumping" sports, basketball and volleyball being most commonly implicated.

Extrinsic Factors

- Hard playing surfaces: cement 38%, parquet 4%, linoleum 23%
- Length of training sessions
- Sinding-Larsen-Johansson disease is a condition of adolescence (10 to 14 years). Especially predisposed to this condition are children with cerebral spasticity.
- A long inferior patellar pole may produce impingement and result in this condition.
- In the absence of sporting activities, blunt trauma is rarely implicated.

Pathophysiology

There is a spectrum of injury encompassing the following:

- The changes that occur with shearing of the tendinous fibers from repeated microtrauma can progress to significant degeneration and increase the risk of tendon rupture.
- Traction with or without contusion and subsequent tendinitis: chronic degeneration eventually disrupts the intratendinous architecture tendon, with a matching increase in pain and activity limitation.
- In the appropriate age group (i.e., before physeal closure), the patellar component of the lesion is secondary to microavulsions of the epiphyseal cartilage, described by some authorities as evidence that the condition represents a variant of an osteochondrosis affecting the inferior pole of the patella (SLJ).

Clinical Findings

The mean age of presentation of patellar tendinosis is 20 years, with a marked male preponderance. Chronic localized pain, which can be debilitating in the athletic population, who often persist with activities despite ongoing pain, lasts for many years (averaging 3 years in one study) in some cases.

The symptoms of jumper's knee are

- Chronic anterior knee pain
- Pain on climbing stairs, long walks, or sitting with the knees bent

The physical signs of jumper's knee are

- Localized swelling over the apex of the patella (found in only 5% of patients)
- Patellar hypermobility, quadriceps wasting, and local tenderness
- The intensity of pain and the extent of activity limitation reflect the degree of tendinous degeneration.

Complications

- Exertional avulsion of the inferior patellar pole
- Recurrent patellar subluxation and dislocation

Stages of Disease

Phase I Pain only after activity
Phase II Pain/discomfort during activity, but does not interfere with participation
Phase III Pain both during and after participation, which interferes with competition
Phase IV Complete tendon disruption

Pathology

GROSS

Operative studies demonstrate that the epitendineum is typically intact, with degenerate or necrotic tissue identified within the tendon immediately caudad to the patellar apex. The superficial tendon fibers are grossly normal.

MICROSCOPIC

Histology reflects the presence of chronic degeneration and regeneration. The focal thickening and nodularity, evident grossly, is demonstrable histologically to be secondary to pockets of mucoid degeneration (this latter finding present in only 8% of cadaveric tendons), edema, fibrinous necrosis, and associated debris.

The increased interfascicular distance is seen to correlate with the rupture of cross-links between collagen fibers, which, when extensive, can disrupt the gross internal architecture of the tendon. Early in the process, this disruption is evident as clefts and microtears interspersed with areas of regeneration (granulation and scar tissue).

Areas of abnormal signal intensity on MRI have been shown to correspond to tissue containing tenocyte hyperplasia, prominent angiogenesis with endothelial hyperplasia, loss of longitudinal collagenous architecture, and microtears with collagen fiber separation.

Hyaline degeneration is present in all examined surgical specimens.

Imaging Findings

RADIOGRAPHY

Radiographs will demonstrate an ill-defined thickened soft-tissue density in the expected position of the patellar tendon, with or without the presence of calcific/ossific fragments if an associated avulsion is also present at the lower pole of the patella.

ULTRASOUND

A normal tendon should have uniform thickness and homogeneous echogenicity throughout its length. Mild "flaring" proximally and distally is seen in the majority of asymptomatic subjects.

- Focal thickening and nodularity of the tendon are seen near the apex of the patella in over 90% of cases.
- Widening of the distance between the longitudinal fascicles is secondary to edema.
- Global tendon thickening is seen in long-standing disease and is thought to be a precursor to rupture.
- Focal hypoechoic areas may also be present.
- Hypoechoic foci may be demonstrated around the tendon (fibromyxoid tissue).
- The fat with the postpatellar space (Hoffa's fat pad) is likely to have an increased echogenicity.
- Calcium is infrequently demonstrated within the actual tendon but may be seen at the tendon insertion site as small fragments of cartilage avulse from the epiphysis. These fragments will become hyperechoic secondary to necrotic ossification.
- Bony enthesophytes may be demonstrated at the patellar insertion site.

A cone-shaped, poorly echogenic area exceeding 0.5 cm in length in the center of the patellar tendon in combination with its localized thickening proved to be a reliable indicator of jumper's knee.

MAGNETIC RESONANCE IMAGING

- A hypointense area on T1 images and hyperintense on T2 images can be seen in the inferior pole of the patella and surrounding soft tissues.
- Intermediate signal intensity on T1 reflects the presence of blood products.

- Focal eccentric thickening (2 to 4 times as thick as normal, which is ~3 mm) can be identified involving the proximal third of the tendon and affecting the medial aspect to a greater extent than the lateral.
- The posterior tendon margin is usually indistinct and may be associated with edema in Hoffa's fat pad, similar to that seen in Kager's fat pad in association with Achilles peritendinitis.
- The anterior fibers of the patellar tendon are typically spared, proving a useful discriminator in deciding between chronic tendinosis and an acute tear.
- There will be altered signal intensity within the proximal patellar tendon, with areas of intermediate signal intensity on proton density and T2-weighted images.
- If the degeneration is significant, it may, in fact, progress to cyst formation, which will be highlighted on fluid-sensitive sequences.
- On proton density-weighted images, abnormal signal intensity is seen in the proximal one third of the patellar tendon.
- On T2-weighted MRI, abnormal signal intensity is seen, most cases being isointense or hyperintense to the signal seen on proton density-weighted images.
- A poorly defined patellar tendon is seen in the posterior margin.
- Chronic tendon tears are intratendinous areas of increased signal.

Treatment

PHYSICAL THERAPY

Specifically, exercise therapy to strengthen the quadriceps is often prescribed, though its efficacy is still debated.

REHABILITATION

- RICE: Rest, ice, compression, and elevation
- Anti-inflammatories

SURGERY

Surgery may be indicated in the professional athlete under these conditions:

- Failure of 6 months' nonoperative therapy
- Tendon rupture

OPEN TENDON DÉBRIDEMENT

- Multiple longitudinal tenotomies
- Avoidance of competition for 4 to 6 months
- Patelloplasty by excising the inferior pole and reinserting the tendon
- Arthroscopic tendon and fat pad débridement
- Débridement of enthesis and inferior pole of the patella

Prognosis

In severe cases, surgical débridement of the degenerated tissue and multiple longitudinal tenotomies are said to be associated with a good symptomatic response.

The results of a study of open and arthroscopic operations revealed that 80% of patients with pain at exercise preoperatively showed complete relief by 12 months. When the open and arthroscopic groups were compared, there was similar symptomatic relief and outcome and a 50% return to the prior level of competition in each group. Patients undergoing arthroscopy returned to their sport earlier than those undergoing open débridement.

PEARLS

- The anterior fibers of the patellar tendon are typically spared, proving a useful discriminator in deciding between chronic tendinosis and an acute tear.
- There will be altered signal intensity within the proximal patellar tendon, with areas of intermediate signal intensity on proton density and T2-weighted images.
- If the degeneration is significant, it may, in fact, progress to cyst formation, which will be highlighted on fluid-sensitive sequences.
- The symptoms of SLJ usually resolve with progressive skeletal maturation, but this may take well over 1 year, compared with the multiple years patients with patellar tendinitis usually suffer.

PITFALL

- On gradient-echo sequences, focal increased signal intensity in the superior part of the patellar tendon may be seen in as many as 75% of asymptomatic subjects, and in the inferior part in 43%, potentially leading to a false-positive diagnosis if the high signal on gradient sequences is not matched by high signal on fluid-sensitive sequences.

Suggested Readings

Bodne D, Quinn SF, Murray WT, et al. Magnetic resonance images of chronic patellar tendinitis. Skeletal Radiol 1988;17:24–28

Kalebo P, Sward L, Karlsson J, Peterson L. Ultrasonography in the detection of partial patellar ligament ruptures (jumper's knee). Skeletal Radiol 1991;20:285–289

Khan KM, Bonar F, Desmond PM, et al. Patellar tendinosis (jumper's knee): findings at histopathologic examination, US, and MR imaging. Victorian Institute of Sport Tendon Study Group. Radiology 1996;200:821–827

Reiff DB, Heenan SD, Heron CW. MRI appearances of the asymptomatic patellar tendon on gradient echo imaging. Skeletal Radiol 1995;24:123–126

Yu JS, Popp JE, Kaeding CC, Lucas J. Correlation of MR imaging and pathologic findings in athletes undergoing surgery for chronic patellar tendinitis. Am J Roentgenol 1995;165:115–118

CASE 11

Anthony G. Ryan and Peter L. Munk

Clinical Presentation

An 18-year-old girl presented with intermittent locking of her knee after gymnastics training.

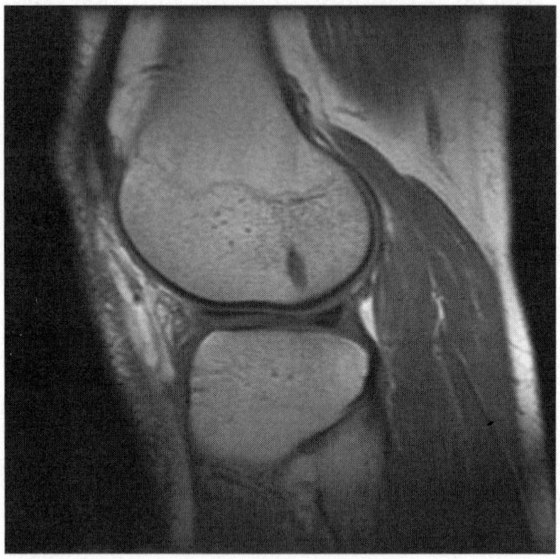

Figure 11A

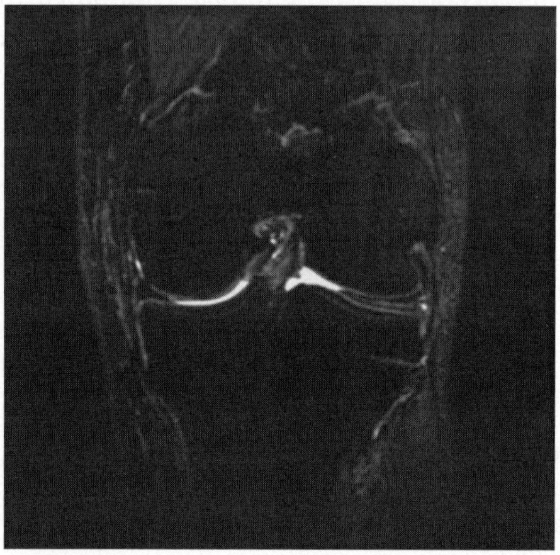

Figure 11B

Radiologic Findings

A sagittal T1-weighted image (**Fig. 11A**) through the lateral aspect of the knee joint shows intermediate/high signal within the anterior horn of the lateral meniscus, reaching the surface in two locations. The high signal also extends into the posterior horn. The anterior horn is considerably bigger than the posterior horn.

A coronal short tau inversion recovery (STIR) image (**Fig. 11B**) shows intrameniscal high signal intensity across the horizontal width of the visible lateral meniscus. The meniscus extends more centrally than the medial meniscus at the same level.

Diagnosis

Torn discoid meniscus.

Differential Diagnosis

None.

Discussion

Background

Discoid meniscus is a relatively common variant of the menisci, present in ~1 in 20 pediatric knees imaged. Discoid menisci are seen far more frequently affecting the lateral meniscus than the medial meniscus, the reported ratio of lateral to medial ranging from 15:1 to 4:1. When present, it is bilateral in 20% of cases.

Discoid meniscus is seen more frequently in children and adolescents; thus, some authors suggest it may regress in maturity.

Etiology

The configuration has been presumed to be congenital; however, recent embryologic studies have not upheld this hypothesis, suggesting the lesion is acquired and that discoid menisci may develop when abnormal attachments to the meniscofemoral ligaments of Humphrey and Wrisberg are present (see Wrisberg's variant below).

Pathophysiology

Discoid meniscus is thought to arise secondary to an abnormal inferior fascicular attachment of the posterior horn, resulting in additional central meniscal growth and subsequent discoid configuration.

Morphologically, there is poor constriction of the central portion and thickening of the free end.

The abnormal extension centrally predisposes it to trauma between the femoral condyle and the tibial plateau.

Clinical Findings

- Usually presents in childhood or adolescence
- In addition to an increased risk of tear, it is said it can be symptomatic even in the absence of trauma.
- Pain
- Snapping or clunking
- Reduced mobility
- Locking
- Giving way

Stages of Disease

Discoid meniscus can adopt many different shapes: lens-shaped, wedged, flat, and so on.

Six subtypes have been described, based on morphology and the presence or absence of tear:

1. Thick, rounded slab with parallel superior and inferior surfaces
2. Biconcave
3. Wedge (smaller than type 1)
4. Asymmetric (anterior greater than posterior)
5. Less bulky than type 1
6. Any of the above with an associated tear

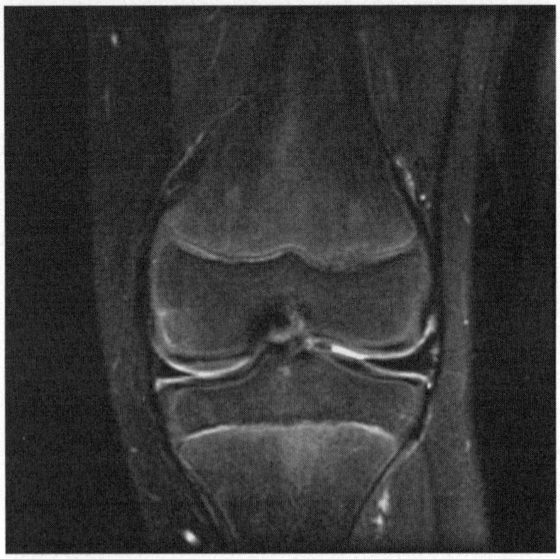

Figure 11C Coronal T2-weighted fat-saturated image of a 14-year-old ballet dancer shows the lateral meniscus to be more substantial than the medial in all dimensions (i.e., height and width), while extending more centrally than the equivalent medial meniscus wedge.

Complications

- Tears are of increased incidence in comparison to nondiscoid menisci.
- Displacement of the torn segments occurs in as many as 70% of cases.
- Four meniscal cysts

Imaging Findings

RADIOGRAPHY

Rarely, plain film findings may be those of hypoplasia of the lateral femoral condyle and a fibular head that is higher than normal.

Widening of the lateral joint space may be seen, and reputedly there is decreased height of the lateral intercondylar tibial spine.

MAGNETIC RESONANCE IMAGING

MRI is the investigation of choice, demonstrating the presence, site, and pattern of a discoid lateral meniscal tear, including the type of displacement of the torn segment.

- Continuity of the anterior and posterior horns of the lateral meniscus is expected laterally on two consecutive 5-mm slices (so-called bow ties). If three or more bow ties are present, discoid meniscus is diagnosed.
- The lateral meniscus is bulkier than a normal or medial meniscus (**Fig. 11C**).
- In comparison to the normal meniscus, the measurable height difference is typically greater than or equal to 2 mm.
- Discoid menisci are clearly demonstrated on coronal images identifying meniscal tissue approaching or extending to the intracondylar region.
- On T1- and T2-weighted images, the meniscal signal is typically increased heterogeneously, in a central, horizontal, linear fashion in 50%, diffusely in 33%, and in a partly linear, partly diffuse fashion in 17% of cases.
- Occasionally, patients may present with an untorn meniscus, producing snapping on flexion and extension. The whole meniscus or only a portion of it may be discoid.

Treatment

As with other meniscal injuries, peripheral tears may be treated surgically by arthroscopic "tacking."

Resection of the unstable free ends and loose fragments may be required for pain relief, to restore full range of motion, and to prevent the later development of osteoarthrosis.

Prognosis

If not treated, these menisci may recede with age. In the absence of an osteochondral defect, the prognosis is expected to be good postsurgery.

PEARLS

- Discoid menisci are clearly demonstrated on coronal images identifying meniscal tissue approaching or extending to the intracondylar region.
- If three or more sagittal images show bridging between the anterior and posterior horns (three or more bow ties), a discoid meniscus may be diagnosed.
- An isolated tear of the lateral meniscus should prompt consideration of the possibility of a discoid meniscus, as this injury occurs at least twice as often in the discoid variant.

PITFALLS

- A meniscus may appear discoid on the coronal images on the most posterior slices (the so-called pseudodiscoid meniscus); therefore, correlation with the sagittal images is mandatory.
- Occasionally, patients may present with an untorn meniscus, producing snapping on flexion and extension. The whole meniscus or only a portion of it may be discoid; consequently, even if no tear is identified, the possibility of a discoid meniscus should be considered, as it may be symptomatic in the absence of a tear.
- Although it is suggested that discoid menisci may be symptomatic even in the absence of a tear, they may be asymptomatic. The exception to this is the Wrisberg's variant of discoid meniscus. In this variant, seen most frequently in children, the posterior horn of the discoid meniscus is not attached to the joint capsule, with the result that it is sufficiently mobile to sublux into the joint, may be pinched between the articulating bones, causing pain, and, if sufficiently mobile, may cause the joint to lock. The presence of a free-floating or unattached posterior horn of a discoid meniscus on MRI should raise suspicion that this is the cause of the patient's pain, especially in the absence of a tear.

Suggested Readings

Lee MJ, Munk PL. Musculoskeletal case 1: lateral discoid meniscus. Can J Surg 1998;41:424, 466

Rohren EM, Kosarek FJ, Helms CA. Discoid lateral meniscus and the frequency of meniscal tears. Skeletal Radiol 2001;30:316–320

Ryu KN, Kim IS, Kim EJ, et al. MR imaging of tears of discoid lateral menisci. Am J Roentgenol 1998;171:963–967

CASE 12

Hema N. Choudur, Anthony G. Ryan, Peter L. Munk, and Laurel O. Marchinkow

Clinical Presentation

An elderly woman presented complaining of long-standing anterior knee pain, especially when descending stairs and rising from a chair.

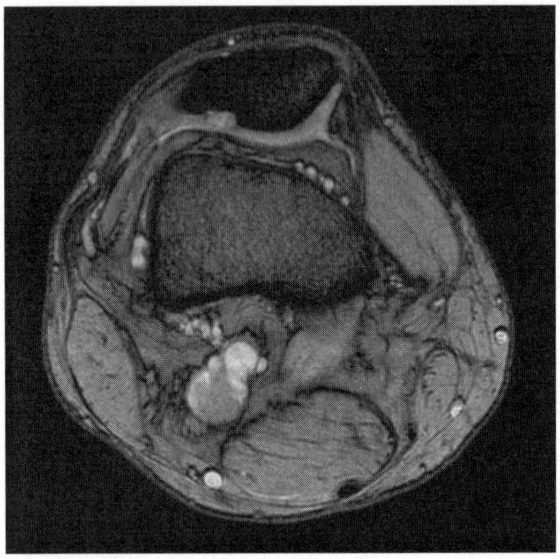

Figure 12A

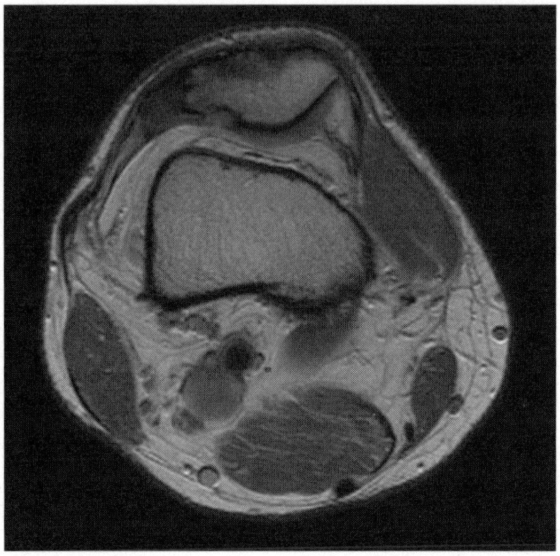

Figure 12B

Radiologic Findings

Axial MPGR (**Fig. 12A**) and axial proton density (**Fig. 12B**) images of the knee reveal a focal increase in signal intensity and a defect in the lateral articular cartilage of the patella with subjacent bony changes, including erosion and sclerosis.

Irregularity of the articular surface of the patella with bony erosion of the lateral patellar surface was demonstrated on an accompanying skyline view.

Diagnosis

Chondromalacia patella.

Differential Diagnosis

- Osteoarthritis
- Peripatellar tendinitis/bursitis
- Patellar fracture
- Subluxation/dislocation of the patella

Discussion

Background

Softening or wearing away of the patellar articular cartilage (chondromalacia patella) causes varying degrees of inflammation and pain. The underlying bone becomes involved when the entire thickness of articular cartilage is destroyed. Severity is graded on a scale from 1 to 4.

Etiology

The patella serves primarily to increase the leverage and therefore the efficiency of the quadriceps muscle. Considerable retropatellar forces are present throughout the entire range of motion of the knee. The articular cartilage is thus compressed against the femoral condyles, exacerbated by acute trauma or chronic overuse.

Other anatomical factors causing excessive compression forces are

1. *Patellar malalignment* This can result from an increased Q angle (line of action of the quadriceps force to the line of patellar motion). This angle lies between a line drawn from the anterior superior iliac spine to the center of the patella and a line from the tibial tuberosity to the center of the patella. With anteversion of the femur and tibial torsion, the angle increases. With the quadriceps relaxed, the normal angle is ~13 to 18 degrees.
2. *Sulcus angle* An increase in this angle (formed by lines drawn from the apices of the femoral condyles to the nadir of the condylar sulcus) causes excessive patellar motion, secondary to the resulting shallow trough.
3. *Position of the patella relative to the femoral condyle* If the patella is high-placed (patella alta) or low-placed (patella baja), there is an alteration of the normal biomechanical forces.
4. *Strength of the quadriceps* An imbalance of patellar tracking can occur secondary to eccentric contraction of the separate components of the quadriceps. The patellar retinaculae and iliotibial tracts may also contribute to patellar maltracking. Atrophy of the vastus medialis (congenital or secondary), reflex inhibition due to pain, and a dystrophic medial mass are potential causes.
5. *Patellar facets* An alteration of the facet surfaces, as compared with the normal, also leads to chondromalacia patella. As per Wilberg's classification, a small convex (type 3) medial facet tends to cause chondromalacia.
6. *Trauma* Ten percent of chondromalacic knees are due to sports injuries, especially football and soccer, where the quadriceps is overused. Abnormal patellar tracking also occurs in running around a bend, especially on a chamfered surface.

Pathophysiology

The articular cartilage of the patella consists of collagen fibers oriented tangentially from the articular surface to the subchondral bone; these fibers are disrupted to varying degrees secondary to applied compressive forces. Most of the resulting changes occur at the median ridge of the patella, where the cartilage is thickest. Associated microfractures and sclerosis of the subchondral bone occur in association.

Clinical Findings

Pain along the anterior aspect of the knee while walking, running, or jumping is the usual complaint. It is often aggravated while descending or ascending stairs. Swelling of the knee with crepitus occurs with chronicity.

Pain elicited on examination when the quadriceps is contracted against a fixed patella is characteristic. Tenderness of the patellar borders and undersurface is another characteristic. A degree of genu valgum is often present. Clinically, it is difficult to differentiate osteoarthritis, patellar tendinitis/bursitis, fat pad syndrome, sympathetic dystrophy, and vasculitis.

Stages of Disease

Chondromalacia patella is graded based on the depth of cartilage thinning and associated subchondral bony changes.

Grade 1 There is softening and swelling of the articular cartilage. The cartilage is spongy on arthroscopy.

Grade 2 Cartilaginous fissures affecting less than 1.3 cm^2 in area with no extension to the subchondral bone

Grade 3 Fissuring, fragmentation, and fibrillation of cartilage extending to the subchondral bone but affecting less than 50% of the patellar articular surface

Grade 4 More than 50% of the patellar articular surface is exposed, with sclerosis and erosions of the subchondral bone. Osteophyte formation also occurs at this stage.

Complications

Patellofemoral osteoarthritis in the later stages of this disease.

Pathology

GROSS

On arthroscopy, cartilage edema, fissures, thinning, and subchondral bony changes can be seen.

MICROSCOPIC

In grade 1, small cartilage fissures with normal chondrocytes are seen. In grade 3, the chondrocytes are affected, becoming hyperactive and degenerative. This is the onset of cartilage necrosis, with some chondrocytes even becoming fibrous.

Imaging Findings

RADIOGRAPHY

- Skyline views are the most appropriate to visualize the femoral sulcus and articular surface of the patella (taken with 20 degrees or greater [45 to 55] of flexion).
- A lateral view will show the position of the patella with respect to the femoral condyle and helps to rule out a patella alta/baja. A standing AP view is necessary to comment on the presence or absence of genu valgus.
- The Q angle can be drawn accurately on a standing scanogram, including the pelvis and entire lower limbs.

COMPUTED TOMOGRAPHY

- In the absence of MRI, an air contrast CT-arthrogram will accurately depict irregularity and thinning of the patellar articular cartilage in the axial plane. Additionally, the presence of structures such as synovial plicae and cysts, intra-/extra-articular calcifications, and subchondral bony changes is well demonstrated on CT.
- Patellofemoral tracking can also be assessed with CT.

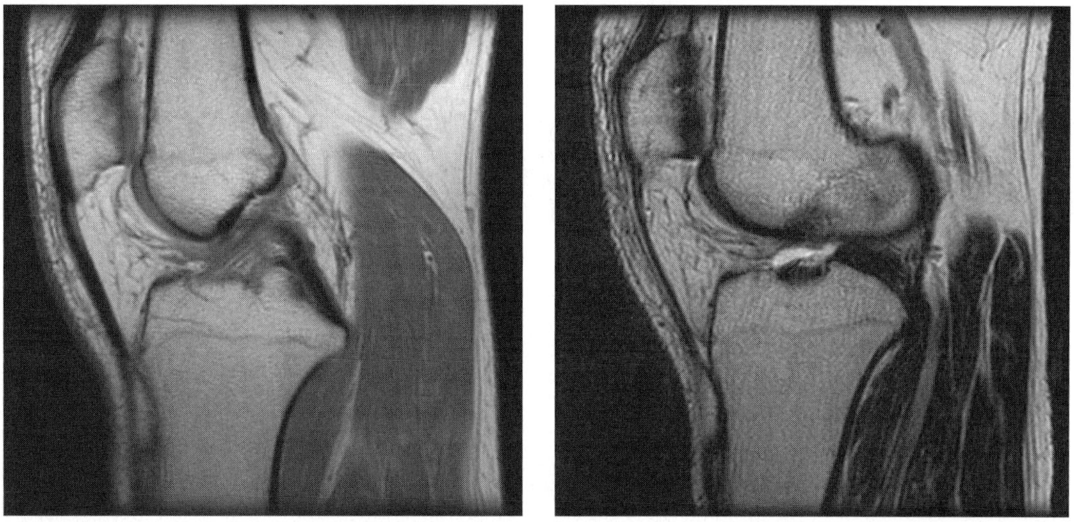

C D

Figures 12C and **12D** Sagittal T1 (**12C**) and T2 (**12D**) demonstrate severe cartilage loss with marked subchondral sclerosis and geode formation.

MAGNETIC RESONANCE IMAGING

- Axial gradient echo images with fat saturation (spoiled GRASS) are the most useful of all sequences to grade chondromalacic changes.
- Proton density fat-saturated axial images have also been shown to be useful in the evaluation of early chondromalacia.
- Routine sagittal T1-weighted, T2-weighted, and gradient images will depict the extensor mechanism in addition to patellar cartilage and bony changes, helping to evaluate for the presence of tendinitis, avulsion injuries, and patellar fractures (**Figs. 12C,12D**). Inversion recovery sequences show patellar edema and pre-/infrapatellar bursitis.

The grading of chondromalacia patella on MRI is as follows (see **Figs. 12E–12I**, line diagrams depicting the staging of chondromalacia patella):

Grade 1 Foci of altered signal intensity as compared with the rest of the cartilage. This signifies focal edema and is the earliest sign on MRI. The cartilage is of normal thickness (**Fig. 12J**).

Grade 2 Foci of cartilage thinning but not reaching the deeper layers adjacent to bone. There could be multiple such foci but each less than 1.3 cm^2 in area. This is the stage when cartilage fissures occur (**Fig. 12K**).

Grade 3 The cartilage thinning extends to the subchondral bone but involves less than 50% of the articular surface of the patella (**Fig. 12L**).

Grade 4 Chondromalacic changes extend to the subchondral bone and involve more than half of the patellar articular surface. Sclerotic changes of the subchondral bone with erosions are clearly visualized, and osteophytes are also noted (**Fig. 12M**).

Treatment

In the earlier stages, treatment consists of conservative measures, such as activity modification, patellar taping/strapping, quadriceps-strengthening exercises, nonsteroidal anti-inflammatory drugs (NSAIDs), and rest. Orthotic inserts to correct tibial torsion/femoral anteversion may help.

Surgical measures are undertaken when symptoms are persistent. Surgical débridement to the level of normal cartilage or anthroscopic drilling helps facilitate growth of healthy tissue in the holes.

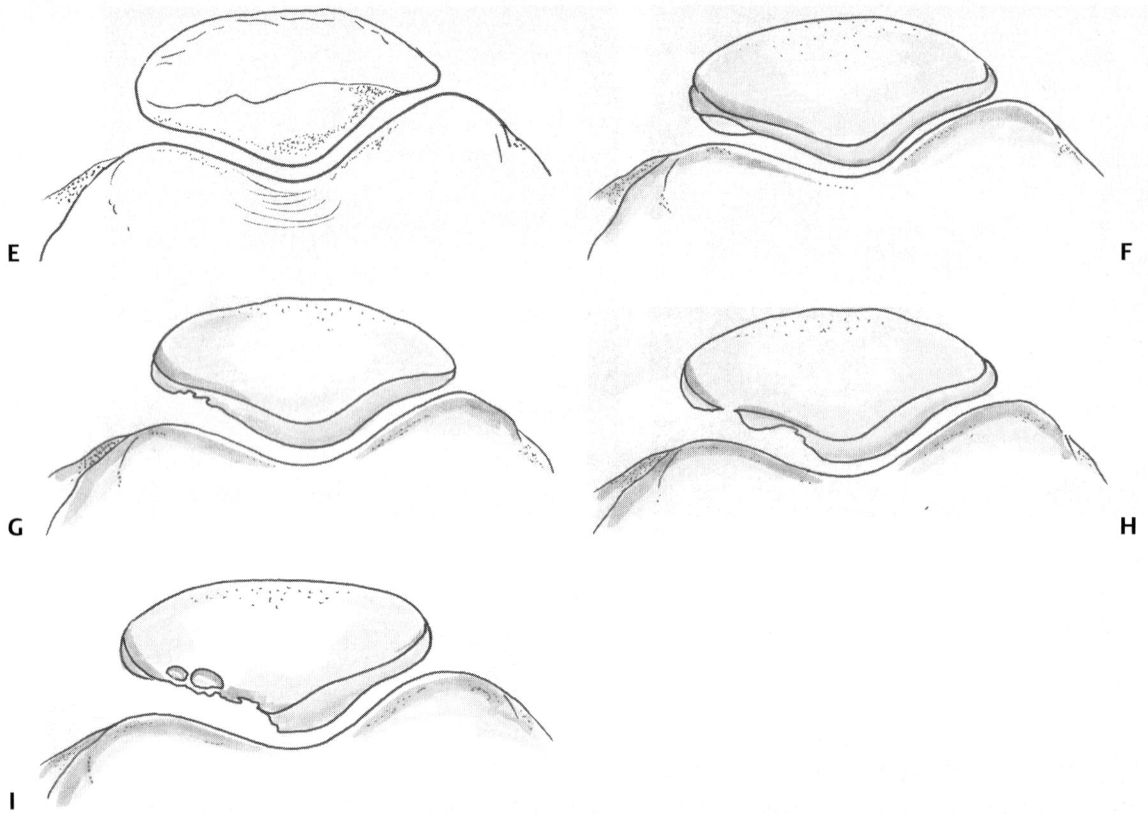

Figures 12E–12I Line diagrams depict the grading of chondromalacia patella. **12E** Normal smooth posterior patellar surface with no signal changes. **12F** Grade 1: The cartilage is of normal thickness; foci of altered signal intensity as compared with the rest of the cartilage. This signifies focal edema and is the earliest sign on MRI. **12G** Grade 2: Foci of cartilage thinning but not reaching bone; there could be multiple such foci but each less than 1.3 cm^2 in area. This is the stage when the cartilage fissures occur. **12H** Grade 3: The cartilage thinning extends to the subchondral bone but involves less than 50% of the articular surface of the patella. **12I** Grade 4: Chondromalacic changes extend to the subchondral bone and involve more than half of the patellar articular surface. Sclerotic changes of the subchondral bone with erosions are clearly visualized, and osteophytes are noted too.

Realignment procedures include tightening of the medial capsule.

Medial shift of the tibial tubercle (so that the quadriceps pulls more directly on the patella), releasing the lateral retinaculum, chondrectomy, and partial patellectomy are other surgical options. A full patellectomy results in persistent quadriceps weakness.

Success has been reported with two new potential treatments:

- Replacement of damaged cartilage by polyethylene cap prosthesis
- Autologous chondrocyte transplantation under a tibial periosteal patch

Prognosis

Early chondromalacia responds favorably if treated appropriately; however, later stages frequently require surgical management.

PEARLS

- Foci of altered signal intensity within cartilage signifies focal edema and is the earliest sign on MRI.
- Proton density fat-saturated axial images have been shown to be especially useful in the evaluation of early chondromalacia.

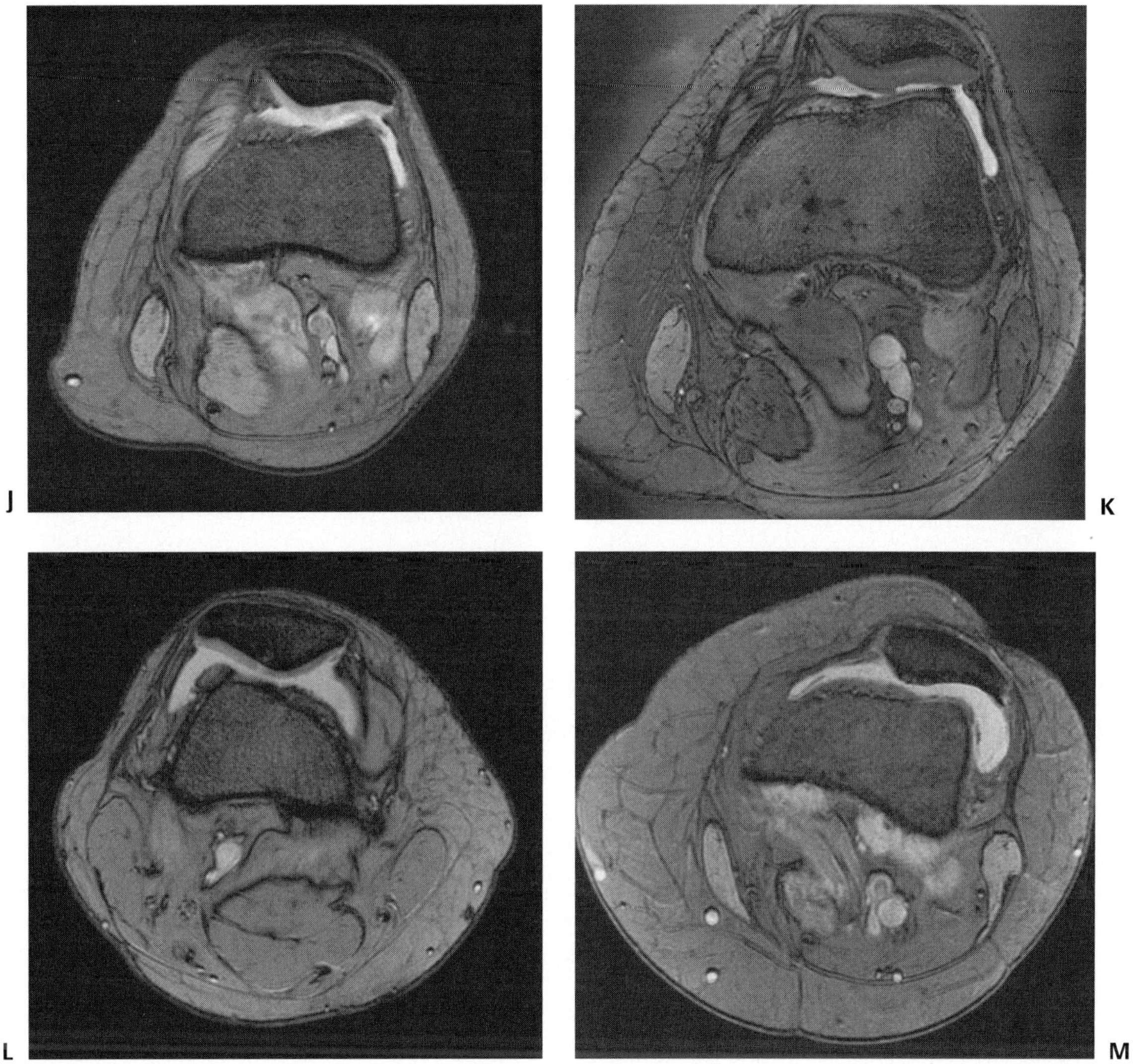

Figures 12J–12M MRI of chondromalacia patellae. **12J** Transaxial MPGR shows focal high signal intensity in the lateral patellofemoral articular cartilage (grade 1). **12K** Axial MPGR shows focal articular cartilage thinning (grade 2). **12L** MRI axial MPGR shows cartilage loss involving the entire lateral patellar articular cartilage extending to the subchondral bone (grade 3). **12M** Axial MPGR image shows absence of the entire patellar articular cartilage with subchondral changes (grade 4).

- The Q angle can be drawn accurately on a standing scanogram, including the pelvis and entire lower limbs.

PITFALLS

- A standing (as opposed to supine) AP view is necessary to comment on the presence or absence of genu valgus.
- In the absence of MRI, an air-contrast CT arthrogram will accurately depict irregularity and thinning of the patellar articular cartilage in the axial plane; however, care must be taken not to injure the cartilage on injection of the joint, as this may induce artifactual abnormalities and lead to a false-positive diagnosis.
- The omission of sagittal acquisitions (to expedite the study) risks missing other pathology, such as extensor mechanism abnormalities, tendinitis, avulsion injuries, and patellar fractures.

Suggested Readings

Boven F, Bellemans MA, Geurts J, et al. The value of computed tomography scanning in chondromalacia patellae. Skeletal Radiol 1982;8:183–185

Burstein D, Gray M. New MRI techniques for imaging cartilage. J Bone Joint Surg Am 2003;85:70–77

McCauley TR, Kier R, Lynch KJ, Jokl P. Chondromalacia patellae: diagnosis with MR imaging. Am J Roentgenol 1992;158:101–105

Rose PM, Demlow TA, Szumowski J, Quinn SF. Chondromalacia patellae: fat-suppressed MR imaging. Radiology 1994;193:437–440

CASE 13

Kevin Rowan, Anthony G. Ryan, Peter L. Munk, and Bruce B. Forster

Clinical Presentation

A 60-year-old woman presented with chronic shoulder pain associated with loss of power and decreased range of motion.

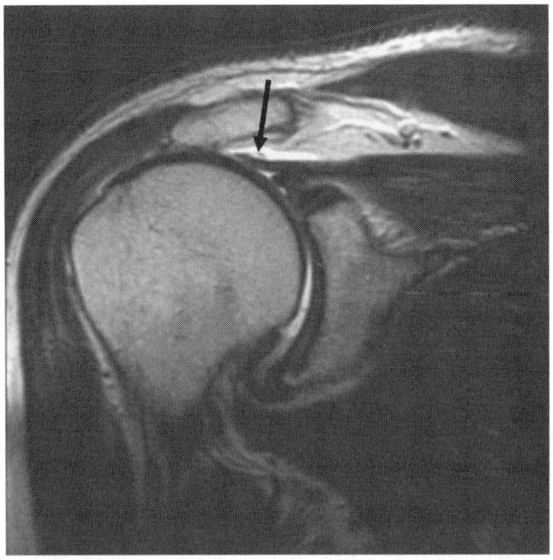

Figure 13A

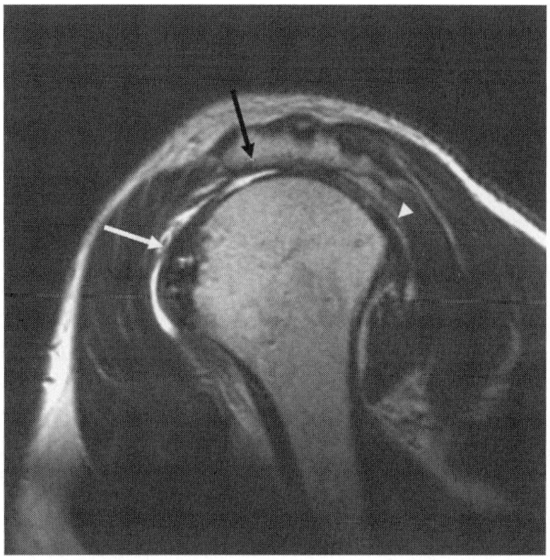

Figure 13B

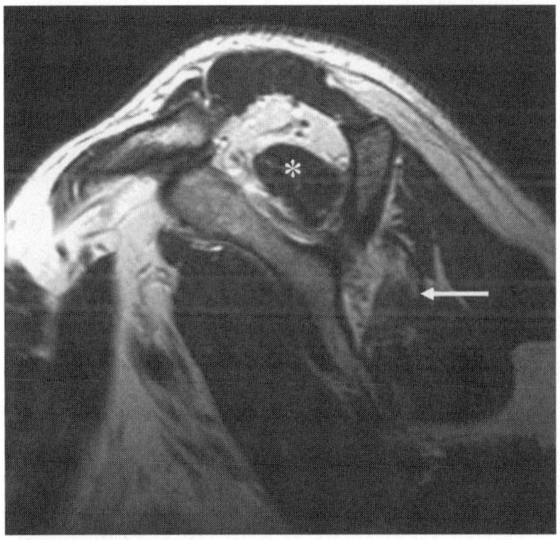

Figure 13C

Radiologic Findings

A coronal oblique FSE T2-weighted MRI (**Fig. 13A**) shows a full-thickness tear of the supraspinatus tendon (arrow). A sagittal oblique T2-weighted image (**Fig. 13B**) shows absence of the supraspinatus tendon in its expected location (black arrow) between the tendons of the infraspinatus (white arrowhead) and subscapularis (white arrow) muscles. The acromiohumeral space is markedly narrowed. A more medial sagittal oblique image (**Fig. 13C**) shows atrophy of the supraspinatus (*) and, to a lesser extent, infraspinatus (arrow) muscles, indicating that the tear is likely chronic in nature.

Diagnosis

Full-thickness supraspinatus tendon tear.

Differential Diagnosis

None: this is a pathognomonic appearance.

Discussion

Background

Shoulder pain is a common clinical complaint, and one of the most frequent causes in patients over 40 years is a rotator cuff tear. The rotator cuff is composed of the tendons of supraspinatus, infraspinatus, subscapularis, and teres minor. Most rotator cuff tears involve the supraspinatus tendon. The etiology of rotator cuff tear is thought to be a combination of intrinsic degenerative change and extrinsic impingement as the tendon passes through the acromiohumeral space. A relative region of hypovascularity—the "critical zone"—is present ~1 cm medial to the insertion on the greater tuberosity. This is a common site of both tendinopathy and full-thickness tears.

Clinical Findings

Rotator cuff tears usually present as chronic shoulder pain, especially with shoulder abduction, associated with loss of power and range of motion. Patients will often report pain being worse at night.

Imaging Findings

ULTRASOUND

- Discontinuity of supraspinatus tendon

MAGNETIC RESONANCE IMAGING

- Discontinuity of the supraspinatus tendon with high signal equal to that of fluid between the tendon fragments
- MR arthrogram images show intra-articular gadolinium flowing freely into the subacromial/subdeltoid bursa through the gap between the torn fragments.
- Chronic tears demonstrate retraction of the torn tendon and atrophy of the supraspinatus muscle.

Treatment

Arthroscopic repair of full-thickness rotator cuff tears is now the treatment of choice. Partial thickness tears are treated conservatively but can progress to full-thickness and complete tears.

Prognosis

Prognosis following surgical repair correlates with several preoperative factors, including

- The amount of retraction and degeneration of the torn supraspinatus tendon (If the tendon is retracted proximal to the glenoid margin, repair is unlikely to be successful.)
- Atrophy of the supraspinatus muscle
- Acromiohumeral distance

- Arthropathy of the glenohumeral joint
- Patient age

Surgical repair is usually successful in relieving patient pain and can improve power and range of motion.

PEARLS

- The most common site of supraspinatus tendon tear is at the critical zone, ~1 cm medial to the tendinous insertion on the greater tuberosity.

PITFALLS

- High signal in the supraspinatus tendon on short TE (T1-weighted or gradient echo) images may be due to the "magic angle" phenomenon, which is seen at the point within the tendon at which the fibers are at 55 degrees to the magnetic field. High signal due to the magic angle will disappear on sequences obtained with a longer TE, such as T2-weighted sequences. High signal related to pathology will remain evident on T2-weighted images.

Suggested Readings

Munk PL, Vellet AD, Levin MF, Bell DA, Marth MM, McCain GA. Intravenous administration of gadolinium in the evaluation of rheumatoid arthritis of the shoulder. Can Assoc Radiol J 1993;44:99–106.

Van Linthoudt D, Deforge J, Malterre L, Huber H. Rotator cuff repair: long-term results. Joint Bone Spine 2003;70:271–275

Villet AO, Munk PL, Hanks P. Imaging techniques of the shoulder: present prospectives. Clin Sports Med 1991;10:721–756

CASE 14

Kevin Rowan, Anthony G. Ryan, Peter L. Munk, and Bruce B. Forster

Clinical Presentation

A 22-year-old man presented with recurrent instability of the right shoulder.

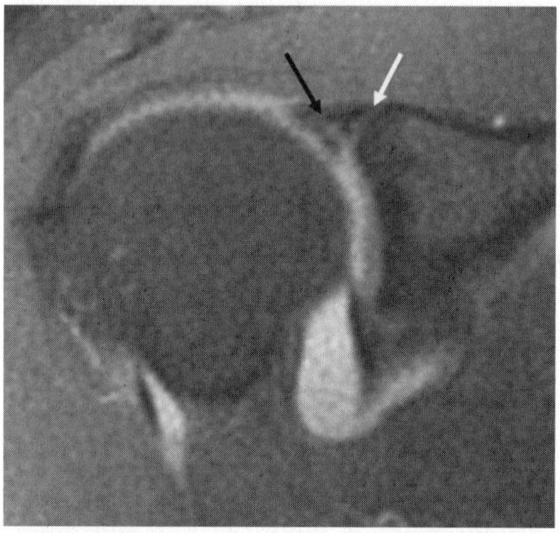

Figure 14A

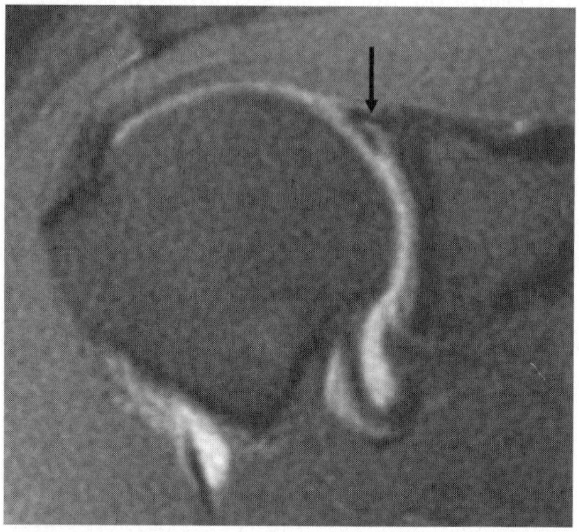

Figure 14B

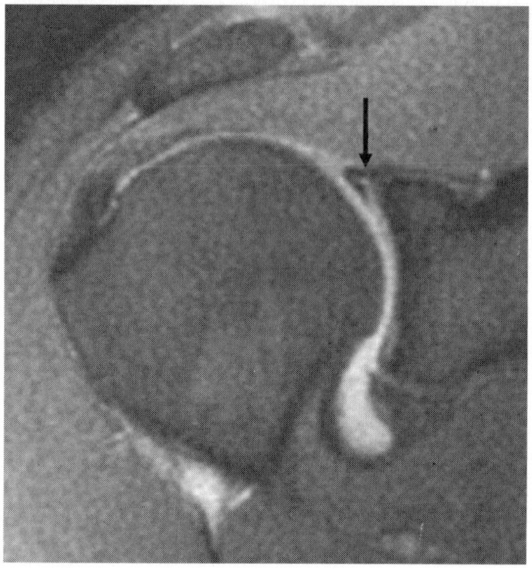

Figure 14C

Radiologic Findings

Coronal oblique T1-weighted fat-saturated images from an MR arthrogram (**Figs. 14A–14C**) show curvilinear high signal within the superior labrum, coursing from the glenoid attachment in a posterolateral direction (black arrows). The superior sublabral recess (**Fig. 14A**, white arrow), a normal anatomic variant, is situated at the 12 o'clock position adjacent to the biceps anchor and follows the superior rim of the glenoid in a medial direction, more medially than the adjacent high signal labral tear.

Diagnosis

Superior labrum anterior-posterior (SLAP) tear, type II.

Differential Diagnosis

Sublabral foramen.

Discussion

Background

MR arthrography, performed with intra-articular injection of dilute gadolinium, is required for definitive diagnosis of most tears of the glenoid labrum, although T2 fat-saturated coronal oblique imaging demonstrates reasonable sensitivity and specificity for types II through IV SLAP lesions. Such tears of the superior labrum are known as SLAP tears. Four types of SLAP tears were originally described, although up to six types have now been identified. The most common tear is the type II lesion, in which the superior labrum is torn and remains minimally displaced. A type III lesion is a bucket handle tear, type IV is a bucket handle tear with extension into the biceps tendon, and a type I SLAP represents degeneration and fraying of the superior labrum.

Clinical Findings

Superior labral tears are often seen in athletes who throw and are a common cause of shoulder pain and instability. Patients are unable to continue with activities that elicit symptoms.

Imaging Findings

MAGNETIC RESONANCE IMAGING

- Coronal oblique MR arthrogram images show intra-articular contrast extending from the articular surface into the superior labrum in a lateral direction.
- A type II SLAP tear represents minimally displaced stripping of the superior labrum from the bony glenoid.

Treatment

Types II, III, and IV are considered surgical lesions. Type I is a degenerative lesion and is treated conservatively.

Prognosis

Surgical repair of SLAP lesions usually provides relief of symptoms related to instability and allows return to activity.

PEARL

- Identification of a paralabral cyst suggests the presence of a labral tear, even if the latter is not clearly demonstrated.

PITFALL

- Discrimination between a sublabral recess and a SLAP II tear is often difficult. A tear will often appear irregular or stellate, as opposed to the smooth sublabral recess. A sublabral recess is oriented in a superomedial direction, as opposed to a true labral tear, which is oriented in a lateral direction. Extension of the curvilinear abnormality posterior to the biceps anchor is also suggestive of a labral tear.

Suggested Readings

De Maeseneer M, Van Roy F, Lenchik L, et al. CT and MR arthrography of the normal and pathologic anterosuperior labrum and labral-bicipital complex. Radiographics 2000;20:S67–S81

Jee WH, McCauley TR, Katz LD, Matheny JM, Ruwe PA, Daigneault JP. Superior labral anterior posterior (SLAP) lesions of the glenoid labrum: reliability and accuracy of MR arthrography for diagnosis. Radiology 2001;218:127–132

Munk PL, Holt RG, Helms CA, Genant HR. Glenoid labrum: preliminary work with the use of radial-sequence MR imaging. Radiology 1989;173:751–753

CASE 15

Kevin Rowan, Anthony G. Ryan, Peter L. Munk, and Bruce B. Forster

Clinical Presentation

A 53-year-old man was admitted to the emergency department with bilateral shoulder pain following a grand mal seizure.

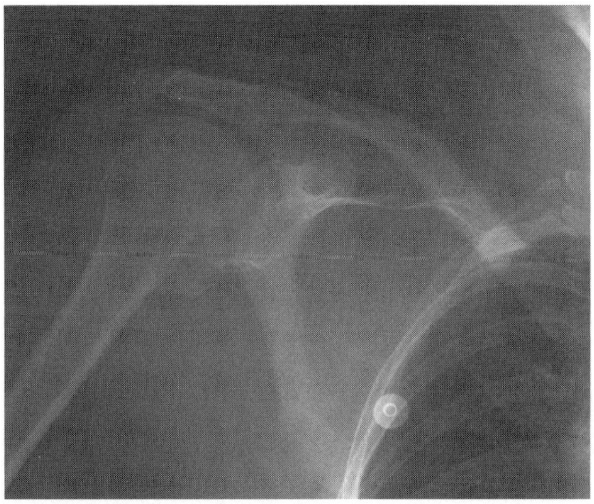

Figure 15A

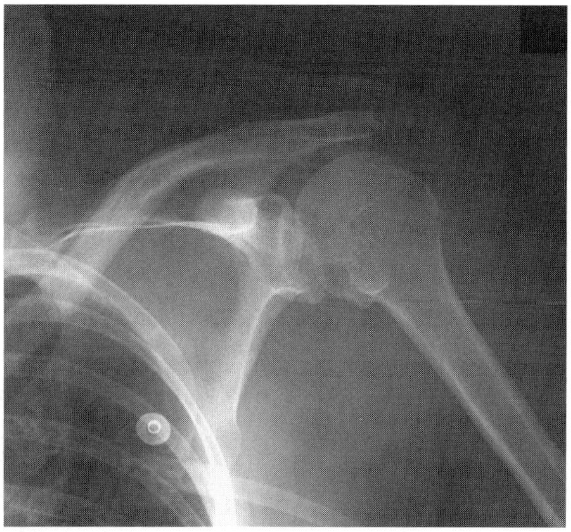

Figure 15B

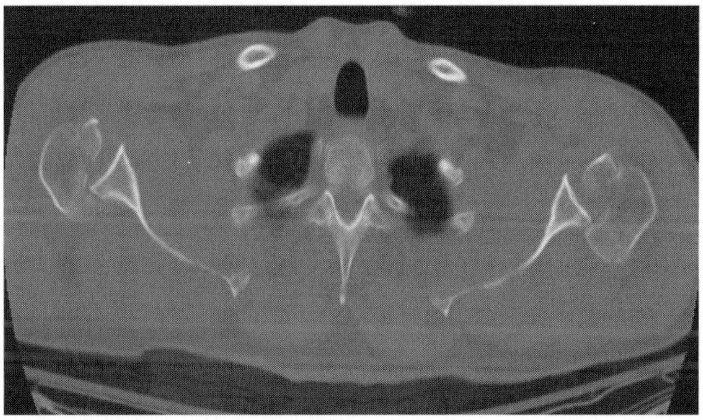

Figure 15C

Radiologic Findings

AP radiographs of the right and left shoulders (**Figs. 15A,15B**) show bilateral fractures of the medial humeral heads and abnormal glenohumeral articulation, with both humeri noted to be in internal rotation. An image from a subsequent CT scan (**Fig. 15C**) shows bilateral posterior glenohumeral dislocations with bilateral impaction fractures of the medial humeral heads.

Diagnosis

Bilateral posterior shoulder dislocations with reverse Hill-Sachs (McLaughlin) fractures.

Differential Diagnosis

None: this is a pathognomonic appearance.

Discussion

Background

Bilateral posterior shoulder dislocation is a rare entity, almost invariably associated with a history of seizures, electrocution, or severe trauma. The muscular forces exerted on the proximal humerus during a seizure or during a convulsion related to electrocution can be powerful enough to dislocate and fracture the humeral head. Posterior shoulder dislocations are rare in comparison to anterior dislocations, and the diagnosis is frequently missed if only a frontal radiograph is obtained. An axillary view or CT scan will provide the correct diagnosis.

Clinical Findings

A history of shoulder pain following grand mal seizure or electrocution should raise suspicion for posterior dislocation. A fall on an outstretched hand can result in unilateral posterior dislocation, although in the setting of trauma, this is a rare injury.

Complications

Posterior glenohumeral dislocation can result in a fracture of the posterior glenoid, termed a reverse Bankart lesion, or an impaction fracture of the anteromedial humeral head, known as a reverse Hill-Sachs or McLaughlin fracture. Injuries to the glenohumeral labroligamentous structures can result in chronic posterior instability.

Imaging Findings

RADIOGRAPHY

- On an AP film, internal rotation of the humerus places the greater tuberosity directly in front of the humeral head. The greater tuberosity is seen en face and simulates the appearance of a light bulb (the "light bulb" sign).
- The "trough line" sign is seen as two parallel cortical lines in the medial aspect of the humeral head, one line representing the medial humeral head cortex and the second representing the troughlike impaction fracture.
- Posterior dislocation is confirmed on axillary or transscapular views.

COMPUTED TOMOGRAPHY

- Posterior displacement of the humeral head in relation to the glenoid
- Humeral or glenoid fractures related to the direction of dislocation

Treatment

- Closed reduction
- Chronic instability is treated with arthroscopic repair of the posterior capsulolabral complex.
- Associated humeral head fractures are treated with open reduction and fixation (**Fig. 15D**).

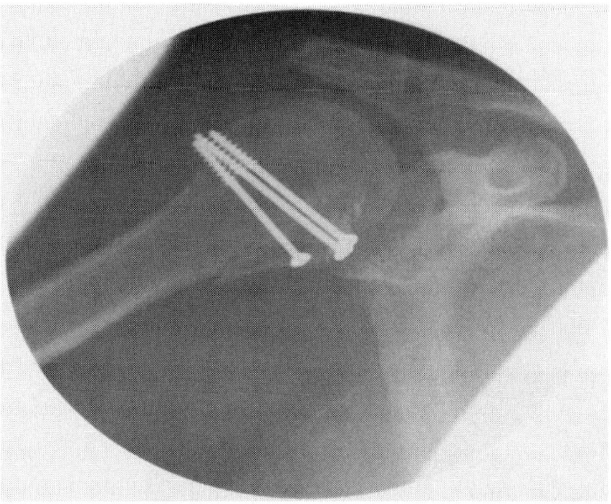

Figure 15D Humeral head fracture reduced with screws. Anteroposterior projection from intraoperative fluoroscopy demonstrating completion of open reduction and fixation of a right glenohumeral fracture dislocation.

PEARLS

- For plain film assessment of the shoulder, always obtain orthogonal views to rule out anterior or posterior dislocation. If such views are not possible because of patient discomfort, have a low threshold for CT assessment.
- Bilateral posterior shoulder dislocations are almost invariably related to seizures, electrocution, or extreme trauma.

PITFALLS

- Posterior dislocation is easily missed on an AP radiograph of the shoulder. The above-mentioned plain film findings are neither highly sensitive nor specific.
- Always obtain orthogonal views or a CT scan.

Suggested Readings

Brackstone M, Patterson SD, Kertesz A. Triple "E" syndrome: bilateral locked posterior fracture dislocation of the shoulders. Neurology 2001;56:1403–1404

Tung GA, Hou DD. MR arthrography of the posterior labrocapsular complex: relationship with glenohumeral joint alignment and clinical posterior instability. Am J Roentgenol 2003;180:369–375

CASE 16

Kevin Rowan, Anthony G. Ryan, Peter L. Munk, and Bruce B. Forster

Clinical Presentation

A 55-year-old man presented to us with chronic shoulder pain, decreased range of motion, and decreased power.

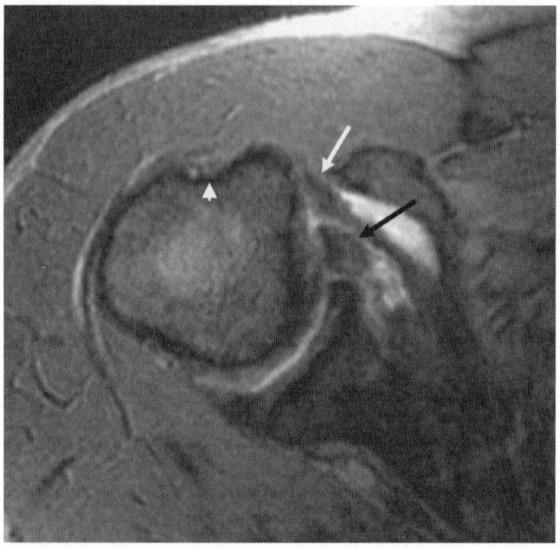

Figure 16A

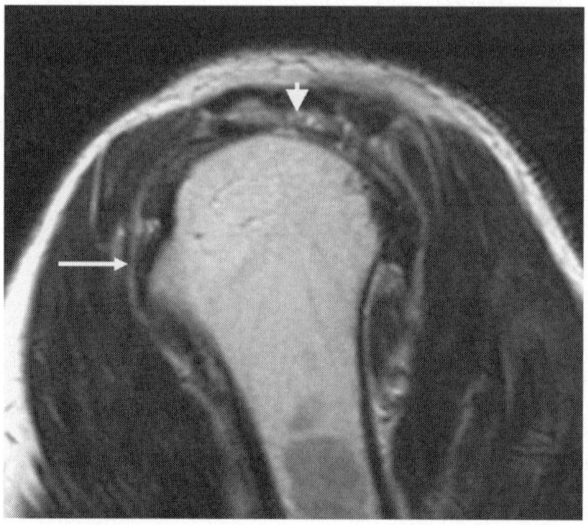

Figure 16B

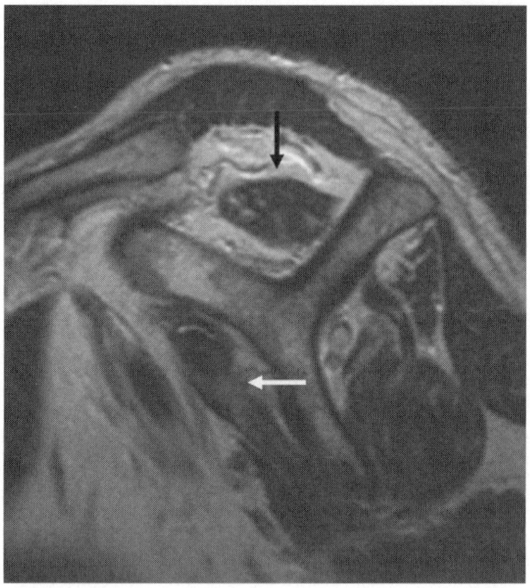

Figure 16C

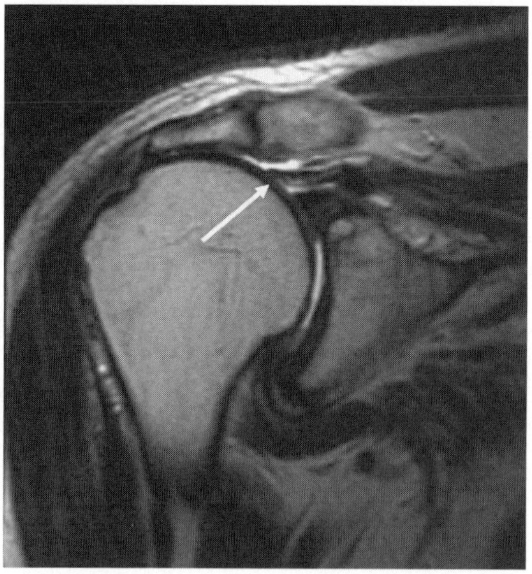

Figure 16D

Radiologic Findings

An axial T2-weighted gradient recalled echo (GRE) image (**Fig. 16A**) shows a medially dislocated long head of the biceps tendon (black arrow) anterior to the glenohumeral joint. The bicipital groove is empty (white arrowhead). The subscapularis tendon (white arrow) is torn from its attachment to the lesser tuberosity. A sagittal oblique T2-weighted image at the level of the humeral head (**Fig. 16B**) shows absence of the subscapularis (white arrow) and supraspinatus (arrowhead) tendons, consistent with full-thickness tears of both tendons. A sagittal oblique T2-weighted image at the level of the scapula (**Fig. 16C**) shows marked atrophy of the supraspinatus (black arrow) and subscapularis (white arrow) muscles. A coronal oblique T2-weighted image (**Fig. 16D**) shows a complete tear of the supraspinatus tendon (arrow) with retraction from the humeral insertion site.

Diagnosis

Medial dislocation of the long head of the biceps tendon, with associated subscapularis and supraspinatus tendon tears.

Differential Diagnosis

The dislocated biceps tendon itself can constitute a glenoid labral ovoid mass (GLOM), which has the differential diagnosis listed below.

- An avulsed labral fragment or other intra-articular loose body
- Thickened middle glenohumeral ligament (as in a Buford complex)

Discussion

Background

The long head of the biceps tendon contributes to the stability of the glenohumeral joint. The tendon is situated in the bicipital groove of the humerus and is held in place by the subscapularis tendon and transverse humeral ligament. Biceps tendon dislocation usually requires an associated tear of the subscapularis tendon to exit the bicipital groove. The tear is not necessarily complete, as the biceps tendon may be interposed into the space between the fibers of a partially torn subscapularis. The biceps tendon almost invariably dislocates medially, due to the orientation of forces acting on the tendon. Subscapularis tears are generally degenerative in nature, and in many cases a degenerative tear of the supraspinatus will also be identified.

Clinical Findings

Patients often present with symptoms related to associated rotator cuff tendon tears, including shoulder pain, weakness, and loss of mobility. Shoulder impingement is a common presentation.

Complications

None.

Imaging Findings

MAGNETIC RESONANCE IMAGING

- Axial images demonstrate an empty bicipital groove and medial displacement of the biceps tendon.
- Partial or complete subscapularis tendon tear can be identified on axial images.

Treatment

Conservative treatment is rendered if there are minimal symptoms; arthroscopic or open repair is offered if tendon dislocation is associated with a severe rotator cuff tear.

Prognosis

Surgical outcome is related to multiple factors, particularly the severity of the associated rotator cuff tear.

PEARLS

- The biceps tendon almost invariably dislocates medially, due to the orientation of forces acting on the tendon.
- A dislocated long head of the biceps tendon (**Fig. 16E**) may appear on an axial MRI as a GLOM (arrow). Assessment of serial axial images inferiorly (**Figs. 16F,16G**) will allow differentiation of a dislocated biceps tendon (arrow) from other sources of GLOM lesions.
- Bicipital tendon dislocations are frequently associated with rotator cuff tears, which should be looked for carefully. The presence of such tears has a large impact on the outcome of treatments directed at the biceps tendon.

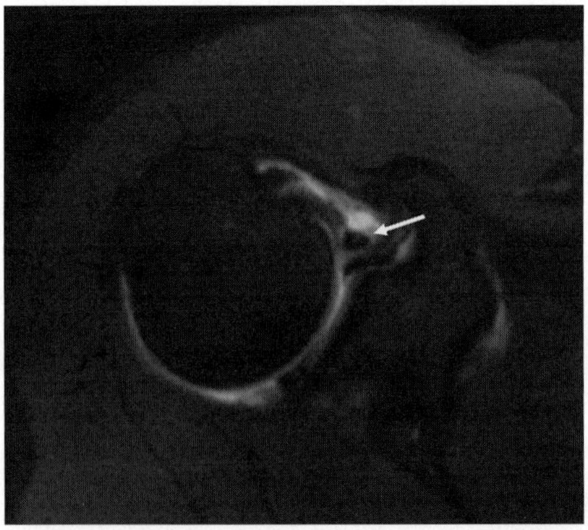

Figure 16E A dislocated long head of the biceps tendon may appear on an axial MRI as a glenoid labral ovoid mass (arrow).

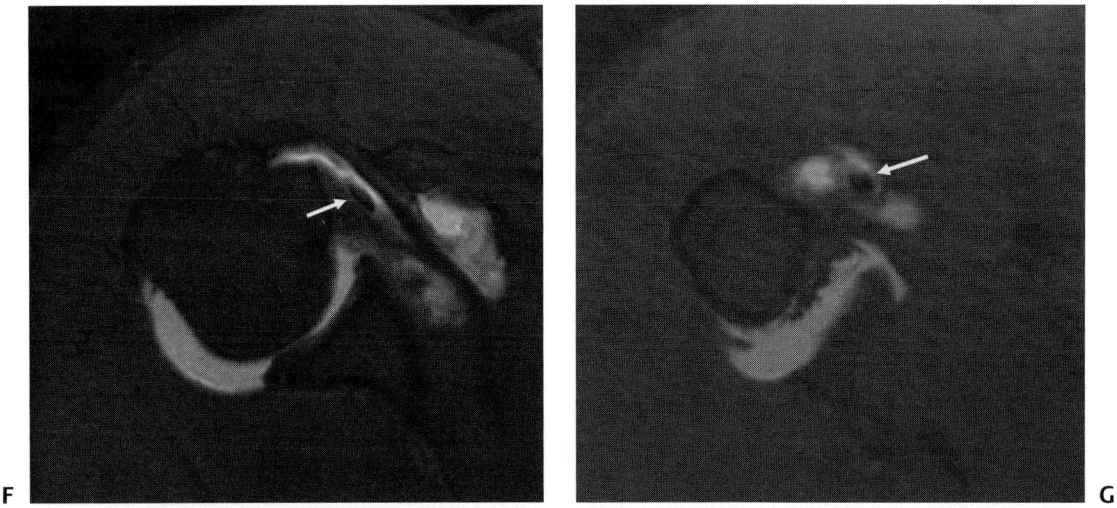

Figures 16F and **16G** Assessment of serial axial images inferiorly will allow differentiation of a dislocated biceps tendon (arrows) from other sources of glenoid labral ovoid mass lesions.

PITFALLS

- The long head of the biceps tendon should be systematically assessed in all cases of suspected rotator cuff tear. When reading these cases, if the search stops on finding a cuff tear, this may result in missing a concomitant bicipital tendon tear or dislocation.
- An empty bicipital groove can also be seen with a full thickness tear of the long head of the biceps, with retraction of the free edge proximally. The presence of the dislocated biceps tendon medially allows differentiation from this entity.
- Occasionally, bicipital dislocation may be associated with labral injuries (due to associated shoulder dislocation). Such injuries may easily be missed if not looked for specifically, particularly when intra-articular contrast is not employed.

Suggested Readings

Chan TW, Dalinka MK, Kneeland JB, Chervrot A. Biceps tendon dislocation: evaluation with MR imaging. Radiology 1991;179:649–652

Li XX, Schweitzer ME, Bifano JA, Lerman J, Manton GL, El-Noueam KI. MR evaluation of subscapularis tears. J Comput Assist Tomogr 1999;23:713–717

Tuckman GA. Abnormalities of the long head of the biceps tendon of the shoulder: MR imaging findings. Am J Roentgenol 1994;163:1183–1188

CASE 17

Peter L. Munk, Anthony G. Ryan, and Laurel O. Marchinkow

Clinical Presentation

A 23-year-old woman presented with a $1^1/_2$-year history of left-sided preauricular pain accentuated by mouth opening and chewing. The patient also reported clicking noises on opening of the mouth.

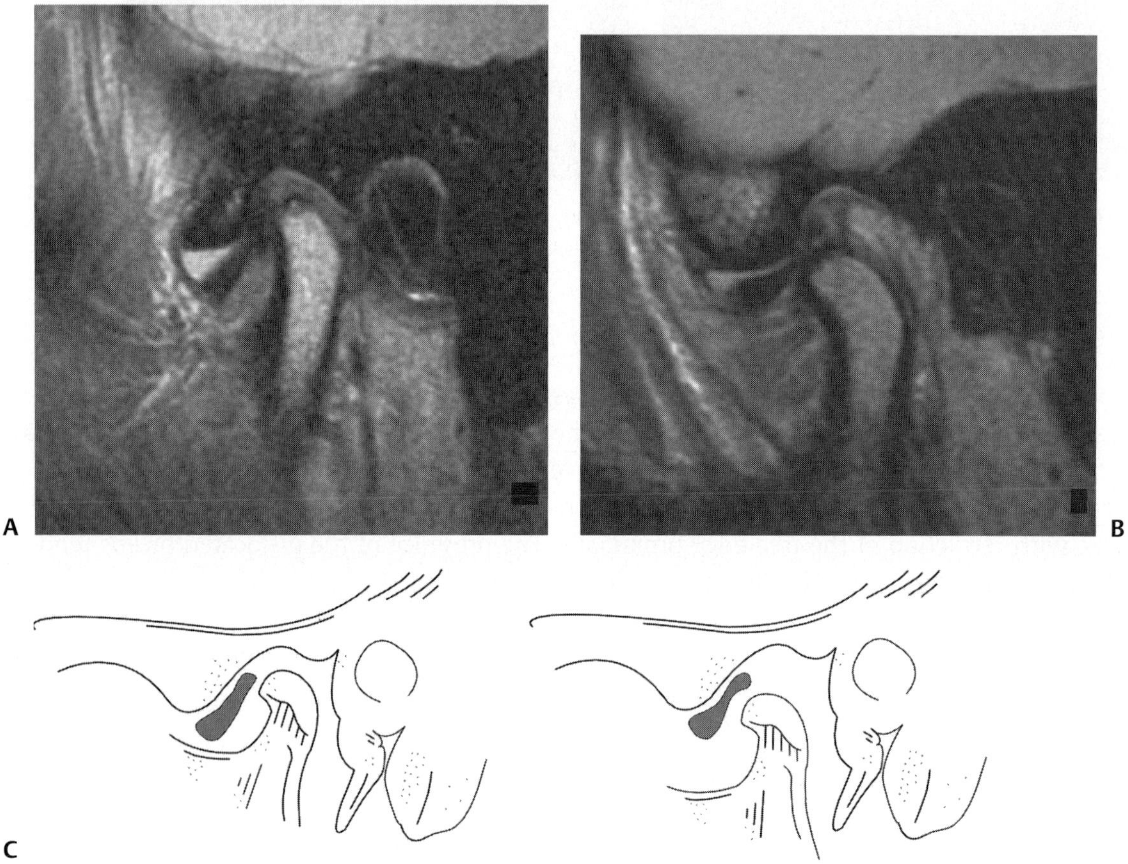

Figures 17A–17C

Radiologic Findings

T2-weighted MRIs show the fibrocartilaginous disk to be displaced, such that its posterior band is anterior to the condyle, that is, dislocated (**Fig. 17A**). On opening the mouth, the condyle has moved anteriorly and regained its normal relationship with the concave undersurface of the disk, which is then said to be "recaptured" (**Fig. 17B**). The accompanying line diagrams (**Fig. 17C**) demonstrate the open-mouth view left (the recapture position) and the closed-mouth view right (showing the disk anterior to the head of the condyle).

Diagnosis

Anterior dislocation of the temporomandibular joint (TMJ) meniscus with reduction on mouth opening.

Discussion

Background

The TMJ is a two-compartment joint, with the segments of the joint separated by a fibrous disk or meniscus. These two compartments do not normally communicate; however, if the disk is damaged or perforated, communication may occur. The meniscus has a donut-shaped elliptical contour and normally travels with the condyle as the mouth opens and the condyle rotates slightly and slides forward over the condylar eminence. Normally, the thin region, known as the intermediate zone, is interposed at the narrowest portion of the joint space between the condylar process and the condylar eminence.

In some cases, the posterior soft tissues (bilaminar zone) that tether the meniscus and prevent it from sliding excessively anteriorly over the condyle may become stretched or disrupted. In these situations, the meniscus may sublux or frankly dislocate anteriorly. When the mouth is opened, the disk may be recaptured and the normal relationship between the disk and the condyle restored. It is in this situation that a palpable clunk may be detected as the mouth opens. A normal disk position is far more frequent in adults than children.

Temporomandibular disorder (TMD) is a collective term used to describe a remarkably common but disparate group of conditions affecting the TMJ and surrounding structures. The pathology responsible may arise in the joint (arthrogenic), the muscles (myogenic), or both.

Clinical Findings

The most common symptoms include pain, crepitus, locking, and trismus. On physical examination, the crepitus and clunking reported when the mouth is opened can frequently be palpated.

Etiology

A history of previous trauma, bruxism, orthodontic manipulation, or malocclusion can often be elicited.

Complications

Chronic disk dislocation may result in the condylar process and condylar eminence articulating directly for prolonged periods of time, and in this situation degenerative changes may evolve, including flattening of the condylar process and development of sclerosis, fibrosis, and osteophytes. As these progress, debris may accumulate within the joint with an accompanying effusion, and eventually the TMJ meniscus may be severely damaged.

Imaging Findings

ARTHROGRAPHY

Displacement of the meniscus may be demonstrated by injecting contrast directly into the joint, although this technique is now infrequently utilized and has been largely replaced by cross-sectional methods.

COMPUTED TOMOGRAPHY

CT has a useful role in the evaluation of the integrity of bony structures due to its ability to show fine bony detail.

MAGNETIC RESONANCE IMAGING

MRI is now the preferred method for evaluation of internal joint derangement, given the superb soft-tissue resolution.

Treatment

Conservative measures are the mainstay of treatment, including physical therapy and oral splints. In severe, chronic cases of TMJ pain and dysfunction, joint reconstruction with bone graft or prosthetic material has been employed, frequently with poor results.

For chronic pain, believed myogenic in origin, botulinum toxin has been proposed as an effective treatment.

Prognosis

When conservative measures are tolerated by the patient, symptoms may resolve over time such that treatment may be discontinued. Only when conservative options fail should surgery be considered.

PEARLS

- The thinnest portion of the disk, known as the intermediate zone, should be interposed at the narrowest portion of the joint space between the condylar process and the condylar eminence; if not, subluxation or dislocation should be suspected.
- Dislocation is defined as displacement of the posterior band of the fibrocartilaginous disk anterior to the mandibular condyle.
- When degenerative joint disease has occurred, particularly postoperatively, the superior fine osseous detail demonstrated by CT makes it of greater utility compared with MRI, which demonstrates the initial dislocation to better effect.

PITFALLS

- The TMJ is a two-compartment joint, and thus examination via arthrography requires a two-compartment injection as, even in the presence of a perforated disk, flow through the defect may be unidirectional.
- The position of the disk displays far greater variability in children than in adults.
- As a synovial joint, the TMJ may be affected by any of the arthritides, and evidence of this should be sought on each examination.

Suggested Readings

Hayt MW, Abrahams JJ, Blair J. Magnetic resonance imaging of the temporomandibular joint. Top Magn Reson Imaging 2000;11:138–146

Munk PL, Lee MJ, Struk DW, Marchinkow LO, Wambeek N. CT and MRI of the temporomandibular joint. J Hong Kong Col Radiol 2000;3:125–135

Schwartz M, Freund B. Treatment of temporomandibular disorders with botulinum toxin. Clin J Pain 2002;18(6 Suppl):S198–S203

CASE 18

Anthony G. Ryan and Peter L. Munk

Clinical Presentation

A patient reported recent onset of hip pain and "clicking" after a forceful twisting injury.

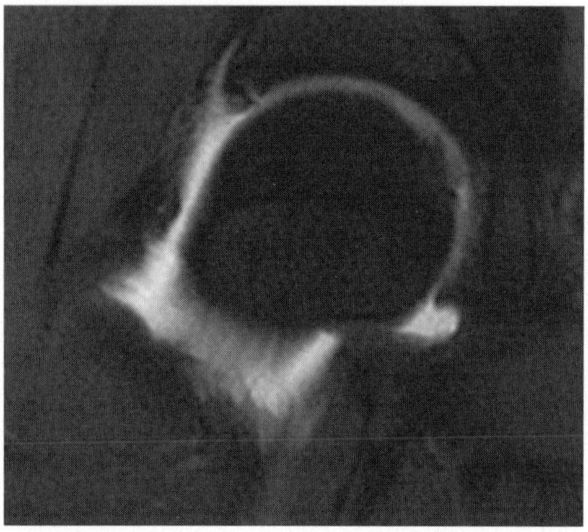

Figure 18A

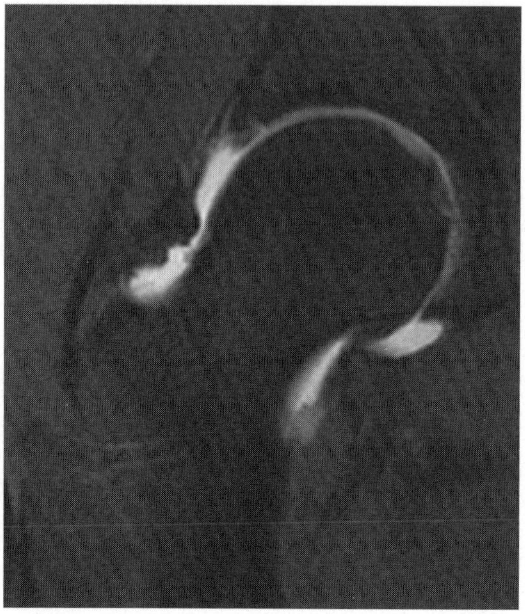

Figure 18B

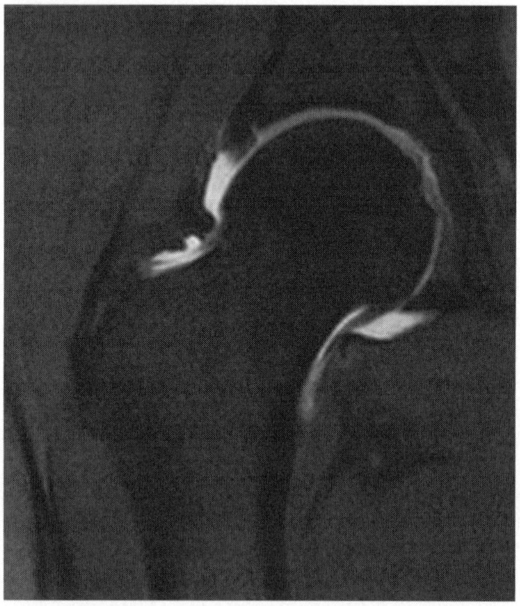

Figure 18C

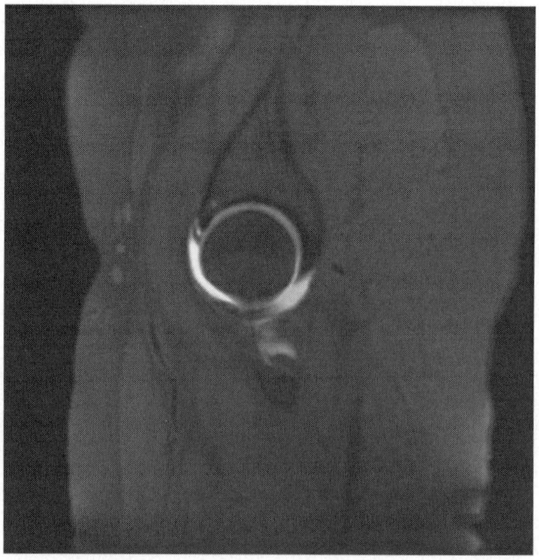

Figure 18D

Radiologic Findings

T1-weighted coronal oblique (**Figs. 18A–18C**) and sagittal (**Fig. 18D**) images after intra-articular injection of dilute gadolinium show linear high signal intensity extending from within the anterosuperior labrum to the surface, present over a series of contiguous slices.

Diagnosis

Acetabular labral tear.

Differential Diagnosis

The clinical presentation has a differential diagnosis, including

- Snapping iliopsoas tendon
- Osteonecrosis
- Intra-articular disorders, such as pigmented villonodular synovitis (PVNS) and synovial osteochondromatosis

The imaging appearance has no differential diagnosis.

Discussion

Background

The acetabular labrum is a fibrocartilaginous ring applied to the outer acetabular fossa margin, serving to increase hip joint stability by deepening the fossa. The increased depth promotes development of negative hydrostatic pressure within the joint, further increasing the "hold" of the acetabulum on the femoral head. Injuries to this structure therefore have significant effects on the stability of the joint.

Etiology

Although trauma is the unifying cause in all cases, certain conditions predispose to developing early or severe labral tears, including femoral acetabular impingement, congenital/developmental hip dysplasias (**Figs. 18E,18F**) and following posterior hip dislocation (**Figs. 18G,18H**). In dysplasias, it is thought that tears occur as a degenerative phenomenon secondary to abnormal force redistribution within the joint.

The causative trauma is not necessarily severe, often involving a simple twisting or slipping mechanism, such as occurs when one tries to catch one's balance on ice or a slippery floor, or recurrent low-grade trauma at the extremes of hip flexion.

Pathophysiology

The labrum is well enervated and thus is very painful when injured or chronically irritated. In addition to the physical instability induced by a defect in the labrum and consequent loss of uniform intra-articular pressure, injury to the abundant proprioceptive supply decreases the stability of the joint.

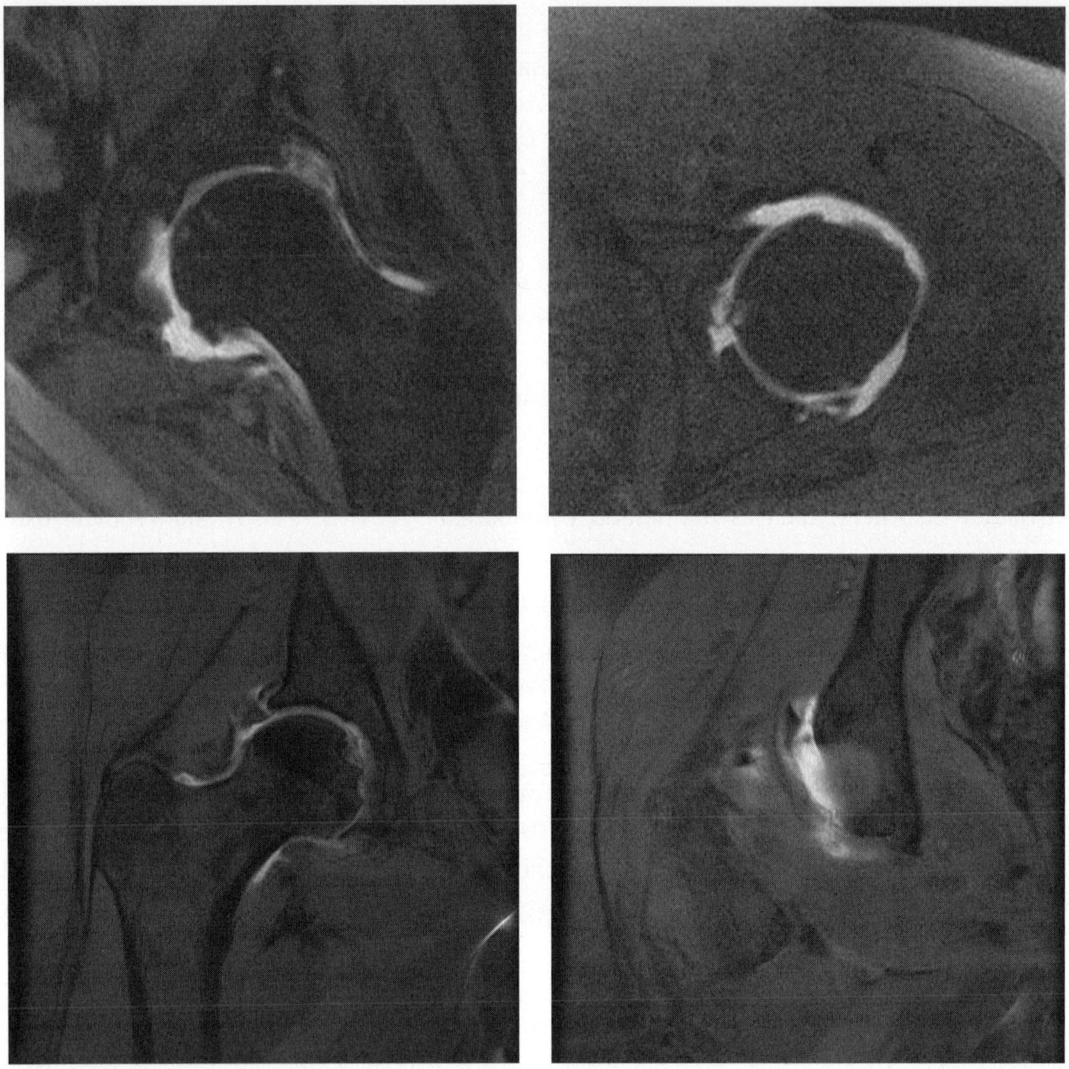

E F G H

Figures 18E and **18F** Coronal oblique (**18E**) and transaxial (**18F**) T1-weighted images of the left hip after intra-articular injection of gadolinium in a patient with congenital hip dysplasia, consequent joint degeneration and labral tears, demonstrating femoral head surface irregularity and truncation, and diffuse high signal intensity of the anterosuperior labrum and a more clearly defined linear high signal intensity tear extending to the surface of the midportion of the posterolateral labrum. **18G** and **18H** Coronal oblique (**18G**) and sagittal oblique (**18H**) T1-weighted images of the right hip after intra-articular injection of gadolinium in a patient after posterior hip dislocation shows a combined labral tear with a fracture of the underlying acetabular margin seen extending from the anterosuperior labral margin to the posterior margin, with a bony fragment projected posterior to the bony acetabulum.

The anterosuperior portion of the labrum is torn most frequently. The labrum is most commonly avulsed from the bony acetabulum rather than a true intrasubstance labral tear.

Clinical Findings

Patients typically complain of hip pain that "catches" them and stops them in their tracks. The pain may be associated with a click, a snapping, or a painful giving way. Occasionally, the joint may lock. On examination, pain is classically elicited by passive flexion and internal rotation of the hip.

Stages of Disease

- Labrum torn from acetabulum
- Intrasubstance labral tear
- Tear with avulsion of bony fragment

Complications

- The femoral articular cartilage is prone to erosion at its site of articulation with the torn labrum.
- Labral cyst formation

Labral tears are frequently associated with cysts around the hip. These cysts, described collectively as "labral cysts," may be intraosseous or within the soft tissues (ganglia or synovial cysts).

Because of the predisposition of dysplasia to both labral tears and early osteoarthrosis, labral cysts are frequently found in this group where a geode (subchondral cyst) may extend through the lateral cortex of the acetabulum and produce a soft-tissue cyst.

The proposed mechanism of action for generating these cysts is that, following the tear, the loss of congruency promotes an increased intra-articular pressure and joint effusion, which may then extrude through the labral defect into the para-acetabular soft tissue.

Imaging Findings

RADIOGRAPHY

- Juxta-articular soft-tissue mass (in the presence of a labral cyst)
- Gas within the mass (gas within the cyst)
- Well-defined erosions of the lateral margins of the acetabulum
- Evidence of osteoarthrosis

ULTRASOUND

- The normal labrum appears as a hyperechoic triangle along the acetabular margin.
- A labral tear will appear anechoic or hypoechoic; if cysts are present, these will be uniformly hypoechoic.

COMPUTED TOMOGRAPHY

- Multislice CT with or without arthrography has been proposed as an alternative to MR arthrography, with spatial resolution adequate to assess articular cartilage. This is potentially useful if access to MRI is an issue.

MAGNETIC RESONANCE IMAGING

MR arthrography is the investigation of choice where a labral tear is suspected on clinical grounds, as its sensitivity is 90% and its accuracy is 91%, compared with MRI without intra-articular gadolinium (sensitivity 30%, accuracy 36%), using surgery as the gold standard.

Normal variants seen on MRI include the following:

- The normal labrum is typically triangular in the coronal plane, although this becomes less common with age.

- The normal labrum has homogeneous low signal intensity (heterogeneity increasing with age).
- A labrum is not demonstrated in as many as 14% of individuals with increasing age; however, an absent labrum in a symptomatic individual is assumed to be pathological.
- Eleven percent of labra are round; 9% are flat. These findings do not vary with age.
- The hyaline cartilage of the acetabular roof may extend beneath the labrum and thus "undercut" the base.
- Signal alterations at the labral base may be due to fibrovascular tissue. Irregular insertion, fissures, or small vessels may easily be mistaken for labral degeneration or detachment.
- A sulcus is frequently seen at the anterosuperior acetabular-labral junction and is thus thought to be a normal variant.

On MRI, labral degeneration, tears, and detachments can be distinguished as follows:

- Degenerative labra
  - Labral degeneration is presumed in the presence of irregular margins, global thickening, and diffuse intrasubstance intermediate signal, although it has been shown that intrasubstance signal abnormality/alteration does not correlate well with histologic degeneration.
- Labral tears
  - Labral tears are suspected in the presence of blunting and absence.
  - A visibly displaced labrum in a symptomatic individual is indicative of a tear.
  - Absent labral tissue and an irregular remnant are good evidence of a tear.
  - The extension of intralabral signal intensity changes to the labral surface is highly suggestive of a labral tear, although these findings occur more frequently with advancing age.
  - A tear may be confined to the labral substance.
- Labral cysts
  - Paralabral cysts are well visualized on MRI and are found in the posterosuperior aspect of the hip joint three times as often as on the anterior aspect.
  - Subchondral cyst formation may be demonstrated in acetabulae affected by osteoarthritis.
  - On transaxial images, labral cysts may be easily differentiated from iliopsoas bursal fluid.

If a labral cyst is the first finding, or is found incidentally, further imaging should be undertaken with MR arthrography to rule out an associated labral tear.

ARTHROGRAPHY

The introduction of dilute gadolinium solution (2 mmol/L) into the hip joint significantly increases the conspicuity of the acetabular labrum and associated tear.

T1-weighted spin-echo (intra-articular gadolinium) or T2-weighted gradient-echo (intra-articular normal saline) images are obtained in the transaxial, sagittal, and coronal planes. In particular, the 3D gradient-echo sequences in the coronal and sagittal oblique planes are reported to have a sensitivity of 90% and an accuracy of 91% in characterizing labral abnormality.

The joint distention inherent in the arthrographic approach facilitates the demonstration of labral detachments and intrasubstance tears and the differentiation from the varied appearances of the asymptomatic labrum.

MR arthrography findings include the following:

- On MR arthrography, labral detachments and tears are recognized by the demonstration of contrast material insinuated at the acetabular-labral interface or imbibed within the substance of the labrum.

- The hyaline cartilage of the acetabular roof may extend beneath the labrum and thus undercut the base. Hyaline cartilage is of lower signal intensity compared with gadolinium insinuated into the tear, facilitating the differentiation of these two entities.
- The sensitivity for detection and correct staging of labral lesions with MR arthrography has been shown to be 91%; the specificity, 71%; and the accuracy, 88%.

Treatment

- Conservative management: initially, partial weight-bearing exercises
- If unresponsive, excision of the torn portion of the labrum is required, which may be performed either arthroscopically or via an open operation.
- Paralabral cysts may be treated using either MRI or ultrasound guidance to aspirate and inject steroids and long-acting local anesthetic.

Prognosis

- In an athlete, repair may be required to provide the best chance of returning to full activity.
- Minor tears heal reasonably well, and, in the absence of athletic activity, a patient can expect to return to full activities.
- Long-term development of osteoarthrosis remains a significant risk.

PEARLS

- The presence of a labral cyst should serve as a "red flag" to investigate for the presence of an underlying tear if not previously demonstrated.
- An absent labrum in a symptomatic individual is pathological, and a sulcus at the anterosuperior acetabular-labral junction may be a normal variant.
- The hyaline cartilage of the acetabular roof may extend beneath the labrum and thus undercut the base. Hyaline cartilage is of lower signal intensity compared with gadolinium insinuated into the tear, facilitating the differentiation of these two entities.

PITFALLS

- MRI without intra-articular gadolinium has very limited exclusionary value for labral pathology (sensitivity 30%, accuracy 36%).
- The frequency of the normal triangular configuration of the labrum decreases with age, and an increase in labral absence (14%) is demonstrated with increasing age.
- Intrasubstance signal abnormality/alteration does not correlate well with histologic degeneration, particularly at the labral base where signal alterations may be due to fibrovascular tissue. Irregular insertion, fissures, or small vessels may easily be mistaken for labral degeneration or detachment, especially without the use of intra-articular gadolinium.

Suggested Readings

Czerny C, Hofmann S, Neuhold A, et al. Lesions of the acetabular labrum: accuracy of MR imaging and MR arthrography in detection and staging. Radiology 1996;200:225–230

Lecouvet FE, Vande Berg BC, Malghem J, Lebon CJ, Moysan P, Jamart J, Maldague BE. MR imaging of the acetabular labrum: variations in 200 asymptomatic hips. Am J Roentgenol 1996;167:1025–1028

Petersilge CA. MR arthrography for evaluation of the acetabular labrum. Skeletal Radiol 2001;30:423–430

CASE 19

Anthony G. Ryan and Peter L. Munk

Clinical Presentation

A 34-year-old amateur tennis player complained of pain on the inside of his elbow, which he noticed particularly when making a forearm smash. Point tenderness over the medial epicondyle was elicited on physical examination. Pain on resisted pronation of the forearm was evident.

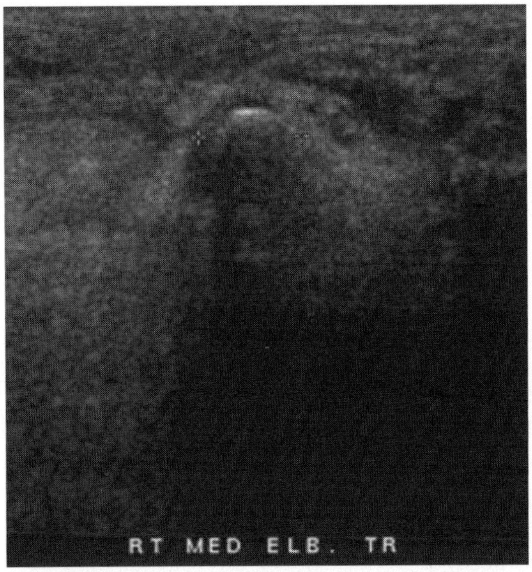

Figure 19A

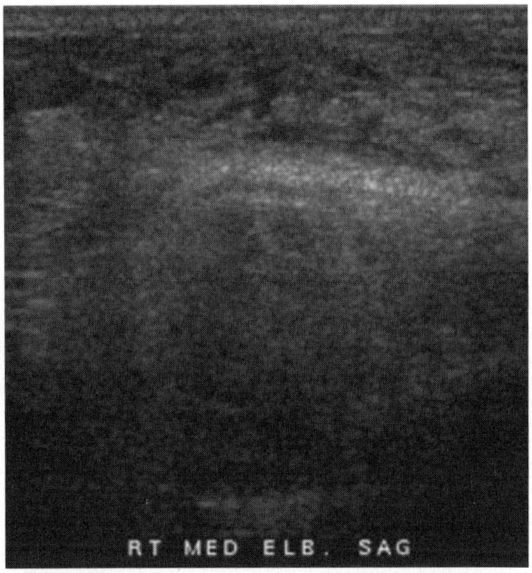

Figure 19B

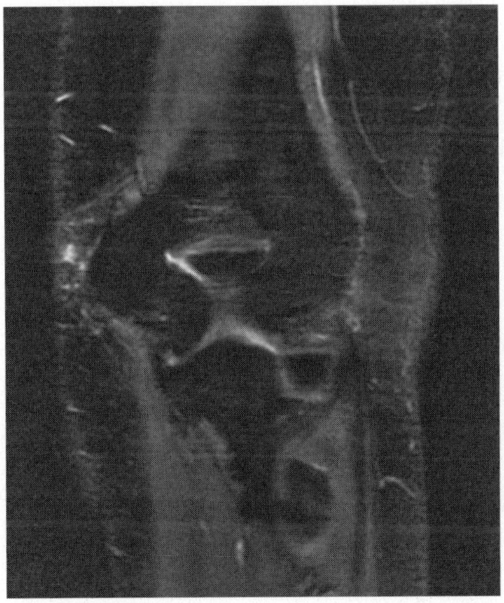

Figure 19C

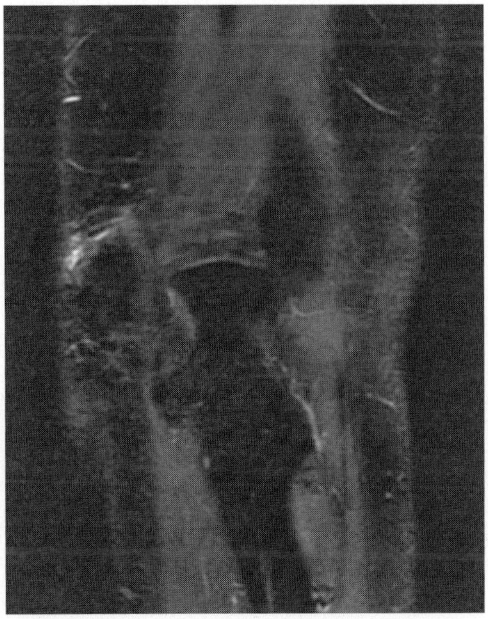

Figure 19D

Radiologic Findings

Ultrasound of the medial epicondyle and overlying soft tissues (**Figs. 19A,** transverse, and **19B,** sagittal) reveals a focal area of hypoechogenicity within the common flexor tendon and edema at the musculotendinous junction. Coronal T2-weighted fat-saturated MRIs (**Figs. 19C,** elbow joint, and **19D,** further posteriorly at the level of the olecranon) show diffuse high signal intensity overlying the medial epicondyle with laxity and partial discontinuity of the common flexor tendon.

Diagnosis

Medial epicondylitis.

Differential Diagnosis

Ulnar collateral ligament tear.

Discussion

Background

MEDIAL EPICONDYLITIS

Also known as golfer's elbow, pitcher's elbow, or medial tennis elbow, medial epicondylitis is caused by degeneration of the common flexor tendon secondary to overload of the flexor/pronator muscle group arising from the medial epicondyle.

LATERAL EPICONDYLITIS

Lateral epicondylitis, commonly referred to as tennis elbow, occurs more frequently than medial epicondylitis and is caused by degeneration of the common extensor tendon with or without the presence of tears.

Etiology

Most patients give a history of overuse. Degenerative tendinosis is common around the elbow, leading to a predisposition to tendon rupture. It was previously thought that a cycle of repetitive overuse led to recurrent and chronic inflammation, leading to the formation of scar tissue that is prone to further tears. However, repeated studies of tendons excised or débrided at surgery show no evidence of inflammatory cells but of degeneration only.

Pathophysiology

Overuse syndromes produce repetitive microtrauma. Although typically thought of as an overuse syndrome secondary to tennis, lateral epicondylitis is actually seen more frequently in nonathletes.

The tendon of the extensor carpi radialis brevis is typically degenerate and is usually partially avulsed from the lateral epicondyle. Lateral epicondylitis is frequent in tennis players because of the forcible pronation and supination involved in forearm and backhand plays.

In the preadolescent age group, instead of a tendon tear, children are more likely to avulse the unfused medial epicondylar apophysis, this being the weak link in the muscle-tendon-bone chain. This is one variant of Little Leaguer's elbow, the others comprising a stress fracture or delayed closure of the medial epicondyle apophysis.

Clinical Findings

The patient typically complains of pain on the inside or outside (sometimes both) of the elbow, with point tenderness elicited directly over the affected epicondyle. Reproduction of the patient's pain with resisted pronation (medial epicondylitis) or supination (lateral epicondylitis) is typical.

Stages of Disease

Mild, moderate, or severe.

Complications

- Lateral collateral ligament (LCL) injury (in association with lateral epicondylitis)
- Associated tears of the LCL are clearly seen. Lateral epicondylitis and LCL tears frequently occur together; however, LCL tears may be iatrogenic, secondary to surgery performed for lateral epicondylitis, further contributing to postoperative instability.
- Ulnar nerve neuritis (in association with medial epicondylitis)
- Delayed fusion of an avulsed fragment
- Stress fracture

Pathology

GROSS

The majority of cases of lateral epicondylitis demonstrate scarring, edema, and macroscopic tears at surgery.

- Focal areas of degeneration
- Discrete tears: partial (1 in 4) and complete (1 in 36)
- LCL involvement is seen in 1 in 6 cases.
- Calcification and bony changes may be noted.
- Ulnar neuritis

MICROSCOPIC

Focal areas of apparent degeneration identified at surgery corresponded to collagen degeneration with fibroblastic proliferation and neovascularization (fibroangiomatous hyperplasia). Disruption of collagen and mucoid/hyaline degeneration are all demonstrated without evidence of inflammatory markers.

Imaging Findings

RADIOGRAPHY

A periosteal reaction is frequently seen in combination with avulsions but not simple tendinosis. Chronically, this may be evinced by enthesopathy and epicondylar cortical irregularity (**Fig. 19E**).

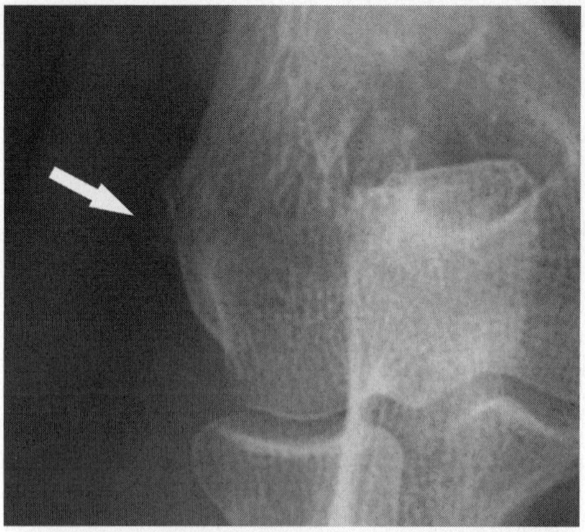

E

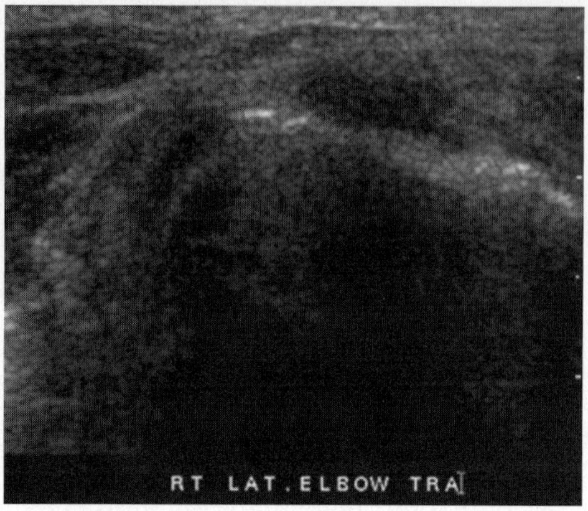

F

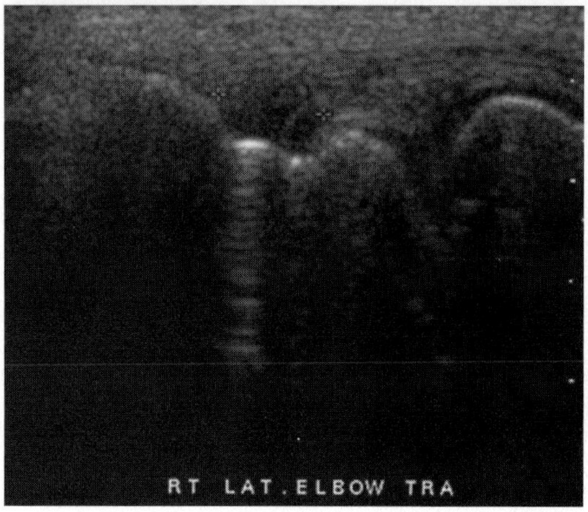

G

Figures 19E Enthesopathy (*white arrow*) at the site of a healing lateral epicondylar avulsion. **19F** and **19G** Ultrasound oriented coronally over the lateral epicondyle shows a hypoechoic region where the normal longitudinal fibrillar pattern is lost, indicative of a complete tear of the deep portion of the tendon (extensor carpi radialis).

ULTRASOUND

- The normal common extensor origin is composed of closely bound longitudinal fibrils. The extensor carpi radialis brevis constitutes most of the deep fibers, with the extensor digitorum making up the superficial component.
- Point tenderness will be elicited during the ultrasound examination over the affected epicondyle.
- The tendon origin will be demonstrated to be thickened and hypoechoic (corresponding to foci of degeneration) in comparison to the contralateral side.
- The most common appearance of lateral epicondylitis is a focal hypoechoic area in the deep part of the tendon (**Figs. 19F,19G**, both in the coronal plane).
- Partial thickness tears may be demonstrated as disruption of the normal fibers, with some fibers remaining contiguous.
- Discrete cleavage tears may be evident (**Figs. 19F,19G**).
- Foci of calcification may be demonstrated, as may an underlying epicondylar bone spur.
- The LCL can be identified as a discrete and separate band and is seen to be affected in one in every six instances of lateral epicondylitis.

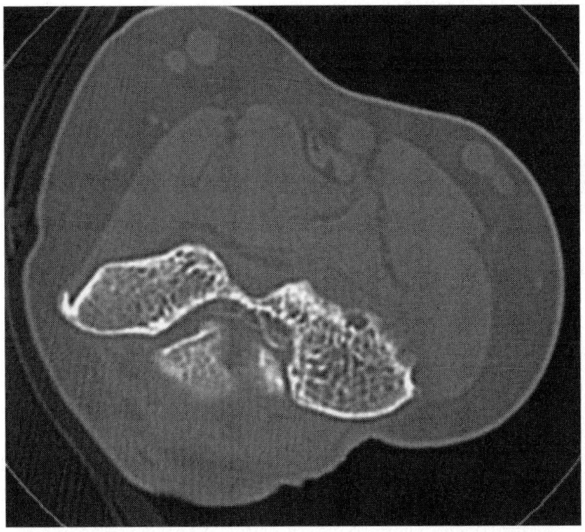

H

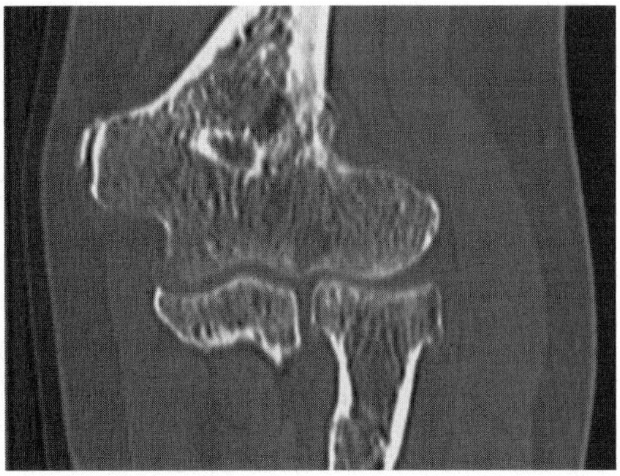

I

Figures 19H and **19I** Transaxial (**19H**) and coronal (**19I**) reformats show a bony spur/enthesophyte arising from the medial epicondyle (same patient as **19E**). A degree of irregularity is evident on the common extensor origin in addition in this patient with both medial and lateral epicondylitis.

- Ultrasound helps differentiate medial epicondylitis from a tear of the underlying ulnar collateral ligament, which is part of the differential, particularly in a professional athlete.

COMPUTED TOMOGRAPHY

Bony changes such as periostitis, acute avulsions, and chronic bony spurs/enthesophytes (**Figs. 19H, 19I**) will be clearly evident, in the absence of conventional radiographic evidence, or in cases where the radiographic evidence is subtle (**Fig. 19E**).

MAGNETIC RESONANCE IMAGING

In MRI, scanning at 1.5 T using axial T1-weighted, axial fat-saturated FSE T2-weighted, and coronal or sagittal STIR sequences will demonstrate the range of injuries from muscle strain, tendinosis, and tendon rupture.

- High signal intensity on T1 and T2 corresponds to areas of intratendinous degeneration.
- Marrow edema (increased T2 signal) may be demonstrated in the adjacent epicondyle.
- Increased signal intensity may be due to the underlying process or changes secondary to the biomechanical effect of pain in the tendon, resulting in altered elbow motion.
- In the presence of an acute avulsion, there will be significantly increased signal intensity within the surrounding supporting tissue.
- Lateral epicondylitis is evinced by increased signal intensity of the extensor tendons close to their insertion on the lateral epicondyle.

In cases of degenerative tendinosis,

- The tendon may be normal or thickened in tendinosis.
- It will be thinned in the case of partial tears.

- It can be absent in a complete tear with increased signal on fat-saturated FSE and fast STIR images.
- Tears of the common flexor tendon, medical collateral ligament (MCL) of the elbow, and neuritis of the adjacent ulnar nerve may be evident as increased signal intensity along the path of any of these structures.

Severe lateral epicondylitis frequently shows abnormalities of the lateral ulnar collateral ligament on MRI.

- If involved, the lateral ulnar collateral ligament will be thickened.
- Partial or complete tears may be present.
- Tendinosis and superimposed tears of the extensor carpi radialis brevis are usually demonstrated anteriorly within the common extensor tendon.
- Anconeus muscle edema and distention of the radial head bursa are infrequent findings.
- MRI may help to detect evidence of delayed fusion or stress fracture, prompting a period of rest to promote healing.

Treatment

- The majority of patients respond to conservative therapy consisting of rest, nonsteroidal anti-inflammatory drugs, and immobilization.
- High-grade partial tears and complete tears are likely to require surgery.
- Surgical treatments include longitudinal tenotomy and tendinous releases.
- Ulnar nerve transposition may be required in the presence of ulnar neuritis.

Prognosis

- Good, if rested adequately and tears are managed appropriately.

PEARLS

- Although typically thought of as an overuse syndrome secondary to tennis, the condition is actually seen more frequently in nonathletes.
- On ultrasound, the most common appearance of lateral epicondylitis is a focal hypoechoic area in the deep part of the tendon.
- Tendinosis and superimposed tears of the extensor carpi radialis brevis are usually demonstrated anteriorly within the common extensor tendon.

PITFALLS

- Increased signal intensity may be the result of the underlying process (epicondylar trauma) or edema due to abnormal elbow motion. Clinical correlation is necessary.
- The tendon may be normal or thickened in the presence of tendinosis.
- One should actively look for evidence of ulnar nerve neuritis manifested as increased signal intensity in the surrounding soft tissues. Early recognition is important, as it may obviate later transposition if treated appropriately in the early stages.

Suggested Readings

Bredella MA, Tirman PF, Fritz RC, Feller JF, Wischer TK, Genant HK. MR imaging findings of lateral ulnar collateral ligament abnormalities in patients with lateral epicondylitis. Am J Roentgenol 1999;173:1379–1382

Connell D, Burke F, Coombes P, et al. Sonographic examination of lateral epicondylitis. Am J Roentgenol 2001;176:777–782

Coel M, Yamada CY. Ko J. MR imaging of patients with lateral epicondylitis of the elbow (tennis elbow): importance of increased signal of the anconeus muscle. Am J Roentgenol 1993;161:1019–1021

Martin CE. Schweitzer ME. MR imaging of epicondylitis. Skeletal Radiol 1998;27:133–138

Potter HG, Hannafin JA, Morwessel RM, DiCarlo EF, O'Brien SJ, Altchek DW. Lateral epicondylitis: correlation of MR imaging, surgical, and histopathologic findings. Radiology 1995;196:43–46

CASE 20

Anthony G. Ryan, Peter L. Munk, and Laurel O. Marchinkow

Clinical Presentation

A 35-year-old male amateur bodybuilder presented with sudden pain in front of his elbow and a marked loss of power on elbow flexion. He claimed to have heard a pop and felt a tearing sensation while performing fast repeated biceps curls.

On examination, there was obvious subcutaneous bruising and a visible mass just cephalad to the elbow joint that was accentuated on active flexion of the joint. The mass was tender, and elbow flexion against resistance was very painful.

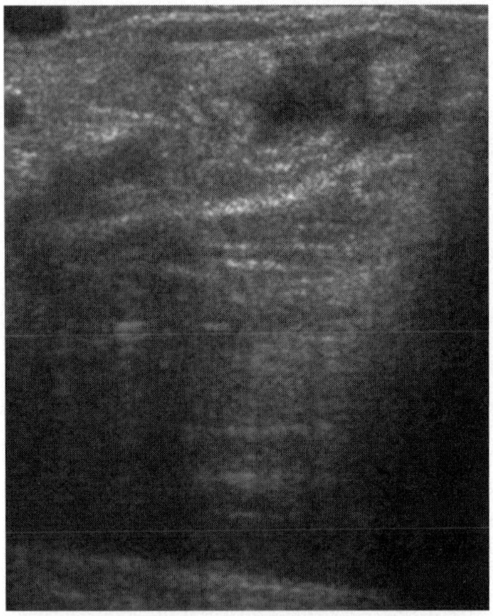

Figure 20A

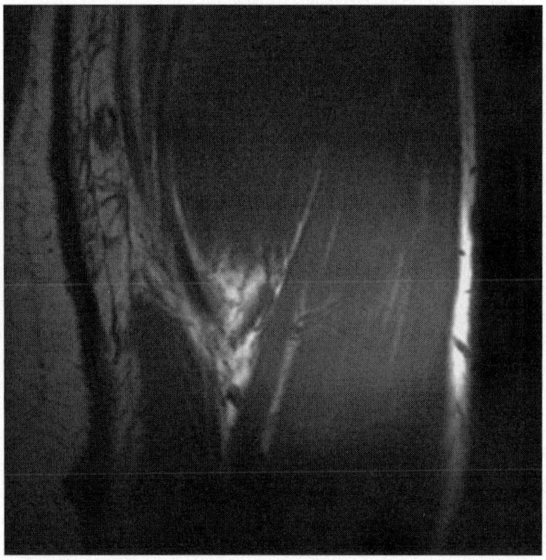

Figure 20B

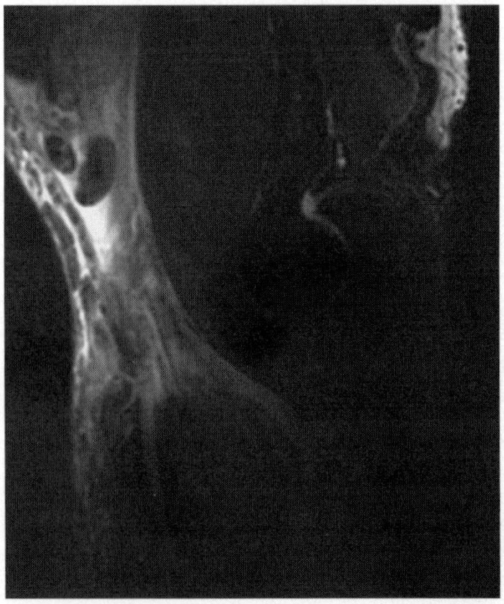

Figure 20C

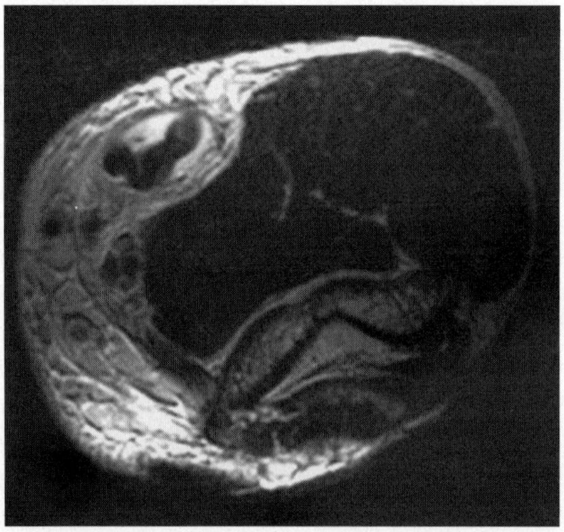

Figure 20D

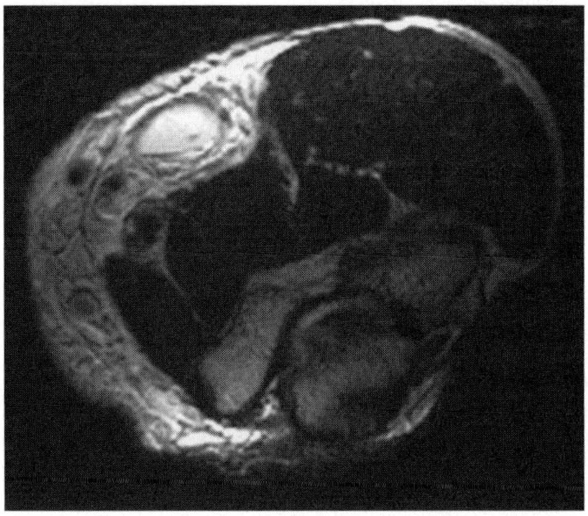

Figure 20E

Radiologic Findings

Sagittal linear ultrasound (**Fig. 20A**) of the painful lump mass demonstrates an irregular heterogeneous lesion consisting of multiple round/oval hyperechoic foci and a wavy, discontinuous fibrillar structure surrounded by anechoic material.

A coronal T2-weighted image (**Fig. 20B**) shows marked high signal intensity and loss of definition in the expected position of the distal biceps tendon. The high signal intensity extends cephalad into the body of the biceps muscle. Discontinuous low signal intensity bands are visible within the heterogenous high signal. A sagittal T2-weighted fat-saturated image (**Fig. 20C**) at the same level shows two heterogeneous round/oval predominantly low signal intensity structures at the cephalad extent of a poorly marginated high signal intensity area. An axial T2-weighted image (**Fig. 20D**) at the level of the low signal intensity structures shows a wavy, nodular structure surrounded by high signal intensity that appears confined within an ovoid space configuration. An axial T2-weighted image (**Fig. 20E**) caudad to **Fig. 20D** shows the same ovoid space to be empty.

Diagnosis

Biceps tendon rupture.

The ovoid high signal intensity collection is the empty tendon sheath at the level of the completely torn tendon. The wavy/nodular structures are the free ends of the tendon, retracted superiorly with muscle spasm and contraction.

Differential Diagnosis

None—the appearances are pathognomonic.

Discussion

Background

The long head of the biceps takes its origin from the supraglenoid tuberosity and inserts on the radial tuberosity, fanning out to form the bicipital aponeurosis attaching to the fascia of the forearm. It acts as a flexor of both the arm and the forearm. The two heads of the biceps join to form a common muscle belly, ending in a flattened, horizontally oriented distal tendon, typically measuring 7 cm in length. The distal biceps ruptures the dominant arm in 80% of cases and usually occurs in men.

Etiology

If no predisposing cause is identifiable, the typical age of rupture is 55. However, in bodybuilders or weight lifters, the injury occurs at a younger age, with abuse of anabolic steroids being a predisposing factor.

In common with injuries at other tendon sites, tears usually occur secondary to acute trauma or overuse injury in athletes or, in the elderly and unconditioned, degenerative tendinopathy.

Pathophysiology

The distal biceps tendon is covered by an extrasynovial paratenon, and the tendon is separated from the radial tuberosity by the radiobicipital bursa.

Bursitis may accompany tendinosis and bicipital tear, the bursa enlarging as much as 5 cm when inflamed.

The blood supply to the distal tendon is relatively poor 1 cm proximal to its insertion. This area, in addition, is prone to impingement between the radius and the ulna during pronation.

The degenerated tendon is liable to become thickened, enlarged, and irregular with inflammation of the adjacent bursa. These factors will make further contributions to impingement likely, leading to further degeneration of the tendon. Bicipital tendinosis is relatively common (**Figs. 20F,20G**) and usually precedes tendon rupture. Almost 50% of patients on direct questioning give a history of chronic and recurrent “ache” before the tear actually occurs.

Clinical Findings

There may or may not be a history of trauma with

- Pain in the front of the elbow
- A marked loss of power in elbow flexion and arm supination
- Infrequently, a reported audible “pop”
- A tearing sensation

The results on examination will be the following:

- Obvious subcutaneous bruising
- Palpable and/or visible antecubital mass that becomes more conspicuous on active flexion of the joint
- The mass is tender, and elbow flexion against resistance is very painful.
- If no discrete mass is present, there is diffuse tenderness in the antecubital fossa.
- There may be visible proximal retraction of the biceps muscle bulk with elbow flexion.
- Weakening of elbow flexion and supination
- Partial tears do not declare themselves as obviously as acute complete ruptures, usually occurring on a background of degeneration. Clinically, patients show little functional deficit, and very few provide a history of trauma or a sudden onset.

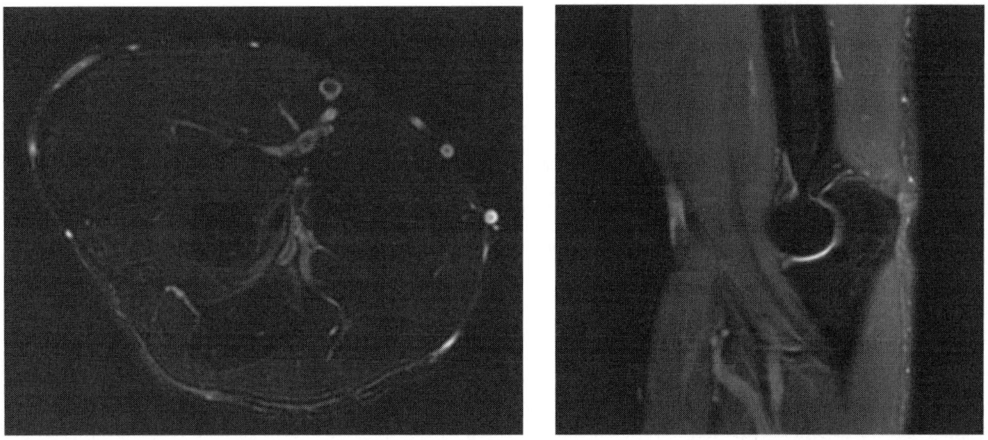

F G

Figures 20F and **20G** Transaxial (**20F**) and sagittal (**20G**) T2 fat-saturated images show intrasubstance high signal intensity and loss of definition of the biceps tendon just proximal to its insertion with surrounding high signal intensity, consistent with tendinosis, peritendinitis, and edema within the adjacent muscle.

Stages of Disease

Patterns of injury include

- Complete rupture of the tendon from its insertion
- Complete tear of the tendon
- Partial tear

Complications

- If untreated, the muscle belly and tendon will retract proximally, making subsequent attempts at repair more difficult and less successful.
- Loss of power of elbow flexion and forearm supination

Imaging Findings

RADIOGRAPHY

- The radial tuberosity may be irregular and hypertrophic (**Fig. 20H**).
- Chronic inflammation of the adjacent radiobicipital bursa (separating the tendon from the underlying proximal radius) may be evident.

ULTRASOUND

- Ruptured tendon (**Figs. 20A** and **20I**)
- Partial tears

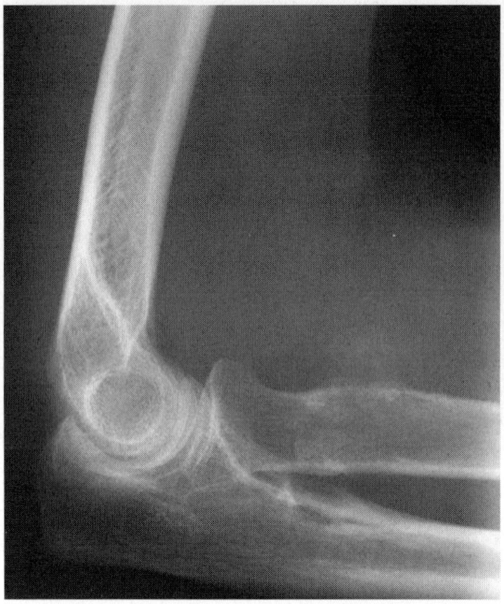

Figure 20H Radiograph of the elbow shows a very prominent, hypertrophied radial tuberosity, secondary to prior biceps tendon avulsion and subsequent healing.

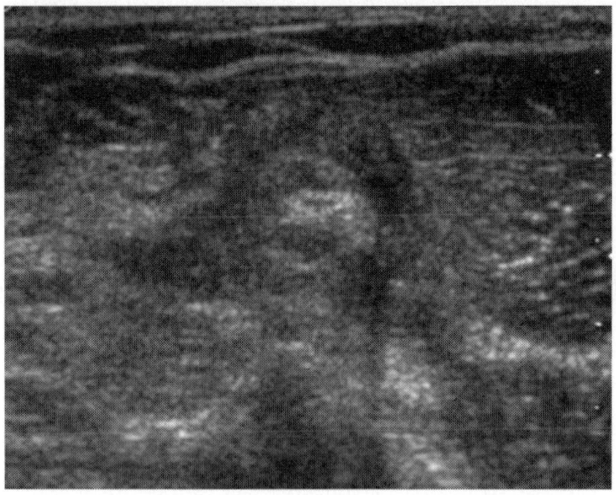

Figure 20I Axial ultrasound image of the distal biceps tendon shows thickening and heterogeneity; the hypoechoic clefts represent partial tears. Hypoechoic fluid is seen within the tendon sheath.

- Tenosynovitis
- Cubital bursitis: fusiform anechoic or hypoechoic lesion

COMPUTED TOMOGRAPHY

CT demonstrates the bony changes to best effect, but occasionally it can demonstrate tendon pathology:

- Radial tuberosity hypertrophy
- Radial tuberosity irregularity
- Radial tuberosity avulsion (**Fig. 20J**)
- Tendon swelling and fluid within the tendon sheath (**Fig. 20K**)

MAGNETIC RESONANCE IMAGING

Complete ruptures

- Absence of the tendon distally (100%)
- Fluid-filled tendon sheath (90%)
- Small fluid collections at the site of a tear at the insertion of the tendon onto the radial tuberosity
- Antecubital fossa mass (30%)

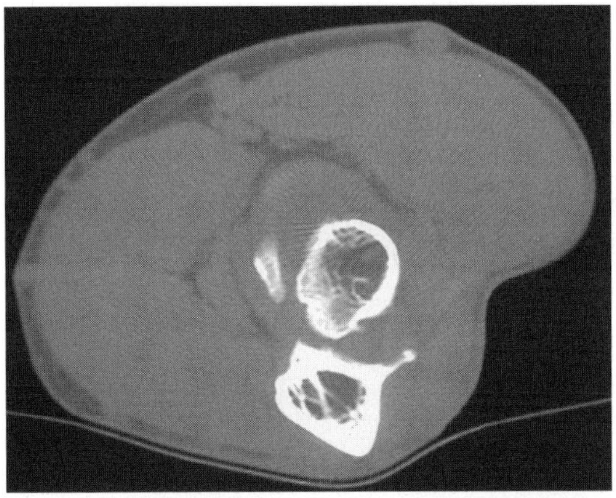

Figure 20J Transaxial CT (bone windows) of the elbow showing avulsion of the radial tuberosity.

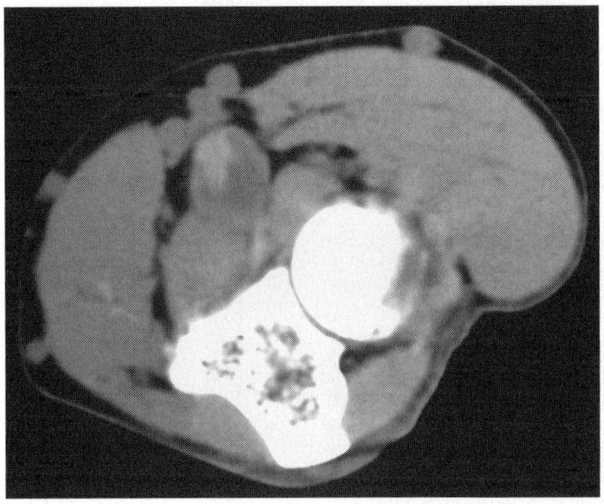

Figure 20K Transaxial CT (soft-tissue windows) of the elbow at the level of the radial head shows the relatively high-density retracted end of the avulsed tendon and surrounding low-density fluid within the distal tendon sheath.

- Muscle edema (30%)
- Muscle atrophy (20%)
- On MRI, the fluid-filled gap between the avulsed tendon and the tuberosity is usually best seen on sagittal images (**Fig. 20C**).

Partial biceps tendon tears

- High tendon intrasubstance signal intensity (100%) (**Fig. 20L**)
- Fluid in the biceps tendon sheath (60%) (**Fig. 20M**)
- Bicipitoradial bursitis and bony microavulsive injury of the radial tuberosity may be seen in as many as 50 to 55% of cases of partial tear. The bicipitoradial bursa has a smooth outline and a wide base along the superficial aspect of the radius and may completely surround the biceps tendon with or without internal septations (**Figs. 20N,20O**).
- Thinning (30%) of the distal tendon
- Thickening (30%) of the distal tendon (**Fig. 20L**)
- T1-weighted transaxial images are especially useful for determining the degree of tendon rupture and evaluation of the bicipital aponeurosis.
- Intravenous gadolinium typically demonstrates peripheral rim enhancement, permitting differentiation from a solid neoplasm.

Acute tendinitis

- Tendon enlargement
- Fluid in the synovial sheath when there is accompanying tenosynovitis and abnormal intrasubstance signal (degeneration or partial tear)

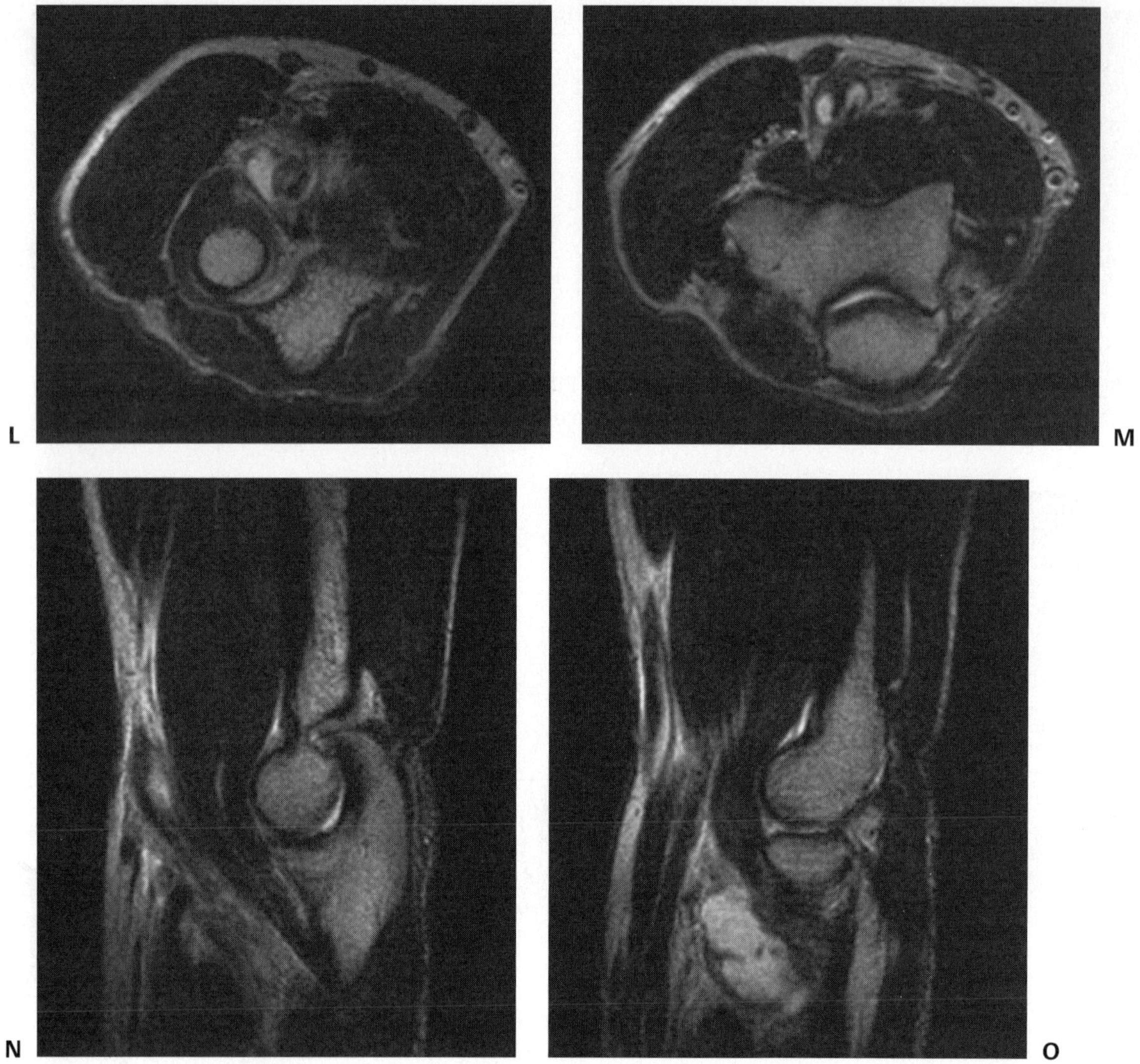

Figures 20L to **20O** T2-weighted images of the elbow. **20L** A transaxial T2-weighted image shows thickening of the distal tendon, heterogeneous intrasubstance high signal, and fluid in the tendon sheath. **20M** demonstrates the tendon at a more cephalad level to have a longitudinal split type injury. **20N** A sagittal T2-weighted image shows the intrasubstance high signal, loss of definition of the posterior margin, and fluid within the bicipitocubital bursa. **20O** A sagittal T2-weighted image at the level of the radial head of the same patient as in **20L** through **20N** shows heterogeneous intrasubstance high signal intensity loss of definition of the anterior margin and a partially septated fluid collection almost completely surrounding the tendon, consistent with bicipitocubital bursitis.

Chronic tendinitis

- The tendon may be thinned or thickened.

Rupture mimics

- Tendinosis
- Tenosynovitis
- Biceps hematoma
- Brachialis contusion, brachialis rupture
- Ganglion
- Antecubital bursitis
- Thinning of the tendon and fluid within the tendon sheath

Treatment

- Rupture requires surgical repair and reattachment to the radial tuberosity.
- Reattachment of the avulsed tuberosity if present
- Early reattachment is stressed because, if diagnosis is delayed, the tendon will retract, with resultant functional disability.

Prognosis

- If complete tears are repaired acutely, a good functional result is expected.
- If untreated, the tendon will proceed to retract, with resultant functional disability.

PEARLS

- To differentiate a partial or complete tear from mucoid degeneration, high signal on T1 will decrease on T2 imaging.
- The tendon will not retract significantly unless there is a concomitant tear of the bicipital aponeurosis; lack of retraction does not exclude a complete tear of the tendon proper. This can give rise to a false-negative clinical exam.
- Although elbow flexion may be maintained if the bicipital aponeurosis is not torn, supination of the forearm will be at least weakened if the tendon is ruptured.

PITFALLS

- The bicipitoradial bursa and interosseous bursae, which lie at the distal biceps tendon insertion on the radial tuberosity, may uncommonly become inflamed, giving rise to cubital bursitis, which presents as a large, painful, tender antecubital swelling.
- Loss of function is more dramatic with tendon tear. The history tends to be more acute with tear and more chronic with bursitis.
- Ultrasound is the investigation of choice if cubital bursitis is suspected and may facilitate treatment by decompression and injection of steroids. Ultrasound may also be useful in the identification of an elbow joint ganglion, another clinical mimic of distal biceps tendon pathology.

Suggested Readings

Falchook FS, Zlatkin MB, Erbacher GE, Moulton JS, Bisset GS, Murphy BJ. Rupture of the distal biceps tendon: evaluation with MR imaging. Radiology 1994;190:659–663

Logan PM, Janzen DL, Connell DG. Tear of the distal biceps tendon presenting as an antecubital mass: magnetic resonance imaging appearances. Can Assoc Radiol J 1996;47:342–346

Williams BD, Schweitzer ME, Weishaupt D, et al. Partial tears of the distal biceps tendon: MR appearance and associated clinical findings. Skeletal Radiol 2001;30:560–564

CASE 21

Anthony G. Ryan and Peter L. Munk

Clinical Presentation

A 41-year-old man heard a snapping sound in his ankle while stretching for a lob shot during a tennis game. He developed an immediate painful limp with reduced plantar flexion. Squeezing his calf musculature while in the prone position (the Thompson test) did not produce the expected plantar flexion. Direct questioning revealed a long history of intermittent pain and discomfort at the back of his ankle.

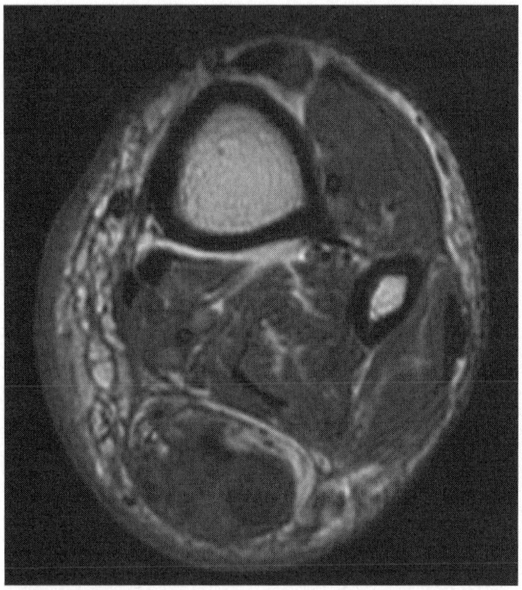

Figure 21A

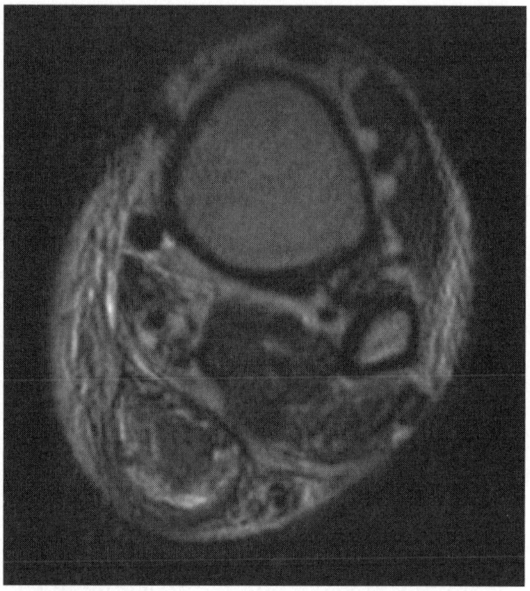

Figure 21B

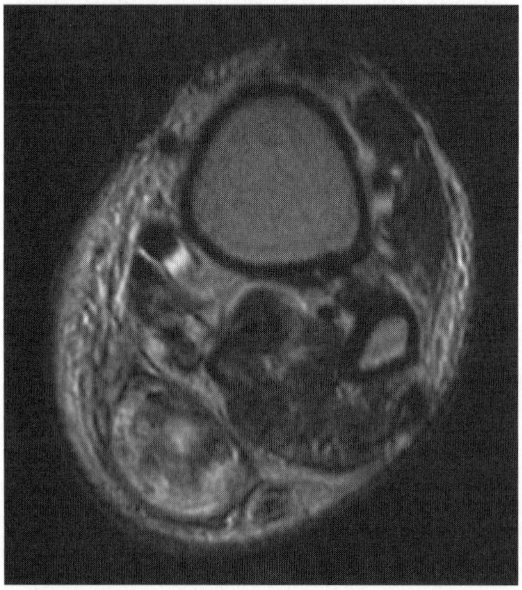

Figure 21C

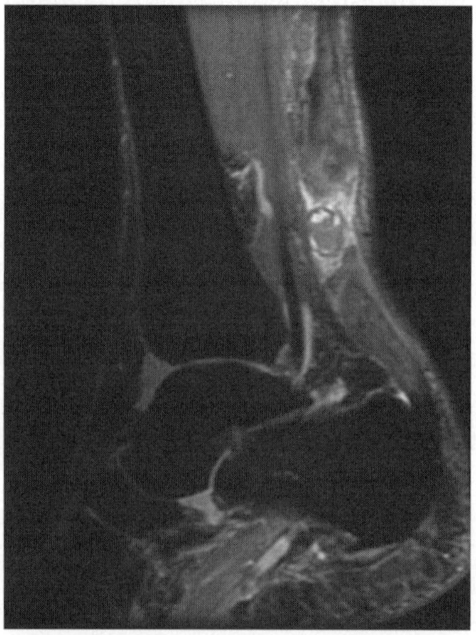

Figure 21D

Radiologic Findings

An axial T1-weighted image (**Fig. 21A**) shows dramatic thickening of the Achilles' tendon close to its calcaneal insertion. There is heterogeneous intratendinous signal consistent with internal architectural disorganization. An axial T2-weighted image (**Fig. 21B**) shows heterogeneous intrasubstance signal, again consistent with internal architectural disorganization. High signal intensity material is shown surrounding the tendon consistent with either edema or hemorrhage. An axial T2-weighted image (**Fig. 21C**), adjacent to **Fig. 21B**, shows heterogeneous, high signal intensity contained within the paratenon with no definite tendon identified: the "absent tendon" sign. A sagittal STIR (**Fig. 21D**) shows a complete tear of the tendon with laxity of each torn end, intervening high signal intensity consistent with edema and/or hemorrhage. The tendon on either side of the tear is markedly abnormal, being thickened with heterogeneous internal signal consistent with chronic tendinosis ± chronic partial tear.

Diagnosis

Torn Achilles' tendon on a background of chronic tendinitis.

Differential Diagnosis

None—the appearance is pathognomonic.

Discussion

Background

Although the Achilles' is the thickest and strongest tendon in the body, it is also the most frequently injured. Formed by the coalescence of the gastrocnemius and soleus, the tendon measures approximately 10 to 15 cm in length and has an anteroposterior (AP) diameter of 7 mm or less in men and less than 6 mm in women. In cross section, the anterior border of the tendon should be concave and parallel the posterior border, except immediately above the calcaneal insertion, where it becomes elliptiform.

The tendon is surrounded by a thin film of connective tissue, the paratenon, which, in addition to lubricating the tendon's motion, serves as a source of auxiliary blood supply. Despite this, the supply to the Achilles' tendon remains relatively deficient between 2 to 6 cm proximal to its calcaneal insertion, resulting in a zone of vulnerability.

There is a fat pad anterior to the tendon, eponymously known as Kager's fat pad.

There are two bursae in relation to the tendon: a retrocalcaneal bursa, anterior to the tendon at the level of the insertion, and a retrotendo-Achilles' bursa, which is an acquired bursa between the tendon and skin at the level of the insertion.

Etiology

This condition is typically secondary either to acute trauma, including severe strain and penetrating injuries, or to overuse in athletes or the elderly (degenerative tendinopathy). Male long-distance runners are particularly susceptible.

Pathophysiology

Rupture may be spontaneous or secondary to acute trauma (sudden excess tensile force or laceration) or chronic trauma (overuse resulting in repeated microtrauma), leading, over time, to degenerative tendinosis. The coalescence of foci of mucoid degeneration can lead to interstitial tears, gross partial tears, and eventually complete rupture.

Spontaneous ruptures occur in those patients with underlying systemic illnesses predisposing to tendinopathy:

- Inflammatory arthropathies (rheumatoid arthritis, gout)
- Collagen vascular disorders
- Crystal deposition diseases
- Hyperlipidemia
- Hyperparathyroidism
- Drugs (steroids, fluoroquinolones)
- Long-term dialysis
- Infectious etiologies such as gonorrhea

It has been calculated that stretching a tendon to between 4 and 8% of its original length causes irreversible disruption of the collagen cross-link structures. This is potentially reparable, unless the inciting activity is continued.

Clinical Findings

- Occurs in unconditioned athletes, mean age 36, usually male
- Sudden posterior heel pain and variable inability to plantar flex, typically following a push-off or rapid directional change with a planted foot
- Sudden snapping associated with pain, swelling, and inability to stand on toes
- On examination, the Thompson test may be false-negative in up to 25% of partial tears.
- It may not be possible to palpate the gap between the torn fibers, as the acute swelling and tissue induration that accompany a tear can mimic the tendon in its expected location.
- Isolated tendinosis in the absence of a tear typically causes pain and consequent limitation of participation in the inciting sport, while often having very little effect on day-to-day activities.

Stages of Disease

- *Type I* Inflammatory reaction
- *Type II* Degenerative changes
- *Type III* Partial rupture
- *Type IV* Complete rupture

Complications

- Painful plantar flexion
- Varying degrees of loss of plantar flexion

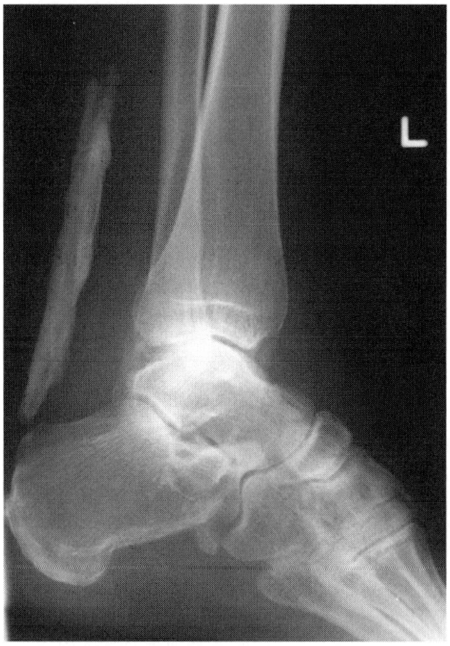

Figure 21E A lateral radiograph shows ossification along the length of the tendon in association with a chronic partial tear.

- Limp
- Ankle, knee, and, consequently, hip osteoarthrosis if untreated

Pathology

GROSS

Studied tendons are swollen, with varying degrees of replacement by degenerative and scar tissue.

MICROSCOPIC

Foci of mucoid degeneration can become coalescent, leading to interstitial tears, gross partial tears, and eventually complete rupture.

Imaging Findings

RADIOGRAPHY

- Tendon swelling
- Loss of definition and increase of radiodensity in Kager's fat pad
- Bursitis of the retrocalcaneal and pre-Achilles' bursae, producing soft-tissue swelling anterior and posterior to the tendon at the level of insertion
- A defect may be evident if the tear is complete and there is retraction of the torn ends.
- Chronic tears may exhibit calcification and occasionally ossification (**Fig. 21E**).

ULTRASOUND

The patient is scanned prone with the feet hanging over the table edge, facilitating comparison with the other side. Scanning while having the patient attempt to plantar flex frequently yields findings not evident on static scanning alone.

Rupture

- Partial or complete interruption of echogenic fibers
- Clefts filled with anechoic/hypoechoic material representing blood or edematous fluid

- The balled-up retracted ends of the tendon should be seen acutely, but their conspicuity fades with time. This retraction is often more evident on dynamic scanning.
- Artifactual acoustic shadowing at the torn tendon edges helps to define the margins of the tear.
- Minimal surrounding hematoma
- The echogenicity of Kager's fat pad is increased as a result of the tendon's absence, reducing the amount of overlying normal attenuation.
- If there is a significant amount of fluid, through transmission is enhanced.

Tendinitis/partial tear

- There is considerable overlap between the findings of tendinitis and partial tear, particularly if the latter is chronic.
- Tendinitis may be diagnosed if the longitudinal fibers are pushed apart by interfibrillar echo-poor fluid. When compared with the other side, a 2-mm disparity in the AP diameter is considered diagnostic.
- Loss of definition and loss of the anterior concavity of the tendon on transverse section
- The loose hypoechoic areolar connective tissue of the paratenon may become visible.
- Increased echogenicity of Kager's fat pad
- Fibromyxoid change is hypoechoic.

Chronic rupture

- Thickened tendon with possibly normal echogenicity or with hyperechoic foci corresponding to calcifications may be seen in either the tendon itself or the surrounding fat.

Subacute tendinitis

- Thickened tendon with reduced echogenicity

MAGNETIC RESONANCE IMAGING

- Normal tendons should be uniformly hypointense on all sequences.
- The Achilles' tendon should have a concave or flat anterior border and a convex posterior border, except just above the insertion, where it assumes an elliptiform shape.
- Maximal normal AP thickness is 7 mm.

Complete tear

- Fiber discontinuity with intervening high signal on T2 and intermediate on T1, typically 2 to 6 cm proximal to the calcaneal insertion
- Fraying ± retraction of the torn ends may be evident.
- If a complete tear is diagnosed remote to the initial injury, the ends are likely to have retracted and fatty atrophy of the muscle bellies of the soleus and gastrocnemius.

Partial tear

- Some mild partial tears are seen as linear high signal on T2 parallel to the long axis of the tendon. Residual continuous tendon fibers should be visible.
- More extensive partial tears have heterogeneous signal intensity, reflecting intratendinous hemorrhage, and diffuse thickening of the tendon. They may be associated with subcutaneous edema and hemorrhage within Kager's fat pad.
- Both healed tears and chronic tendinopathy produce circumferentially thickened fusiform tendons.

Chronic rupture

- Scar or fat may replace the tendon.
- Eventually, although thickened, no abnormal intrasubstance signal abnormality is evident.

Acute tendinitis

- Enlargement > 6 mm in AP.
- Loss of anterior concavity, with a resulting flat or convex anterior margin
- Foci of intrasubstance increased signal intensity

Chronic tendinosis

- The tendon may be thinned or thickened.
- Fusiform thickening is best seen sagittally (**Fig. 21F**).
- Minimal or no hyperintensity on T2-weighted images (**Figs. 21G,21H**)

Achilles' peritendinitis

Tendon sheath fluid, typically seen in association with acute tenosynovitis, is not seen in the Achilles' tendon, as there is no tendon sheath (in common with the patellar tendon). The Achilles' tendon has a paratenon, however, a loose connective tissue covering, although closely applied to the tendon surface, reduces friction between the tendon and its surroundings, allowing up to 1.5 cm of gliding.

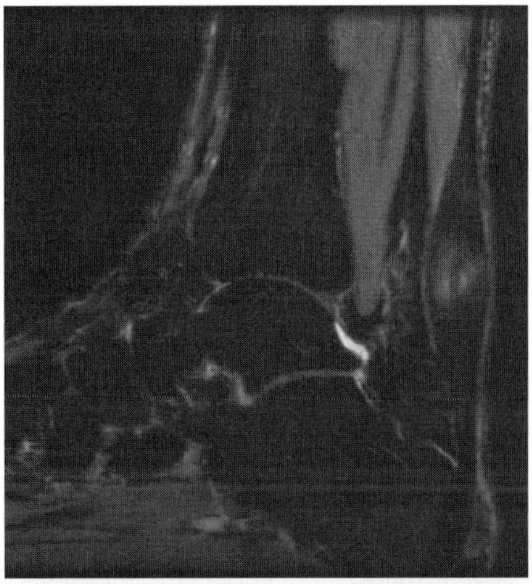

F

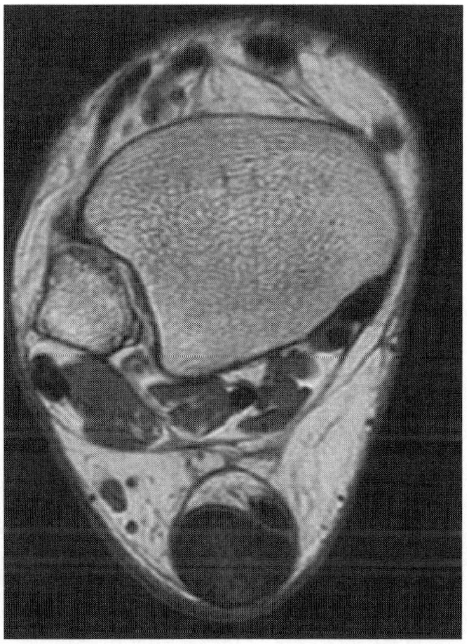

G

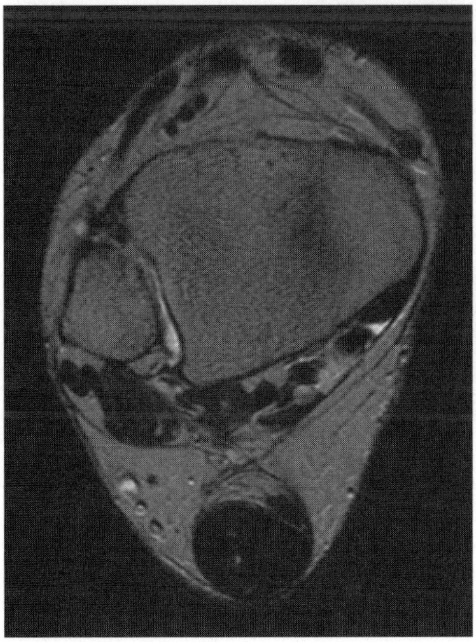

H

Figures 21F A sagittal STIR image shows fusiform thickening of the tendon and focal intermediate signal intensity (less than the fluid seen posterior to the talus) with fuzzy margins consistent with intrasubstance mucoid degeneration and a chronic partial tear. Note the characteristic location of the high signal, that is, 5 to 6 cm above the insertion. **21G** and **21H** The same case as in **21F**, chronic partial tear on T1 (**21G**) and T2 (**21H**). Massive thickening of the tendon shows subtle intrasubstance heterogeneity, but with no increased intrasubstance signal on the corresponding T2 images.

The Achilles' tendon may thus experience peritendinitis but not tenosynovitis.

- Linear, reticular areas of altered signal intensity in the Kager's fat pad are seen, representative of edema.
- If chronic irritation is present, the paratenon may become thickened by successive layering of fibrin, which is subsequently low signal on all sequences.
- Because the dark, thickened paratenon will have the same signal intensity as the underlying tendon, the two cannot be distinguished, so the MRI will simply show a markedly thickened tendon.

POSTOPERATIVE IMAGING

- Evaluate the extent of tendinous union and healing.
- Intratendinous high signal is expected to resolve with successive studies.
- Chronic tendinosis will result in chronic thickening but will be replaced by scar tissue/fatty degeneration.

Normal variants include the following:

- Plantaris tendon, seen in 90% of cases, courses medial to the Achilles' tendon and inserts into the posterior calcaneus or the Achilles' tendon itself. Deep to Kager's fat pad is the flexor hallucis longus muscle.
- The accessory soleus muscle (**Figs. 21I** and **21J**) lies posteromedially, posterior to the distal tibia, and may fill most of Kager's triangle; it is sometimes misinterpreted as a space-occupying lesion. The appearance of the muscle fibers in the supracalcaneal region should make the diagnosis.

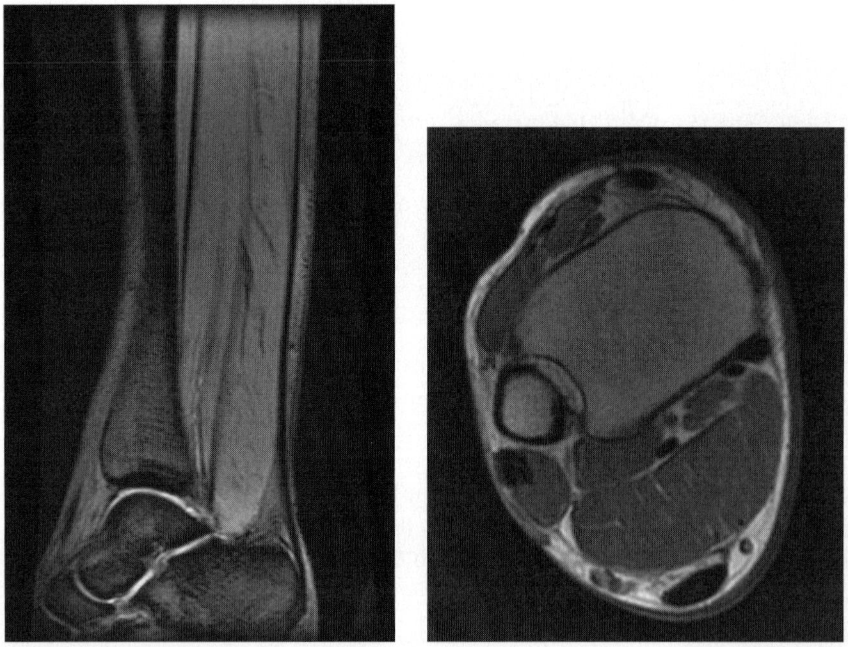

I J

Figures 21I and **21J** Accessory soleus muscle. A sagittal T2 image (**21I**) shows a bulky longitudinal structure anterior to the Achilles' tendon, seen on axial T2 image (**21J**) to have a typically muscular fascicular internal structure and to be of the same signal intensity as adjacent muscles. Interposed between the Achilles' tendon posteriorly and the flexor hallucis longus anteriorly, this is typical of an accessory soleus muscle.

- Haglund's syndrome: Frequently seen thickening of the distal tendon, representing chronic irritation secondary to prominent heel cups as found in hockey skates, golf shoes, and high-heeled shoes (when it is described as a "pump bump")

Treatment

- If the tear is complete or more than 50% of the fiber is torn, surgical repair is indicated.
- Surgical repair is mandated in tears secondary to penetrating injuries.
- For partial tears, use a cast with the ankle in marked plantar flexion (the equinus position) for 3 months.
- Ultrasound-guided steroid injection of the paratenon may be beneficial in peritendinitis.

Prognosis

- The degree of separation of the torn ends can be assessed at MRI; if significant retraction has occurred acutely, surgery is recommended, with an expected return to normal levels of activity.
- If a tear goes undetected, retraction and consequent atrophy of the soleus and gastrocnemius muscles make surgical repair difficult, sometimes requiring tendon transfer.

PEARLS

- On ultrasound examination, a fusiform configuration of the distal tendon should prompt a careful search for a more proximal site of the tear before making a diagnosis of uncomplicated tendinitis.
- Artifactual acoustic shadowing at the torn tendon edges helps to define the margins of the tear.
- The anterior border should be concave and parallel to the posterior border.

PITFALLS

- On ultrasound, anisotrophy may induce echo-poor foci within the tendon, which may be mistaken for a partial tear. This is avoided by ensuring the incident beam is perpendicular to the tendon. Scanning in the orthogonal plane should make any anisotrophic artifact disappear.
- Scan tendon under tension, as bow stringing may be misinterpreted as tendinitis.
- The magic angle phenomenon, more prominent on short TE (0 to 40 msec) spin-echo and gradient sequences, can produce artifactual intrasubstance high signal if the tendon is oriented at ~55 degrees to the main magnetic field.
- Clinically, it may not be possible to palpate the gap between the torn fibers, as the acute swelling and tissue induration that accompany a tear can mimic the tendon in its usual location.
- If chronic irritation is present, the paratenon may become thickened by successive layering of fibrin, which is subsequently low signal on all sequences. Because the dark, thickened paratenon will be the same signal intensity of the underlying tendon, the two cannot be distinguished, so the MRI will simply show a markedly thickened tendon.

Suggested Readings

Fessell DP, van Holsbeeck MT. Foot and ankle sonography. Radiol Clin North Am 1999;37:831–858

Harcke HT, Grissom LE, Finkelstein MS. Evaluation of the musculoskeletal system with sonography. Am J Roentgenol 1988;150:1253–1261

Jacobson JA. Musculoskeletal sonography and MR imaging: a role for both imaging methods. Radiol Clin North Am 1999;37:713–735

Schweitzer ME, Karasick D. MR imaging of disorders of the Achilles tendon. Am J Roentgenol 2000;175:613–625

Weinstali R, Stiskal ZM, Neuhold A, Aamlid B, Hertz H. Classifying calcaneal tendon injury according to MRI findings. J Bone Joint Surg [Br] 1991;73:683–685

CASE 22

Anthony G. Ryan and Peter L. Munk

Clinical Presentation

A middle-aged diabetic woman presented with pain and swelling on the medial aspect of her ankle and progressive flatfoot.

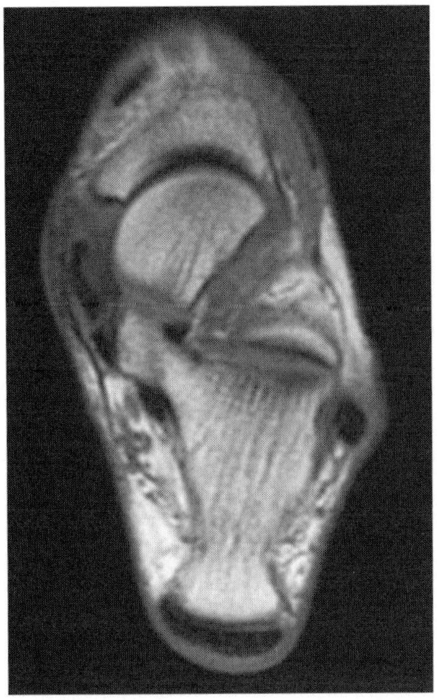

Figure 22A

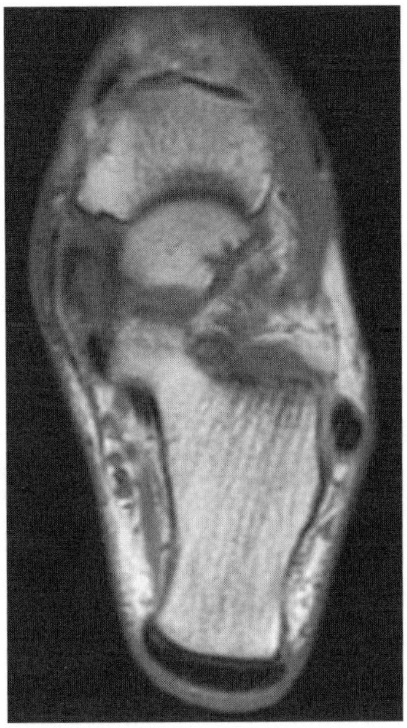

Figure 22B

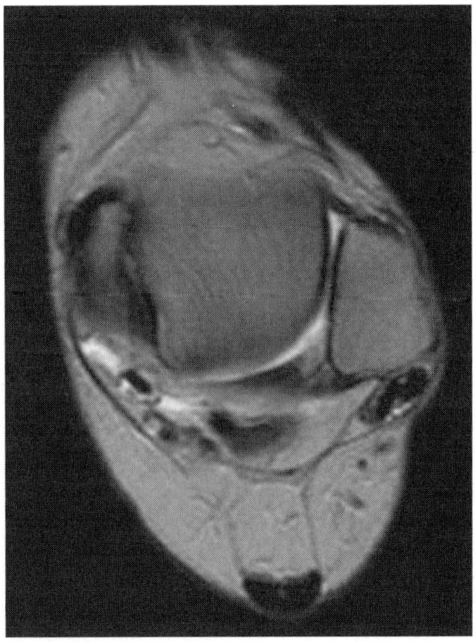

Figure 22C

Radiologic Findings

An axial T1-weighted image (**Fig. 22A)** shows internal signal heterogeneity within the tibialis posterior tendon and intermediate signal intensity material surrounding the tendon within the tendon sheath. There is focal tendon discontinuity evident medially. Low signal intensity is visible within the overlying subcutaneous fat.

An axial T1-weighted image (**Fig. 22B**) more caudad **Fig. 22A** shows the same findings with more extensive tendon disruption visible medially, the intermediate signal intensity within the tendon occupying ~80% of its cross-sectional diameter.

An axial T2-weighted image (**Fig. 22C**) at a level more cephalad **Figs. 22A,22B** shows the "empty sheath" sign, in which no tendon is visible within the tibialis posterior tendon sheath, seen anteromedial to the normal tendon of the flexor digitorum.

Diagnosis

Torn tibialis posterior tendon

Differential Diagnosis

None.

Discussion

Background

The tibialis posterior muscle takes its origin from the posterior surface of the intraosseous membrane, the posterior shaft of the tibia, and the upper shaft of the fibula. Its tendon inserts onto the navicular tuberosity with additional slips to the sustentaculum tali, the cuneiforms, the cuboid bone, and the bases of the second, third, and fourth metatarsals.

The tibialis posterior tendon runs in a groove behind the medial malleolus deep to the flexor retinaculum and anterior to the tendon of the flexor digitorum longus. The tendon lies superficial to the deltoid ligament and deep to the calcaneonavicular ligament.

Its main actions are plantar flexion, adduction, and inversion of the foot, while also serving as a plantar arch support.

Etiology

Posterior tibial tendinitis and rupture are common occurrences in association with rheumatoid arthritis. Women in their fifth or sixth decades, especially if diabetic, are most at risk.

Other clinical associations include

- Hypertension
- Obesity
- Diabetes
- Inflammatory arthropathies: rheumatoid arthritis, ankylosing spondylosis, Reiter's syndrome, and psoriasis
- Increasing age
- In the younger age group, it is typically athletes who injure the tendon secondary to sports such as basketball where standing/springing off one's toes puts tibialis posterior tendon under significant strain. Track athletes may also injure the tendon as a result of running on a chamfered surface (e.g., a sloping track), whereby the foot is continuously everted while running.

Pathophysiology

The most commonly torn of the flexor tendons, the tibialis posterior is the second-most commonly torn ankle tendon after the Achilles' tendon. The loss of the tibialis posterior tendon itself leads to minimal loss of plantar flexion; however, its loss as an arch support leads to a cascade of hindfoot dysfunction.

Acute complete tibial tendon rupture leads to an acute flatfoot. If a partial tear goes untreated, over time it is likely to result in a progressive flatfoot. Longitudinal arch collapse produces secondary heel valgus. Hindfoot valgus collapses the sinus tarsi, which, in turn, is a further source of chronic hindfoot pain.

Conversely, if there are problems in the arch or plantar fascia, this can adversely affect the posterior tibial tendon, leading to tendinitis and/or rupture.

If an acute tibialis posterior tendon injury is severe, injury to the spring ligament is a frequent accompanying feature. In the case of a chronic partial tear, excess strain is placed on the spring ligament over time, which may thus become attenuated.

Clinical Findings

The typical patient is a middle-aged diabetic woman presenting with medial hindfoot pain, swelling, and progressive loss of function secondary to acquired flatfoot, including difficulty standing on "tiptoes."

If an acute injury occurs, pain with an accompanying tender swelling on the medial aspect of the foot is the typical presentation, with reduced adduction that is painful against resistance.

In assessing a patient's ability to stand on his or her toes, the heel of a patient with an intact posterior tibial tendon will rotate inward; if the tendon is torn, the heel will not rotate inward and may in fact turn out.

If a tear has been progressive or present for some time, hindfoot valgus, midfoot abduction at the midtarsal joints, and forefoot pronation may all be evident. Pain on the lateral aspect of the foot may become superimposed.

Rarely, the tibialis posterior tendon may be involved in fractures of the medial malleolus.

Stages of Disease

The staging is based on a combination of clinical and MRI findings:

Stage 1 Medial pain and edema; normal MRI

Stage 2 Increasing pain; "too many toes" sign (this is present when the examining physician sees "too many toes" when looking at the patient from behind; that is, the foot is pointing more laterally than normal); the deformity is reducible; partial tears evident on MRI

Stage 3 Fixed hindfoot deformity; complete tear on MRI

Stage 4 End-stage; pes planus; degenerative joint disease on MRI

Complications

The loss of normal tendon function results in

- Acute or progressive flatfoot
- Hindfoot valgus
- Mid/forefoot abduction
- Lateral navicular subluxation
- Forefoot pronation
- Sinus tarsi collapse
- Reactive tibial periostitis
- Spring ligament injury/strain (acute or chronic secondary to excess strain)
- Tendon subluxation
- Tendon tenosynovitis

All of the above may lead eventually to rigid flatfoot and hindfoot arthritis.

Imaging Findings

RADIOGRAPHY

- Erect anteroposterior (AP) and lateral views of the feet, supplemented with AP views of the ankles (to evaluate valgus tilt), are standard if tibialis posterior tendon dysfunction is suspected.

- In the presence of an acute tear, radiographs are typically normal, as acute flatfoot is rarely evident secondary to spasm. If there is a complete tear, the unopposed pull of the peroneus brevis eventually overcomes the spasm, resulting in forefoot abduction and lateral navicular subluxation. This may be measured by assessing the degree of uncovering of the talar head (normally 95% covered by the navicular).
- Differentiating calcification secondary to chronic tear from an os tibiale externum sesamoid within the tibialis posterior tendon should be straightforward, as the sesamoid is 2 to 6 mm, round, and well corticated.

Radiographs are expected to be abnormal in at least 50% of patients in the presence of a chronic tear, including one or more of the following:

- Progressive flatfoot
- Longitudinal arch collapse
- Secondary hindfoot/heel valgus
- Sinus tarsi collapse
- Decreased calcaneal plantar angle (50%)
- Increased lateral talometatarsal angle (47%)
- Increased anterior talocalcaneal angle (43%)
- Increased lateral talocalcaneal angle (13%)
- Uncovering of the talar head (which should be 95% covered by the navicular)
- Forefoot abduction

Associated abnormalities include

- Medial soft-tissue swelling (27%)
- Tarsal osteoarthritis (20%)
- Distal tibial proliferative changes (7%); "spurring" secondary to reactive periostitis adjacent to the tendon
- Osteoporosis (37%)

Evidence of predisposing factors may be seen:

- The presence of accessory navicular bones (17%), particularly a type 2 accessory (triangular or heart-shaped lying over the medial pole of the navicular to which it is connected by a cartilaginous bridge)
- A cornuate navicular; prominent medial pole
- Secondary findings suggestive of a predisposition to a tibialis posterior tendon tear, such as inflammatory arthropathy, may be evident.

ULTRASOUND

The normal tibialis posterior tendon should demonstrate homogeneous longitudinal echogenic fibers with no Doppler flow in or around the tendon.

Ultrasound findings of a tear include the following:

- Discontinuity of the normal fibrillar pattern is best appreciated sagitally.
- The synovial sheath may be intact despite the presence of a full-thickness tendon tear. The sheath is seen to collapse when the tendon retracts on dynamic scanning when the patient is asked to plantar flex the foot.

Ultrasound findings of tendinopathy include

- Increased AP diameter with consequent rounding of the tendon
- Tendon inhomogeneity
- Intratendinous flow on color Doppler sonography (seen in 35% of cases)

Ultrasound findings of peritendinosis include

- Flow on color Doppler sonography

COMPUTED TOMOGRAPHY

The sensitivity and specificity of CT in the detection of tibialis posterior tendon tears is high. Particularly with the advent of multidetector CT, there may be an increasing role for CT in the evaluation of the ankle tendons, given the increased spatial and improving soft-tissue contrast resolution.

CT is superior to MRI in showing associated bone abnormalities such as

- Acute fractures
- Periostitis
- Subtalar osteoarthritis
- Subtalar dislocation

MAGNETIC RESONANCE IMAGING

Normal

- The normal tendon should be elliptic on cross section and return low signal intensity on all sequences.
- The normal tendon flares and demonstrates increased signal intensity ~1 cm proximal to its navicular insertion secondary to the magic angle phenomenon.
- Minimal peritendinous enhancement and fluid may be seen in relation to the normal tibialis posterior tendon.

MRI staging of tears

- *Type 1* Partial tear, longitudinal splitting of the tendon resulting in a tendon 4 to 5 times thicker than normal with heterogeneous (high) signal intensity secondary to hemorrhage and, if chronic, fibrous tissue
- *Type 2* Partial tears, whereby the tendon is attenuated or atrophied, usually with concomitant enlargement of the remainder of the tendon. Signal intensity may be normal or increased.
- *Type 3* Complete tendon disruption and retraction with a gap filled by fat or fluid between the torn margins. Fatty atrophy of the muscle belly, if chronic, is seen.

Partial tears are seen in **Figs. 22D–22F**.

- Partial tears may be seen as clefts extending into the synovial surface of the tendon.
- Tendon retraction results in increased tendon girth. Tendons may appear bilobed in coronal or sagittal orientation as a result of attenuation secondary to a partial tear.
- Linear striated increased signal intensity may be evident, representing longitudinal splits or partial tears.
- Chronic partial tears may demonstrate hyperemia.

Complete tears/ruptures show tendon discontinuity with a fluid-filled tendon sheath (**Fig. 22C**).

Associated findings

- If the posterior tibial tendon is ruptured, chronic excess strain is placed on the spring ligament (normally 5 mm thick on T2 transverse), which may thus become attenuated or heterogeneous. It has been estimated that the spring ligament is abnormal in as many as 92% of patients with a posterior tibial tendon injury.
- If longitudinal arch collapse is present, the resultant secondary heel valgus is best seen on coronal sequences. The secondary sinus tarsi collapse produces abnormal signal intensity within the sinus. Pes planus may be evident (**Figs. 22G–22I**).

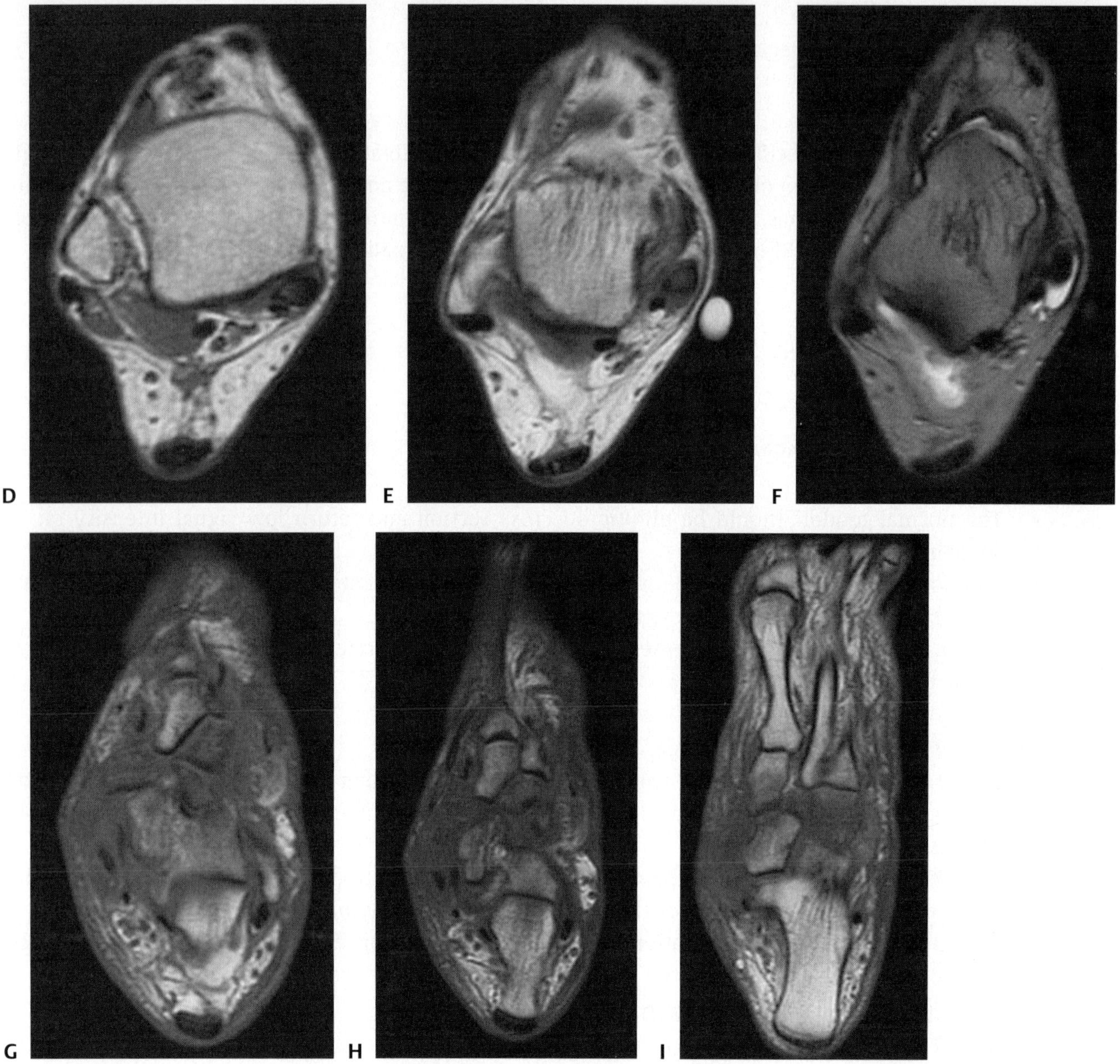

Figures 22D and **22E** Axial T1-weighted images show a swollen but intact tibialis posterior tendon with focal intratendinous high signal intensity consistent with a partial tear. A capsule attached to the overlying skin marks the site of a clinically palpable swelling and the site of maximal pain. **22F** An axial T2-weighted image shows fluid within the tendon sheath surrounding the grossly intact tendon. This, in association with the findings in **Figs. 22D** and **22E**, is diagnostic of a partial tear. **22G–22I** Axial T1-weighted images show a combined injury of the flexor digitorum and tibialis posterior, resulting in pes planus. There is marked swelling and internal signal heterogeneity of the tibialis posterior tendon which cannot be clearly defined as a distinct structure. Pes planus is evinced by the presence of the full length of metatarsal and cuneiform on the same slice as the length of calcaneus: findings not seen in the presence of an intact longitudinal arch.

- Sinus tarsi abnormalities occur in as many as 72% of patients with tibialis posterior tendon injury.
- Tears of the anterior talofibular ligament are found relatively frequently (43% of cases).
- If the patient has significant pain, abnormal marrow signal may be demonstrated in the tibia adjacent to the tendon; however, this is seen more commonly in those with inflammatory arthritides.

- MRI studies have found the presence of medial tubercle hypertrophy (sensitivity, 89%; specificity, 75%) and an accessory navicular bone (sensitivity, 20%; specificity, 100%) to be useful secondary signs of a complete tibialis posterior tendon tear.

Although the MRI characteristics of severe tendinosis and partial tear may overlap, tendinopathy is characterized by

- Increased AP diameter, causing a rounding of the tendon
- Intratendinous signal inhomogeneity
- Enhancement of the tendon after intravenous gadolinium

The characteristics of peritendinosis are

- Fluid within the tendon sheath in the presence of a normal tendon
- Pronounced peritendinous enhancement

Treatment

TEARS

- Complete disruption requires repair, particularly to prevent long-term flatfoot deformity. Tears up to a few centimeters in length are reparable by direct end-to-end suturing.
- If the tear is long-standing, tendon retraction into the muscle belly may render end-to-end repair impossible, and tendon grafting utilizing the flexor digitorum will be required.

TENDINOSIS

- Nonsteroidal anti-inflammatories and immobilization of the foot for 6 to 8 weeks with a rigid below-knee cast, followed by orthotics as necessary
- In the treatment of tendinosis, steroids may be injected into the tendon sheath just proximal to the medial malleolus. Steroids must be avoided, however, in the presence of a partial tear, as they predispose to completion of the tear.
- Tenosynovectomy is occasionally required.

Prognosis

If treatment is initiated before progressive deformity has commenced, a good functional result can be expected.

PEARLS

- The three flexor tendons line up behind the medial malleolus in this order, from anterior to posterior: tibialis posterior, flexor digitorum, and flexor hallucis longus, remembered by the mnemonic Tom, Dick, and Harry.
- On MRI, the tibialis posterior tendon usually measures twice the diameter of the flexor digitorum at the level of the ankle joint.
- The finding of abnormal signal intensity within the sinus tarsi on MRI should alert the radiologist to potential abnormalities of the tibialis posterior tendon.
- Differentiating calcification secondary to chronic tear from an os tibiale externum sesamoid within the tibialis posterior tendon should be straightforward, as the sesamoid is 2 to 6 mm, round, and well corticated.

PITFALLS

- The flexor digitorum may be used as a graft. It is important not to mistake this for an intact tibialis posterior tendon.
- The normal tendon flares and demonstrates increased signal intensity ~1 cm proximal to its navicular insertion, which is classically secondary to the magic angle phenomenon.
- In the acute tear, radiographs are typically normal, and flatfoot is rarely evident secondary to spasm.

Suggested Readings

Karasick D, Schweitzer ME. Tear of the tibialis posterior tendon causing asymmetric flatfoot: radiologic findings. Am J Roentgenol 1993;161:1237–1240

Khoury NJ, El-Khoury GY, Saltzman CL, Brandser EA. MR imaging of tibialis posterior tendon dysfunction. AJR Am J Roentgenol 1996;167:675–682

Ohashi K, El-Khoury GY, Bennett DL. MDCT of tendon abnormalities using volume-rendered images. AJR Am J Roentgenol 2004;182:161–165

Rosenberg ZS, Cheung Y, Jahss MH, Noto AM, Norman A, Leeds NE. Rupture of tibialis posterior tendon: CT and MR imaging with surgical correlation. Radiology 1988;169:229–235

CASE 23

Anthony G. Ryan and Peter L. Munk

Clinical Presentation

A 26-year-old woman presented, having twisted her ankle playing tennis, with acute focal pain on the lateral aspect of her hindfoot just distal to the tip of the lateral malleolus.

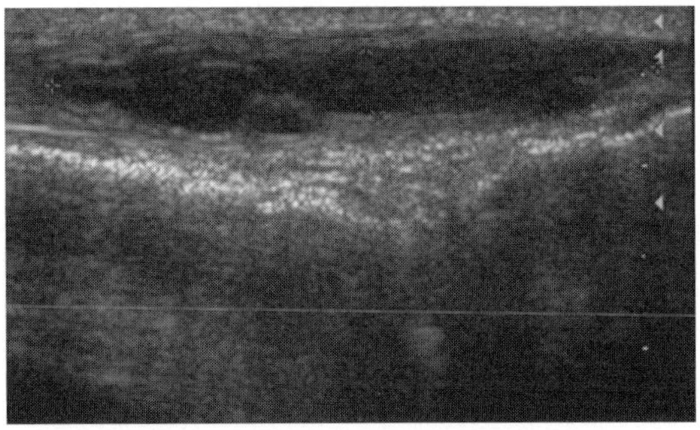

Figure 23A

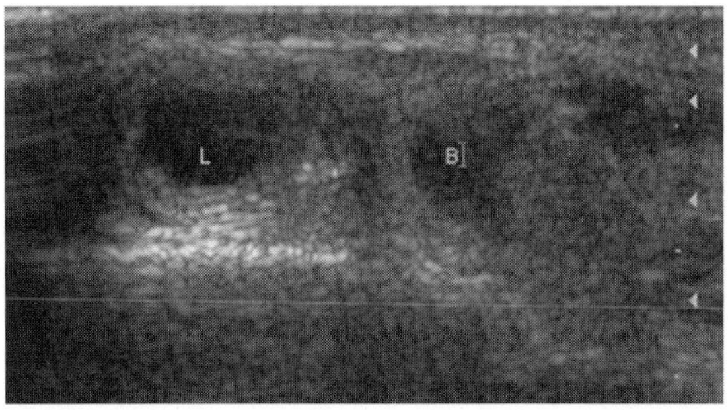

Figure 23B

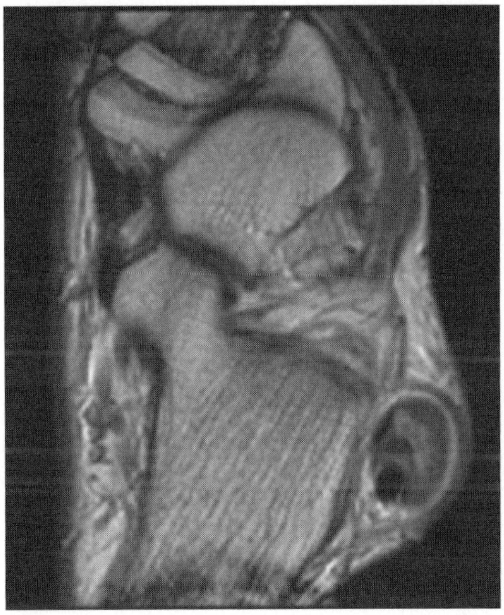

Figure 23C

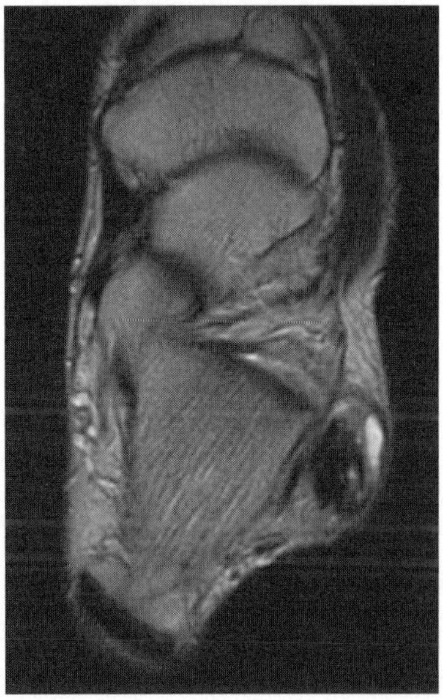

Figure 23D

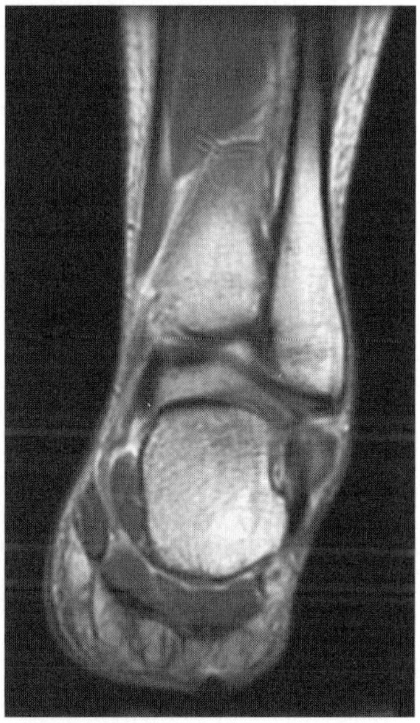

Figure 23E

Radiologic Findings

A sagittal ultrasound of the peroneus longus tendon (**Fig. 23A**) over the region of maximal pain and tenderness shows an irregular tubular anechoic collection within the peroneus longus tendon. Discontinuity of the internal fibrillar architecture is evident. Residual fibers are visible at the cephalad extent of the tendon (to the diagrammatic left of the image). The calcaneocuboid joint is visible deep to the tendon. Transaxial scanning at the same level (**Fig. 23B**) shows the tendons of the peroneus longus and brevis (labeled *L* and *B*) and an equivalent round anechoic defect within the substance of the peroneus longus.

Transaxial T2-weighted images (**Figs. 23C** and **23D**) through the same region show the tendon of the peroneus longus (anterolateral) to be 5 to 6 times the size of the adjacent tendon of the peroneus brevis. The internal architecture is disrupted, with a portion of normal (black) tendon visible on the deep/medial aspect and intermediate signal intensity rim surrounding an amorphous central higher signal component. The more caudad image (**Fig. 23D**) shows further disruption, including splitting of the tendon of the peroneus longus and high signal intensity fluid on the superficial aspect of the tendon.

A coronal T2-weighted image (**Fig. 23E**) shows focal swelling and high signal intensity within the peroneus longus tendon. Deep to the obvious swelling, the normal peroneus brevis tendon is seen adjacent to the underlying calcaneus.

Diagnosis

Peroneus longus tear.

Differential Diagnosis

None.

Discussion

Background

The peroneal tendons are the principal everters of the ankle, coursing behind the lateral malleolus in a common tendon sheath, the latter extending to the level of the fibular tip. They run together in the retromalleolar fibular notch and are covered superiorly by the superior peroneal retinaculum, which resists tendon subluxation.

In addition to ankle eversion, the peroneus longus is a flexor of both the ankle and the first digit (great toe). There are several acute bends on its course to the first metatarsal: at the retromalleolar fossa at the tip of the lateral malleolus, the peroneal tubercle of the calcaneus, and the cuboid notch. The tendons of longus and brevis separate at the peroneal tubercle, the latter serving to direct the peroneus longus tendon inferiorly and medially toward the cuboid notch.

The bend at the cuboid notch coincides with the entry of the peroneus longus tendon to the plantar tunnel (cuboid tunnel) inferior to the cuboid bone. A fibrocartilage sesamoid, the os peroneum, is frequently present within the tendon at this site, protecting the tendon in its gliding motion over the peroneal tuberosity. The sesamoid is ossified in 20% of adults and, when present, is bipartite in 30% and bilateral in 60%.

The peroneus longus continues across the sole of the foot to insert onto the lateral aspect of the first metatarsal.

The peroneus brevis tendon everts the subtalar joint. It has two turns as opposed to the three of the longus, initially turning anteroinferiorly within the fibular groove at the tip of the lateral malleolus, with a second turn at the level of the peroneal tubercle, from which it courses anteriorly into its insertion at the base of the fifth metatarsal.

Etiology

As with injuries to other tendons, the presence of rheumatoid arthritis, diabetes, obesity increasing age, and hypertension all predispose to tendon tears.

In younger patients, tears of the peroneal tendons typically occur secondary to sports involving a rapid change in direction (e.g., in soccer, tennis, and basketball), resulting in a longitudinal split as opposed to a transaxial tear.

Avulsion fractures of the posterolateral fibula, such as in skiing, are occasionally complicated by disruption of the superior peroneal retinaculum. This leads to dislocation of one or both of the tendons. The peroneal tendons may also become entrapped between fragments of fibular or calcaneal fractures.

Pathophysiology

The frequent bends, routes deep to retinacula and over osseous prominences, place the peroneal tendons at particular risk for the development of degeneration and tendinopathy, as well as subsequent tear as a "wear and tear" phenomenon.

The peroneus brevis has a relatively greater predisposition to injury, however, as it is compressed to a greater extent between the more lateral peroneus longus and the stiff edge of the retromalleolar fibular notch. This compression predisposes the tendon to tendinosis, tenosynovitis, and consequent rupture. Tendinopathy at the level of its insertion on the fifth metatarsal is much less common.

Peroneus brevis tendon tears are usually partial, in a longitudinal orientation, and centered at the tip of the lateral malleolus.

Disruption of the superior retinaculum is frequently seen secondary to trauma with associated fibular fractures. When the superior peroneal retinaculum is torn, the tendons will tend to slip anteriorly out of the retromalleolar groove. A shallow retromalleolar sulcus (20% of individuals) predisposes to peroneal subluxation. The superior peroneal retinaculum extends from the posteroinferior margin of the fibula to the adjacent supralateral calcaneus. The inferior peroneal retinaculum runs from the inferolateral aspect of the calcaneus across the bony peroneal tubercle to the lateral rim of the sinus tarsi.

Tendon dislocation may occur in the absence of a fracture with forceful plantar flexion and inversion or dorsiflexion and eversion.

Clinical Findings

Patients tend to complain either of a sudden acute event, such as a severe ankle sprain (the younger sporting group), or of chronic worsening pain (older deconditioned group).

Physical examination reveals a focal, tender swelling in the line of the affected tendon and pain that is worsened when ankle eversion is attempted against resistance. The pain and tenderness tend to be more diffuse in the presence of tendinopathy or tenosynovitis. If the latter is present, crepitus may be palpated.

The clinical findings in peroneal tendon dislocation are very similar to those of ankle strain and are thus frequently underdiagnosed.

Complications

- Ankle instability
- Peroneal compartment syndrome
- Entrapment if a fracture is present
- Paratendinitis
- Stenosing tenosynovitis

Painful os peroneum syndrome is characterized by the following:

- Fracture and avulsion of the os peroneum with peroneus longus tears and stenosing tenosynovitis.
- If the os peroneum is fractured, callous formation may interrupt the peroneus longus tendon. If the peroneal tubercle of a calcaneus is hypertrophied, this may present a further restricting obstacle to the peroneus longus tendon.
- Fractures of the os peroneum commonly occur secondary to a direct blow to the lateral aspect of the foot, crushing it against the cuboid bone. A retracted os peroneum may be detected radiographically, indicative of a peroneus longus tendon tear.

Imaging Findings

RADIOGRAPHY

In the absence of an accompanying fracture (fibula, calcaneus, cuboid), radiographs are typically normal, other than variable soft-tissue swelling over the lateral hindfoot.

Secondary radiographic signs of morphology predisposing to subluxation/dislocation may be present, including flat or convex retromalleolar grooves, lateral fibular spurs, and abnormal lateral ligaments.

In the presence of a superior peroneal retinaculum injury, the lateral malleolus may be stripped of periosteum and may have a variable bone fragment from the distal fibula. This fragment will be seen in up to 50% of patients with acute peroneal dislocations and is best seen immediately posterior to the fibula on an internal rotation ankle mortise view.

A normal os peroneum should have a smooth, well-corticated margin and be at the level of the calcaneocuboid joint and the adjacent cuboid bone. The normal os may be anywhere from 7 mm proximal to 8 mm distal to the calcaneocuboid joint on a lateral radiograph.

On radiographs, proximate retraction of the whole os (10 mm or more proximal to the calcaneocuboid joint) and fracture or diastasis (6 mm or more) of the cephalad fragment of the os peroneum are secondary signs of a peroneus longus tendon tear.

In the presence of a bipartite os peroneum, fragment separation of 2 mm or less is acceptable; more than 2 mm indicates tendon injury.

ULTRASOUND

- A normal tendon should have a uniform hyperechoic fibrillar pattern.
- Tendinosis is characterized by diffuse hypoechoic swelling.
- Partial tears are characterized by hypoechoic swelling with variable hypoechoic clefts.
- Complete tears are characterized by complete disruption of the normal fibrillar pattern, with the gaps filled with anechoic fluid representing blood and tissue edema (**Figs. 23A** and **23B**).

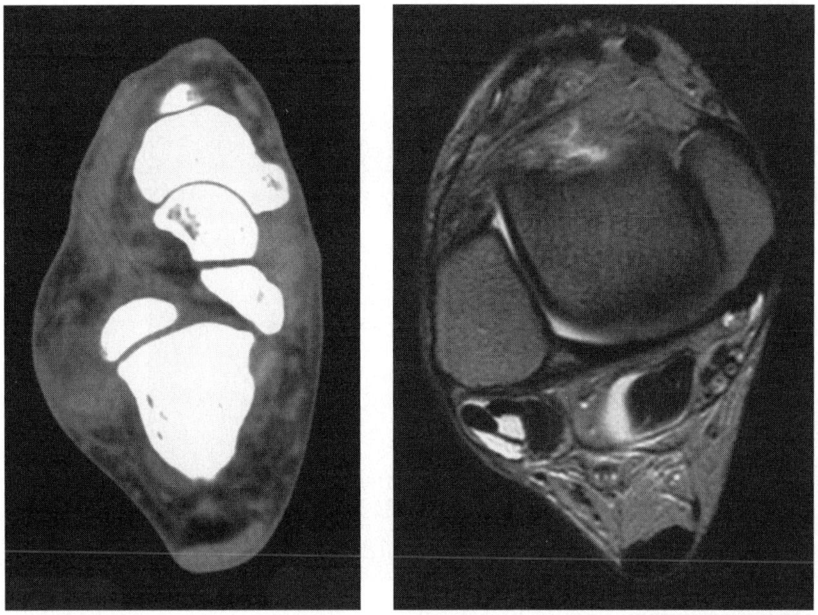

F G

Figures 23F A transaxial CT performed to exclude a fracture shows intermediate density (less than muscle) within the substance of the peroneus brevis tendon and associated surrounding fluid density. The tendon of the peroneus longus is seen as a uniform hyperdense oval structure at ~9 o'clock within the common sheath. **23G** A transaxial T2 fat-saturated image at the level of the lateral malleolus shows a significant volume of fluid within the common tendon sheath and a (reversed) "C-shaped" peroneus brevis tendon, typical of the configuration in the presence of a longitudinal split.

- When present, an os peroneum should be hyperechoic and show acoustic shadowing. If bipartite, both fragments should be hyperechoic, in close proximity to each other with well-defined margins, and each fragment should cause posterior shadowing.

COMPUTED TOMOGRAPHY

Although performed most commonly to assess bony injuries, CT can frequently demonstrate tendon tears and secondary evidence of same, that is, soft-tissue swelling and stranding (**Figs. 23F** and **23G**). In the presence of a calcaneal fracture, tendon entrapment is best demonstrated by CT.

MAGNETIC RESONANCE IMAGING

Above the tip of the fibula, the tendons are best visualized in the transaxial plane, and best visualized more distally in the coronal plane. Additional coronal obliques across the ankle may be necessary, given the multiple direction changes of each tendon. If present, an os peroneum should appear as a well-defined, fat-containing ossicle within the longus tendon. To image the entirety of the peroneus longus tendon, the region covered should be extended to the first metatarsal.

Tears

Partial tears are more common than complete tears. Complete tears will be seen as a tendon defect, with the gap filled by fluid or fat. Because tears are commonly found at those sites, subject to the most biomechanical stress, these sites must be scrutinized closely.

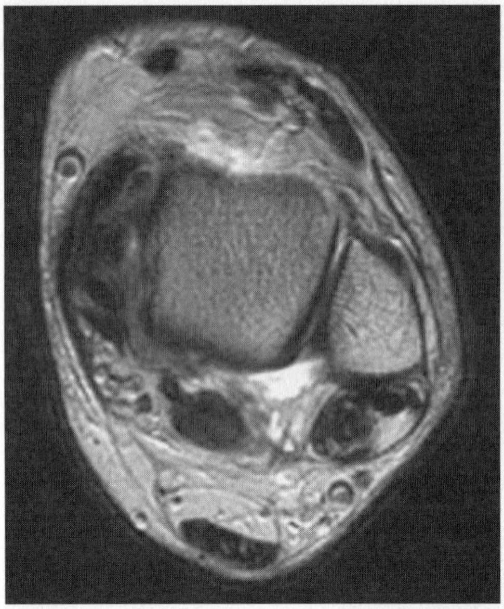
H

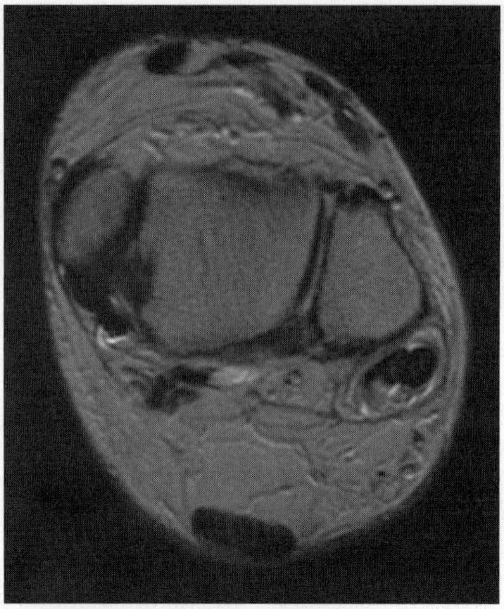
I

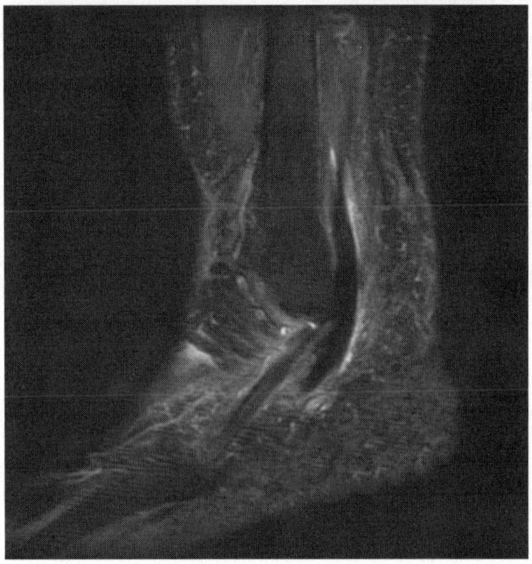
J

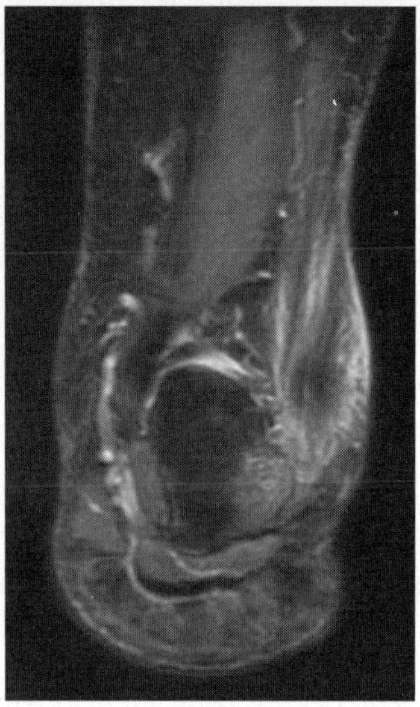
K

Figures 23H A transaxial T2-weighted image at the level of the lateral malleolus shows a further example of a split peroneus tendon, seen "saddlebagged" over the tendon of the peroneus longus. The medial portion of the peroneus brevis shows intrasubstance disruption in addition to the central split. Additional findings in this injury include an ankle effusion and a torn anterior talofibular ligament (focal discontinuity and laxity). **23I** A transaxial T2-weighted image shows patchy high signal within both peroneal tendons and a trace of fluid within the common sheath. **23J** A sagittal STIR image shows fusiform swelling of the peroneus longus tendon, which has an essentially uniform internal architecture. Intermediate signal is seen along the length of the peroneus brevis tendon to its insertion onto the base of the fifth metatarsal. High signal fluid is seen within the tendon sheath. Edema is also present within the subcutaneous tissues posteriorly and anteriorly. The findings are consistent with chronic tendinopathy of the peroneus longus tendon and a partial tear of the peroneus brevis tendon. **23K** A coronal STIR image shows marrow edema within the calcaneus subjacent to the torn peroneus brevis tendon, most likely secondary to the same inciting event. Marrow edema may also be seen as a reactive phenomenon in the presence of overlying acute tenosynovitis or secondary to the altered mechanics secondary to a tear.

Table 23–1 Normal Variants: Permissible Depth of Fluid in Relation to Tendon Sheaths around the Ankle

< 3 mm of fluid is permissible within the common peroneal tendon sheath
≤ 4 mm is permissible in relation to the posterior tibial tendon (posterior to the tendon and inferior to the medial malleolus, but not extending to the navicular insertion)
Anterior ankle joint < 3 mm
Retrocalcaneal bursa < 2.5 mm
Flexor hallucis longus: trace fluid
If normal, no detectable fluid should be present in relation to the flexor digitorum, anterior tibial tendon, Achilles' tendon, or the posterior ankle joint

Complete tears are characterized by

- Tendon discontinuity
- Foci of increased signal intensity in the distal tendon
- Fluid in the tendon sheath
- Enlarged peroneal tubercle

Partial tears are characterized by

- Heterogeneous signal intensity
- The peroneus tendon may demonstrate thickening of the tendon in association with a typical C-shape (**Figs. 23H** and **23I**).

Marrow edema in the lateral calcaneus and peroneal tubercle is a frequent attendant to either complete or partial tears, secondary to either the inciting incident or marrow edema induced secondary to altered biomechanics by the painful tendon (**Figs. 23J** and **23K**).

Chronic tears of either tendon result in a fusiform thickening of the tendon (**Figs. 23J** and **23K**).

Normal variants: Small amounts of fluid can be seen around the tendons (see **Table 23–1**).

Treatment

- Conservative treatment
  - Rest
  - Nonsteroidal anti-inflammatories
  - Orthotics
  - Steroid injection in the presence of stenosing tenosynovitis
- Surgical repair
  - A single longitudinal tear is repaired with a running suture.
  - If multiple degenerative tears are present, they are débrided with an eventual attempt to tubularize the remaining tendon.
  - *Peroneus brevis tendon injuries* If less than one third of the thickness of the peroneus brevis tendon remains, the residual is usually sutured to the adjacent peroneus longus tendon.
- Surgical approaches to tenosynovitis
  - Isolated tenosynovitis: common sheath division
  - Tendon débridement
  - Removal of inciting osseus morphology, such as peroneal tubercle smoothing or excision of os peroneum

Prognosis

Adequate immobilization postrepair (cast for 6 weeks, weight-bearing exercises after 4 weeks, followed by use of a boot for an additional 4 weeks) should result in a good functional outcome.

- Untreated injuries can lead to recurrent/chronic peroneal tendon dislocation.
- Missed peroneal tendon entrapment will lead to chronic disability.

PEARLS

- In association with a superior peroneal retinaculum injury, the lateral malleolus may be stripped of periosteum, giving rise to a variable associated bone fragment. This fragment will be seen in up to 50% of patients with acute peroneal dislocations and is best seen on an internal rotation mortise view just posterior to the fibula. This can be differentiated from a lateral ligament injury with an associated avulsion, as in this case, the avulsed fragment is anteroinferior and is best seen on an AP projection.
- A retracted os peroneum $\geq$ 10 mm indicates a ruptured peroneus longus tendon. Diastasis of a bipartite os peroneum $\geq$ 2 mm is highly suggestive of a rupture.
- The relationship between the peroneal tendons at the level of the distal fibula may be remembered by the fact that the peroneus longus is posterolateral, a mnemonic being PLPL. Thereafter, the longus tendon curves inferiorly and maintains a superficial relation to the brevis tendon throughout the remainder of its course.

PITFALLS

- Failing to look for accompanying peroneal tendon injuries in the presence of a distal fibular fracture or calcaneal fracture can result in missing entrapped tendons—a crucial finding in deciding between an operative and a nonoperative approach.
- A significantly retracted os peroneum, (e.g., at the level of the tibiotalar joint) may be mistaken for an os trigonum or mimic other bone fragments around the ankle joint.
- If the full length of the peroneus longus tendon is not visualized, tears may be missed.
- Normal variants: Permissible volume of fluid in relation to tendon sheaths around the ankle

Suggested Readings

Brigido MK, Fessell DP, Jacobson JA, et al. Radiography and US of os peroneum fractures and associated peroneal tendon injuries: initial experience. Radiology 2005;237:235–241

Khoury NJ, El-Khoury GY, Saltzman CL, Kathol MH. Peroneus longus and brevis tendon tears: MR imaging evaluation. Radiology 1996;200:833–841

Peterson JJ, Bancroft LW. Os peroneal fracture with associated peroneus longus tendinopathy. Am J Roentgenol 2001;177:257–258

Rademaker J, Rosenberg ZS, Delfaut EM, Cheung YY, Schweitzer ME. Tear of the peroneus longus tendon: MR imaging features in nine patients. Radiology 2000;214:700–704

CASE 24

Anthony G. Ryan and Peter L. Munk

Clinical Presentation

A 30-year-old man presented to us with complaints of chronic wrist pain and weakness since a motorcycle accident 18 months previously.

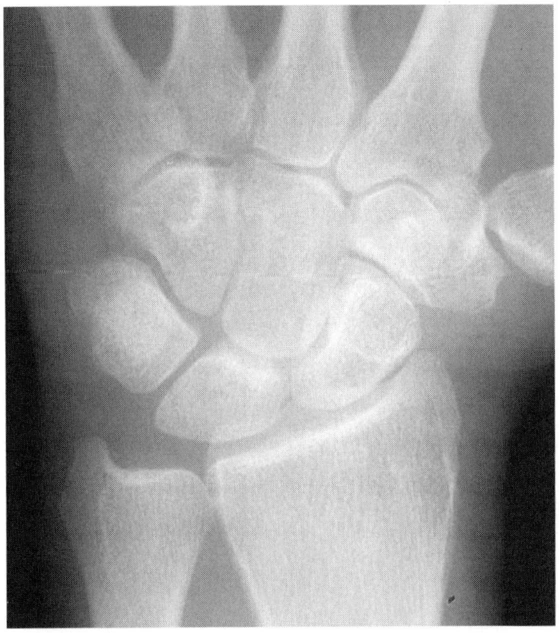

Figure 24A

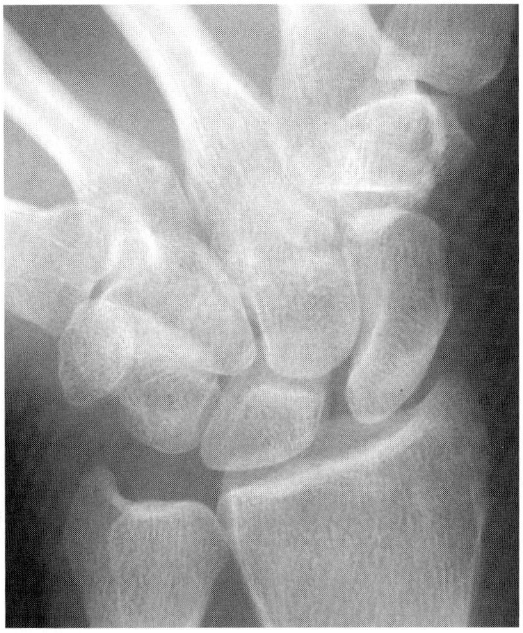

Figure 24B

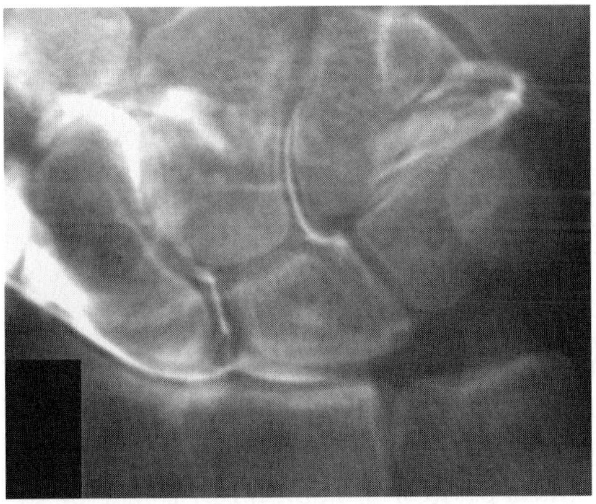

Figure 24C

Radiologic Findings

An AP radiograph with the wrist in the neutral position (**Fig. 24A**) appears unremarkable initially; however, the scaphoid is foreshortened, and the distal pole appears more prominent than usual, projected as a ring through the distal body of the scaphoid. The arcs of the wrist (arcs of Gilula) are intact. An AP radiograph with the wrist in ulnar deviation shows an increase in the scapholunate (SL) interval (**Fig. 24B**). An exposure from an arthrogram (**Fig. 24C**) shows contrast insinuating into the SL interval.

Diagnosis

Scapholunate ligament tear with rotary subluxation of the scaphoid.

Differential Diagnosis

Normal variant of ligamentous anatomy, that is, congenital absence of the SL ligament.

Discussion

Background

The SL ligament is typically composed of a dense fibrous volar trapezoidal component; a thin, filmy middle triangular component; and a dorsal component, composed of a dense fibrous band. The dense volar and dorsal components are attached directly to bone and provide the majority of the biomechanical stability of the joint, whereas the thinner middle portion attaches to hyaline cartilage.

The SL ligament may be congenitally absent. Through acute trauma, chronic repetitive trauma, or wear and tear, the ligament may become stretched and elongated or perforated. Degenerative perforations tend to involve the thinner central section and are thus rarely mechanically significant.

Etiology

Trauma or degeneration, the latter most commonly secondary to rheumatoid arthritis or calcium pyrophosphate deposition disease.

Pathophysiology

The ligament may stretch and tear in isolation or occur in combination with a scaphoid fracture. In combination with the lunatotriquetral ligament, the SL ligament is responsible for the mechanical and rotational stability of the proximal carpal row. The disassociation of the scaphoid and lunate thus results in altered biomechanics and disrupts carpal stability.

SL instability occurs secondary to a tear of the ligament and is frequently associated with a scaphoid fracture. Carpal instability may be either static or dynamic, the latter producing abnormal intercarpal motion.

SL ligament tears are almost unheard of in children.

Rotary subluxation of the scaphoid may occur after a fall on the outstretched hand, whereby subsequently, on dorsiflexion of the wrist, the scaphoid cannot maintain its normal relationship with the radius.

For SL dissociation to occur, the dorsal SL ligament must be torn in addition to a tear of the interosseous SL ligament.

In dorsal intercalated segment instability (DISI), the lunate undergoes palmar translation and dorsal angulation, the capitate is dorsally subluxed, and the scaphoid moves in a volar direction.

In volar intercalated segment instability (VISI), the scaphoid and lunate are palmar-flexed with a decreased SL angle ($<$ 30 degrees), a normal or increased capitolunate angle ($>$ 30 degrees), and palmar subluxation of the capitate. VISI is usually associated with lunatotriquetral instability, rather than with SL instability.

Clinical Findings

Findings include wrist pain and disability, including loss of grip strength, which may hinder a return to normal occupation in skilled manual workers and limit participation in certain sporting pursuits, such as weightlifting.

Complications

- Carpal instability, pain, and disability
- Degenerative arthritis
- When SL instability is established, it may result in collapse of the scaphoid and a so-called SLAC wrist (SL advanced collapse).

Imaging Findings

RADIOGRAPHY

- In an adult, an intercarpal interval greater than 2 to 4 mm is suggestive of a ligament injury.
- Static carpal instability is suggested on a static posteroanterior (PA) film of the wrist by loss of congruity of the carpal arcs: the proximal line of the proximal carpal row, the distal line of the proximal carpal row, and the line formed by the proximal margins of the capitate and hamate (also known as arcs of Gilula).

In choosing patients for a dedicated fluoroscopic wrist examination looking for instability, patients should have

- SL ligament or joint pain
- Reproducible popping or clunking
- Abnormal carpal alignment on routine radiography
- Positive capitolunate instability on clinical examination

Rotary subluxation of the scaphoid (RSS)

- Results in an increased SL interval (> 4 mm). The scaphoid is palmar-flexed and consequently appears foreshortened on a PA wrist, bringing the distal pole in line with the main axis of the scaphoid body, producing the so-called ring sign.
- On a lateral neutral radiograph, the SL angle measures > 70 degrees (normal should be between 30 and 60 degrees).

In scapholunate disassociation (SLD),

- The findings of RSS are present; in addition, there is usually a widened SL gap on a neutral PA radiograph.

In the presence of DISI,

- Palmar-flexion of the scaphoid and an SL angle greater than 60 degrees and an increased capitolunate angle greater than 30 degrees on a neutral lateral radiograph.

In the presence of VISI,

- The scaphoid and lunate are palmar-flexed with a decreased SL angle (< 30 degrees), a normal or increased capitolunate angle (> 30 degrees), and palmar subluxation of the capitate.

In both DISI and VISI on a posteroanterior (PA) wrist radiograph, the tilted lunate appears triangular with a rounded distal margin instead of its usual trapezoidal shape.

ARTHROGRAPHY

- Controversy exists regarding the correct arthrographic protocol, with various authorities proposing bilateral tricompartmental (radiocarpal, midcarpal, and distal radioulnar injections) arthrography in all cases of suspected intercarpal ligament and triangular fibrocartilage complex tears. The reasoning behind performing multicompartmental injections is that flow from one compartment to another may be unidirectional (by a valve-type action), and thus a false-negative may be reported on a single compartment injection.
- The value in performing these examinations has been called into question, however, as intercompartmental communication has been shown to correlate very poorly with clinical symptoms. Degenerative tears and perforations are common and can occur as early as 15 years of age. The examination is time-consuming and invasive, and carries risks of contrast allergy and septic arthritis. We generally reserve arthrography to resolve questions raised by MRI or immediately preceding MR arthrography.

ULTRASOUND

- Limited experience suggests that, compared with conventional tricompartmental arthrography, high-resolution ultrasound (9 to 13 MHz) had a sensitivity and specificity of 100% for SL tears.

COMPUTED TOMOGRAPHY ARTHROGRAPHY

- CT arthrography may be more sensitive (100%) than MRI in the detection of palmar tears and significantly better in the detection of dorsal segment tears.
- When compared with arthroscopy and standard arthrography, high-resolution CT after tricompartment arthrography has brief sensitivity and specificity in the detection of SL ligament tears. In addition, CT arthrography shows the site of tears or perforation with greater precision in comparison to the indirect demonstration of standard arthrography.

MAGNETIC RESONANCE IMAGING

- The SL ligament is demonstrated on MRI to be composed of three intermediate signal structures: a volar trapezoidal component, a middle triangular component, and a dorsal component, essentially composed of a simple band. Studies performed on normal volunteers demonstrate a "delta" configuration in over 90% of cases and linear in the remainder. In these normal volunteers, there was absent signal intensity in 63% or intermediate signal intensity traversing all or part of the SL ligament in 37%.
- Full-thickness tears are shown as ligamentous discontinuity. Examining the wrist with ulnar deviation in the coronal plane is said to increase the sensitivity in the detection of full-thickness tears.
- A ridge of soft tissue covers the articular ridge of the distal radial articular surface (between the scaphoid and lunate fossae), which, when seen adjacent to the margin of the SL ligament, may simulate discontinuity in the latter.
- MRI is estimated as having a sensitivity of between 50 and 93% and a specificity of between 86 and 100% for SL ligament perforations.
- Indirect MR arthrography significantly improves sensitivity in the evaluation of the SL ligament when compared with unenhanced MRI of the wrist. In addition, the diagnostic performance of MRI in suspected lesions of the SL and lunotriquetral ligaments is improved by adding MRI after tricompartmental arthrography, that is, direct MR arthrography.

In the presence of a partial tear, the ligament may be thinned or irregular, or abnormal high signal intensity may be demonstrated in the substance of the ligament. Partial tears are frequently very difficult to identify on unenhanced MRI, so three secondary signs have been described to aid in their detection:

- Carpal bone malalignment
- Disruption of the carpal arcs
- Evidence of focal osteoarthritis

Treatment

Arthroscopic repair is recommended as a minimally invasive treatment to avoid the sequela of severe degenerative change.

For arthroscopic débridement:

- Formal repair may not be necessary, as it has been shown that surface débridement of the torn margins of the ligaments results in almost complete resolution of symptoms in 66% of wrists with a complete SL ligament tear and 85% of wrists with a partial SL ligament tear. In addition to pain relief, grip strength improves in 23% postoperatively.

Prognosis

Untreated, these injuries lead to degenerative arthritis.

PEARLS

- Degenerative perforations tend to involve the thinner central section and are thus rarely mechanically significant.
- In an adult, an intercarpal interval > 2 mm is suggestive of a ligament injury.
- The dynamic nature of arthrography gives it an advantage over static unenhanced MRI, given the ability to visualize early passage of contrast via the SL interval.

PITFALLS

- The SL ligament may be congenitally absent.
- Perforations may develop in the ligament secondary to aging; thus, the passage of contrast through the SL interval does not necessarily indicate the source of pain, particularly in an older patient.
- Similarly, dynamic screening is vital on arthrography, as contrast may gain access to the intercarpal row and back into the SL interval, leading to a false-positive diagnosis of an SL tear. For this reason, all wrist arthrograms are videotaped in our institutions.
- A ridge of soft tissue covers the articular ridge of the distal radial articular surface (between the scaphoid and lunate fossae), which, when seen adjacent to the margin of the SL ligament, may simulate a tear in the latter.

Suggested Readings

Finlay K, Lee R, Friedman L. Ultrasound of intrinsic wrist ligament and triangular fibrocartilage injuries. Skeletal Radiol 2004;33:85–90

Haims AH, Schweitzer ME, Morrison WB, et al. Internal derangement of the wrist: indirect MR arthrography versus unenhanced MR imaging. Radiology 2003;227:701–707

Schmid MR, Schertler T, Pfirrmann CW, et al. Interosseous ligament tears of the wrist: comparison of multi-detector row CT arthrography and MR imaging. Radiology 2005;237:1008–1013

Smith DK. Scapholunate interosseous ligament of the wrist: MR appearances in asymptomatic volunteers and arthrographically normal wrists. Radiology 1994;192:217–221

Zanetti M, Bram J, Hodler J. Triangular fibrocartilage and intercarpal ligaments of the wrist: does MR arthrography improve standard MRI? J Magn Reson Imaging 1997;7:590–594

CASE 25

Peter L. Munk and Anthony G. Ryan

Clinical Presentation

A 46-year-old man presented with chronic pain on the inside of his wrist, exacerbated while performing home improvements, particularly when hammering and when lifting his toolbox by the handle. Years previously he had sustained a fracture of the distal radius.

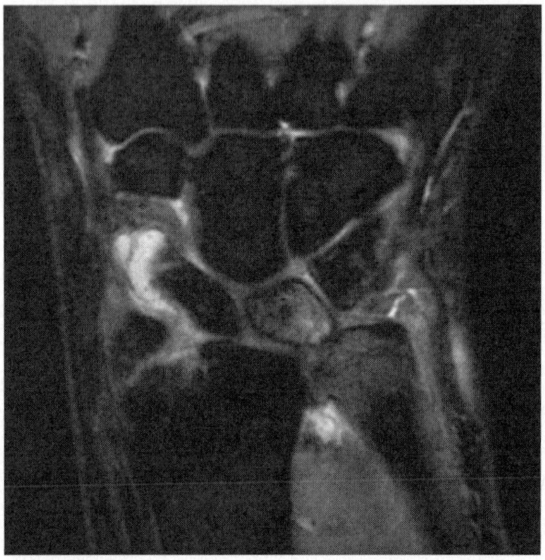

Figure 25A

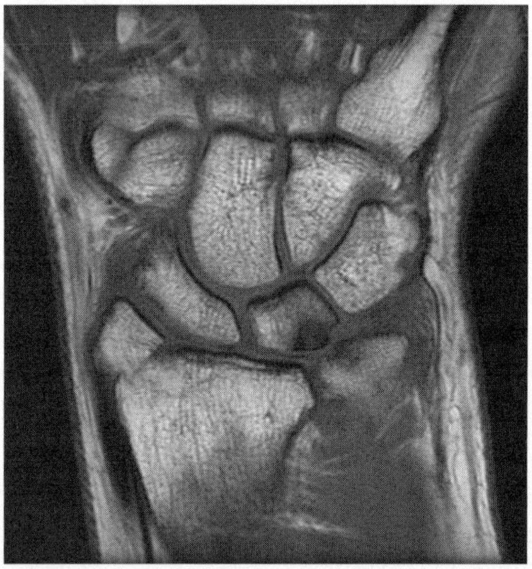

Figure 25B

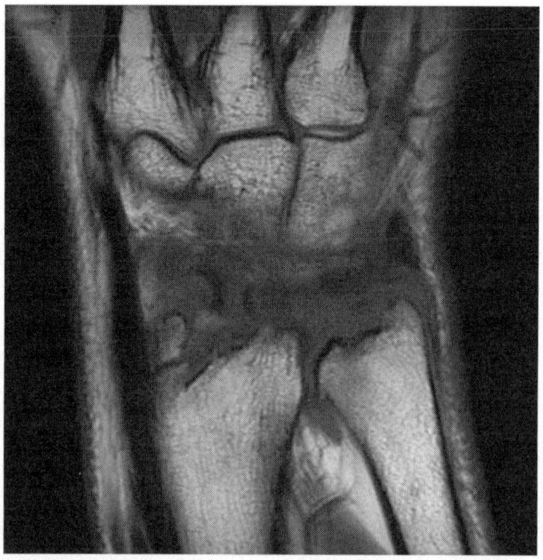

Figure 25C

Radiologic Findings

A coronal STIR image (**Fig. 25A**) shows high signal intensity in the head of the ulna and in the ulnar aspect of the lunate. The distal lateral aspect of the ulnar head abuts the lunate. There is loss of contiguity of the radial and ulnar carpal articular surfaces. An essentially free portion of the triangular fibrocartilage (TFC) is seen just distal to the ulnar head. A bony fragment is projected distal to the distal radius in the expected position of the radial styloid. A ganglion is seen in relation to the radial aspect of the scaphoid.

A coronal T1-weighted image (**Fig. 25B**) volar to the STIR image shows a low signal intensity focus on the ulnar aspect of the lunate and a corresponding low signal intensity focus on the adjacent ulnar head. Bony irregularity of the radial styloid process is evident.

A coronal T1-weighted image (**Fig. 25C**) dorsal to the STIR image shows an irregular radial styloid process, distal radius, and ulna, as well as an osteophyte on the ulnar aspect of the distal radioulnar joint.

Diagnosis

Ulnar impaction syndrome with TFC complex tear.

Differential Diagnosis

- *Intraosseus lunate ganglion or lunate cyst* Both of these entities appear on the radial aspect of the lunate, have sharp margins, and demonstrate no corresponding changes in the ulna or triquetral.
- *Kienböck's lunatomalacia* More diffuse or radial sided findings, with no corresponding ulnar or triquetral findings

Discussion

Background

Proper functioning of the wrist requires smooth articulation of the proximal carpal row with the distal radius and ulnar. The TFC complex plays a crucial role in this regard.

Most commonly, patients demonstrate what is referred to as positive ulnar variance (although this is not a sine qua non for degenerative ulnar impaction syndrome). Ulnar variance refers to the relative lengths of the distal articular surfaces of the radius and ulna. With positive ulnar variance, the ulna is longer than the radius; in particular, the carpal articular surface of the ulnar projects more distally than the radial carpal articular surface. Because ulnar variance can depend on the position of the wrist, that is, supination versus pronation, variance is usually measured in neutral rotation using a posteroinferior (PA) projection, the elbow flexed to 90 degrees and the shoulder abducted by 90 degrees. When present, pronation of the forearm and gripping both exacerbate the degree of positive variance.

Etiology

Ulnar impaction syndrome is a degenerative process that involves limited motion at the wrist associated with wrist pain at the ulnar aspect. It should be cautioned that because of the position assumed in MRI, accurate determination of ulnar variance is often not possible using this imaging technique.

Other than degeneration, the other major predisposing cause is previous trauma resulting in fractures that have produced malunion and disturbed the normal articulation between the radius, ulna, and carpus. Radial shortening after fractures can produce a relative positive ulnar variance.

Developmental abnormalities such as early physeal closure can also occasionally have a similar effect.

Pathophysiology

The primary abnormality consists of excessive weight bearing at the ulnar aspect of the wrist, which leads to development of a TFC tear. The ulnar aspect of the carpal joint usually accommodates only ~20% of the forces transmitted across the wrist. Increases in ulnar positivity cause a disproportionate increase in forces transmitted across this compartment; for example, an increase of 1 mm yields an increase of force of 25%.

Eventually, due to abnormal weight bearing by the lunate, chondromalacia develops, which can also affect the triquetral bone or the ulna.

Clinical Findings

- Medial wrist pain exacerbated by activities involving wrist motion or gripping objects tightly (including a painful handshake)
- Limitation of wrist adduction
- Weakened grip
- Focal tenderness on the medial aspect of the wrist, especially just distal to the ulnar styloid
- Painful resisted wrist adduction

Stages of Disease

The Palmer classification describes the combinations of ligament injuries and bony changes found in the TFC complex. Class I injuries are traumatic in origin, whereas class II are degenerative. The subclasses describe the anatomic findings.

CLASS I TFC INJURIES (SECONDARY TO TRAUMA)

- Central perforation of the TFC complex
- Ulnar avulsion with or without distal ulnar fracture
- Distal avulsion (carpal attachment)
- Radial avulsion with or without sigmoid notch fracture

CLASS II TFC INJURIES (SECONDARY TO DEGENERATION)

- TFC complex wear
- TFC complex wear, lunate or ulnar chondromalacia
- TFC complex perforation, lunate or ulnar chondromalacia
- TFC complex perforation, lunate or ulnar chondromalacia, lunatotriquetral ligament perforation
- Ulnocarpal osteoarthritis

Complications

- Chondromalacia affecting the lunate, triquetral bone, or ulna
- Lunatotriquetral ligament tears further disturbing the normal biomechanics of the joint
- Degenerative osteoarthritis eventually affects the involved joints.

Imaging Findings

RADIOGRAPHY

- Positive ulnar variance on the conventional projection, that is, a PA projection, with the elbow flexed to 90 degrees and the shoulder abducted by 90 degrees
- If operative repair is considered, specific views in pronation with and without a "gripped" fist should be performed, bearing in mind the latter makes ulnar positivity more pronounced.
- Bony deformity, such as an impacted distal radial fracture
- Once the process is well advanced, subchondral sclerosis, loss of mineralization, and cyst formation in the ulnar head, lunate, and triquetrum may become evident.

COMPUTED TOMOGRAPHY

Bony changes will be elegantly demonstrated by CT; however, MRI is the investigation of choice.

MAGNETIC RESONANCE IMAGING

MRI is able to detect more subtle disease, directly imaging the soft tissues of the wrist.

- Bone marrow edema, particularly in the lunate, may be evident on MRI without any radiographic changes being present.
- Fat-suppressed inversion recovery or T2-weighted images are particularly helpful in picking up early edematous changes.
- The TFC is often perforated, particularly at its midportion or radial insertion.
- The lunatotriquetral ligament and associated tears may be demonstrated.
- With more advanced disease, areas of low signal on all sequences representing the development of sclerosis and fibrosis, and high signal cystic changes on T2-weighted imaging, may be present.
- Although other abnormalities, such as osseous ganglia and avascular necrosis of the lunate, may mimic this condition, the configuration of associated findings usually allows a differentiation between these other entities. For instance, avascular necrosis is more prone to affect the radial side of the lunate than the ulna.
- In the case of ulnar impaction following a distal radial fracture, MRI changes may be apparent as early as 4 months after the injury; the presence of unresolving pain should prompt consideration of the condition, as the MRI findings correlate well with the degree of persistent pain.
- In such cases, MRI has been shown to be more sensitive than arthroscopy in detecting lunate changes, particularly when the overlying cartilage remains intact.

Treatment

Treatment typically involves some sort of ulnar shortening procedure that may require a wedge osteotomy or direct burring of the distalmost 2 to 3 mm of the ulna. The latter may be performed arthroscopically if the TFC is torn—the so-called arthroscopic wafer procedure.

When ulnocarpal osteoarthrosis is present, a complete or partial resection of the ulnar head or arthrodesis of the distal radioulnar joint with distal ulnar pseudoarthrosis may be required.

Prognosis

The wafer procedure, particularly when performed arthroscopically, permits an early return to normal activities.

PEARLS

- Avascular necrosis of the lunate (Kienböck's lunatomalacia) may mimic this condition; however, avascular necrosis is more prone to affect the radial side of the lunate than the ulna, permitting differentiation between these other entities.
- An intraosseus lunate ganglion or lunate cyst may mimic the lunate changes; however, both these entities appear on the radial aspect of the lunate, have sharp margins, and have no corresponding changes in the ulna or triquetral.
- The geographic nature of the associated changes aids in the diagnosis of the syndrome, that is, changes centered on the distal ulnocarpal articulation.

PITFALLS

- Because of the position assumed in MRI of the wrist, determination of ulnar variance is unreliable using this imaging technique.
- Although the ulnar impaction syndrome is frequently used interchangeably with ulnar impingement, the latter is a different entity. Typically, with impingement, the ulna is appreciably shorter than the radius, and the distal radioulnar joint is abnormally articulated. Symptoms may sometimes be similar, contributing to the confusion.
- In posttraumatic cases, such as distal radial fracture, MRI has been shown to be more sensitive than arthroscopy in detecting lunate changes, particularly when the overlying cartilage remains intact.

Suggested Readings

Cerezal L, del Pinal F, Abascal F, Garcia-Valtuille R, Pereda T, Canga A. Imaging findings in ulnar-sided wrist impaction syndromes. Radiographics 2002;22:105–121

Escobedo EM, Bergman AG, Hunter JC. MR imaging of ulnar impaction. Skeletal Radiol 1995;24:85–90

Imaeda T, Nakamura R, Shionoya K, Makino N. Ulnar impaction syndrome: MR imaging findings. Radiology 1996;201:495–500

Steinborn M, Schurmann M, Staebler A, et al. MR Imaging of ulnocarpal impaction after fracture of the distal radius. Am J Roentgenol 2003;181:195–198

CASE 26

Anthony G. Ryan, Peter L. Munk, and Laurel O. Marchinkow

Clinical Presentation

A 5-year-old boy presented with a 3-month history of a limp.

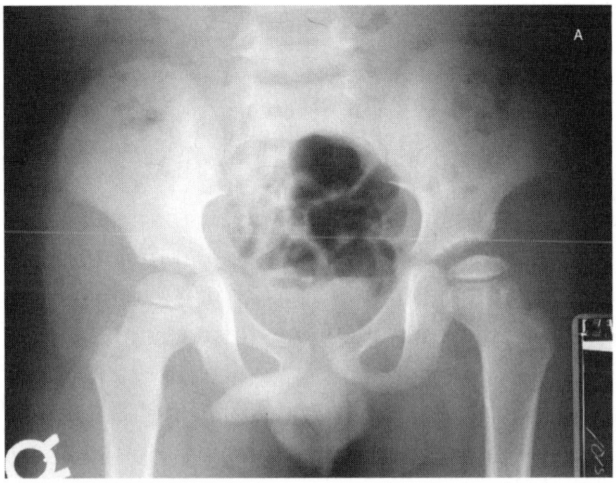

Figure 26A

Radiologic Findings

A flattened irregular left capital femoral epiphysis is shown in **Fig. 26A**.

Diagnosis

Legg-Calvé-Perthes disease.

Discussion

Background

Otherwise known as coxa plana, Legg-Calvé-Perthes disease is avascular necrosis of the femoral head in children, most common between the ages of 4 and 8, with a male (5:1) and Caucasian preponderance. The condition occurs bilaterally in 15%.

Etiology

The condition is most commonly idiopathic, but in 30% of cases, it is secondary to trauma.

Clinical Findings

Hip pain and limp, lasting between 1 week and 6 months (mean = 2.7 months).

Stages of Disease

- I No radiographic findings; abnormal radionuclide bone scan (2 weeks)
- II Osteoporosis, sclerosis with or without cystic changes with normal femoral head contour (5 months)
- III Crescent sign and subchondral femoral head collapse (10 months)
- IV Femoral head flattening (18 months)
- V Acetabular collapse and reduced joint space (chronic) (24 months and later)

Complications

Early severe degenerative hip joint disease.

Pathology

Legg-Calvé-Perthes disease is one of a heterogeneous group of disorders known as the osteochondritides, characterized radiologically by fragmentation, collapse, sclerosis, and eventual reossification of the involved bone, and pathologically by osteonecrosis. The femoral head is at particular risk for this latter process by virtue of the tenuous blood supply to the femoral epiphysis via the medial circumflex and lateral epiphyseal arteries.

If the blood supply is disrupted by trauma or other causes (e.g., intravascular), 6 to 12 hours of anoxia leads to death of the hematopoetic cells. Twelve to 48 hours of anoxia is required for bone cell death. Forty-eight to 60 hours of anoxia leads to death of the marrow fat cells. This results in loss of fat cell nuclei and the formation of fat cysts, both of which are taken as pathological features of established osteonecrosis.

Surrounding the central zone of cell death is a zone of ischemic injury, and at the margin of this is an advancing hyperemic zone as a result of recanalization of thrombosed vessels and neovascularity.

Imaging Findings

The radiologic findings parallel the evolution of the disease process. Thus, at the time of cell death, conventional radiographs will be normal, as will radionuclide studies.

RADIOGRAPHY

With subsequent ischemia and reactive hyperemia, osteopenia will be evident, but it takes between 2 and 5 months for this to be demonstrable radiographically. At this stage, cysts and sclerosis may become evident.

At 9 to 10 months, the "crescent" sign (see below) becomes visible, often with associated subchondral collapse. Femoral head remodeling (e.g., resulting in flattening) becomes evident at 18 months. Early degenerative changes may become evident, for example, by the presence of reduced joint space.

During the early phase,

- Femoral epiphysis smaller than on the contralateral side (in 98% of cases)
- Widened joint space secondary to joint effusion or synovial swelling
- The "crescent sign" (i.e., a curvilinear subcortical lucency) corresponding to the presence of a subchondral fissure fracture is best seen in the frog-leg view (**Fig. 26B**).

During the intermediate phase,

- The femoral epiphysis becomes fragmented (**Figs. 26B–26D**).
- Variable femoral head sclerosis as reossification occurs

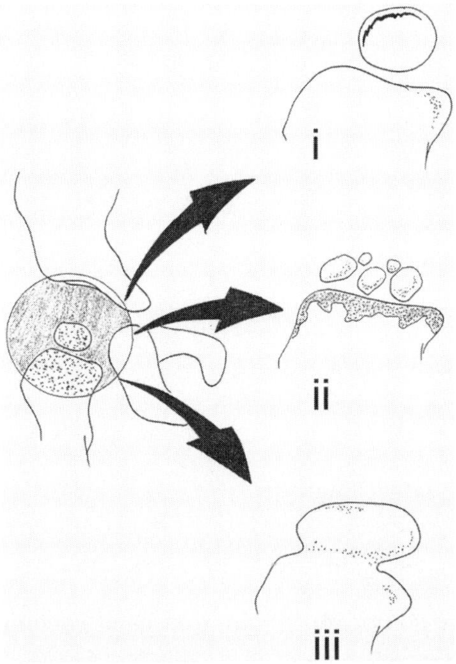

B

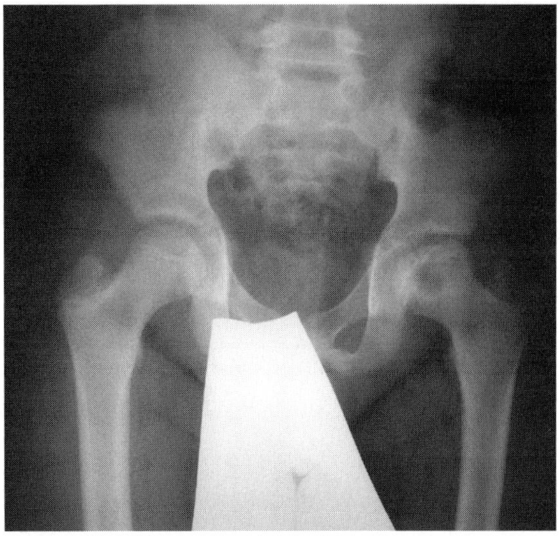

C

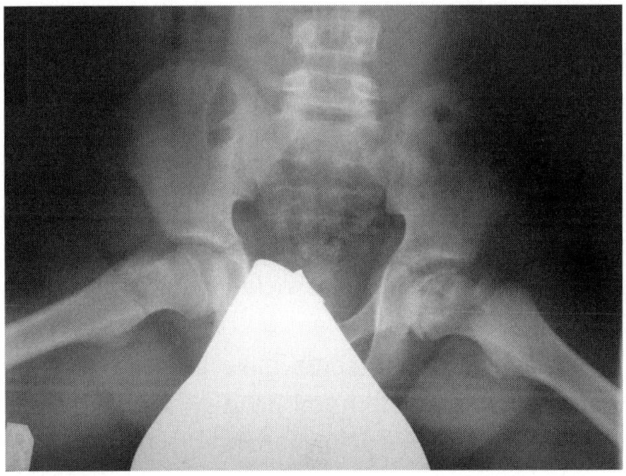

D

Figures 26B Line diagram shows the three main stages of Legg-Calvé-Perthes disease: (i) the typical subchondral lucency seen in association with a subchondral fracture, (ii) the fragmentation of the epiphysis, and (iii) the typical appearance of the resulting chronically deformed femoral head. **26C** and **26D** Anteroposterior frog-leg lateral images show flattening and fragmentation of the femoral head with associated cystic change in the subjacent femoral metaphysis (the latter associated with a poor prognosis).

- Calcification within the devascularized cartilage
- Demineralization cysts, seen in the lateral metaphysis in one third of cases

During the late phase,

- Flattened, deformed femoral head (**Fig. 26B**)
- Early degenerative disease

RADIONUCLIDE STUDIES

- Reduced uptake may be evident in the blood pool phase in the initial stages of the disease, reflecting the reduced blood supply.
- In the later stages, there is increased uptake, reflecting remodeling osteoblastic activity.
- Later still, increased uptake in both the femoral head and the acetabulum may be demonstrated if the disorder is complicated by secondary degenerative disease.

ULTRASOUND

- Synovial swelling and increased joint space may be identifiable acutely.

MAGNETIC RESONANCE IMAGING

- Greater sensitivity for the earlier changes of the disease, permitting earlier diagnosis
- Permits direct assessment of articular cartilage
- Useful in the evaluation of femoral head coverage

T1-weighted images

- Irregular, subchondral low signal
- Low-signal foci or linear signal within the epiphysis, which extends to the subchondral bone

T2-weighted images

- The "double line" sign: an inner hyperintense line corresponding to acute granulation tissue and an outer hypointense line corresponding to developing fibrosis and sclerosis

T2 gradient images

- Initially, increased cartilage thickness, which decreases in later stages

T2 STIR/fat-saturated images

- Increased physeal signal
- The coronal and sagittal planes are useful in assessing the congruity of joint and head coverage.

Treatment

- Abduction bracing
- Varus derotation osteotomy

Prognosis

The prognosis depends on the amount of femoral head involved; if more than 20% of the head is extruded laterally, the prognosis is poor. A metaphyseal abnormality is associated with a poor outcome. The younger the child at presentation (< 8 years), the better the outlook.

Numerous combined clinical and radiographic classification systems have been proposed to predict outcome in Legg-Calvé-Perthes: Catterall, Salter-Thompson, femoral head sphericity, and the Herring grouping. The Herring grade and arthrographic sphericity have proved to be the best predictors of final outcome.

The use of subtraction gadolinium-enhanced MR angiography to evaluate femoral head vascularity has been proposed as a potentially useful early predictor of outcome.

PEARLS

- The "crescent" sign (i.e., a curvilinear subcortical lucency corresponding to the presence of a subchondral fissure fracture) is best seen on the frog-leg view.
- On MRI, the coronal and sagittal planes are most useful in the assessment of joint congruity and femoral head coverage (of prognostic significance).

PITFALLS

- Conventional radiographs are normal during the initial months of the disease, so a high degree of clinical suspicion must be maintained in the presence of ongoing hip pain in this age group. Further imaging investigations are recommended.
- The hip joint space may be either widened (in the presence of an acute effusion) or narrowed (in the case of early degenerative disease).

- Depending on the timing of MRI, the thickness of the cartilage may be thicker (early phase) or narrowed (late phase); in the intermediate phase, the cartilage may appear of normal thickness, potentially leading to a false-negative diagnosis.

Suggested Readings

Hubbard AM, Dormans JP. Evaluation of developmental dysplasia, Perthes' disease, and neuromuscular dysplasia of the hip in children before and after surgery: an imaging update. Am J Roentgenol 1995;164:1067–1073

Ismail AM, Macnicol MF. Prognosis in Perthes' disease: a comparison of radiological predictors. J Bone Joint Surg Br 1999;81:179–180

Lamer S, Dorgeret S, Khairouni A, et al. Femoral head vascularisation in Legg-Calvé-Perthes disease: comparison of dynamic gadolinium-enhanced subtraction MRI with bone scintigraphy. Pediatr Radiol 2002;32:580–585

Lecuire F. The long-term outcome of primary osteochondritis of the hip (Legg-Calvé-Perthes disease). J Bone Joint Surg Br 2002;84:636–640

CASE 27

Anthony G. Ryan and Peter L. Munk

Clinical Presentation

A 21-month-old girl was noted to have a waddling gait and, on physical examination, was found to have a shorter left leg.

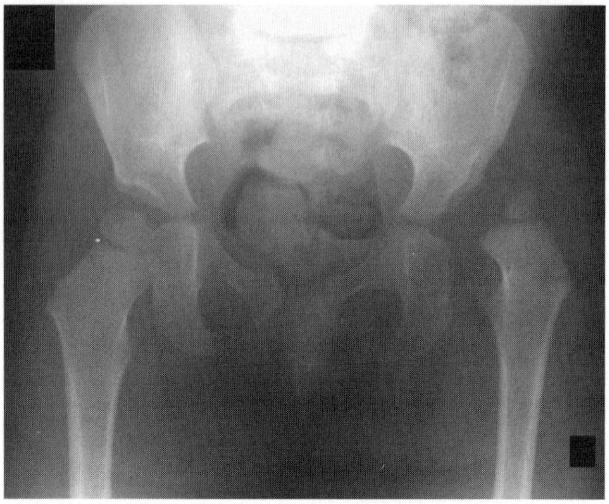

Figure 27A

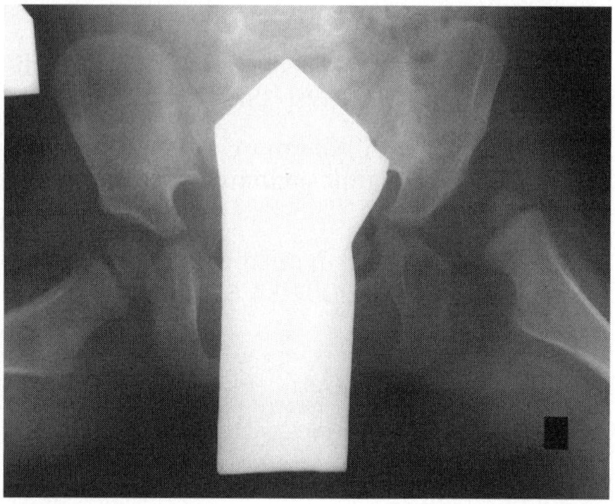

Figure 27B

Radiologic Findings

The anteroposterior (AP) (**Fig. 27A**) and Von Rosen (with 45-degree abduction and internal rotation) (**Fig. 27B**) projections show Putti's triad: the left proximal femur is dislocated superolaterally, the acetabular angle is steep, and the capital femoral epiphysis is smaller than on the contralateral side.

Diagnosis

Congenital dysplasia of the hip.

Discussion

This is a relatively common condition, affecting 0.15% of newborns, with a marked female (8:1) and left-sided (11:1) preponderance. In the majority of cases, the cause is a combination of ligamentous laxity (secondary to maternal estrogens) and acetabular dysplasia, whereby the acetabulum is steeper and more shallow than normal. The femoral head is thus predisposed to fall out of the acetabulum, putting the hip at risk of subluxation/dislocation when exposed to mechanical stress, for example, breech birth.

Clinical Findings

The hip is "dislocatable" on provocation, or the hip is already dislocated. When the hip is dislocatable, the head of the femur jerks in and out of the acetabulum with posterior pressure applied along the length of the femur.

When already dislocated, a positive Ortolani's click describes the snapping of the femoral head back into the acetabulum.

If relocation is not possible, the Ortolani will be falsely negative, in which case other signs may be indicative of the condition:

- Limited abduction
- Asymmetry with apparent shortening
- Deeper skin creases on the affected side (not appreciable if the condition is bilateral)

If the child is walking, the gait will be abnormal, with a positive Trendelenburg's sign: the contralateral pelvis drops when the child stands on the affected limb.

Imaging Findings

RADIOGRAPHY

On the Von Rosen view, femoral head location is usually self-evident when ossified. Acetabular assessment on conventional radiographs is based on the angle that a line drawn from the superolateral acetabular margin to the iliac margin of the triradiate cartilage makes with the horizontal (Hilgenreiner's line: a line drawn between the superior edges of the capital epiphyses). This angle should be between 15 and 30 degrees, with angles > 30 degrees resulting in greater susceptibility to dislocation (**Fig. 27C**). During the course of normal development, this angle tends to decrease in the first year of life, with the relative risk decreasing accordingly.

ULTRASOUND

Because both physical examination and radiography are unreliable as screening tests in the newborn, ultrasound is now the method of choice in assessing the hip joint for the presence of hip dysplasia.

Ultrasound has the obvious advantage over radiography in its ability to assess the acetabular cartilage, the acetabular labrum, and the unossified capital femoral epiphysis, while avoiding the risks associated with the use of ionizing radiation in this age group.

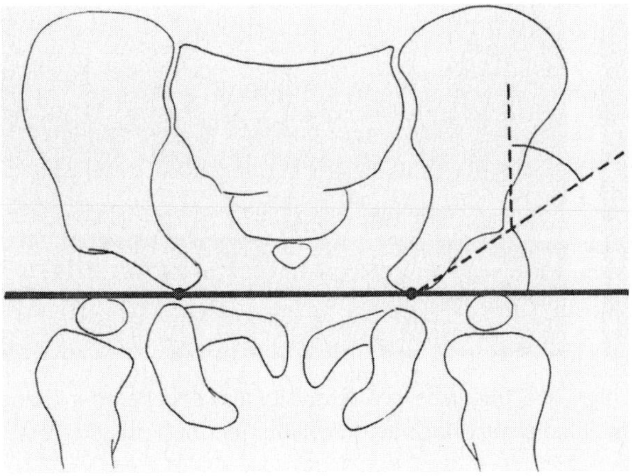

Figure 27C Diagram showing Graf's α angle between the vertical line subtended from the superior margin of the acetabulum (Perkin's line) and a line drawn between the acetabular margins. The smaller the angle, the greater the risk of subluxation/dislocation. Hilgenreiner's line is the horizontal line drawn between the superior edges of the capital epiphyses.

Dynamic maneuvers may be performed, as in the Ortolani and Barlow clinical tests, and the degree of instability should be assessed. The degree of femoral head coverage (< 50% suggests a congenital dislocated hip) and the presence of an abnormal labrum (e.g., inversion) may be evaluated. Graf's α angle is the angle created by a vertical line subtended from the superior margin of the acetabulum and a line drawn between the acetabular margins. An angle < 45 degrees correlates with subluxation/dislocation (see **Fig. 27C**).

Complications

- If untreated, chronic dislocation leads to abnormal development of both the femoral head and the acetabulum, which leads to further malformation and consequent early advanced degeneration (**Fig. 27D**, bilateral severe untreated dysplastic hips).
- Chronic dislocation can lead to the formation of a pseudoacetabulum (**Fig. 27E**).
- There may be delayed ossification of the femoral head.
- The acetabulum itself may become abnormally sclerotic.
- There is an increased risk of femoral head avascular necrosis (AVN).

Treatment and Prognosis

If the hip is dislocatable:

- Abduction splinting: the hips are flexed and abducted (not more than 60 degrees, so that AVN of the femoral head does not occur)

For a dislocated hip:

- Between birth and 18 months: Closed reduction with spica cast is usually successful.
- 18 months to 4 years: Traction followed by open reduction; 90% of patients do well if reduction is successful.
- Older children/adults: Iliac osteotomies to improve acetabular coverage
- Total hip replacement is usually required over the long term.

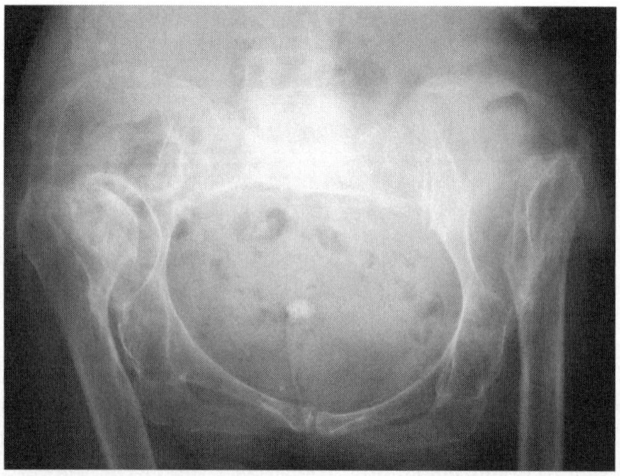
D

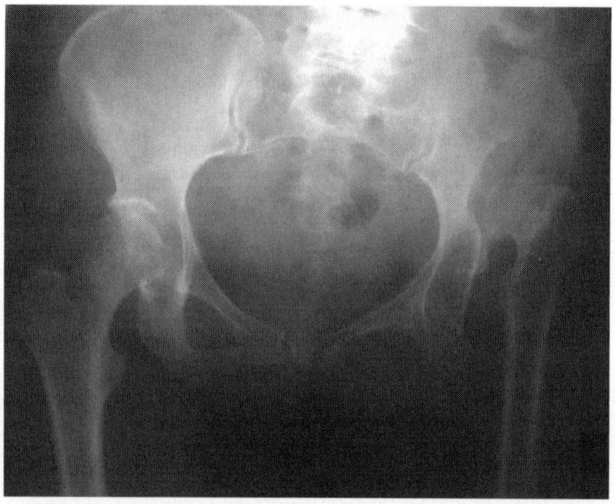
E

Figures 27D An AP radiograph shows untreated dysplastic hips, resulting in severe deformity and degenerative changes bilaterally. **27E** Untreated congenital dysplasia resulting in dramatic deformity, including development of a pseudoacetabulum on the lateral aspect of the ilium.

PEARLS

- The acetabular angle should be between 15 and 30 degrees, with angles > 30 degrees resulting in greater susceptibility to dislocation.
- If congenital dysplasia is suspected, the Von Rosen view should be performed.
- Ultrasound has an advantage over radiography in its ability to assess the acetabular cartilage, the acetabular labrum, and the unossified capital femoral epiphysis while avoiding the risks associated with the use of ionizing radiation in this age group.

PITFALLS

- The hip joint reduces in the frog-leg view, potentially leading to a false-negative result.
- Ultrasound should be delayed until the third week of life, as up to 6 mm of subluxation is within normal limits for a newborn.
- Conventional radiographs cannot exclude congenital dislocated hip until the femoral head is ossified, which does not occur before 6 months and which is further delayed by the presence of dysplasia.

Suggested Readings

Gerscovich EO. A radiologist's guide to the imaging in the diagnosis and treatment of developmental dysplasia of the hip: 1. General considerations, physical examination as applied to real-time sonography and radiography. Skeletal Radiol 1997;26:386–397

Schlesinger AE, Hernandez RJ. Diseases of the musculoskeletal system in children: imaging with CT, sonography, and MR. Am J Roentgenol 1992;158:729–741

Walter RS, Donaldson JS, Davis CL, et al. Ultrasound screening of high-risk infants: a method to increase early detection of congenital dysplasia of the hip. Am J Dis Child 1992;146:230–234

CASE 28

Brian Edward Reeves, Anthony G. Ryan, Peter L. Munk, and Thomas Pope

Clinical Presentation

A 16-year-old girl presented with back pain. Physical exam revealed that she has short arms and legs and macrocephaly, and she is bowlegged.

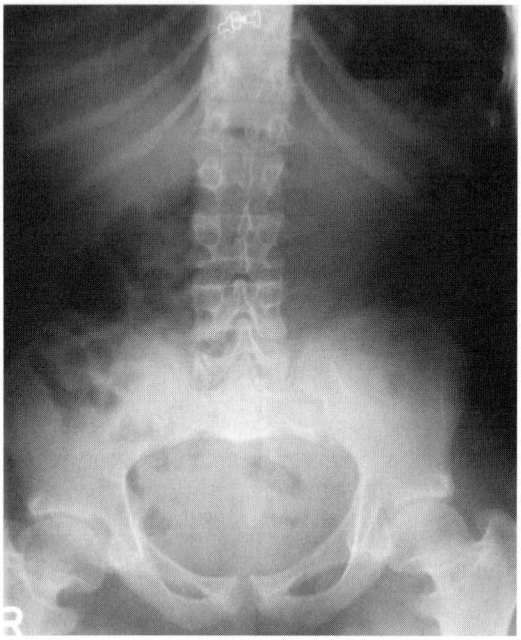

Figure 28A

Radiologic Findings

A lumbar spine anteroposterior (AP) radiograph (**Fig. 28A**) shows lumbar spinal stenosis with a gradual decrease in interpedicular width cranially to caudally. Squaring of the iliac wings and bilateral coxa vara deformities are also seen. The femoral necks are short and thick bilaterally.

Diagnosis

Achondroplasia.

Differential Diagnosis

Although other rhizomelic short-limbed dwarf syndromes may have similar radiographic findings, the combination of the typical phenotype and radiographic findings makes no other diagnosis admissible.

Discussion

Background

Achondroplasia, affecting ~1 in every 25,000 to 40,000 births, is the most common short-limbed dwarf syndrome. The characteristic features of achondroplasia are present at birth, and diagnosis is made by physical examination and the characteristic skeletal radiographic findings.

Etiology

Affecting all races and both sexes, achondroplasia is transmitted as an autosomal dominant disorder with complete penetrance. Eighty percent of achondroplasia cases are caused by mutations in the gene for fibroblast growth factor receptor-3, whose primary function is to limit osteogenesis. These mutations severely limit enchondral ossification. Advanced paternal age (> 40 years old) is identified as a major risk factor.

Pathophysiology

Achondroplasia is due to a defect in enchondral bone formation, with a resulting decrease in the rate at which epiphyseal cartilage cells convert to bone. This results in shortening of the long bones and a decrease in vertebral body and posterior arch diameters.

Clinical Findings

Gross motor development is frequently delayed, and head control, standing, and ambulation can lag behind by 6 months. Speech and language problems may occur because of the abnormal maxillomandibular relationship. Cognitive skills are preserved.

Physical examination findings may include macrocephaly, frontal bossing, flattening of the nasal bridge, midface hypoplasia, and prominent mandibles. Recurrent otitis media is common due to poor drainage of the eustachian tube from underdevelopment of the midface, hypertrophy of the tonsils, and temporal bone abnormalities.

Standing height is below the third percentile, and sitting height is normal, consistent with rhizomelia. There is lack of full elbow extension, and a trident hand, characterized by a persistent space between the long and ring fingers, is often present. Hip flexion contractures, ligamentous laxity, and genu varum deformities can also be seen in the lower extremities and result in a waddling gait.

Spinal deformities are the most common and potentially debilitating features. Spinal and intervertebral foraminal stenosis may lead to back pain, leg pain, paresthesias, incontinence, dyesthesias, and neurogenic claudication. More than 50% of patients experience symptoms of lower extremity radiculopathy. The mean age of onset of back pain is 26 years; one third of patients are younger than 15 years of age at onset.

A small foramen magnum at the base of the skull may compress the cervicomedullary junction, causing symptoms of respiratory insufficiency, apnea, cyanotic episodes, feeding problems, quadriparesis, and sudden death.

Upper airway obstruction, a small chest wall, and pectus excavatum can reduce the vital capacity, leading to an increased incidence of pneumonia, cyanotic spells, and apnea.

Complications

Recurrent otitis media, hearing loss, hypotonia, respiratory insufficiency, apnea, cyanotic episodes, feeding problems, sudden death, upper airway obstruction, pneumonia, hydrocephalus, obesity, spinal canal stenosis, genu varum, and/or cardiovascular complications may develop.

Imaging Findings

RADIOGRAPHY

- A lateral skull may show midface hypoplasia, enlarged calvaria, frontal prominence, and shortening of the skull base.

- The frontal view of the lumbar spine often shows narrowing of the interpedicular widths cranially to caudally. The lateral lumbar spine view shows shortening of the pedicles and vertebral bodies with prominent posterior scalloping. The vertebral bodies are characteristically bullet-shaped in infancy and become mildly flattened in adulthood.
- Thoracolumbar kyphoscoliosis may also be present. The ribs are shortened, and the extremities will demonstrate metaphyseal flaring and be short and thick.
- The pelvis will be broad and short, with squaring of the ilii and narrow pelvic inlet.
- The distal femoral physes often have an inverted–V-shaped configuration, which is secondary to the central portion of the epiphyseal plate, being affected more than the periphery. Bowing deformities affect the tibia more than the femur, and the fibula is usually longer than the tibia.
- The radial head is frequently dislocated, and the distal ulna is usually shorter with a long styloid process. The proximal and middle phalanges of the hand are shorter and broader than the distal phalanges and metacarpals relative to normal.

COMPUTED TOMOGRAPHY

- The sizes of the foramen magnum and spinal canal are frequently narrowed. This is easily measured by CT.

MAGNETIC RESONANCE IMAGING

- MRI may show myelomalacia, intramedullary cysts, or angulation at the craniocervical junction. A baseline craniocervical MRI during infancy will be helpful if neurological symptoms develop later on.

Treatment

- There is no way to normalize skeletal development of children with the disorder. Growth hormone is currently being used to augment the height in people with achondroplasia. The greatest acceleration in growth velocity is seen during the first year of treatment and in those with the lowest growth velocities before treatment. Initiation of treatment before the age of 6 is recommended for maximum benefit.
- Leg-lengthening procedures using distraction osteogenesis have been performed. With the current techniques, 30 cm of length can be gained. Complications with the procedure have been reported in up to 35% of patients and include foot drop, vascular compromise, soft-tissue contractures, loss of motion, knee subluxation, and infection.
- Suboccipital decompressions and laminectomies may be performed for craniocervical compression and spinal stenosis, respectively.

Prognosis

- The standardized mortality ratio is increased for all age groups by a factor of 2.27 over that of the general population.
- In children younger than 4 years, death most commonly occurs due to brainstem compression, with sudden death.
- In individuals ages 5 to 24 years, central nervous system and respiratory abnormalities are the common causes of death.
- In persons ages 25 to 54 years, cardiovascular problems are the most frequent cause of death.

PEARLS

- The frontal view of the lumbar spine often shows narrowing of the interpedicular widths cranially to caudally.
- The lateral lumbar spine view shows shortening of the pedicles and vertebral bodies with prominent posterior scalloping.
- The vertebral bodies are characteristically bullet-shaped in infancy and become mildly flattened in adulthood.

PITFALLS

- The clinical phenotype is so characteristic, that false diagnoses are not encountered. Imaging is directed at demonstrating the complications of the condition, as outlined above.
- A baseline craniocervical MRI during infancy will be helpful if neurological symptoms develop later on; however, this is not routinely performed in many centers.
- Leg-lengthening procedures are associated with their own significant complications, including foot drop, vascular compromise, soft-tissue contractures, loss of motion, knee subluxation, and infection.

Suggested Readings

Lachman RS. Neurologic abnormalities in the skeletal dysplasias. Am J Med Genet 1997;69:33–43

Macpherson RI, Pai GS. Evaluation of newborns with skeletal dysplasias. Indian J Pediatr 2000;67:907–913

Takata S, Ikata T, Yonezu H, Inoue A. Effects of lower leg lengthening on bone mineral density and soft tissue composition of legs in a patient with achondroplasia. J Bone Miner Metab 2000;18:339–341

Thomeer RT, van Dijk JM. Surgical treatment of lumbar stenosis in a patient with achondroplasia. J Neurosurg 2002;96(3 Suppl):292–297

CASE 29

Anthony G. Ryan and Peter L. Munk

Clinical Presentation

A child presented with increasing irritability over the previous several weeks with marked swelling and tenderness in both lower extremities. Birth history was unavailable, as the child was adopted shortly after birth. Clinical examination demonstrated pain in both lower extremities affecting both thighs and legs. Examination was otherwise unremarkable apart from bilateral sport affecting the sclera of both eyes.

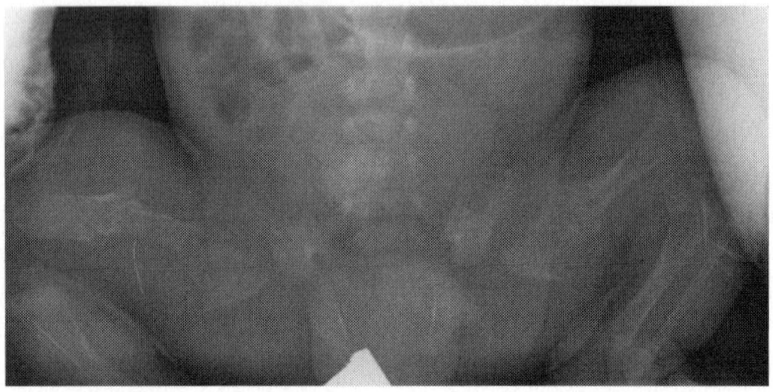

Figure 29A

Radiologic Findings

A frog-leg view of the hips and thighs (**Fig. 29A**) shows bilateral partially healed fractures. Two fractures are noted on the left with a single fracture distally on the right. The fractures appear subacute.

Diagnosis

Osteogenesis imperfecta.

Differential Diagnosis

- Nonaccidental injury. Although the pattern is not classic for nonaccidental injury (that is, metaphyseal corner injuries), this must be considered.
- Menkes' kinky hair syndrome

Discussion

Background

Osteogenesis imperfecta describes a group of genetic conditions of varying severity resulting in multiple pathologic fractures in the fetus, neonatal period, or childhood, the diagnosis of which is made from clinical, genetic, and radiographic features.

Radiologists are frequently called as expert witnesses and asked to distinguish osteogenesis imperfecta from child abuse to avoid an improper accusation of child abuse in a child with obvious osteogenesis imperfecta.

Etiology

- *Type 1* Autosomal dominant inheritance
- *Type 2* Autosomal recessive inheritance
- *Type 3* Autosomal recessive inheritance
- *Type 4* Autosomal dominant inheritance (latent)

Pathophysiology

This disorder of connective tissue, found in 1 in 40,000 births, affects the synthesis and quality of fibrillar collagen, resulting in congenital osteoporosis secondary to inadequate osteoid formation with normal mineralization. Inadequate amounts of osteoid are produced to balance physiological osteolysis.

The bones are osteoporotic, gracile, and, consequently, extremely fragile, causing bowing and fractures. Excessive callus formation is characteristic and may involve the entire length of the bone. Some fractures may heal with a pseudoarthrosis.

Depending on the subtype, at presentation deformities from previous fractures may be dominant, or the bones may be bowed secondary to microfractures.

Clinical Findings

Osteogenesis imperfecta may be diagnosed antenatally by chorionic villus sampling.

Type 1

Also known as osteogenesis imperfecta tarda, patients are typically of normal birth weight and length. The first fracture typically occurs in the second or third year of life, although presentation may be as early as delivery (intrapartum fractures in 20%) or as late as 6 years of age.

On examination, blue sclerae (found in 90%) and presenile deafness (20% secondary to otosclerosis and auditory nerve impingement) will be seen. There are variable dental findings (30%) secondary to dentin dysplasia. Joint hypermobility may be evident secondary to ligamentous laxity.

Type 2

These children are frequently stillborn or die soon postnatally secondary to pulmonary hypoplasia.

- Blue sclera, loose skin, and ligamentous laxity are typical.
- The limbs may be shortened and obviously deformed.
- Polyhydramnios may be clinically evident antenatally.

Type 3

- This is a progressively deforming disorder that is compatible with life.
- The sclerae, blue at birth, usually turn pale with time. The vertebrae and pelvis are typically normal. The deformities of the limbs and spine are progressive. Children have normal hearing.
- Fractures are present at birth in over 60% of cases. These fractures heal well, although they tend to lead to progressive limb deformity during childhood and adolescence. There may be occasional subsequent fractures.

Type 4

This is the mildest form with the best prognosis.

- The sclerae are normal.
- Deafness is rare.
- The teeth are discolored.
- The bones are fragile, however; genu valgum and coxa vara are the most frequent deformities secondary to bowing, and deformities become evident when the child begins to walk.

Stages of Disease

The condition is classified into four major types.

- *Type 1* Also known as osteogenesis imperfecta tarda or Ekman-Lobstein syndrome. It is a more benign form with a normal life expectancy.
- *Type 2* Also known as osteogenesis imperfecta congenita or Vrolik-type, this has the worst prognosis, resulting in severe hypomineralization. This is the most frequent variety and usually results in death in utero or in the neonatal period usually due to intracranial hemorrhage. Typically, it is detected prenatally on antenatal ultrasound.
- *Type 3* This is a progressively deforming disorder compatible with life.
- *Type 4* This is the mildest form with the best prognosis.

Types 1 and 2 account for the vast majority of cases; both types 3 and 4 are rare. Types 1 and 4 are frequently classed together as osteogenesis imperfecta tarda.

Complications

Type 1

- Presenile deafness found in 20% secondary to otosclerosis and auditory nerve impingement
- 30% demonstrate variable dental findings secondary to dentin dysplasia.
- Early degenerative joint disease secondary to ligamentous laxity
- Osteoporosis and bowing of the long bones; may experience fractures during delivery

Type 2

- Frequently stillborn or die soon postnatally secondary to pulmonary hypoplasia or from intracranial hemorrhage secondary to abnormal platelet function
- Multiple fractures
- The long bones may be shortened, broad, and crumpled.
- Bone angulation, bowing, and demineralization will be seen.
- Platyspondyly secondary to spinal osteopenia
- Mitral valve prolapse or aortic regurgitation may occur secondary to the abnormal collagenous structure of the valves.

Type 3

- Fractures are present at birth in over 60% of cases.
- Progressive deformities of the limbs and spine during childhood and adolescence

Type 4

- Osteoporosis resulting in widespread cortical thinning, bone fragility, and frequent fractures
- Severe kyphoscoliosis
- Discolored dentition
- Ligamentous laxity predisposes to premature degenerative joint disease.
- A case of osteosarcoma complicating osteogenesis imperfecta has been reported.

Pathology

GROSS

Abnormalities, primarily a global weakening, may be evident in bones, organ capsules, fascia, cornea, sclera, tendons, cardiac valves, meninges, and dermis.

MICROSCOPIC

The underlying disorder is evident as a defect in the conversion of procollagen to type I collagen with abnormal cross-linking. There are, however, normal osteoblastic function and intramembranous bone formation.

Imaging Findings

RADIOGRAPHY

Type 1

- Osteoporosis
- The first fracture typically occurs in the second or third year of life, although presentation may be as early as delivery (intrapartum fractures in 20%) or as late as 6 years of age (**Fig. 29B**).
- Bowing of the long bones may be seen (**Fig. 29C**).
- There are variable dental findings (30%) second to dentin dysplasia.
- Ligamentous laxity is common, leading to early degenerative joint disease.

Type 2

- Bone angulation, bowing, and demineralization are common.
- The long bones may be shortened, broad, and crumpled.
- Localized bone thickening may be seen secondary to callus formation.
- The ribs are typically thin and beaded with a concave superior margin, abnormal rotation, and curvature as a result of multiple fractures, producing a bell-shaped chest.
- The skull is typically poorly ossified.
- There is spinal osteopenia and platyspondyly.

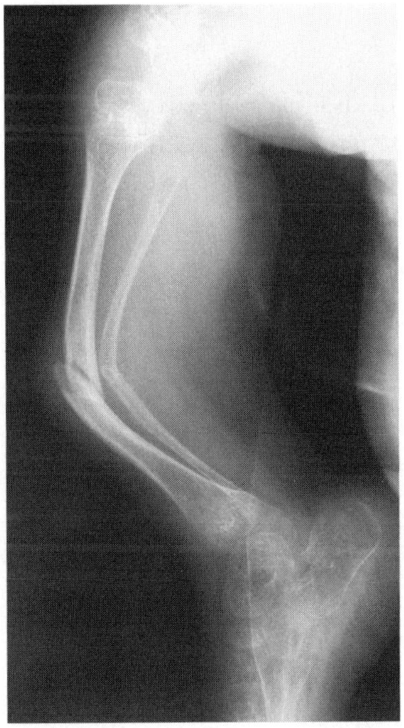
B

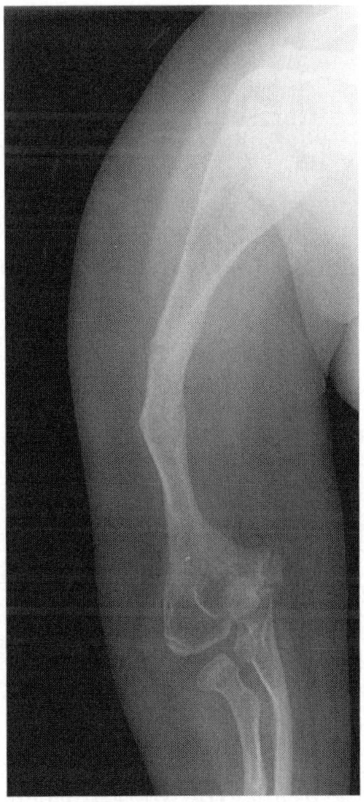
C

Figures 29B Midshaft fracture of the tibia and fibula with angulation at the fracture site. Note the diffuse diminished mineralization. **29C** Right humeral radiograph shows a partially healed midshaft fracture. Deformity with bowing is noted.

Type 3

- Fractures are present at birth in over 60% of cases. These fractures heal well, however.
- The vertebrae and pelvis are typically normal at birth.
- The deformities of the limbs and spine are progressive during childhood and adolescence.
- Elongated lumbar pedicles may become evident over time.

Type 4

- Osteoporosis
- Skull: platybasia, basilar invagination. Wormian bones are frequently found in the skull.
- Abnormal dentition
- The vertebral bodies become biconcave, and intervertebral disk height increases. Schmorl's nodules develop, and vertebral scalloping become evident. These features collectively result in severe kyphoscoliosis.
- Protrusio acetabuli (arthrokatadysis) is common.
- The tubular bones are of normal length; however, mild femoral bowing may occur resulting in genu valgum or coxa vara.
- There is an increase in the diameter of the proximal ends of the humeri and femora with multiple cystlike areas demonstrated throughout.
- 52% of patients with type IV osteogenesis are said to have "popcorn" calcifications (a collection of scalloped radiolucencies, each with a sclerotic margin) at one or more sites, which are observed only during active skeletal growth. They are not present at birth, occur predominantly around the knees and ankles, and are associated with irregularity or absence of the normal horizontal growth plate. These calcifications appear to result from fragmentation and disordered maturation of the physis, and their presence indicates a disturbance in enchondral ossification.

ANTENATAL ULTRASOUND

Type 1

- On antenatal ultrasound, bowing of the long bones may be seen; however, no intrauterine growth retardation is demonstrated.

Type 2

- There may be increased through transmission of the skull secondary to lack of ossification with enhanced visualization of the intracranial contents. The skull vault may be paper thin and seen to be compressed by the transducer.
- The skeleton is less well seen than expected.
- There may be multiple in utero fractures with long bone angulation and thickening.
- Polyhydramnios is a frequent finding.
- A normal antenatal ultrasound after 17 weeks excludes the diagnosis.

Type 3

- Short and bowed long bones ± accompanying fractures
- The humerus tends to be less severely involved than the femur.

Type 4

On antenatal ultrasound, the criteria of diagnosis are

- Multiple fractures
- Demineralization of the calvaria
- Femoral length more than 3 standard deviations below the mean for gestational age

However, not all the criteria are necessary for diagnosis. In the absence of fractures, bowing of the long bones may be evident.

Treatment

Skin biopsy for collagen analysis may be needed to aid in the diagnosis in confusing or mild cases.

MEDICAL THERAPY

Various therapies have been utilized, including oral 3-amino-1-hydroxypropylidene-1,1-bisphosphonate (APD), in a regime of 250 mg daily, for periods of 2 months, alternating with periods of 2 months of abstinence for a year, with striking radiological and clinical improvement. Post-treatment radiographs demonstrated large, metaphyseal parallel radio-opaque striae, corresponding to the periods of therapy.

INTERVENTIONAL RADIOLOGY

Percutaneous vertebroplasty has been used in a patient with a vertebral body compression fracture secondary to osteogenesis imperfecta.

Prognosis

- *Type 1* This is a more benign form with a normal life expectancy.
- *Type 2* This subtype has the worst prognosis, resulting in severe hypomineralization. It usually results in death in utero or in the neonatal period.
- *Type 3* This is a progressively deforming disorder compatible with life.
- *Type 4* This is the mildest form with the best prognosis.

PEARLS

- A normal antenatal ultrasound after 17 weeks excludes the diagnosis of type 2 osteogenesis imperfecta.
- Although osteogenesis imperfecta may be implicated, nonaccidental injury should be considered in all cases of pediatric rib fracture, particularly fracture of the first rib. Mechanisms for the latter include impact or compressive forces and shaking or acute axial load (slamming), which cause an indirect fracture.
- 52% of patients with type 4 osteogenesis imperfecta have "popcorn" calcifications at one or more sites.

PITFALLS

- The exuberant callus formation may produce bizarre deformities and simulate an osseous malignancy.
- Pseudoarthroses may arise secondary to abnormal joint fracture healing.
- The abnormally wide cranial sutures may simulate increased intracranial pressure.

Suggested Readings

Ablin DS. Osteogenesis imperfecta: a review. Can Assoc Radiol J 1998;49:110–123

Devogelaer JP, Malghem J, Maldague B, Nagant de Deuxchaisnes C. Radiological manifestations of bisphosphonate treatment with APD in a child suffering from osteogenesis imperfecta. Skeletal Radiol 1987;16:360–363

Gagliardi JA, Evans EM, Chandnani VP, Myers JB, Pacheco CM. Osteogenesis imperfecta complicated by osteosarcoma. Skeletal Radiol 1995;24:308–310

Goldman AB, Davidson D, Pavlov H, Bullough PG. "Popcorn" calcifications: a prognostic sign in osteogenesis imperfecta. Radiology 1980;136:351–358

Munoz C, Filly RA, Golbus MS. Osteogenesis imperfecta type II: prenatal sonographic diagnosis. Radiology 1990;174:181–185

Pretorius DH, Rumack CM, Manco-Johnson ML, et al. Specific skeletal dysplasias in utero: sonographic diagnosis. Radiology 1986;159:237–242

Rami PM, McGraw JK, Heatwole EV, Boorstein JM. Percutaneous vertebroplasty in the treatment of vertebral body compression fracture secondary to osteogenesis imperfecta. Skeletal Radiol 2002;31:162–165

CASE 30

Peter L. Munk and Anthony G. Ryan

Clinical Presentation

A 32-year-old woman presented with left shoulder pain after a fall, which also resulted in left femoral neck fracture. She has a long history of fractures and is also anemic.

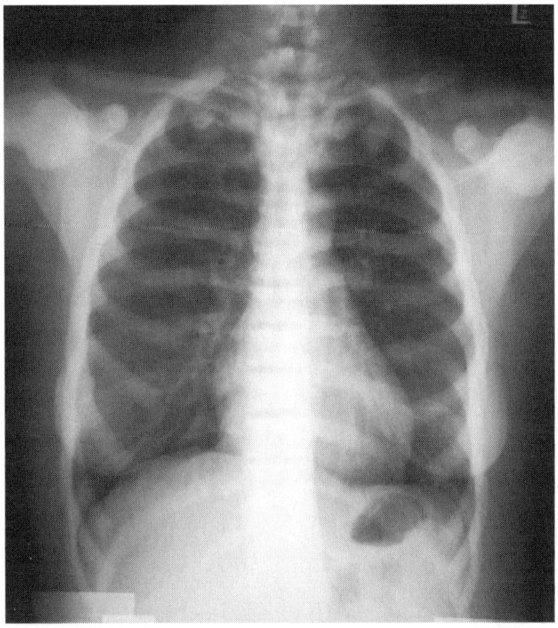

Figure 30A

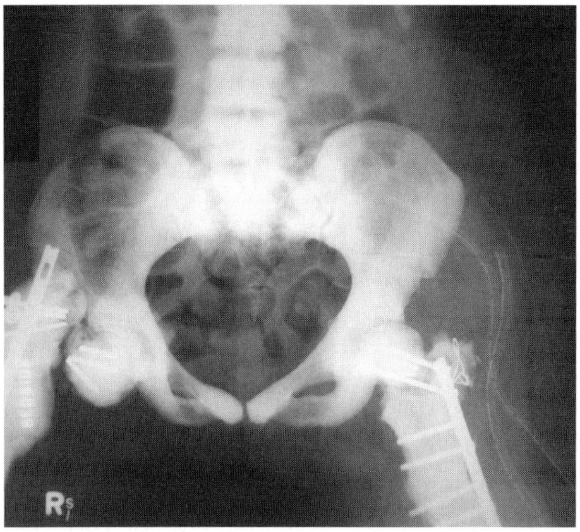

Figure 30B

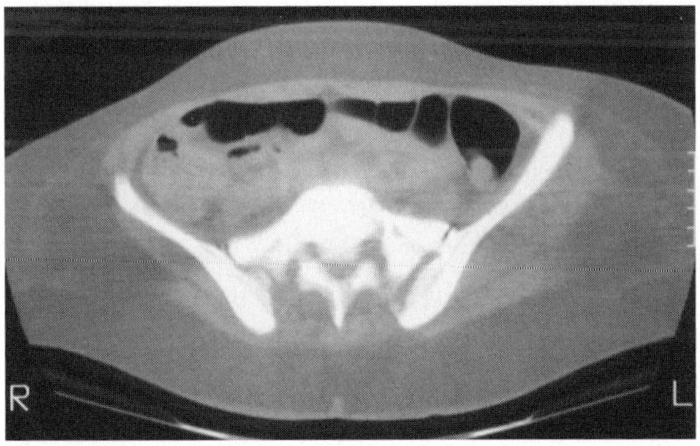

Figure 30C

Radiologic Findings

All images from this 32-year-old woman show a generalized increase in bone density. The chest film (**Fig. 30A**) shows that all osseous elements are sclerotic and that, in addition, the left clavicle is fractured. The pelvic film (**Fig. 30B**) was obtained immediately after surgery to repair a left femoral neck fracture. All the bones are dense, and an old unhealed right hip fracture is present. A lamellated/arcs pattern is present within the iliac wings (bone within bone). The CT of the pelvis (**Fig. 30C**) once again shows diffuse increased density and no obvious marrow space.

Diagnosis

Osteopetrosis.

Differential Diagnosis

The appearance is usually characteristic; however, the differential includes

- Myelofibrosis
- Renal osteodystrophy
- Mastocystosis
- Fluorosis

Discussion

Background

Osteopetrosis is a bone dysplasia associated with deficient osteoclast activity and consequent increased bone density. Abnormal remodeling results in brittle bone that is prone to fracture. In addition, the marrow cavity becomes extremely narrowed, resulting in deficient bone marrow and secondary bone marrow failure.

Etiology

A variety of different subtypes exist with differing severity, depending on the means of transmission and penetrance. There are infantile and adult forms; the infantile severe autosomal recessive osteopetrosis (ARO) is, in part, due to mutations in the *Atp6a3* (*TCIRG1*) and *ClCN7* genes in 60% and 13%, respectively; whereas the adult autosomal dominant osteopetrosis (ADO) form (also known as tarda) is thought to be secondary to *ClCN7* mutation. The degree of dominant interference with chloride channel function varies widely even in patients with identical genetic makeup. Mutations in the gene coding for an osteoclast-specific vacuolar pump have also been described, contributing to osteoclast dysfunction.

Pathogenesis

- Bony encroachment on the optic nerve in the optic foramen causes progressive visual loss.
- A combination of auditory nerve compression, ossicle sclerosis, and/or chronic middle ear effusion results in a third of patients having some degree of hearing loss.
- Bony pressure at the nerve root in rare instances results in peripheral motor nerve dysfunction.
- Chronic anemia, feeding problems caused by bulbar nerve involvement, nasal congestion, and recurrent infections result in failure to thrive in affected infants.
- In addition to the changes in bone composition, leukocyte superoxide generation is defective, resulting in an increased susceptibility to infection, especially viral respiratory infections. Pneumonia and septicemia are thus frequent causes of death in the severe infantile form.
- Abnormal dentinogenesis, in combination with the predisposition to infection, leads to frequent dental problems, failure of tooth eruption, and recurrent caries. In the adult form, this is occasionally the presentation that leads to the delayed diagnosis.
- Rarely, neurodegeneration results in developmental delay or regression or seizures.

Clinical Findings

The most severe form is seen in infants and significantly diminishes life expectancy, usually due to bone marrow failure and infection. Affected children usually present within the first year of life; poor vision (usually noticed by parents) is the most common presenting complaint, followed by failure to thrive and recurrent infection. In older children, the typical triad of fractures, visual impairment, and bone marrow failure occurs regularly.

Adults have a delayed type or an intermediate recessive type. Although some patients may have minimal symptomatology, patients with this disease are often detected because of pathologic fractures or difficulties with dentition and tooth extraction.

Pathology

GROSS

- Thickened sclerotic bones with a severely limited marrow cavity

MICROSCOPIC

- Persistent areas of primary spongiosa with cores of calcified cartilage within the bone

Imaging Findings

RADIOGRAPHY

On radiography, the bones are noted to be diffusely osteosclerotic and show thickened cortex and abnormal tabulation with loss of the normal corticomedullary differentiation, often having a club-like appearance, particularly in children. A "bone-within-a-bone" appearance is often encountered, most frequently seen in the metacarpals.

A skeletal survey is advised in children to evaluate the extent of disease, skull views often demonstrating craniosynostosis when frontal bossing and macrocephaly are evident clinically.

CROSS-SECTIONAL IMAGING

- Marrow space obliteration will be clearly evident on both CT and MRI.
- Compensatory extramedullary hematopoiesis with hepatosplenomegaly may be demonstrated secondary to severe anemia and thrombocytopenia.
- Neural foraminal narrowing may be evident, for example, of the optic foramina or internal acoustic meatus.
- Pronounced calvarial thickening may result in limitation in intracranial volume in particularly severe cases. MRI of the brain is advised in these cases, as central nervous system involvement is often associated with rapidly progressive disease with a poor prognosis.
- CT may be indicated in cases of craniosynostosis where surgical correction is considered.

Treatment

Therapy has employed symptomatic treatment for fractures and nerve compression (although optic nerve decompression has been shown to be overly risky with unproven benefit), as well as steroids and parathormone in an effort to stimulate osteoclast activity. High-dose calcitriol and recombinant human interferon gamma-1b have also been used with varying degrees of success.

Bone marrow transplantation may be required to ensure hematopoietic competency and improved leukocyte function. Prior to marrow transplant, anemia may require repeated transfusions.

Most fractures are treated with closed methods, and the fracture heals normally but with some delay. Because of the sclerotic bone, open treatment with fixation can be technically demanding, especially intramedullary rod fixation, because of the obliteration of the normal marrow cavity. Furthermore, bleeding and infective complications are common.

Chronic middle ear effusion is treated by ventilation tubes (grommets).

Surgical vault release for craniosynostosis associated with osteopetrosis is fraught with danger, as underlying cerebral venous obstruction at the level of the exit foramina predisposes these patients to severe, sometimes uncontrollable peri- and postoperative hemorrhage.

Prognosis

In the infantile form, there is a high mortality rate in the first 2 years of life (those with severe disease dying before the age of 3 months), secondary to bone marrow failure and overwhelming infection.

Transfusion dependency prior to 3 months of age is an indicator of severe disease and thus a poor prognostic sign. Children surviving past 2 years of age who are not transfusion-dependent have a more favorable prognosis. Bone marrow transplantation significantly alters the course of disease, although patients may still experience orthopedic and dental problems.

PEARLS

- Although some patients may have minimal symptomatology, this disease is often detected because of pathologic fractures or difficulties with dentition and tooth extraction.
- Although there are several rare, genetic conditions associated with osteosclerosis, osteopetrosis is one of the few diseases that are associated with anemia and visual impairment.

PITFALLS

- Although densely sclerosed, abnormal remodeling results in brittle bone that is prone to fracture.
- Maintaining nutrition in affected children may be challenging, as securing nasogastric access can be difficult secondary to choanal narrowing, nasal congestion, and obstructive sleep apnea.
- Gastrostomy (regardless of implantation method: radiological, endoscopic, or surgical) is associated with a higher rate of infection, which may be critical for inpatients awaiting a bone marrow transplant.

Suggested Readings

Curé JK, Key LL, Goltra DD, VanTassel P. Cranial MR imaging of osteopetrosis. Am J Neuroradiol 2000;21:1110–1115

Kocher MS, Kasser JR. Osteopetrosis. Am J Orthop 2003;32:222–228

Stoker DJ. Osteopetrosis. Semin Musculoskelet Radiol 2002;6:299–305

Wilson CJ, Vellodi A. Autosomal recessive osteopetrosis: diagnosis, management, and outcome. Arch Dis Child 2000;83:449–452

CASE 31

Brian Edward Reeves, Anthony G. Ryan, Peter L. Munk, and Thomas Pope

Clinical Presentation

A 55-year-old man presented with right hip pain after a motor vehicle accident. An AP pelvic film and a preoperative chest x-ray were performed.

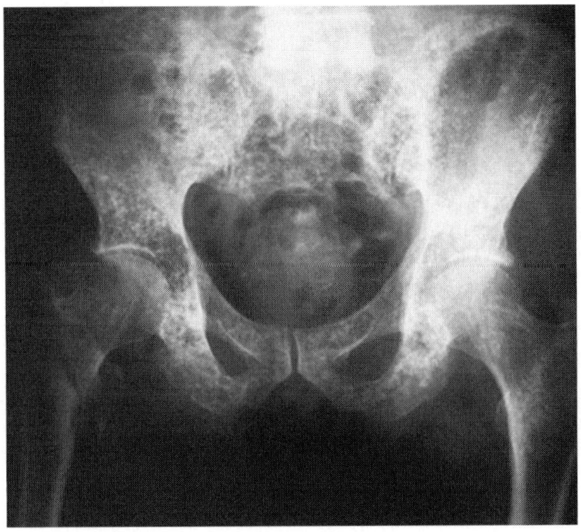

Figure 31A

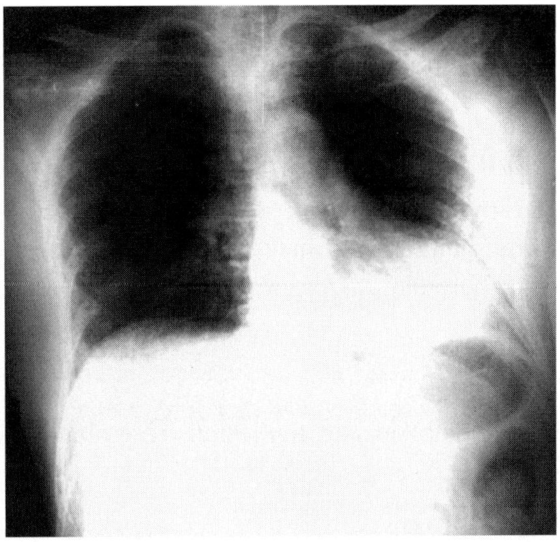

Figure 31B

Radiologic Findings

The pelvic film (**Fig. 31A**) shows a fracture of the right femoral neck. Also noted are several sclerotic bony foci with round to ovoid radiolucent centers. These foci are also diffusely present on the chest film (**Fig. 31B**). The enlarged cardiac silhouette is likely due to poor inspiratory effort.

Diagnosis

Osteopoikilosis.

Differential Diagnosis

- Osteoblastic metastases
- Mastocytosis
- Tuberous sclerosis

Discussion

Background

Osteopoikilosis (literally "spotted bone") is a benign, rare, hereditary bone disorder. Disorders reported to be associated with osteopoikilosis are osteopathia striata, melorheostosis, dermatofibrosis lenticularis disseminata, and subcutaneous fibrous nodules.

Etiology

The disease is inherited as a highly penetrant autosomal dominant trait.

Clinical Findings

Clinically, the patients have no symptoms, and most cases are found incidentally. The condition affects both genders and may be seen at any age; cutaneous lesions may be seen in up to 25% of patients. Laboratory values are normal.

Pathology

Grossly and histologically, the lesions resemble bone islands.

Imaging Findings

The diagnosis of osteopoikilosis is made by its characteristic radiographic appearance. The lesions are round, have uniformly sclerotic density, and vary in size from a few millimeters to several centimeters. They are scattered within cancellous bone, demonstrate continuity with the surrounding trabeculae, and are oriented parallel to the surrounding trabeculae.

The lesions are located symmetrically in the metaphysis and epiphysis of affected bones. The lesions cluster at the end of tubular bones, concentrated near joint surfaces, around the acetabulae, the glenoid, and in the carpus and tarsus of the hands and feet. Involvement of the axial skeleton is usually limited to the pelvis.

These foci may change in size or number, or even disappear during bone growth. The number of lesions often stabilizes at skeletal maturity.

Distinguishing the bone islands in osteopoikilosis from metastases is usually straightforward, as metastases tend to spare the epiphyses, whereas osteopoikilosis is most densely concentrated there.

PEARLS

- *Osteopoikilosis* means "spotted bone."
- Buschke-Ollendorff syndrome describes patients with osteopoikilosis and dermatofibrosis lenticularis disseminata.
- Involvement of the axial skeleton is usually limited to the pelvis.

PITFALLS

- Occasionally, there may be a patient with known malignancy and confusion between this entity and osteoblastic metastases. The study of choice for clarification would be a nuclear medicine bone scan. Bone scan activity is normal in osteopoikilosis and increased in metastatic disease (with the exception of the majority of myelomatous lesions).

- Distinguishing the bone islands in osteopoikilosis from metastases should be straightforward, as metastases tend to spare the epiphyses, whereas osteopoikilosis is most densely concentrated there.

Suggested Readings

Al Attia HM, Sherif AM. Buschke-Ollendorff syndrome in a grande multipara: a case report and short review of the literature. Clin Rheumatol 1998;17:172–175

Calimano M, Acosta A, Neitzschman H. Abnormal bone survey in a cancer patient: osteopoikilosis. J LA State Med Soc 2000;152:321–322

Kim GH, Dy LC, Caldemeyer KS, Mirowski GW. Buschke-Ollendorff syndrome. J Am Acad Dermatol 2003;48:600–601

Rucker PT, Sundaram M. Radiologic case study: osteopoikilosis. Orthopedics 1996;19:357–358

CASE 32

Anthony G. Ryan and Peter L. Munk

Clinical Presentation

A 40-year-old female patient reported chronic discomfort and stiffness in the lower extremities, that had been present for many years and had been slowly progressive.

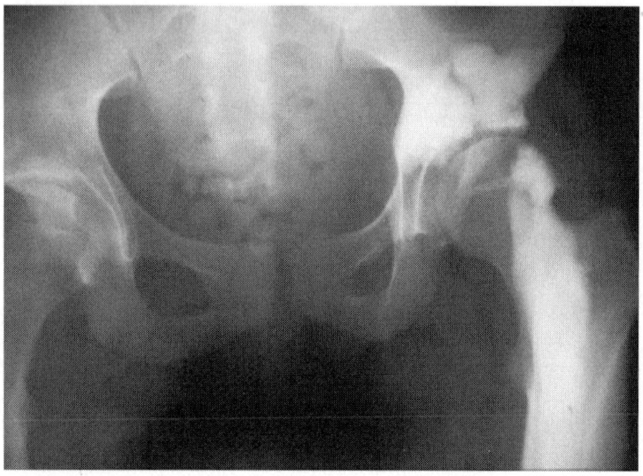

Figure 32A

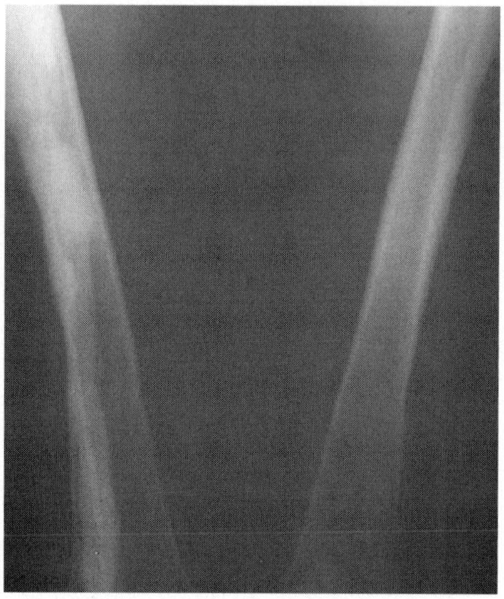

Figure 32B

Radiologic Findings

Radiographs of the pelvis and thighs were obtained. Anteriorposterior views of the pelvis (**Fig. 32A**) and femora (**Fig. 32B**) show areas of strikingly dense ossification involving the acetabulum and femur on the left. The ossification has a strikingly "flowing" pattern especially apparent in the femur. At the lateral aspect of the femur the margin of the ossification has an undulating lobulated appearance in keeping with the classic pattern of dripping candle wax. The changes involve both the cortex and adjacent soft tissue.

Diagnosis

Melorheostosis.

Differential Diagnosis

Other sclerosing bone dysplasias:

- Osteopetrosis (Albers-Schönberg disease)
- Pyknodysostosis (Maroteaux-Lamy syndrome)
- Enostosis (bone island)
- Osteopoikilosis
- Osteopathia striata (Voorhoeve's disease)
- Progressive diaphyseal dysplasia (Camurati-Engelmann disease)

- Hereditary multiple diaphyseal sclerosis (Ribbing disease)
- Four types of endosteal hyperostosis (van Buchem's syndrome, Worth disease, Nakamura disease, and Truswell-Hansen disease)
- Dysosteosclerosis
- Metaphyseal dysplasia (Pyle's disease)
- Craniometaphyseal dysplasia
- Craniodiaphyseal dysplasia

Other sclerosing lesions:

- Neurofibromatosis-associated hyperostosis
- Tuberous sclerosis and hemangiomas
- Pulmonary osteoarthropathy

Discussion

Background

Melorheostosis is a rare nongenetic congenital mesodermal anomaly that gives rise to a sclerosing bone dysplasia, predominantly affecting the long bones of the upper and lower limbs, the short bones of the hand and foot, and, rarely, the axial skeleton. Often diagnosed incidentally in adults, the condition is characterized radiologically by progressive hyperostotic linear densities in bone in a sclerotomal distribution (zones of the skeleton supplied by individual spinal sensory nerves). Multiple sclerotomes may be involved, and if so, the clinical manifestations are correspondingly more severe.

It may coexist in a so-called overlap syndrome known as mixed sclerosing bone dystrophy (MSBD) with osteopoikilosis and osteopathia striata, as well as with tumors, vascular malformations, lymphangiectasis, or fibrolipomatous lesions. Typically, the cutaneous and other clinical features occur in the same sclerotome as the affected bone(s).

Etiology

The etiology is unknown, although it is postulated to be a developmental error secondary to an embryonic metameric abnormality, resulting in disturbances in either enchondral or intramembranous bone formation, or both (abnormalities of the latter dominating).

The sclerotomal distribution has given rise to a theory proposing that melorheostosis may be the late result of a segmental sensory nerve lesion.

Pathophysiology

The developmental disturbances result in defects in bone resorption and/or formation during the processes of skeletal maturation and modeling, resulting in hyperostotic bone.

The abnormal sclerotic bone encroaches and impinges upon neighboring structures, causing severe pain and limited joint motion. The latter, in combination with associated neural involvement, frequently gives rise to muscular atrophy.

Clinical Findings

Chronic progressive pain is typical, with joint stiffness and decreased range of motion contributing to muscular atrophy and weakness. Patients present at any age, and both sexes are affected equally.

Although the condition may be recognized in infancy, onset is usually insidious, with deformity of the extremity, pain, limb stiffness, and limitation of motion in the joints first manifesting in late childhood or early adolescence, which then progress as the patient reaches skeletal maturity.

A scleroderma-type thickening and fibrosis of the overlying skin may be evident.

Complications

- Intolerable pain
- Joint contractures
- Cutaneous/subcutaneous fibrosis and subcutaneous edema
- Bursitis overlying bony spurs
- Varices
- May be associated with fibromatosis (desmoid tumor) of the adjacent soft tissues
- Rarely, superimposed osteosarcoma

Pathology

GROSS

- Bone remodeling leading to deformity in bones and associated joints
- Sclerotic bone encroaching/impinging upon neighboring neurovascular bundles
- Muscular atrophy
- Fibrous masses within the intervening soft tissues
- Scleroderma-type thickening and fibrosis of the overlying skin

MICROSCOPIC

There is a mixture of immature and mature bone with interlacing osteoid and thickening trabeculae that eventually obliterates the haversian system. Fibrous tissue may be seen within the marrow surrounding areas of new bone.

The associated soft-tissue masses are found histologically to be composed of vascularized fibrous tissue with variable collagen content.

Imaging Findings

RADIOGRAPHY

- Although the lesion typically begins as a linear hyperostosis, the characteristic radiographic appearance consists of continuous undulating hyperostotic cortical changes generally on one side of the bone, resembling melted wax dripping down one side of a candle. This appearance gives the anomaly its name, which is taken from the Greek words for *member* (*melos*) and *flow* (*rhein*).
- It may affect the entire cortex or may be limited to one side of the cortex; it also may extend into cancellous bone (**Fig. 32C**).
- The lesions are usually unilateral and diaphyseal with at least two bones involved in a sclerotomal distribution. The cortical new bone appears to accumulate toward the end of the bone, extending from diaphyses to metaphysis and typically from the proximal to the distal portion of the bone. Lesions may cross joints and give rise to an effusion.
- It is more frequent in the lower limb. There may be a discrepant limb length. Flexion contractures may be demonstrated in the hip and knee. Genu valgum or varus may be demonstrated at the knee. The patella may be dislocated.
- Although the axial skeleton is rarely involved, small opacities may be visualized within the scapula and hemipelvis, similar to osteopoikilosis.
- Para-articular ossified soft-tissue masses are found in up to 27% of patients, which may be related to involvement of a corresponding myotome.

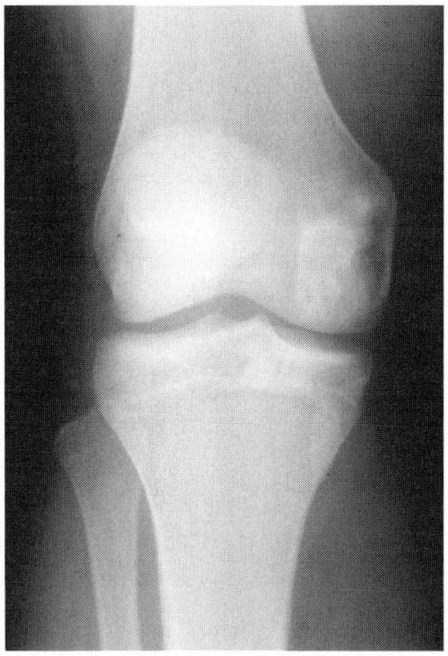

Figure 32C AP view of the knee shows an area of high calcific density that is mainly endosteal.

RADIONUCLIDE IMAGING

- Technetium 99m pyrophosphate bone scintigraphy shows moderate to marked increased focal uptake of tracer in each radiographically abnormal area.

COMPUTED TOMOGRAPHY

- CT demonstrates the cortical and trabecular thickening elegantly as cortical hyperostosis with expected high attenuation. It also aids in the evaluation of associated soft-tissue masses.
- Marrow space encroachment secondary to endosteal involvement is clearly seen.
- Muscular atrophy is usually evident.

Soft-tissue masses

- 50% of cases demonstrate extensive mineralization on CT, and 50% are nonmineralized.

MAGNETIC RESONANCE IMAGING

- Cortical hyperostosis is evident as markedly low signal intensity on all MR pulse sequences.
- Marrow space encroachment is well demonstrated.
- Muscle atrophy is evident as diminished muscle bulk and fatty infiltration.
- In individual cases, MRI is invaluable in evaluating the associated soft-tissue abnormalities, such as thickening of the iliotibial band and fibrosis in the subcutaneous tissues (low signal), that may need to be addressed as part of osseous and joint reconstructive surgery.

Soft-tissue masses

- The extensive mineralization of associated soft-tissue masses is evident as low intensity on all pulse sequences.
- Nonmineralized soft-tissue masses demonstrate intermediate signal intensity on T1-weighted and intermediate to high signal on T2-weighted images. When present, soft-tissue masses have infiltrative margins in 80% of cases.
- The soft-tissue masses enhance after intravenous gadolinium.

Treatment

- Treatment of this chronic and sometimes debilitating condition consists of surgical soft-tissue procedures and, in very severe cases, amputation.
- Early reports of the use of bisphosphonates (e.g., pamidronate infusion) show promise in the treatment of the pain and swelling of the affected limb.

Prognosis

- There tends to be a rapid progression in children, whereas the disease pursues a slow chronic course in adults.

PEARLS

- In melorheostosis, focal increased radiopharmaceutical accumulation appears in each radiographically abnormal area. Technetium 99m pyrophosphate bone images should prove helpful when superimposed osseous disease must be differentiated from osteopoikilosis, osteopathia striata, or melorheostosis.
- In differentiating melorheostosis from osteopoikilosis, the latter is typically much more diffuse and generalized.
- Melorheostosis may be differentiated from fibrous dysplasia because normal bone structure is retained in melorheostosis.

PITFALLS

- Some authors have proposed that the nonmineralized soft-tissue masses seen in association with melorheostosis should simply be recognized as another manifestation of the disease rather than concomitant neoplasia, making biopsy unwarranted; however, each lesion must be examined on its own merits and biopsy pursued if atypical features are present.
- Osteopathia striata is an asymptomatic autosomal dominant or sporadically inherited disorder that causes dense striations at sites of enchondral bone formation, with a predilection for the metaphyses of long bones.
- Pain should be investigated, rather than being ascribed to the bone and joint abnormalities, given the possibility of superimposed osteosarcoma.

Suggested Readings

Brennan DD, Bruzzi JF, Thakore H, O'Keane JC, Eustace S. Osteosarcoma arising in a femur with melorheostosis and osteopathia striata. Skeletal Radiol 2002;31:471–474

Greenspan A. Sclerosing bone dysplasias—a target-site approach. Skeletal Radiol 1991;20:561–583

Judkiewicz AM, Murphey MD, Resnik CS, Newberg AH, Temple HT, Smith WS. Advanced imaging of melorheostosis with emphasis on MRI. Skeletal Radiol 2001;30:447–453

Murray RO, McCredie J. Melorheostosis and the sclerotomes: a radiological correlation. Skeletal Radiol 1979;4:57–71

CASE 33

Hema N. Choudur, Anthony G. Ryan, and Peter L. Munk

Clinical Presentation

A family practitioner incidentally noted the absence of fingernails in a female patient. This raised suspicions of possible nail-patella syndrome, and the patient was investigated further. On clinical examination, her knees were noted to have a squared appearance but no other discernible skeletal abnormality.

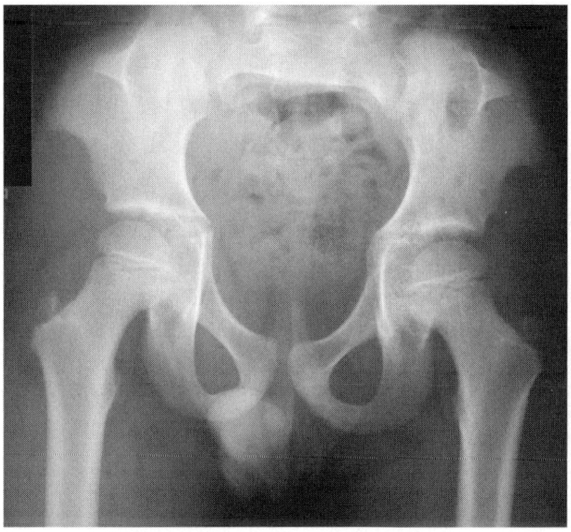

Figure 33A

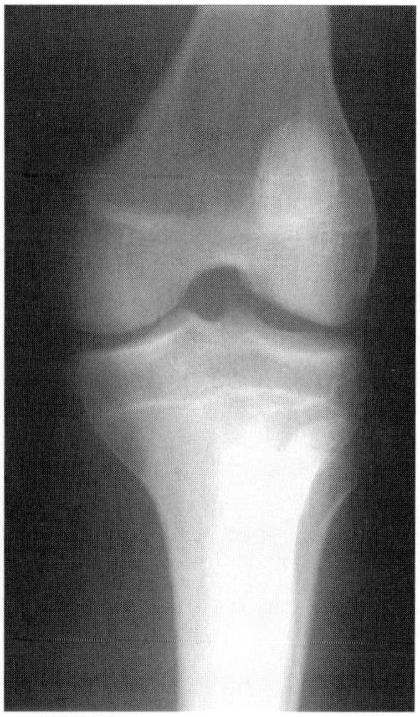

Figure 33B

Radiologic Findings

The plain radiographs of the pelvis (**Fig. 33A**) reveal pathognomonic iliac horns bilaterally. Hypoplastic patellae were noted in the knee radiographs (**Fig. 33B**).

Diagnosis

Nail-patella (Fong's) syndrome (NPS).

Differential Diagnosis

None. Iliac horns are pathognomonic.

Discussion

Background

NPS (Fong's disease or hereditary osteo-onychodysplasia (HOOD) iliac horn syndrome, Turner-Kieser syndrome) is characterized by typical skeletal abnormalities with frequently coexisting glaucoma and kidney disease.

Etiology

NPS has been recognized as a hereditary condition, with an autosomal dominant inheritance in the ABO blood group. The risk of transmission is 50% per pregnancy, irrespective of gender, females being affected ~10% more often than males. About 20% of cases are sporadic, as a result of a new mutation. The incidence is ~1 in 50,000, and the condition occurs in all ethnic groups.

Pathophysiology

The gene for NPS, recently discovered and named *LMX1B*, is located on chromosome 9q34. The pathophysiology underlying NPS is not yet known, but it is clear that the musculoskeletal abnormalities arise from a disorder of collagen synthesis, assembly, or degradation.

Clinical Findings

NAILS

Deformity of the nails is the most noticeable abnormality. The nails are either absent or underdeveloped, especially those of the thumbs, or may be brittle, cracked, concave, or ridged. Often, the lunalae (which are the light parts of the nail near the cuticle) are pointed instead of the usual rounded shape. Abnormality of the nails is seen in 80 to 90% of patients with NPS.

SKIN

The skin may be wrinkled and loose, although there are often no creases over the distal joints of the fingers, resulting in decreased mobility.

KNEES

Squared appearance of the knees is seen due to small or absent patellae and muscle, ligament, and bony abnormalities. Recurrent patellar dislocation is frequent. Hypoplastic patellae are seen in 60% of all NPS cases. Genu valgum may be present.

ELBOWS

The elbow joints and forearm bones are deformed, resulting in bent elbows with frequent dislocations. Tightening of the skin over the elbow with contractures results in a webbed appearance.

FEET

Twisted legs and/or clubfeet are often associated with NPS.

SPINE

Scoliosis worsens with age, and lordosis, which may be severe in children, may be an accompaniment.

KIDNEYS

About 30 to 50% of cases have renal involvement presenting with proteinuria, hematuria, and hypertension or as toxemia/preeclampsia in pregnancy. Some cases may progress to renal failure.

GLAUCOMA

There is a high incidence of glaucoma in families with NPS. This may be due to the fact that the glaucoma gene is similar to the NPS gene.

Other associated abnormalities include digestive/gastrointestinal disorders (e.g., irritable bowel syndrome), tipped uterus, toxemia of pregnancy/preelampsia/eclampsia, abnormal clover pattern pigmentation of the iris, receding hairline at temples, attention deficit hyperactivity disorder/learning disabilities, thyroid disorders, recurrent urinary tract disorders, waddling gait, poor teeth with thin enamel, spina bifida occulta, spinal stenosis, cleft lip and palate, and cataracts.

Soft-tissue abnormalities result from contractures and hypoplastic muscles (deltoid, triceps, and quadriceps).

Complications

A relatively small number of cases can progress to full renal failure and require kidney transplants. However, once a kidney transplant has been performed, it is usually successful, and no further kidney damage occurs.

Pathology

MICROSCOPIC

Renal histology changes by light microscopy are nonspecific, with localized thickening of the capillary wall and focal glomerular deposits of immunoglobulin M (IgM) and C3 demonstrable. The characteristic ultrastructural changes are localized areas of rarefaction of the glomerular basement membrane, with intramembranous deposits having the appearance and periodicity of collagen. On electron microscopy, the "moth-eaten" appearance is pathognomonic.

Imaging Findings

RADIOGRAPHY

Pelvis

Posterior iliac horns or crests are pathognomonic of NPS. This was described by Kieseer in 1939 and Fong in 1946. Bony outgrowths from the posterior ilium may be capped with an epiphysis. Rarely, outgrowths can be unilateral.

The horns themselves are rarely clinically significant. However, the hip joints may be abnormal and result in dislocations. Dysplastic iliac wings are often noted on plain radiographs.

Knees

Absence or hypoplasia of the patellae (**Fig. 33A**) is a characteristic finding that is a cause of recurrent patellar dislocation. Asymmetric development of the femoral condyles, with hypoplastic lateral condyles and true or apparent enlargement of the medial condyles, and sloping tibial plateau with a prominent tibial tubercle are the other features.

Spine

Scoliosis and lordosis are associated deformities and are often first detected on plain radiographs incidentally.

Elbows

Aplasia, hypoplasia, or a posterior process of the distal humerus with an increased carrying angle, limited extension and supination, hypoplastic capitulum, abnormal radioulnar articulation, and hypoplastic radial heads are often evident radiographic abnormalities.

Ankle and subtalar joints (talipes), shoulder, and wrist abnormalities can also occur.

Treatment

No definite treatment is known. Multidisciplinary management with a focus on the prevention and treatment of renal complications is recommended.

Prognosis

NPS is usually benign, but 10% of all NPS patients can develop end-stage renal failure, with either dialysis or transplantation becoming necessary.

Because the gene has been mapped (chromosome 9), it is possible to perform prenatal diagnosis for couples who do not wish to pass the syndrome to their children. This diagnosis requires a chorionic villus sample to be taken at ~10 weeks of gestation. However, it is not possible to determine how severe NPS would be relative to the affected parent or other children.

PEARLS

- Iliac horns are pathognomonic of NPS.
- Abnormality of the nails is seen in 80 to 90% of NPS.
- Hypoplastic patellae and abnormality of the nails are associated findings.
- The goal of treatment is to prevent renal complications.

Suggested Readings

Fong EE. "Iliac horns" (symmetrical bilateral central posterior iliac processes): a case report. Radiology 1946;47:517–518

Garces MA, Muraskas JK, Muraskas EK, Abdel-Hameed MF. Hereditary onchyo-osteo-dysplasia (HOOD syndrome): report of two cases. Skeletal Radiol 1982;8:55–58

Goshen E, Schwartz A, Zilka LR, Zwas ST. Bilateral accessory iliac horns: pathognomonic findings in nail-patella syndrome: scintigraphic evidence on bone scan. Clin Nucl Med 2000;25:476–477

Karabulut N, Ariyurek M, Erol C, Tacal T, Balkanci F. Imaging of "iliac horns" in nail-patella syndrome. J Comput Assist Tomogr 1996;20:530–531

Yarali HN, Erden GA, Karaarslan F, Bilgic SC, Cumhur T. Clavicular horn: another bony projection in nail-patella syndrome. Pediatr Radiol 1995;25:549–550

CASE 34

Anthony G. Ryan and Peter L. Munk

Clinical Presentation

A 22-year-old woman presented with chronic, worsening pain in her midfoot, exacerbated by, and now limiting participation in, recreational dance classes.

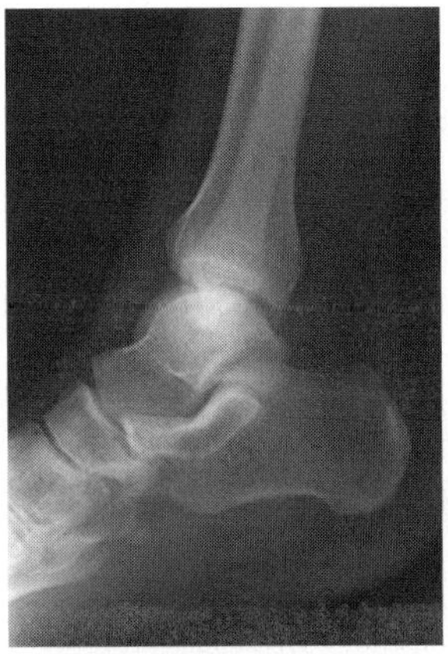

Figure 34A

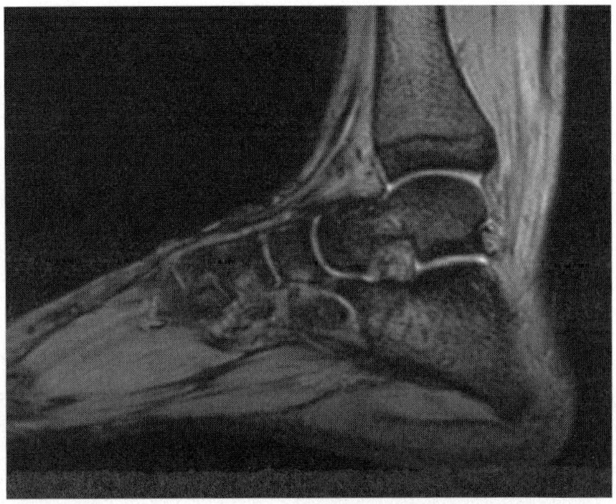

Figure 34B

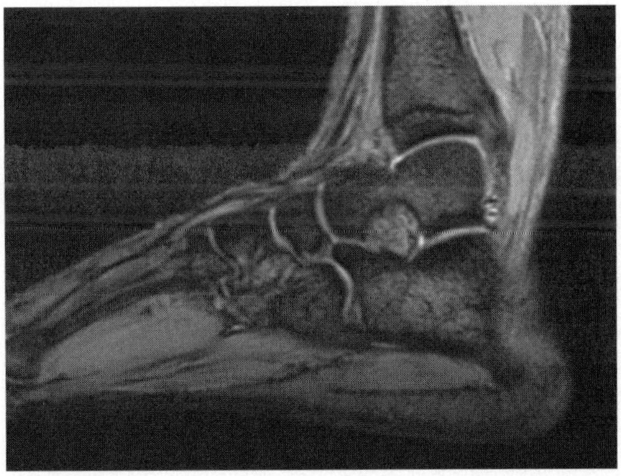

Figure 34C

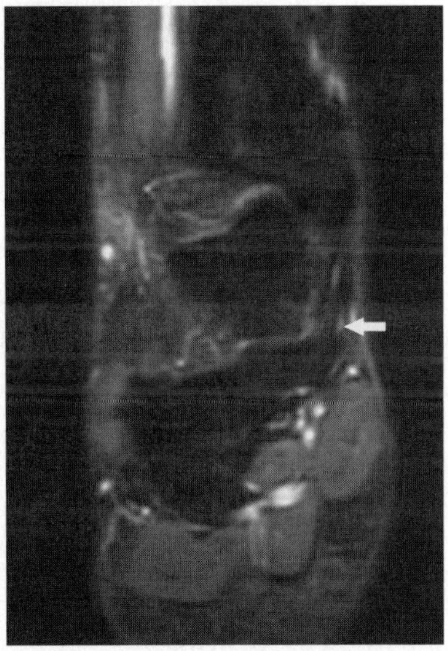

Figure 34D

Radiologic Findings

A lateral foot radiograph (**Fig. 34A**) demonstrates loss of definition of the posterior navicular wall and an elongated anterior process of the calcaneum, with an apparent bony bar extending between the two bones. Sagittal MPGR images (**Figs. 34B,34C**) demonstrate a clear union between the anterior calcaneum and posterior navicular. The junction between the two bones is of higher signal intensity than the adjacent cortex. The margins of the junction demonstrate irregular low signal intensity encroaching on the higher signal region. The higher signal intensity does not reach that of cartilage. A coronal T2-weighted fat-saturated image (**Fig. 34D**) shows contiguity of the calcaneum and navicular at this site (arrow).

Diagnosis

Calcaneonavicular coalition (partially ossified fibrous union).

Differential Diagnosis

Acquired intratarsal ankylosis secondary to infection, trauma, arthritis, or surgery.

Discussion

Background

Tarsal coalition is defined by abnormal fibrous, cartilaginous, or bony fusion of two or more tarsal bones. Bony coalition is characterized by the presence of a bony bar that extends between the involved bones.

Complete fusion, when present, usually occurs by the age of 12.

In the absence of a bony bar, fibrous and cartilaginous coalitions are usually evident by the presence of sclerosis and close approximation of the bones in question.

Etiology

Tarsal coalition is usually sporadic. Talocalcaneal tarsal coalition occurs as a result of failure of tarsal bone segmentation.

Talonavicular coalition is uncommon and may be associated with a genetic hereditary transmission, either dominant or recessive; it has a described association with anomalies of the little finger.

The association of coalition with other malformations suggests that the ball-and-socket ankle joint that can occur in patients with coalition results from a global developmental abnormality of the ankle and foot.

Pathophysiology

At birth, the coalition is liable to be fibrous, with ossification occurring during the second decade of life. The resulting ankylosis leads to abnormal biomechanical forces, which may in turn cause the development of secondary osteoarthritis.

Clinical Findings

The patient may be asymptomatic, and the abnormality may be discovered incidentally at the time of trauma or because of limitation of athletic interests. When symptomatic, the majority of coalitions may present with a painful flatfoot with associated peroneal spasm.

On examination, subtalar movements are limited (inversion/eversion and anterior gliding). A tarsal tunnel syndrome may be present.

Although calcaneonavicular coalition is the most common coalition, including all subtypes, that is, bony, cartilaginous, and fibrous, talocalcaneal coalition accounts for ~60% of bony coalitions and is thus seen more frequently on conventional radiographs. Quoted figures for the incidence of bilaterality vary dramatically from 20 to 80%.

Occasionally, there is more than one type of coalition in the same foot.

TALOCALCANEAL COALITION

- This condition gives rise to a painful peroneal spastic flatfoot, which is relieved by rest. Also seen is a diminished range of motion of the subtalar joints.

CALCANEONAVICULAR COALITION

- Clinical symptoms are usually less severe than with talocalcaneal coalition.
- Rigid flatfoot presenting in adolescence
- Equal sex prevalence

TALONAVICULAR COALITION

This is uncommon and may be associated with a genetic hereditary transmission, either dominant or recessive; it is associated with anomalies of the little finger.

The other tarsal coalitions, such as calcaneocuboid and talonavicular, are very uncommon.

Complications

The major complication is degenerative joint disease affecting not only the articulations of the involved bones but also those joints affected secondarily by the chronically altered biomechanics.

Imaging Findings

RADIOGRAPHY

Talocalcaneal coalition

Direct radiographic visualization of talocalcaneal coalition is more difficult than with other coalitions, and the classic teaching was that an axial (Harris) view of the calcaneum was required. The diagnosis is suggested by the presence of secondary radiographic signs, which have been well described:

- Talar beaking (present in up to 66% of cases, arising from the dorsal aspect of the head of talus)
- The C sign is often quoted as a characteristic finding in talocalcaneal coalition. This is a C-shaped line created by the outline of the talar dome and the inferior margin of the sustentaculum tali on lateral ankle radiographs. Studies differ on how useful the C sign actually is in making the diagnosis. It is specific, but not sensitive, for flatfoot deformity (hence the association with coalition).
- Also seen in the "anteater" sign, whereby the anterior process of the calcaneum is prominent and broad tipped compared with the usual triangular configuration (sensitivity 72%, specificity 94%).
- Broadening of the lateral process of the talus
- Concave undersurface of the talar neck and asymmetry of the talocalcaneal-navicular joint
- Narrowing of the posterior subtalar joint
- Ball-and-socket ankle mortise joint
- Other signs include nonvisualization of the middle facet, whereby the articular cortices and joint space of the middle facet are not visible (sensitivity 100%, specificity 42%); and a dysmorphic sustentaculum tali, which is enlarged with an ovoid shape on the lateral radiograph (sensitivity 82%, specificity 70%).

Calcaneonavicular coalition

Oblique radiographs are utilized, looking for a narrowed calcaneonavicular interval with indistinct articular margins.

The elongated anterior process of the calcaneum seen in coalition has been likened to the snout of an anteater—hence the so-called anteater sign.

Hypoplastic talar head

Crim and Kjeldsberg also described two new signs in relation to calcaneonavicular coalition on the anteroposterior (AP) radiograph of the foot, namely a "wide" navicular (wider than the articulating surface of the adjacent talus) (sensitivity 53%, specificity 98%) and a "laterally tapering" navicular; the lateral navicular is smaller from proximal to distal in comparison to the medial portion (sensitivity 50%, specificity 100%).

Talonavicular coalition

The bony coalition is usually seen clearly on radiography (**Fig. 34A**).

The ball-and-socket ankle joint is a malformation of the ankle in which the articular surface of the talus is hemispherical in both the AP and lateral projections and has a congruent, concave tibial articular surface. However, a ball-and-socket joint is seen in association with congenital malformations, such as short limb, and ray fusion and deletion anomalies or acquired secondary to myelomeningocele, and is thus not specific to coalition.

Joint space irregularity or loss may thus be demonstrated in the other tarsal joints, if there is superimposed osteoarthritis.

RADIONUCLIDE IMAGING

- Increased uptake in the region of the coalition (technetium 99m)

COMPUTED TOMOGRAPHY

Talocalcaneal coalition

CT has been shown to provide the most graphic depiction of bony coalition sites, but it also provides elegant demonstrations of the extent of joint involvement and secondary bony changes in the presence of fibrous coalitions.

- Best depicted on direct coronal or coronal reformats
- When osseous, a bony bar will be shown across the middle facet of the subtalar joint.
- In fibrous coalitions, there may be narrowing of the middle facet with reactive cystic and sclerotic changes of the underlying bone, but these findings may be subtle.
- A useful clue to the presence of a fibrous coalition in these cases is an abnormal orientation of the sustentaculum tali. The latter should normally slope upward medially; however, when coalition is present, it slopes downward (**Fig. 34E**), or, alternatively, the middle facet articular surface may be horizontally oriented.

MAGNETIC RESONANCE IMAGING

- MRI permits the differentiation of osseous from nonosseous coalitions.
- The extent of joint involvement is seen on MRI.
- Secondary degenerative changes are also seen.
- STIR images may demonstrate marrow edema at the margins of the coalition, providing secondary evidence of its presence, particularly when radiographic findings are equivocal.
- Synovitis affecting the subtalar joint has been mistaken for coalition, a potential pitfall in the use of MRI in these circumstances. The addition of gadolinium may be helpful in these cases, however, as synovitis is expected to enhance.

Treatment

- Surgery if the condition is painful and function has been limited

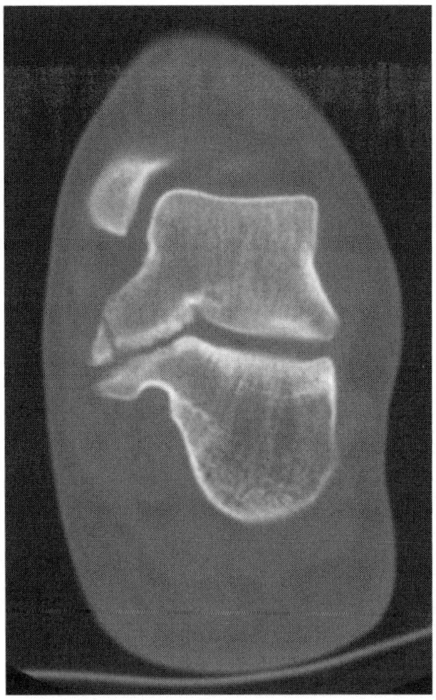

Figure 34E Direct coronal CT shows a downward-sloping sustentaculum, a narrowed joint space, and subtle adjacent sclerotic bony changes. A fibrous talocalcaneal coalition is present. The condition was discovered incidentally when the patient presented with ankle trauma, which caused the visible talar fracture.

Prognosis

A reasonable recovery is expected from surgery, depending on the age of the patient, the degree of ossification of nonosseous coalitions, and the degree of secondary degenerative joint disease present. Young patients with a fibrous coalition that is divided before any degeneration has set in are likely to do best.

PEARLS

- No articulation usually exists between the calcaneus and navicular bone; thus, if they are closely approximated and sclerosis is evident, calcaneonavicular coalition should be suspected.
- On the lateral radiograph, the "anteater" sign, whereby the anterior process of the calcaneum is prominent and broad tipped compared with the usual triangular configuration, is 94% specific for the diagnosis of calcaneonavicular coalition.
- A useful clue to the presence of a fibrous coalition in cases where the bony changes are subtle is the presence of an abnormal orientation of the sustentaculum tali. In the coronal plane, the latter should normally slope upward medially; however, when coalition is present, it slopes downward, or, alternatively, the middle facet articular surface may be horizontally oriented.

PITFALLS

- The absence of flatfoot (defined as the axis of the talus being inferior to the axis of the first metatarsal) does not exclude tarsal coalition, as flatfoot is present in just under half of all cases.
- The presence of a ball-and-socket talus does not imply tarsal coalition, as the former is more frequently found in other causes of flatfoot.
- At MRI, proliferative synovitis may be characterized as a fibrous coalition. Intravenous gadolinium may be necessary to distinguish between these entities.

Suggested Readings

Crim JR, Kjeldsberg KM. Radiographic diagnosis of tarsal coalition. Am J Roentgenol 2004;182:323–328

Munk PL, Vellet AD, Levin MF, Helms CA. Current status of magnetic resonance imaging of the ankle and the hindfoot. Can Assoc Radiol J 1992;43:19–30

Sakellariou A, Sallomi D, Janzen DL, Munk PL, Claridge RJ, Kiri VA. Talocalcaneal coalition: diagnosis with the C-sign on lateral radiographs of the ankle. J Bone Joint Surg Br 2000;82:574–578

CASE 35

Brian Edward Reeves, Anthony G. Ryan, Peter L. Munk, and Thomas Pope

Clinical Presentation

A 30-year-old man presented with a history of flushing, nausea, and emesis. Physical exam revealed urticaria pigmentosa.

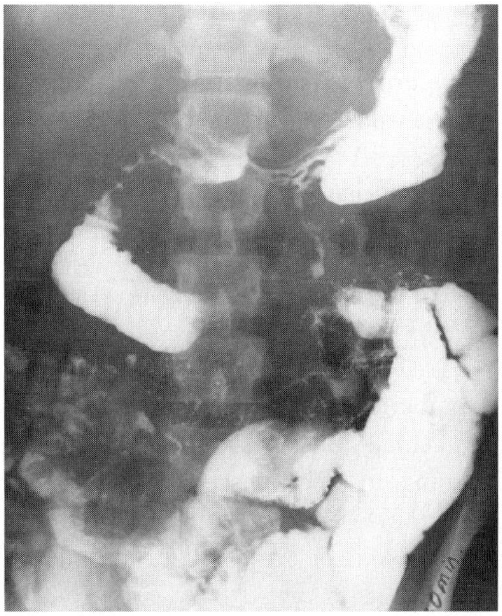

Figure 35A

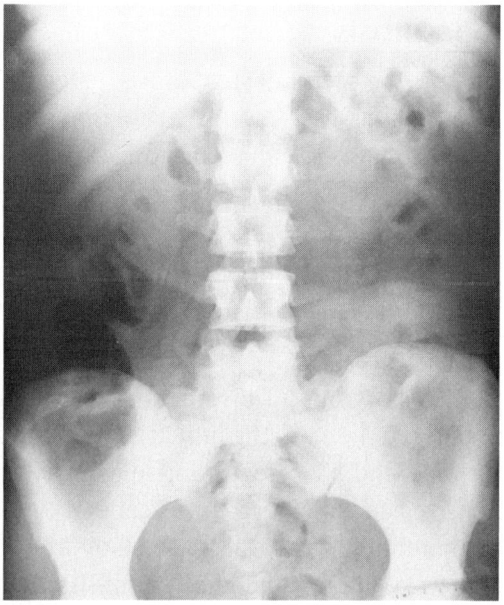

Figure 35B

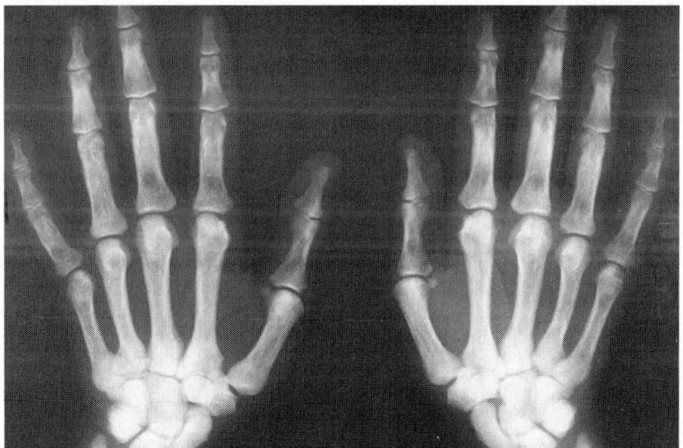

Figure 35C

Radiologic Findings

An anteroposterior (AP) radiograph of the abdomen from a small bowel follow-through (SBFT) study (**Fig. 35A**) shows small mucosal nodules and diffuse thickening of the valvulae conniventes throughout the proximal small bowel.

The AP lumbar spine radiograph (**Fig. 35B**) shows diffuse osteosclerosis throughout the lumbar spine.

A radiograph of the hands (**Fig. 35C**) shows diffuse osteosclerosis throughout.

Diagnosis

Mastocytosis.

Differential Diagnosis

Diffuse osteopenia may be seen in osteoporosis, osteomalacia, hyperparathyroidism, and plasma cell myeloma. Multiple osseous lytic lesions may simulate the appearance of osteoporosis, sickle cell anemia, and Gaucher's disease. Diffuse osteosclerosis may be observed in fluorosis, renal osteodystrophy, osteopetrosis, myelofibrosis, metastatic disease, and Paget's disease.

Discussion

Background

Mastocytosis comprises a group of disorders caused by an overabundance of mast cells, which are located predominantly in the skin, the linings of the stomach and small intestine, and the lungs. Mast cells release histamine and play important roles in wound healing, in blood vessel growth, and in the immune defense system. There are two general types of mastocytosis: cutaneous and systemic. Cutaneous is the more common form and mostly affects children. Mastocytosis occurs in children 75% of the time, is usually mild, and is often self-limited.

Systemic mastocytosis is a rare proliferative disorder equally affecting both men and women, typically beginning in the fourth to eighth decades, and most commonly seen in Caucasians. Mast cells may accumulate in the liver, spleen, lymph nodes, and skeleton, although it is the cutaneous involvement that is the most common and characteristic.

Etiology

It is believed that mastocytosis is a hyperplastic response to an unknown stimulus rather than a neoplastic condition.

Pathophysiology

Increased mast cell growth factor is believed to stimulate melanin pigment production, explaining the characteristic hyperpigmentation. Associated systemic manifestations are thought to be secondary to the release of histamine, prostaglandins, heparin, and neutral proteases.

Clinical Findings

Most patients present with pruritic cutaneous lesions and may experience acute systemic symptoms exacerbated by certain activities or ingestion of certain foods. These symptoms include local urticaria, flushing, shocklike episodes, diarrhea, headache, wheezing, rhinorrhea, and vomiting. In severe cases, weight loss, malaise, weakness, hepatosplenomegaly, lymphadenopathy, and peptic ulcer disease are encountered. Bone pain has been observed in as many as 28% of patients. Soft-tissue masses, tenderness, and pathological fractures may occur. Hepatic dysfunction may result from mast cell proliferation and periportal fibrosis.

Laboratory values may show anemia, thrombocytopenia, leukopenia, and eosinophilia. Plasma and urinary histamine levels are usually elevated.

Imaging Findings

RADIOGRAPHY

- The skeletal manifestations of systemic mastocytosis are nonspecific. Diffuse osteopenia, multiple lytic lesions, and diffuse or focal osteosclerosis may be observed.
- Mast cell infiltration, heparin, and prostaglandins are thought to be the cause of diffuse osteopenia.
- Pressure atrophy of bony trabeculae from adjacent mast cell accumulations is hypothesized to be the reason for multiple lytic lesions.
- Osteosclerosis may be due to extensive mast cell proliferation within marrow with associated fibrosis, or it may reflect bone infarction.

FLUOROSCOPY

- Upper gastrointestinal (GI) series with SBFT study may demonstrate thickening of the valvulae conniventes or small nodules within the mucosa of the small bowel or stomach, representing mast cell infiltration and proliferation.

CROSS-SECTIONAL IMAGING

- May show an enlarged liver or spleen

RADIONUCLIDE STUDIES

- Show areas of increased tracer accumulation in regions of osteosclerosis and may be used for assessment of disease progression

Treatment

There is no cure for mastocytosis. Antihistamines can ameliorate pruritis, flushing, and GI symptoms.

Aspirin can inhibit prostaglandin synthesis and may be beneficial to disease resistant to antihistamines.

Cutaneous lesion may be treated with corticosteroids. Patients should avoid activities and food that induce mast cell mediator release.

Prognosis

The prognosis depends on the extent of systemic involvement. If the disease is contained to the skin and skeleton, it runs a mild and protracted course. With extensive involvement of the reticuloendothelial system, death may occur within a few years. Approximately 30% of patients with extensive involvement develop leukemia. Hemorrhage, infection, cachexia, perforated ulcers, gastroenteritis, hepatic failure, and leukemia are common causes of death.

PEARLS

- The multiple lytic lesions are thought to arise from pressure atrophy on bony trabeculae from adjacent mast cell accumulation.

- Radionuclide studies will show areas of increased tracer accumulation in regions of osteosclerosis and may be used for assessment of disease progression.
- Upper GI series with SBFT study may demonstrate thickening of the valvulae conniventes or small nodules within the mucosa of the small bowel or stomach, representing mast cell infiltration and proliferation.

PITFALLS

- The skeletal manifestations of systemic mastocytosis are nonspecific and may include diffuse osteopenia, multiple lytic lesions, and diffuse or focal osteosclerosis.
- Osteosclerosis may be due to extensive mast cell proliferation within marrow with associated fibrosis, or may be due to bone infarction and a combination of clinical findings such as pain. Cross-sectional imaging is required to resolve the issue.
- Although multiple lytic lesions raise the differential of lytic metastases, the clinical setting and the other characteristic findings will typically suggest mastocytosis.

Suggested Readings

Asmis LM, Girardet C. Images in clinical medicine: systemic mast cell disease. N Engl J Med 2002;346:174

Delsignore JL, Dvoretsky PM, Hicks DG, O'Keefe RJ, Rosier RN. Mastocytosis presenting as a skeletal disorder. Iowa Orthop J 1996;16:126–134

Siegel S, Sadler MA, Yook C, Chang V, Miller J. Systemic mastocytosis with involvement of the pelvis: a radiographic and clinicopathologic study. Clin Imaging 1999;23:245–248

CASE 36

Brian Edward Reeves, Anthony G. Ryan, Peter L. Munk, and Thomas Pope

Clinical Presentation

A 1-year-old child developed coarse, thick, facial features, prominent dark eyebrows, cloudy corneas, progressive stiffness, gibbus deformity, and obvious mental retardation. The child had appeared normal at birth. Laboratory values showed increased urinary excretion of dermatan and heparan sulfates.

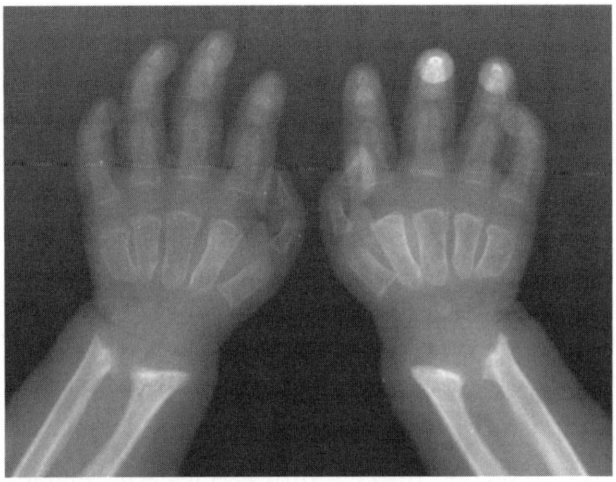

Figure 36A

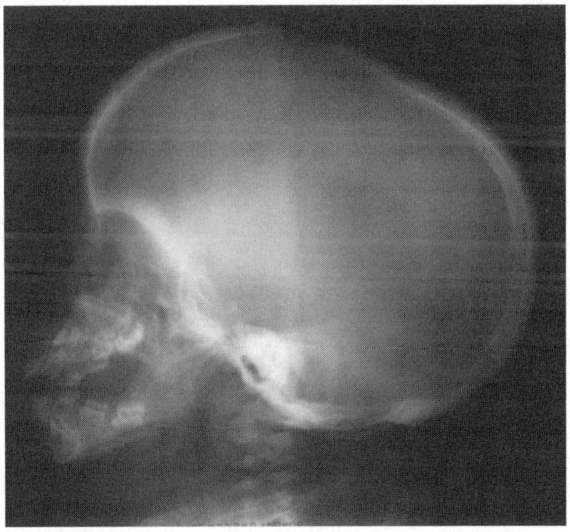

Figure 36B

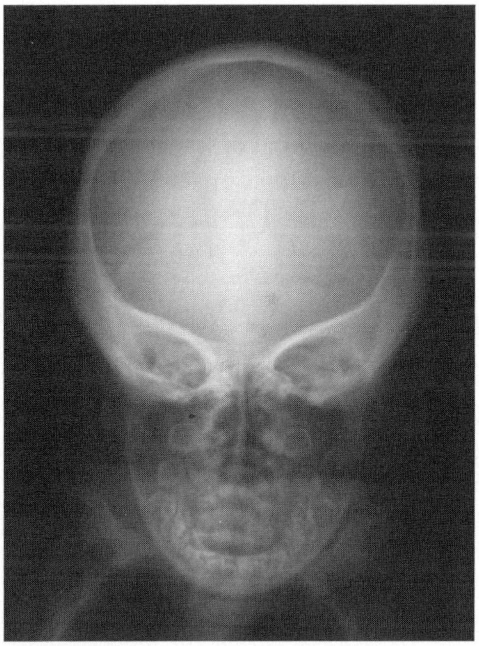

Figure 36C

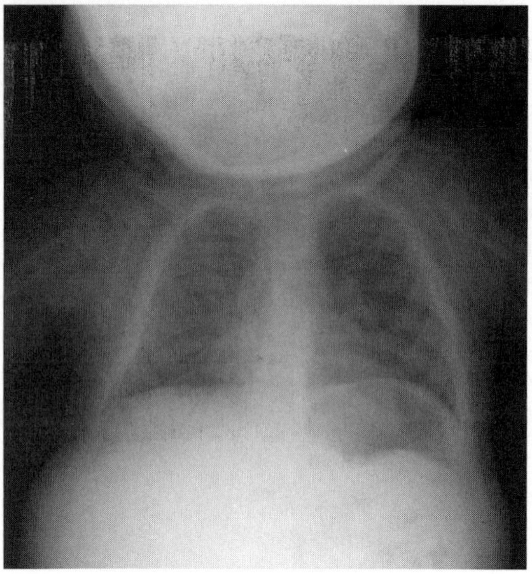

Figure 36D

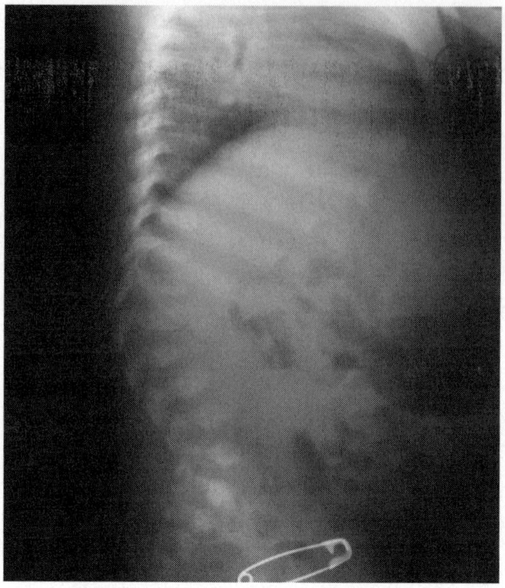

Figure 36E

Radiologic Findings

Hands

Figure 36A shows pointing of the proximal portions of the second through fifth metacarpals, widening of the proximal and middle phalanges, and a V-shaped deformity of the distal radius and ulna.

Skull

Figures 36B and **36C** show macrocephaly, poorly developed mastoids, a prominent forehead, heavy supraorbital ridges, an elongated and J-shaped pituitary fossa, poorly developed paranasal sinuses, a large tongue, and a thick diploic space.

Chest

Figure 36D shows widening of the anterior aspect of the ribs.

Spine

Focal kyphosis at L2 due to the presence of a hypoplastic, bullet-shaped vertebral body is seen in **Fig. 36E**.

Diagnosis

Hurler's syndrome.

Discussion

Background

Hurler's syndrome is an inherited autosomal recessive trait belonging to a group of diseases called the mucopolysaccharidoses. Abnormal quantities of mucopolysaccharide are stored in different body tissues and are responsible for the symptoms and appearance in this disorder. Hurler's syndrome is designated mucopolysaccharidosis type 1H. The specific diagnosis is made according to corneal clouding, age, IQ, urinary excretion of heparan, keratan, and dermatan sulfates, and other clinical findings. Approximately 1/150,000 infants are affected.

Etiology

Hurler's syndrome is a genetic disorder secondary to an inherited autosomal recessive (X-linked) trait.

Pathophysiology

Low or absent levels of the enzyme α-L-iduronidase are responsible for the mucopolysaccharide accumulation in Hurler's syndrome.

Clinical Findings

Newborn infants with this defect appear normal at birth, but by the end of the first year, signs begin to develop. Other signs not shown in this case that may be present include deafness, hirsutism, short stature, full lips, small, malformed teeth, and shortness of breath.

Findings on physical exam may reveal hepatosplenomegaly, inguinal or umbilical hernia, heart murmurs, cardiomegaly, kyphosis, hip dislocation, retinal pigmentation, epicanthal folds, enlarged tongue, and flared nostrils.

Several laboratory tests may also aid in the diagnosis. Urine analysis will show increased excretion of dermatan and heparan sulfate, cultured fibroblasts will show the absence or low levels of α-L-iduronidase, and histologic staining of leukocytes will show metachromasia.

Imaging Findings

RADIOGRAPHY

The diagnosis of Hurler's syndrome is contingent upon the early recognition of the pattern of musculoskeletal abnormalities, which become increasingly pronounced after the sixth month. Cranial abnormalities include macrocephaly, craniostenosis, elongated J-shaped sella turcica, widened diploic space, and poorly developed sinuses.

Spine radiographs will show hypoplastic hook- or bullet-shaped vertebral bodies in the thoracolumbar junction with a gibbus deformity. Atlantoaxial subluxation may also be seen.

Chest radiographs may show widened anterior portions of the ribs and cardiomegaly.

Hypoplasia of the ilia, coxa valga, and shortening/widening of the shafts of the long tubular bones may also be present. Pointing of the proximal portions of the second through fifth metacarpals with a V-shaped appearance to the distal ulna and radius is a common finding, and most patients show diffuse osteopenia.

Complications

There may be cardiac valvular thickening, coronary artery disease, severe mental retardation, deafness, premature death, constipation with alternating diarrhea, and neurological problems.

Treatment

Because of the characteristic progression of neurological and intellectual deterioration found in children with Hurler's syndrome, early diagnosis and treatment are critical to the preservation of long-term intellectual development.

Intravenous enzyme replacement therapy is possible for patients with a defect in α-L-iduronidase. Patients receiving this treatment have shown improved joint mobility, growth, and heart function. Few side effects have been reported, and patients tolerate the medication well. How the enzyme replacement therapy affects neurological function or life span is unproven at this time.

Bone marrow transplantation has increased the survival of patients with Hurler's syndrome. However, this therapy must be performed at a young age to prevent mental retardation and to improve the patient's symptoms.

Prognosis

Hurler's syndrome is a disease with a poor prognosis. Children with this disease have significant progressive physical and mental deficiencies. Death can occur in late childhood, early adolescence, or adulthood.

PEARLS

- The differential of vertebrae with anterior pointing at the lower third includes Hunter's syndrome, achondroplasia and pseudoachondroplasia, congenital hypothyroidism, and Down syndrome.
- Morquio's syndrome (a disorder of keratan sulfate storage) may be differentiated from Hurler's because in the former, the vertebral beak occurs in the middle of the vertebral body.
- The differential for congenital conditions causing a V-shaped appearance of the distal ulna and radius (also known as a Madelung's deformity) includes Leri-Weil syndrome (dyschondrosteosis), diaphyseal aclasia, and Turner's syndrome.

PITFALLS

- Newborn infants with this defect appear normal at birth, but by the end of the first year, signs begin to develop.
- The diagnosis of Hurler's syndrome is contingent upon the early recognition of the pattern of musculoskeletal abnormalities, which become increasingly pronounced after the sixth month. Missing the diagnosis has disastrous implications because the later treatment is instituted, the more severe will be the disease.
- Significant overlap occurs in the axial skeleton findings of the storage diseases, precluding their differentiation on this basis alone.

Suggested Readings

Belmont PJ Jr, Polly DW Jr. Early identification of Hurler's syndrome with the aid of identification of the characteristic gibbus deformity. Mil Med 1998;163:711–714

Field RE, Buchanan JA, Copplemans MG, Aichroth PM. Bone-marrow transplantation in Hurler's syndrome: effect on skeletal development. J Bone Joint Surg Br 1994;76:975–981

Tandon V, Williamson JB, Cowie RA, Wraith JE. Spinal problems in mucopolysaccharidosis 1 (Hurler syndrome). J Bone Joint Surg Br 1996;78(6):938–944

CASE 37

George Nomikos, Brian Edward Reeves, Anthony G. Ryan,
Peter L. Munk, Thomas Pope, and Mark Murphey

Clinical Presentation

A 39-year-old man experienced increasing fullness and pain in his left lower quadrant and left groin. He has a family history of bone tumors.

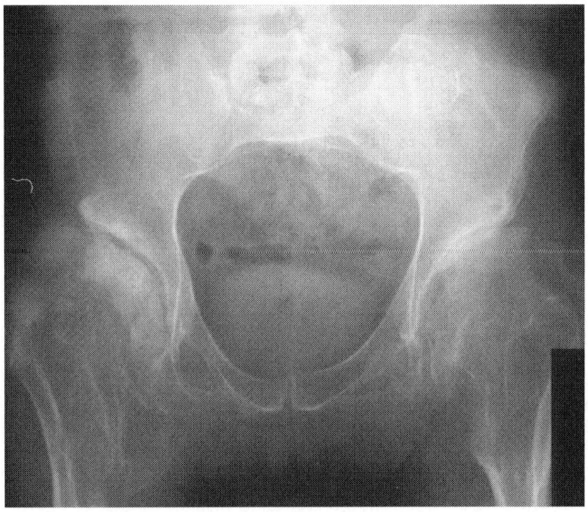

Figure 37A

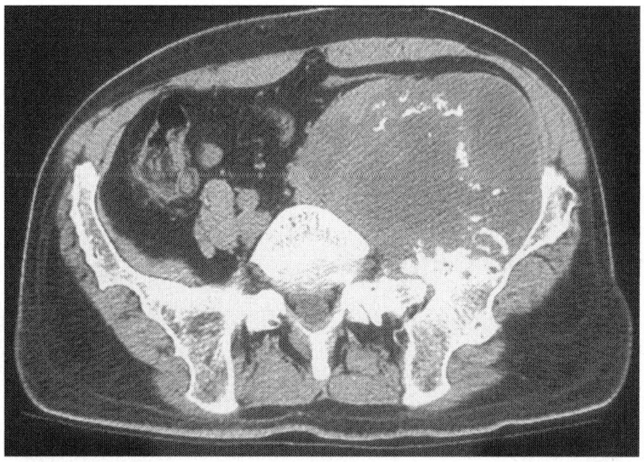

Figure 37B

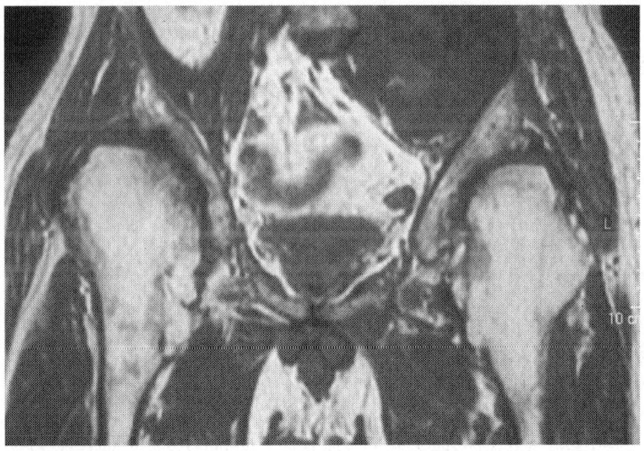

Figure 37C

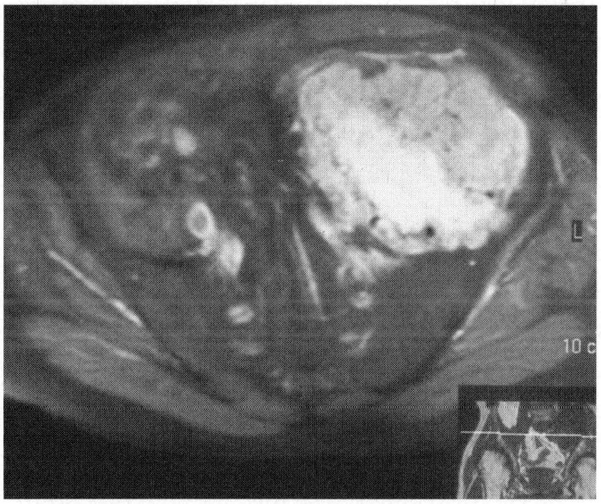

Figure 37D

Radiologic Findings

The radiograph of the pelvis (**Fig. 37A**) shows marked deformity of the proximal femora bilaterally. There is undertubulation of the femora (Erlenmeyer flask deformities), as well as multiple osseous excrescences arising from the femora. These osseous excrescences demonstrate cortical and medullary continuity with the underlying bone and are consistent with multiple osteochondromas. Multiple smaller lesions are identified in the pelvis as well. In addition, there is an area of osseous destruction involving the left periacetabular region. The CT (**Fig. 37B**) shows a large mass arising from an osteochondroma involving the left iliac wing. The lesion demonstrates a chondroid pattern of internal mineralization. Note the low attenuation of the nonmineralized portions of the mass. This attenuation is due to the high water content of hyaline cartilage. Also note the multiple small osteochondromas on the pelvis, producing a "wavy" contour. The T1-weighted MRI (**Fig. 37C**) shows pelvic corticomedullary continuity between the osteochondromas and underlying bone. The large pelvis mass is also seen to be very low signal intensity on the T1-weighted image and high signal intensity on the T2-weighted image (**Fig. 37D**), again because of the high water content of the hyaline cartilage in the low-grade chondrosarcomatous degeneration.

Diagnosis

Hereditary multiple exostoses (familial osteochondromatosis or diaphyseal aclasia) with malignant transformation of one lesion into chondrosarcoma.

Differential Diagnosis

None.

Discussion

Background

Osteochondromas, which represent the most common tumor or tumorlike process of bone, may be solitary or multiple. Solitary lesions are much more common than multiple, with an estimated frequency in the general population of 1 to 2%. Lesions most frequently affect the knee, and the femur is the most commonly involved bone. Lesions may develop, however, in any bone that forms from enchondral ossification.

Etiology

These lesions arise from a fragment of physeal cartilage that separates from the growth plate and extrudes through the periosteal bone cuff encircling the growth plate (zone of Ranvier) into the cortex. This is thought to be related to the process of remodeling occurring in the "cutback" zone of long bones during their growth phase. By the process of enchondral ossification, this intracortical fragment of physeal cartilage develops into an osseous stalk (with cortical and medullary continuity with the underlying bone) with a cartilaginous cap that continues to grow until skeletal maturity is reached.

The development of one or more exostoses with pathology identical to that of de novo osteochondromas has been associated with radiation therapy. These radiation-induced exostoses are usually seen in children who receive radiation between the ages of 8 months and 11 years, often for Wilms' tumor, neuroblastoma, or rhabdomyosarcoma of the bladder, and tend to occur at the periphery of the radiation field. The mean time to development of an osteochondroma after radiation is ~3 to 17 years. Malignant transformation is rare.

Clinical Findings

The most common symptom for a solitary osteochondroma is a painless mass causing an aesthetic deformity. The lesions first appear in childhood as lumps near joints and may produce pain in children if traumatized. The lesions may also compress adjacent nerves and tendons or cause mechanical problems if they grow large enough to impede joint mobility.

Hereditary multiple exostoses (HME) is a familial disorder with autosomal dominant inheritance, secondary to genetic abnormalities involving chromosomes 8, 11, and 19. Cases infrequently arise spontaneously. Because of more severe deformities, diagnosis is usually made early in life (usually by age 5 and rarely after age 12). There is incomplete penetrance in females. People with diaphyseal aclasia may be shorter than average or have bowed extremities, as the proximity of the exostoses to the growth centers can interfere with epiphyseal growth.

Complications

Common complications include mechanical impingement on adjacent joints; formation of a reactive bursa over the lesion; tenosynovitis secondary to mechanical irritation; mechanical irritation of other structures (e.g., bladder, pleura); fracture; vascular sequelae, including pseudoaneurysm formation (particularly in the popliteal artery) and deep venous thrombosis; and neurological disturbances, such as entrapment neuropathies and nerve palsies. Lesions located on the anterior scapula may become caught on chest wall structures and produce the snapping scapula syndrome. A common forearm deformity seen in HME is the pseudo-Madelung's deformity (**Fig. 37E**), in which there is shortening of the ulna and bowing of the radius or radius and ulna. A similar appearance may occur in the lower limb secondary to fibular shortening. Undertubulation deformities of the metaphysis, in which the diametaphyseal junction is abnormally long and widened (Erlenmeyer flask appearance), are common in HME and may be one of the initial manifestations of the disease.

The most worrisome complication is malignant transformation, usually to chondrosarcoma. There is an approximately 1% lifetime risk of malignant transformation in the case of a solitary osteochondroma and an approximately 3 to 5% lifetime risk in the case of HME. Features suggestive of malignant transformation include pain or growth in the lesion after skeletal maturity, focal regions of radiolucency centrally in the lesion, destruction of the adjacent bone, and formation of a significant soft-tissue mass. Lesions located more centrally (e.g., hips, pelvis, shoulders) have a higher propensity for malignant transformation.

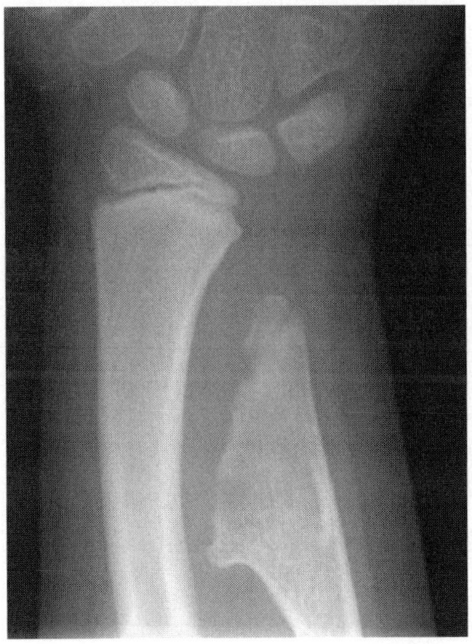

Figure 37E Dramatic shortening and deformity of the ulna with associated bowing of the radius producing the pseudo-Madelung's deformity.

The most important radiologic feature in suggesting malignant transformation is the thickness of the cartilage cap. A cap thickness greater than 1.5 cm in a skeletally mature patient is highly suggestive of malignancy. The cartilage cap may be much thicker in skeletally immature patients, and so this finding should not be taken to suggest malignancy in these patients. Malignant transformation occurs at an average age of 25 to 30 years in the case of HME and at an average age of 50 to 55 years for solitary lesions. Malignant transformation below the age of 20 years is rare. Growth of exostoses after skeletal maturity with pain is a worrisome sign for transformation.

Pathology

GROSS

Pathologically, these lesions are developmental and not neoplastic. They consist of an osseous stalk or base usually containing fatty marrow and an overlying hyaline cartilage cap of variable thickness.

MICROSCOPIC

The cartilage cap has an organization similar to growth plate cartilage and may contain areas of calcification related to the process of enchondral ossification.

Imaging Findings

RADIOGRAPHY

- Lesions in the long bones are most commonly metaphyseal in location (diaphyseal lesions are rare). See **Figs. 37F–37J**.
- Usually point away from the underlying joint due to the pull of the overlying tendons and ligaments (although these are not usually attached to the osteochondroma)
- May have a narrow (pedunculated) or wide (sessile) area of continuity with the underlying cortex and medullary canal
- Cortical and medullary continuity with the underlying bone is pathognomonic and is often demonstrated on radiographs; however, advanced imaging is sometimes required to see this continuity, particularly in the case of flat bones.

COMPUTED TOMOGRAPHY

- May be the best modality to demonstrate cortical and medullary continuity, particularly in flat bones and areas of complex osseous anatomy
- Determination of the thickness of the cartilage cap with CT is often easier if there is some mineralization in the cap; otherwise, differentiation of the cap from the surrounding muscle may be difficult (especially if the cap is between 1.0 and 2.5 cm).

MAGNETIC RESONANCE IMAGING

- Also demonstrates cortical and medullary continuity well
- Probably better than CT at determination of thickness of the cartilage cap
- The cap is usually intermediate to low signal intensity on the T1-weighted image and high signal intensity on the T2-weighted image because of the high water content in the hyaline cartilage (**Fig. 37K**); the signal intensity of the cap in younger patients is often more heterogeneous because of the mixture of calcium, hyaline cartilage, and calcification in the cap in these patients.
- The cartilage cap should be no more than 1 cm in thickness. A thicker cartilaginous cap, soft-tissue mass, and osseous destruction are signs suggesting malignant degeneration, and further evaluation is warranted.
- Peripheral and septal enhancement pattern characteristic of hyaline cartilage cap lesions

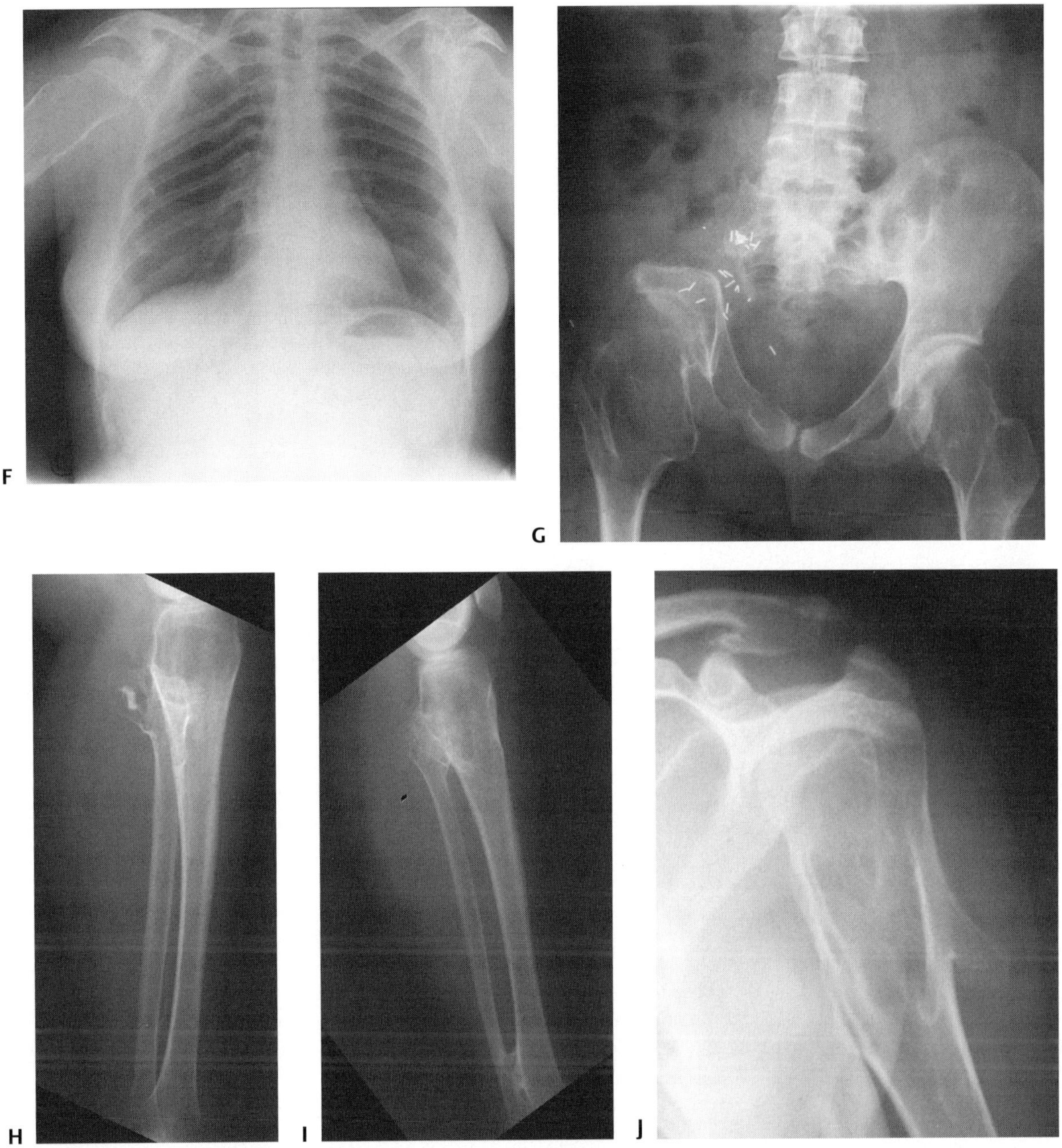

Figures 37F to **37J** A 25-year-old woman presenting with swelling of the knees and shoulders. Radiographs of the chest (**37F**), pelvis (**37G**), tibiae (**37H** and **37I**), and left shoulder (**37J**) demonstrate flaring of the proximal humeral and femoral metaphyses with multiple exostoses in the proximal humeri and tibiae and distal femora and pelvis that are contiguous with the cortex of the bone from which they originate. Partial resection of the right ilium is evident.

Variants

1. Trevor's disease (dysplasia epiphysealis hemimelica) represents an uncommon variant in which an osteochondroma arises from the epiphysis, usually in the lower extremity (**Fig. 37L**). Lesions may be monostotic (usually involving the bones of the hindfoot), may involve several different epiphyses in a lower extremity, or may involve a lower extremity diffusely. Complications include joint abnormalities and deformities and limb length discrepancies. Malignant degeneration has not been reported.

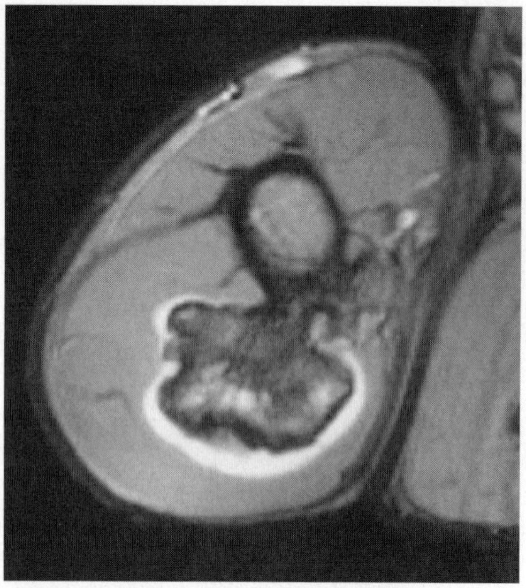
K

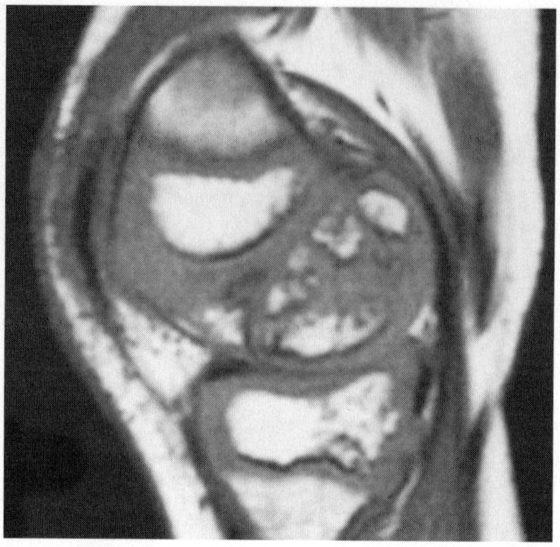
L

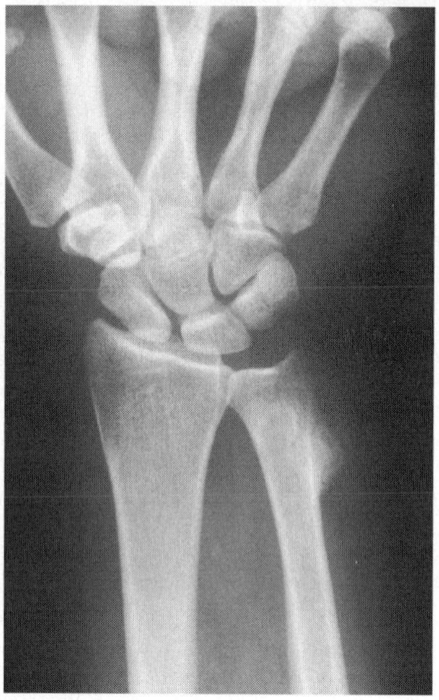
M

Figures 37K The cartilaginous cap demonstrates high signal intensity on the fat-saturated T2-weighted image because of high water content in the hyaline cartilage. **37L** An example of Trevor's disease (dysplasia epiphysealis hemimelica) affecting the epiphyses of the distal femur and proximal tibia. **37M** A broad-based surface lesion is demonstrated on the medial aspect of the ulna: bizarre parosteal osteochondromatous proliferation (Nora's lesion) of the distal ulna. Note the lack of corticomedullary continuity with the underlying bone.

2. A turret exostosis is an area of ossification usually along the dorsal surface of the proximal or middle phalanges of the hand. These lesions are secondary to injury to the digital extensor mechanism that results in subperiosteal hematoma formation and subsequent ossification. They may diminish the ability to flex the involved digit.
3. Subungual (or Dupuytren's) exostoses arise under or adjacent to the nail bed, usually in the toes, and are superficially similar in appearance to osteochondromas. However, these lesions do not demonstrate cortical and medullary continuity with the underlying bone, and the cartilage cap is formed of fibrocartilage, not hyaline cartilage. These lesions are likely related to trauma or chronic infection.
4. Bizarre parosteal osteochondromatous proliferation (BPOP, or Nora's lesion) (**Fig. 37M**) represents a broad-based surface lesion often affecting the small bones of the hands and feet, but also occasionally involving long bones. These lesions demonstrate mature mineralization and lack corticomedullary continuity with the underlying bone. A definite etiology has not been determined, although trauma has been considered as a possible explanation.

Treatment

- For solitary osteochondromas, many patients never require treatment, and observation is all that is required; however, if an exostosis becomes painful, presses on an important structure such as a nerve, or is cosmetically unattractive, resection may be indicated.
- Patients with HME often need correction of deformities related to the disease process in addition to resection of large lesions.
- Malignant lesions are treated with wide resection and limb salvage; chemotherapy and radiation usually are not employed.

Prognosis

- Recurrence rate after osteochondroma removal varies from 2 to 30%. Many osteochondromas, however, do not regrow to a size large enough to be symptomatic again.
- Most chondrosarcomas that develop from a preexisting osteochondroma are low grade, so that long-term survival is high (70 to 90%).
- Patients with higher grade tumors have a worse prognosis.

PEARLS

- An osteochondroma can be differentiated from a parosteal osteosarcoma by the type of matrix and lack of continuity of the cortex and marrow with the host bone seen in osteosarcoma.
- CT may be helpful, when myositis ossificans is adjacent to the cortex, in demonstrating lack of cortical or marrow continuity and in identifying the ossification pattern. In myositis ossificans, the mature calcification is peripheral.
- The most important radiologic feature in suggesting malignant transformation is the thickness of the cartilage cap. A cap thickness greater than 1.5 cm in a skeletally mature patient is highly suggestive of malignancy.
- Malignant degeneration almost always occurs in adulthood after skeletal maturity

PITFALLS

- The radiographic findings may simulate a dysplasia.
- Lesions in the long bones are most commonly metaphyseal in location (diaphyseal lesions are rare).
- Although an osteochondroma variant, BPOP or Nora's lesion does not demonstrate corticomedullary continuity with the underlying bone.

Suggested Readings

Brien EW, Mirra JM, Luck JV Jr. Benign and malignant cartilage tumors of bone and joint: their anatomic and theoretical basis with an emphasis on radiology, pathology, and clinical biology. II. Juxtacortical cartilage tumors. Skeletal Radiol 1999;28:1–20

Carroll KL, Yandow SM, Ward K, Carey JC. Clinical correlation to genetic variations of hereditary multiple exostosis. J Pediatr Orthop 1999;19:785–791

Crandall BF, Field LL, Sparkes RS, Spence MA. Hereditary multiple exostoses: report of a family. Clin Orthop Relat Res 1984;190:217–219

Karasick D, Schweitzer M, Eschelman D. Symptomatic osteochondromas: imaging features. Am J Roentgenol 1997;168:1507–1512

Lee KC, Davies AM, Cassar-Pullicino VN. Imaging the complications of osteochondromas. Clin Radiol 2002;57:18–28

Murphey MD, Choi JJ, Kransdorf MJ, Flemming DJ, Gannon FH. Imaging of osteochondroma: variants and complications with radiologic-pathologic correlation. Radiographics 2000;20:1407–1434

Peterson HA. Multiple hereditary osteochondroma. Clin Orthop Relat Res 1989;239:222–230

Robbin MR, Murphey MD. Benign chondroid neoplasms of bone. Semin Musculoskelet Radiol 2000;4:45–58

Scarborough MT, Moreau G. Benign cartilage tumors. Orthop Clin North Am 1996;27:583–589

Stanton RP, Hansen MO. Function of the upper extremities in hereditary multiple exostoses. J Bone Joint Surg Am 1996;78:568–573

Sundaram M, Wang L, Rotman M, Howard R, Saboeiro A. Florid reactive periostitis and bizarre parosteal osteochondromatous proliferation: pre-biopsy imaging evolution, treatment and outcome. Skeletal Radiol 2001;30:192–198

CASE 38

Anthony G. Ryan and Peter L. Munk

Clinical Presentation

A patient presented with the left hand larger than the right since birth, with associated gross forearm soft-tissue swelling.

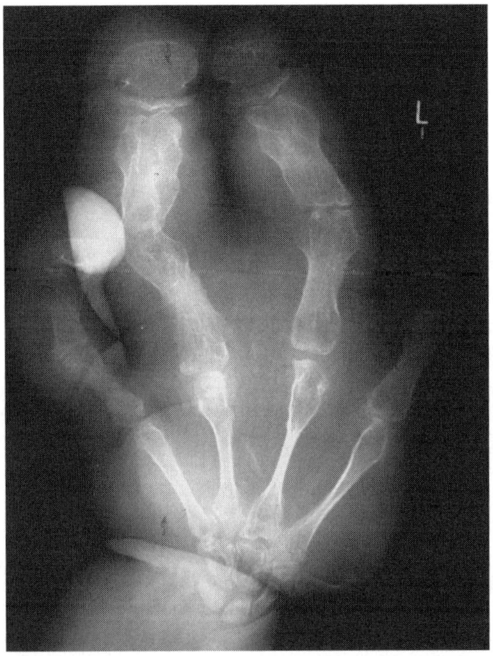

Figure 38A

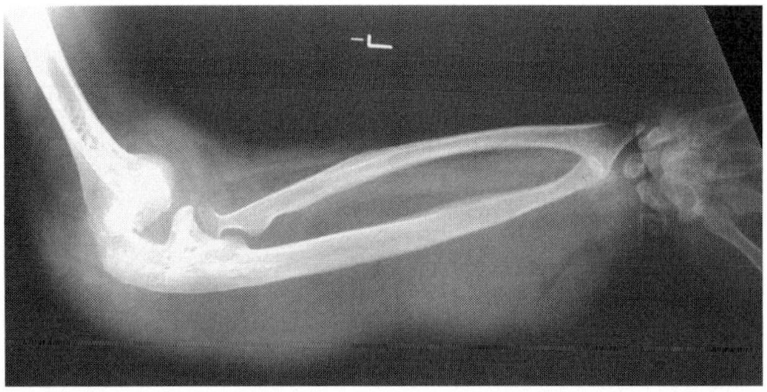

Figure 38B

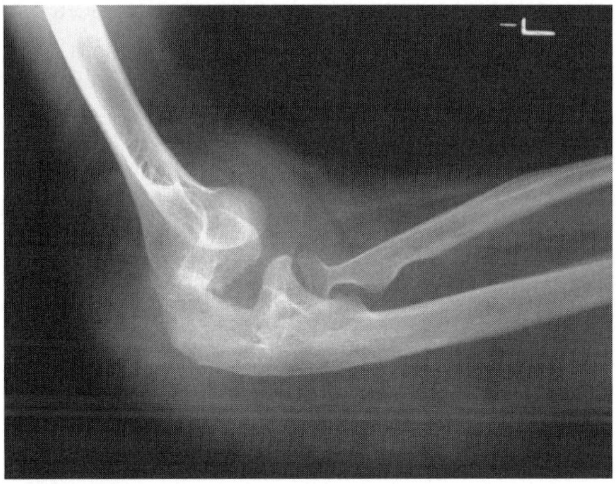

Figure 38C

Radiologic Findings

An anteroposterior radiograph of the left hand (**Fig. 38A**) shows markedly abnormal second and third digits, with an absent fifth digit. The phalanges of the involved digits are massively enlarged in both longitudinal and axial planes, with "splaying" most marked distally. Clinodactyly of the affected digits is present. There is a pathological fracture of the proximal phalanx of the third digit with resultant deformity. Endosteal bone resorption and subsequent remodeling are evident, most marked in the middle phalanx of the third digit.

The forearm radiograph (**Fig. 38B**) and corresponding focused view of the elbow (**Fig. 38C**) show massive soft-tissue swelling with prominent lucent foci, highly suggestive of macroscopic fat within the lesion.

Diagnosis

Macrodystrophia lipomatosa (nerve territory-oriented macrodactyly).

Differential Diagnosis

- Fibrolipomatous hamartoma with associated macrodystrophia lipomatosa
- Neurofibromatosis
- Klippel-Trénaunay-Weber syndrome
- Lymphangiomatosis
- Hemangiomatosis
- Chronic vascular stimulation
- Proteus syndrome

Discussion

Etiology

The condition is congenital but not hereditary; however, the precise etiology of macrodystrophia is unknown. A related condition involves the presence of a fibrolipomatous hamartoma of a nerve that gives rise to an indistinguishable clinical pattern.

Pathophysiology

The neural fibrolipoma causes local gigantism in the affected nerve's territory, resulting in progressive overgrowth of all mesenchymal elements, particularly fibroadipose tissue.

The condition may be associated with other local developmental abnormalities, such as polydactyly.

Clinical Findings

Males and females are equally affected.

The condition is recognizable at birth. The adipose overgrowth is typically greatest at the volar and distal portions of the affected digit/limb; however, when an entire limb is involved (which is unusual), the lateral aspect of the upper limb and the medial aspect of the lower limb are most severely affected.

The second or third digits of either hand or foot are most frequently affected, with the foot more frequently involved than the hand. The condition is usually unilateral and painless.

Although neural involvement may become apparent at any time from birth to 30 years of age, overgrowth typically ceases with the onset of puberty, whereas mechanical problems tend to develop thereafter (i.e., degenerative joint disease with florid osteophyte overgrowth).

STAGES OF DISEASE

Two clinical subtypes exist: static and progressive.

- *Static* Enlarged digit(s) at birth, which grow at the same rate as the nonaffected digits
- *Progressive* Enlarged digit, which grows more rapidly than the nonaffected digits. The overgrowth may cause articular surface slanting and consequent degeneration, the resultant osteophytes being disproportionately large.

Although the changes are most severe distally in both types, they affect the metacarpals more frequently in the progressive type.

Complications

- Dramatic proliferation of fatty tissue
- Local gigantism
- Local pressure symptoms (nerve irritation may occur)
- Osseous erosion
- Joint degeneration secondary to splaying of digits and distortion of affected digits

Pathology

GROSS

Lipomatous proliferation involving periosteum, bone marrow, nerve sheath, muscle, and subcutaneous tissue is demonstrated.

MICROSCOPIC

The nerve itself is distended by interaxonal adipose tissue. The phalanges are enlarged by new bone in endosteal and periosteal locations, the latter frequently studded with nodules consisting of chondroblasts and osteoblasts.

Imaging Findings

RADIOGRAPHY

Bone

- Long, broad, and splayed phalanges (mushroom-shaped) with endosteal and periosteal irregularity secondary to the local pressure of the fibrofatty network and periosteal nodularity
- Normal trabeculae

Soft tissues

- Lucent foci are seen within the abundant soft tissue, reflecting the mature fat content (said to be diagnostic); they are most evident along the volar and distal aspects of the digit. The volar overgrowth causes dorsal deviation of the affected digit.

ULTRASOUND

- High-frequency linear transducers may be useful in identifying the lipomatous proliferation in relation to the affected nerve, seen as alternating hyper- and hypoechoic bands within the nerve.

MAGNETIC RESONANCE IMAGING

The gross fatty proliferation will be elegantly demonstrated by MRI as high signal on both T1- and T2-weighted images, with uniform suppression on fat-saturated sequences.

Medullary cavities will be seen to be filled with fat in addition to the proliferation of subcutaneous and intramuscular fat.

Intermixed low-signal bands corresponding to the nerve fibrils will be evident within the affected nerve sheaths, which will be distended in a fusiform pattern. On transaxial sequences, the appearance is striking: the nerve sheath is seen to be distended, and the individual nerve fibers are seen as black dots admixed within the high-signal fat.

Treatment

Surgical approaches to achieve functional and cosmetic improvements include debulking, amputation, and reconstruction. All operative procedures carry the risk of injury to the involved nerve with subsequent sensory (with or without motor) deficit.

In cases with associated carpal tunnel syndrome, the median nerve may be released.

Prognosis

Growth of the affected digit(s) ceases at adolescence.

- *Static* Enlarged digit(s) at birth that grow at the same rate as the nonaffected digits
- *Progressive* Enlarged digit that grows more rapidly than the nonaffected digits

PEARLS

- Neurofibromatosis will make itself known by the multiplicity of lesions and other associated findings.
- Klippel-Trénaunay-Weber syndrome typically causes gigantism of the entire limb, and the associated vascular abnormalities should be evident.
- Lucent foci visible within the abundant soft tissue are said to be diagnostic.

PITFALLS

- Macrodystrophia lipomatosa is indistinguishable from the macrodactyly found in the distribution of a nerve affected by the presence of a fibrolipomatous hamartoma.
- When examining the affected limb, be sure to include the area proximal to the soft-tissue overgrowth. This will allow the proximal portion of the nerves to be assessed.
- Where diagnostic doubt exists between macrodystrophia and neurofibromatosis, the absence of cutaneous manifestations and the absence of neurofibromas exclude the latter.

Suggested Readings

Boren WL, Henry RE Jr, Wintch K. MR diagnosis of fibrolipomatous hamartoma of nerve: association with nerve territory-oriented macrodactyly (macrodystrophia lipomatosa). Skeletal Radiol 1995;24:296–297

De Maeseneer M, Jaovisidha S, Lenchik L, et al. Fibrolipomatous hamartoma: MR imaging findings. Skeletal Radiol 1997;26:155–160

Resnick D. Diagnosis of Bone and Joint Disorders. 4th ed. Philadelphia, PA: WB Saunders; 2002

CASE 39

Anthony G. Ryan and Peter L. Munk

Clinical Presentation

A 65-year-old woman presented to her family practitioner with a recurrent history of progressive weakness, having particular difficulty climbing stairs. On examination, the patient had a striking violaceous discoloration and puffiness around her eyes and erythematous raised plaques on the skin overlying her knuckles. The practitioner noticed that the patient labored over standing up from the chair to get on the examination couch.

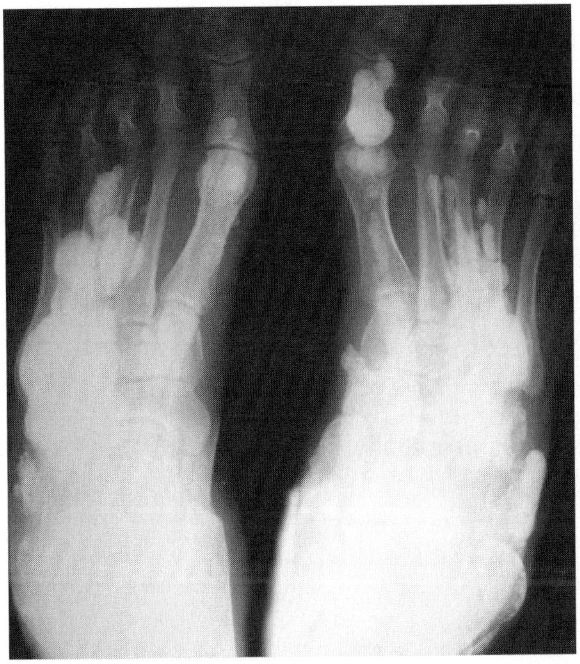

Figures 39A

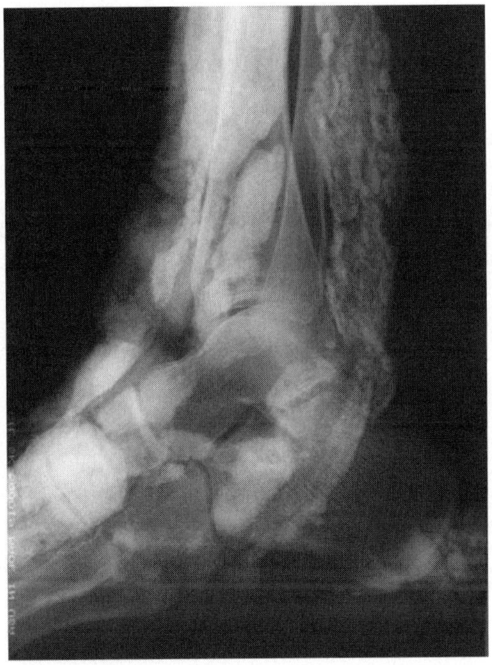

Figures 39B

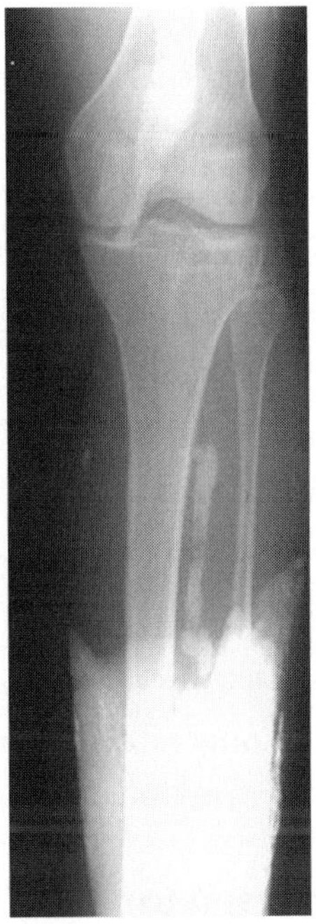

Figure 39C

Radiologic Findings

Conventional radiographs of the feet (**Fig. 39A**), right ankle (**Fig. 39B**), and distal foreleg (**Fig. 39C**) demonstrate sheets and conglomerations of calcification within the subcutaneous soft tissues, some of which assume the configuration of underlying tendons and musculature.

Diagnosis

Dermatomyositis.

Differential Diagnosis

Soft-tissue calcifications

METASTATIC

- High calcium/phosphate
- Hyperparathyroidism/renal osteodystrophy
- Hypo- and pseudohypoparathyroidism

CALCINOSIS (NORMAL CALCIUM)

- Dermatomyositis (universalis/circumscripta)
- Scleroderma/CREST (calcinosis, Raynaud's phenomenon, esophageal dysmotility, scleroderma, telangiectasia)
- Idiopathic tumoral calcinosis (hyperphosphatemic)

DYSTROPHIC

- Calcifications in soft tissues without metabolic disorder

The differential for sheets of calcification within the soft tissues is essentially limited to two entities:

- Congenital myositis ossificans progressiva
- Dermatomyositis

Discussion

Background

Thought of as an idiopathic autoimmune condition affecting the skin and skeletal muscle, dermatomyositis may also affect cardiac muscle, joints, and lungs. It is a rare condition, with only five new cases per million expected per year. It has a bimodal age distribution affecting children (5–14 years) and older middle-aged adults (45–65 years), women twice as often as men. In the childhood group, subcutaneous calcifications and necrotizing vasculitis tend to predominate, whereas in the older age group, there is a well-established association with solid tumors (especially of the stomach, colon, and lung), the risk being 4.4 times that of an age-controlled group. This approximates to 1 in 10 patients with dermatomyositis having an underlying malignancy. The diagnosis of dermatomyositis in a person over 40 should prompt a search for an occult malignancy. Surveillance is also suggested, as the malignancies may take up to 5 years to declare themselves.

Dermatomyositis rarely may be associated with other connective tissue disorders, for example, mixed connective tissue disorder and scleroderma.

Etiology

This is an autoimmune cell-mediated myopathy. The immune component is postulated to have an infectious origin, with protozoa (*Toxoplasma gondii*) and viruses (Coxsackie B RNA has been isolated from muscle biopsy specimens in one study in as many as 50% of dermatomyositis patients) under investigation.

Pathophysiology

Cytotoxic T cells dominate the cellular inflammatory response; however, a humoral contribution is also evident. Microvasculature changes include deposits of immune complexes in vessel walls and the presence of microtubuloreticular structures in endothelial cells consistent with an accompanying vasculitis.

Clinical Findings

The classic presentation is with a symmetric proximal myopathy as evinced by difficulty arising from the seated position and in reaching above the head.

The dermal manifestations are most conspicuous on the eyelids, where a lilac discoloration (heliotrope) with periorbital edema may be evident. In addition, dusky red, raised, scaly plaques may be visible on the bony prominences of the extremities, known as Gottron's papules, most frequently affecting the skin overlying the metacarpophalangeal (MCP) joints.

Dysphagia may occur secondary to striated muscle involvement in the proximal esophagus. Rarely, the diaphragm is affected in advanced cases, resulting in respiratory compromise.

A symmetric polyarthropathy of the small extremity joints affects as many as one quarter to one third of patients. This is rarely aggressive, however, and the cartilage is usually undamaged.

To establish the diagnosis in the appropriate clinical context requires the dermal manifestations plus three of several major criteria, based on the myopathy, elevated skeletal muscle creatine kinase (typically in the thousands compared with a normal value of 25–170 U/L), electromyographic abnormalities, and muscle biopsy.

Complications

Dysphagia may occur secondary to striated muscle involvement in the proximal esophagus. Rarely, the diaphragm is affected in advanced cases, resulting in respiratory compromise. Further contributing to respiratory compromise is interstitial lung disease, which may be superimposed, resulting in a restrictive pattern.

A symmetric polyarthropathy of the small extremity joints affects as many as one quarter to one third of patients. This is rarely aggressive, however, and the cartilage is usually undamaged.

There is an increased risk of developing a neoplasm in all biopsy-proven myositis, which is greatest in dermatomyositis but is also present in polymyositis and inclusion-body myositis. This risk diminishes with time after diagnosis: 4.4% in the first year, 3.4% between 1 and 3 years, 2.2% between 3 and 5 years, and 1.6% beyond 5 years.

Pathology

GROSS

- Gross muscle wasting and fatty atrophy are seen. Sheets of subcutaneous calcifications, some layering along tendons and on muscle belly surfaces, can also be found.

MICROSCOPIC

- Atrophy of type 2 muscle fibers with central nuclei
- Indistinct perifascicular pattern
- Lymphocytes may be evident in the perimysium.
- Perivascular inflammatory changes, but, importantly, no evidence of an actual myositis
- Diagnostic of dermatomyositis are swollen endothelial cells with intracytoplasmic microtubuloreticular aggregates on electron microscopy.

Imaging Findings

RADIOGRAPHY

- Sheetlike calcifications distributed throughout the affected region

ULTRASOUND

- Echogenic foci corresponding to those seen on radiographs in the subcutaneous tissues and in tendons and muscles
- In the acute phase, increased interbundle tissue edema may be evident by hypoechoic fluid spreading the fibers.
- Ultrasound-guided biopsy occasionally is required to confirm the diagnosis.

COMPUTED TOMOGRAPHY

- Rarely, prominence of the thoracoabdominal musculature may be evident.

MAGNETIC RESONANCE IMAGING

- Low signal on T1-weighted sequences and increased signal intensity on water-sensitive sequences, that is, T2-weighted or STIR, reflecting muscle edema (**Figs. 39D,39E**), usually apparent at the time of presentation, permitting an early diagnosis
- A differential of diffuse muscle edema on MRI would include
  - Dermatomyositis, polymyositis
  - Trauma
  - Infectious myositis
  - Radiation therapy
  - Subacute denervation
  - Compartment syndrome
  - Early myositis ossificans
  - Rhabdomyolysis
  - Sickle cell crisis
- In dermatomyositis, the high signal intensity may be diffusely distributed throughout all muscle compartments; however, there is a predominance in the vastus lateralis, with less intense findings in the vastus intermedius and vastus medialis. The degree of signal intensity correlates well with clinical symptoms.

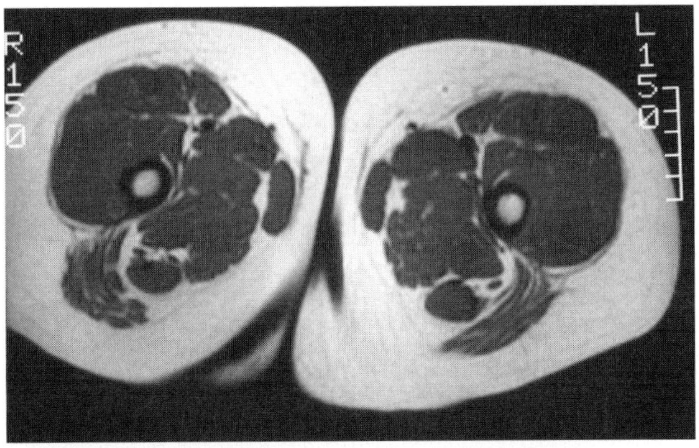

D

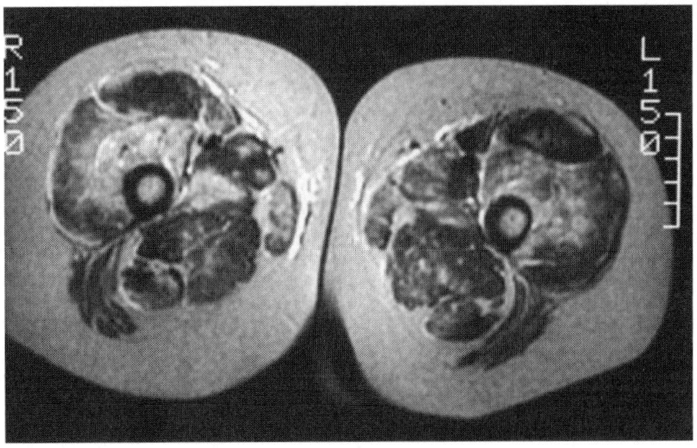

E

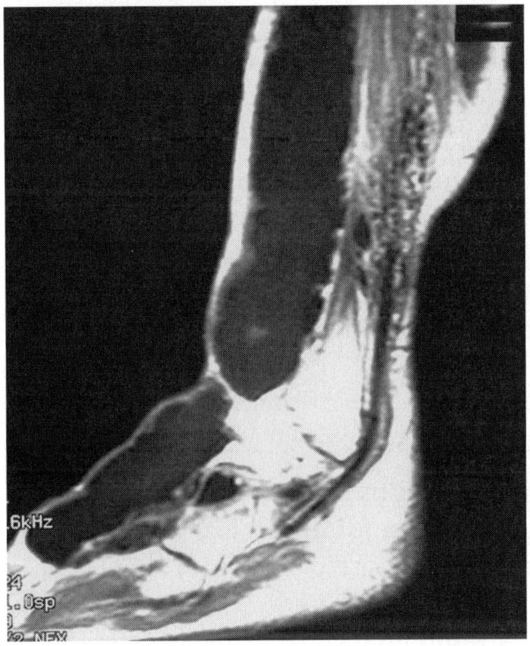

F

Figures 39D Transaxial T1-weighted image shows bilateral low signal intensity throughout and relative swelling of the anterior compartment. **39E** Equivalent transaxial T2-weighted image shows corresponding increased signal intensity within all compartments of the thighs, most pronounced in the vastus lateralis and intermedius. **39F** Sagittal T2-weighted image shows a sheet of low signal intensity on the anterior aspect of the distal foreleg corresponding to the calcifications seen on the radiograph.

- Calcifications present will be very low signal on all sequences (**Fig. 39F**).
- Traditionally, limited scans of the shoulder and lower limb girdles were performed, but there is a recent trend toward whole-body MRI, permitting an assessment of the full extent of involvement and also the potential for identifying gross underlying malignancy.
- P-31 MR spectroscopy obtained during rest, exercise, and in recovery demonstrates concentrations of adenosine triphosphate and phosphocreatine (PCr) in diseased muscles are 30% below normal. The inorganic phosphate/PCr ratios are increased in the patient's muscles at rest and throughout exercise, correlating closely with symptoms and clinical assessment.
- Biopsy may be required to establish the correct diagnosis, and the use of MRI to choose the site of biopsy based on visibly active areas increases the yield. When correlated with the results of such biopsies, MRI has been shown to be 97% specific for inflammatory myopathy.
- MRI may be used to follow the response to treatment, but if the patient is better clinically and the creatine kinase is coming down, repeat MRI is usually not required.
- Fatty infiltration may be seen secondary to steroid treatment, best seen on T1-weighted images.
- T2-weighted fat-suppression sequences are better suited to the examination of children (compared with STIR) when a faster sequence is less likely to be spoiled by motion artifact.

Treatment

- High-dose steroids
- If steroid resistant, more potent immunosuppressives are used, such as azathioprine and methotrexate.

Prognosis

- Steroids usually result in a response in 4 to 5 weeks, as measured by decreasing creatine kinase levels. The clinical response frequently lags behind the biochemical.
- If untreated, progression of the myopathy leads to profound debilitation.

PEARLS

- The recurrence of dermatomyositis in a patient previously treated for a malignancy found in association with dermatomyositis should prompt a search to exclude a recurrence of the malignancy.
- A patient over the age of 40 with a new diagnosis of dermatomyositis should have a chest radiograph, fecal occult blood tests, sigmoidoscopy, gastroscopy, prostate-specific antigen test in a male, abdominopelvic ultrasound, mammography, and Ca-125 levels in a female.
- T2-weighted fat-suppression sequences are better suited to the examination of children (compared with STIR) when a faster sequence is less likely to be spoiled by motion artifact.

PITFALLS

- New onset back pain in a patient on high-dose steroids for dermatomyositis may relate to steroid-induced osteoporotic compression fractures or be a manifestation of an associated malignancy. The imaging should be reviewed carefully to ensure that a malignant cause of back pain is not falsely ascribed to the steroids.
- Respiratory compromise in a patient with dermatomyositis may result from either diaphragmatic involvement or interstitial lung involvement. High-resolution CT may be used to confirm the presence of dermatomyositis usual interstitial pneumonia secondary to dermatomyositis in such a setting.
- If a patient develops worsening proximal myopathy after steroids have been commenced, it may be due to either progression of the disease (steroid resistance) or steroid-induced myopathy. The creatine kinase levels are usually used to assess the response to treatment; if they remain elevated, this is usually indicative of resistance. MRI may assume a role in equivocal cases, where increased signal on T1-weighted imaging may indicate fatty atrophy, suggesting steroid-induced myopathy.

Suggested Readings

Garcia J. MRI in inflammatory myopathies. Skeletal Radiol 2000;29:425–438

O'Connell MJ, Powell T, Brennan D, et al. Imaging in the diagnosis of polymyositis. Am J Roentgenol 2002;179:967–971

Park JH, Vansant JP, Kumar NG, et al. Dermatomyositis: correlative MR imaging and P-31 MR spectroscopy for quantitative characterization of inflammatory disease. Radiology 1990;177:473–479

Young JW, Haney PJ. Case report 314. Diagnosis: juvenile dermatomyositis with changes of the hallux typical of fibrodysplasia (myositis) ossificans progressiva. Skeletal Radiol 1985;13:318–321

CASE 40

Peter L. Munk and Anthony G. Ryan

Clinical Presentation

Our patient was an infant boy in the lowest percentile for height and developmental delay.

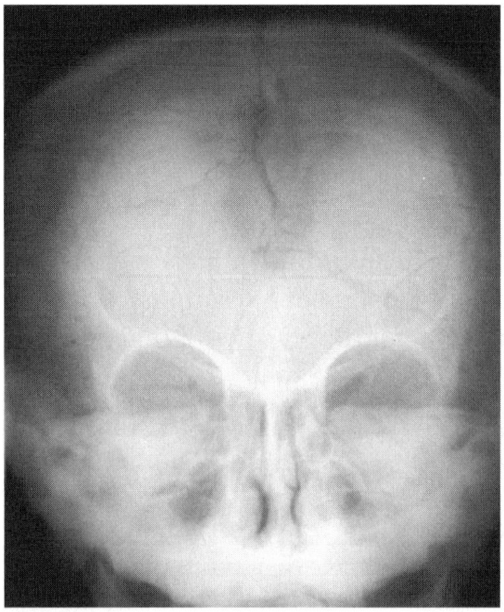

Figure 40A

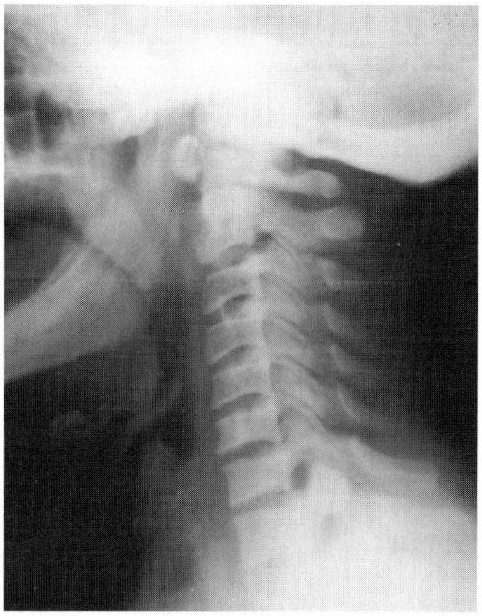

Figure 40B

Radiologic Findings

An anteroposterior image of the skull (**Fig. 40A**) shows multiple wormian bones. A lateral cervical spine radiograph (**Fig. 40B**) demonstrates an obviously flattened and sclerotic skull base. There is basilar invagination (the clivus-canal angle is $<$ 150 degrees). The mandibular angle is obtuse.

Diagnosis

Pyknodysostosis.

Differential Diagnosis

- Osteopetrosis
- Down syndrome

Discussion

Background

Pyknodysostosis is a rare (fewer than 130 cases described) congenital disorder with autosomal recessive transmission, the clinical, and some radiographic, manifestations of which were first described by Maroteaux and Lamy in 1962. Patients with this syndrome have patchy to diffuse osteosclerosis.

Etiology

Pyknodysostosis is an autosomal recessive congenital abnormality resulting in mutations in the *CTSK* gene at 1q21, which codes for cathepsin K.

Pathophysiology

Cathepsin K is a lysosomal cysteine protease that plays a key regulatory role in bone metabolism, abnormalities of which interfere with bone resorption and remodeling. Bone resorption is further compromised by diminished osteoclast activation secondary to a global reduction in interleukin-1 secretion.

Clinical Findings

Males are affected twice as often as females. Patients are generally of short stature, with slightly misshapen skulls that have frontal and occipital bossing. Often the maxilla is small, as is the mandible, giving rise to a typical facial appearance of a receding jaw and a beaked nose. The teeth are frequently stained yellow and malformed (dysodontiasis).

- Reduced mental capacity is present in a minority of cases (10%).
- Broad hands and feet are peripheral features.
- Patients are prone to experience an appreciably increased number of fractures.
- Visceral manifestations such as hepatosplenomegaly are reported but are uncommon.
- Rare manifestations of this condition include extramedullary hematopoiesis and obstructive airways disease.

Complications

- Increased risk of fractures
- Extradural hematoma
- If platybasia is severe, the cervical cord (at the level of the cervicomedullary junction) may be compressed secondary to basilar invagination, whereby the clivus-canal angle is < 150 degrees.
- Diminished immunocompetence is common, evinced by reduced monocyte killing capacity and diminished interleukin function.
- In part, secondary to the abnormal morphology and impaired immunity, suppurative osteomyelitis of the jaws may occur, particularly after dental work.
- Giant-cell granuloma of the maxilla has been described.

Pathology

GROSS

- Sclerotic bones demonstrating undertubulation

MICROSCOPIC

- An accumulation of intracellular lipid has been demonstrated. Structural collagenous abnormalities result in osteocondensation. There may be evidence of chronic osteitis.
- In relation to teeth, there may be a diminishment or loss of the periodontal ligament.

Imaging Findings

RADIOGRAPHY

Skull and spine

- The skull tends to be thicker and more sclerotic than normal (hence the differential of osteopetrosis).
- Multiple wormian bones are common in the skull (**Fig. 40A**).
- Significant delay in closure of sutures is typically observed.
- Brachycephaly (wide skull secondary to premature closure of the coronal and lambdoid sutures)
- Platybasia (flattened) with a thickened skull base (**Fig. 40B**)
- Hypoplastic mandible with obtuse mandibular angle (**Fig. 40B**)
- Hypoplasia and nonaeration of the paranasal sinuses
- The latter two findings give rise to the characteristic facies.
- There may be failure of C1/C2 and L5/S1 to segment.

Periphery

- The bones of the hands and feet are typically short, and the phalanges in particular are hypoplastic or osteolytic, including resorption of the distal portion of the phalanges (acro-osteolysis) (**Fig. 40C**). Dysplasia of the distal clavicles (usually resorption) is sometimes seen (giving rise to the differential of cleidocranial dysostosis).
- Dense, thickened long bones (again giving rise to the differential of osteopetrosis)

ULTRASOUND

- Useful in the confirmation of clinically suspected hepatosplenomegaly

RADIONUCLIDE STUDIES

- Densitometry typically will reveal values of up to 291% of age-matched normal controls; the increased density is evident mainly in trabecular bone.

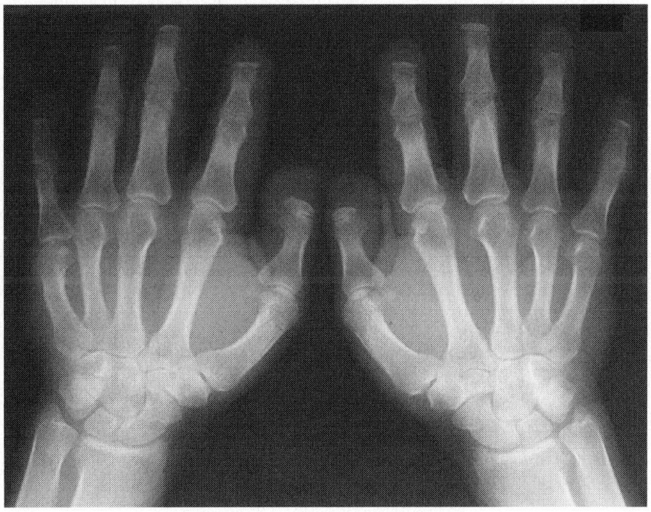

Figure 40C Bilateral hand radiograph shows profound resorption of almost the totality of all the distal phalanges. In addition, an old fracture of the neck of the right fifth metacarpal is evident.

- Techmetium 99m bone scans and SPECT (single photon emission computed tomography) demonstrate an increased uptake of up to 538% of age-matched controls.

COMPUTED TOMOGRAPHY/MAGNETIC RESONANCE IMAGING

- Both CT and MRI will show the cortical bone to be of normal thickness, with an increase in the trabecular bone, the latter limiting the medullary canal volume.

Treatment

- Treatment is primarily directed at managing the complications of the condition, although reconstruction of the mandible may be required if nutrition is impaired or cosmesis is a consideration.
- Genetic counseling

Prognosis

- Although most patients develop fractures and/or infective complications, pyknodystosis does not shorten life.
- The tendency to fracture actually reduces as the patient gets older.

PEARLS

- In differentiating this condition from osteopetrosis, the latter should have no mandibular or skull abnormality or phalangeal dysplasia. Pyknodysostosis does not demonstrate the Erlenmeyer flask deformity or the "bone-within-a-bone" deformity.
- Cleidocranial dysostosis does not share the dense bones or acro-osteolysis seen in pyknodysostosis.
- The artist Henri de Toulouse-Lautrec is said to have had this syndrome.

PITFALLS

- Because the clinical manifestations have considerable overlap with other congenital syndromes, such as osteopetrosis, hemolytic anemia, and other osteochondrodystrophies, the diagnosis may only be secured on the basis of the radiographic signs (in the absence of formal genetic analysis).
- Wormian bones have a long differential, including cleidocranial dysostosis, osteogenesis imperfecta, and Down syndrome.
- A simian crease, wormian bones, and (occasionally) acro-osteolysis may be found in both pyknodysostosis and Down syndrome; the clinical scenario should be obvious, however.

Suggested Readings

Bathi RJ, Masur VN. Pyknodysostosis—a report of two cases with a brief review of the literature. Int J Oral Maxillofac Surg 2000;29:439–442

Karkabi S, Reis ND, Linn S, et al. Pyknodysostosis: imaging and laboratory observations. Calcif Tissue Int 1993;53:170–173

Singh AR, Kaur A, Anand NK, Singh JR. Pyknodysostosis: visceral manifestations and simian crease. Indian J Pediatr 2004;71:453–455

Maroteaux P, Lamy M. La Pycnodysostoge. La Press Medicale 1962;70:999

CASE 41

George Nomikos, Anthony G. Ryan, Peter L. Munk, and Mark Murphey

Clinical Presentation

A 14-year-old boy presented with an enlarging, painful, left distal femoral mass.

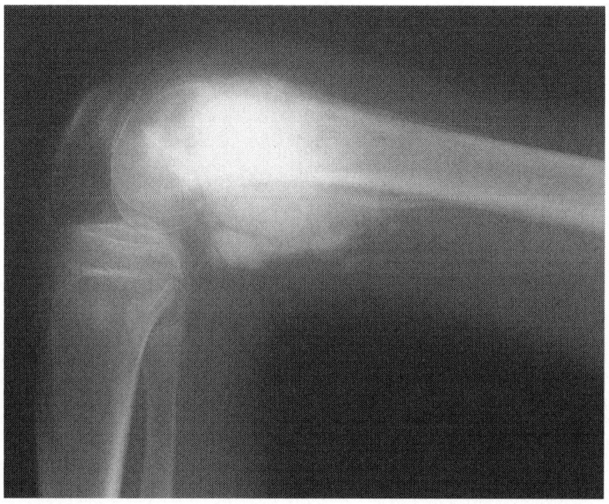

Figure 41A

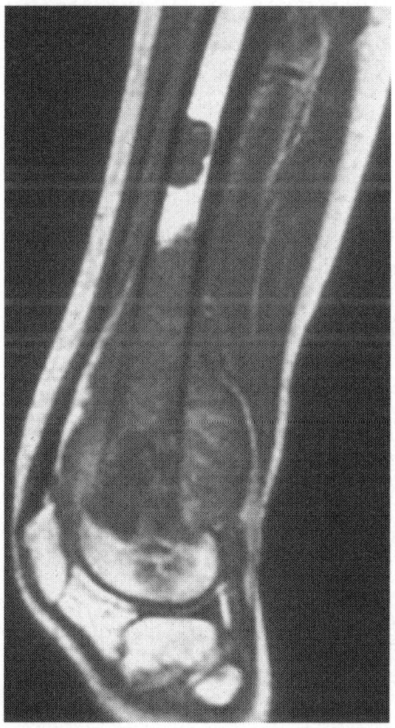

Figure 41B

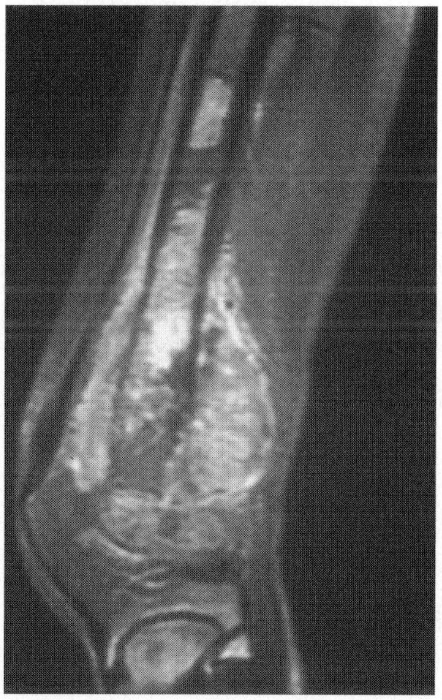

Figure 41C

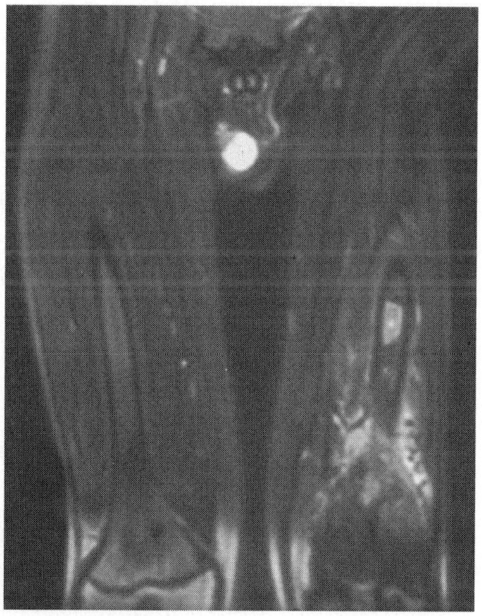

Figure 41D

Radiologic Findings

The radiograph shows a large destructive mass arising from the distal femoral metaphysis (**Fig. 41A**). Dense matrix mineralization is apparent in both the intraosseous and soft-tissue components of the lesion. The pattern of mineralization is cloudlike, compatible with osteoid mineralization. Also note the aggressive-appearing periosteal reaction and Codman's triangle.

Sagittal T1-weighted images before (**Fig. 41B**) and after (**Fig. 41C**) intravenous contrast administration and a T2-weighted image (**Fig. 41D**) show a large area of marrow replacement in the distal femur and the associated soft-tissue component. In addition, there is a second, smaller focus of tumor in the femoral metaphysis separated from the primary tumor by normal intervening marrow.

Diagnosis

High-grade intramedullary (conventional) osteosarcoma with a skip metastasis.

Differential Diagnosis

None.

Discussion

Background

Osteosarcoma is the second most common malignant primary osseous neoplasm following myeloma. Although there are multiple subtypes of osteosarcoma, the conventional (or central intramedullary) type depicted in this case is the most common form. The most common skeletal location of the conventional osteosarcoma is about the knee, accounting for 50 to 55% of cases. Most affected patients are in their teens or twenties and there is a 2:1 male-to-female ratio. Lesions are most commonly metaphyseal, although diaphyseal (2 to 11%) and epiphyseal ($<$ 1%) lesions may occur. Epiphyseal extension of metaphyseal lesions is common.

Pathology

Pathologically, these are malignant tumors of mesenchymal origin whose cells produce osteoid or immature bone. Some lesions contain areas of chondroid (5 to 25%) and fibroblastic-fibrohistiocytic differentiation (7 to 25%); however, most lesions are predominantly osteoblastic (50 to 80%).

Imaging Findings

RADIOGRAPHY

- Although some lesions may be purely lytic or sclerotic, most usually demonstrate mixed lysis and sclerosis.
- Abundant osteoid mineralization with a cloudlike appearance, cortical destruction, soft-tissue mass, and aggressive-appearing periosteal reaction (laminated, Codman's triangle, or sunburst appearance) are common.
- High-grade intramedullary tumors often disrupt the overlying cortical bone without causing osseous expansion, reflecting their aggressive behavior.
- Lesions are often large at the time of presentation, and soft-tissue masses are commonly encountered.

COMPUTED TOMOGRAPHY

- CT may demonstrate internal osteoid matrix mineralization to better advantage than radiographs, especially in lesions with scant mineralization or complex areas of anatomy.
- Cross-sectional imaging is also useful for evaluation of the local extent of tumor spread for purposes of staging.

MAGNETIC RESONANCE IMAGING

- Areas of nonmineralized tumor are predominantly intermediate signal intensity on T1-weighted images and high signal intensity on T2-weighted images.
- Marrow involvement, soft-tissue extension, neurovascular and joint invasion, and epiphyseal spread are all well evaluated on MRI and represent important information in planning limb-salvage surgery.
- Pathological analysis has shown that tumor extension across the physis is relatively common (seen in 75 to 88% of cases), and joint involvement is relatively common also (19 to 24% of cases), particularly around the knee.
- Common routes of intra-articular extension include through the posterior capsule, along the cruciate ligaments, and into the suprapatellar recess anteriorly.
- Joint invasion is usually best assessed on postcontrast T1-weighted images or standard T1-weighted images without fat suppression.
- Although the absence of a joint effusion has a high negative predictive value for tumor extension, the presence of an effusion may indicate tumor extension or may be sympathetic.

Variants

Whereas the high-grade intramedullary, or conventional subtypes, account for 75% of all osteosarcomas, several variants require mention.

The telangiectatic form accounts for 4.5 to 11% of lesions and most commonly occurs about the knee. It is characterized by the presence of large cystic, necrotic, or blood-filled spaces that comprise $> 90\%$ of the lesion volume as well as by the presence of large vessels. It usually demonstrates an aggressive radiologic appearance with marked osseous expansion, similar to that seen in aneurysmal bone cysts. Mineralized osteoid is usually minimal in extent, is usually peripherally located, and can be detected on CT in up to 81% of cases.

Common surface variants of osteosarcoma include the parosteal (**Fig. 41E**) and periosteal (**Fig. 41F**) subtypes.

Parosteal osteosarcoma is usually a low-grade lesion (although high-grade foci may be present) that arises from the outer layer of periosteum and is most commonly found on the posterior metaphysis of the distal femur (50 to 65% of cases). The average age at presentation is about a decade older than that for patients with conventional osteosarcoma, and there is a female predilection. Lesions typically appear as a well-defined mass of densely mineralized osteoid on the metaphyseal surface of the involved bone, often with a stalk of attachment as well as a partial cleavage plane between it and the underlying bone. With growth, the cleavage plane may disappear, and medullary backgrowth may occur (41 to 50%). The pattern of mineralization is more mature-appearing centrally than peripherally, an important difference from myositis ossificans, in which the mineralization is more mature peripherally than centrally. Myositis ossificans is also not usually attached to the underlying osseous cortex as parosteal osteosarcomas are.

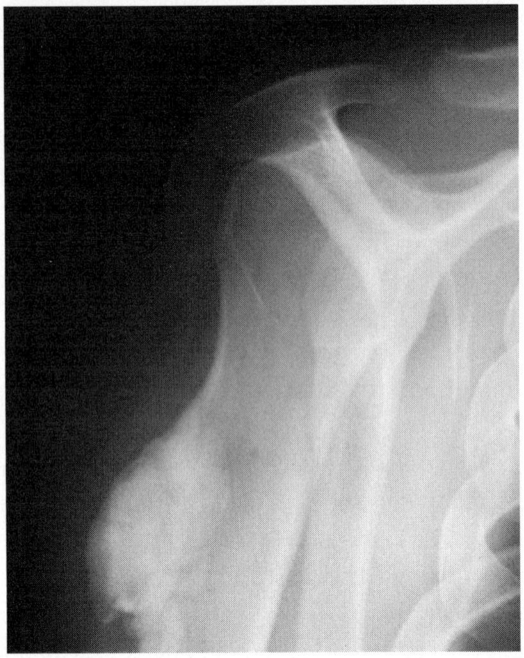

E

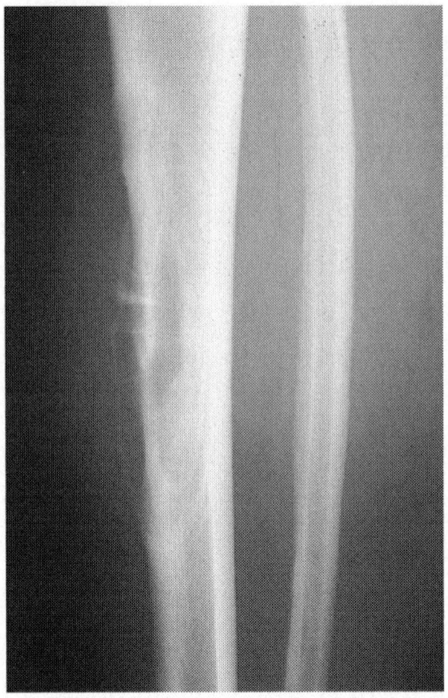

F

Figures 41E An anteroposterior (AP) shoulder radiograph shows a well-defined mass of densely mineralized osteoid on the proximal metaphyseal surface of the posterolateral aspect of the humerus in a 27-year-old woman: biopsy-proven parosteal osteosarcoma. The typical partial plane of cleavage between the lesion and the underlying bone is not clearly seen in this instance. **41F** An AP image of the tibia and fibula shows the characteristic appearances of a periosteal osteosarcoma of the midtibial diaphysis: "hair on end" periosteal reaction perpendicular to the long axis of the underlying bone extending into a large soft-tissue component in association with saucerization of the underlying cortical bone. Codman's triangles are seen at either end of the lesion.

Periosteal osteosarcomas (**Fig. 41F**) represent another surface variant and arise from the deep layer of periosteum. They are intermediate-grade lesions that affect a similar age group as the conventional variant. They most commonly arise on the diaphysis or metadiaphysis of long bones (especially the femur and tibia). Lesions produce cortical scalloping or saucerization of the underlying cortical bone and are only rarely associated with medullary extension. Sunburst or "hair on end" periosteal reaction perpendicular to the long axis of the underlying bone extending into a large soft-tissue component is characteristic. A Codman's triangle is often seen. Lesions are most commonly highly chondroblastic histologically.

An association between certain bone lesions and development of secondary osteosarcoma is well known. These secondary lesions account for 5 to 7% of all osteosarcomas. The most commonly associated preexisting condition is Paget's disease, followed by radiation therapy. Other predisposing conditions include osteonecrosis, fibrous dysplasia, osteogenesis imperfecta, chronic osteomyelitis, and metallic hardware.

Treatment

- Treatment for conventional osteosarcoma currently consists of preoperative neoadjuvant chemotherapy followed by surgical excision with wide margins (limb-salvage surgery when possible).

Prognosis

- The most important prognostic indicator is tumor response to chemotherapy.
- Greater than 90% tumor necrosis (good responder) correlates with a favorable long-term prognosis.

- Overall, the 5-year survival rate is 60 to 80% (up to 80 to 90% for the parosteal variant) for the good responders.
- The lungs, other bones, and regional lymph nodes are common sites of metastatic spread.
- Pulmonary metastases may show ossification and have a well-known association with spontaneous pneumothorax.
- Skip metastases, seen in 1 to 25% of patients with conventional high-grade osteosarcoma, have a similar negative impact on prognosis as distant metastases.

PEARLS

- In osteosarcoma, the pattern of mineralization is more mature-appearing centrally than peripherally, an important difference from myositis ossificans, in which the mineralization is more mature peripherally than centrally. Also, unlike parosteal osteosarcomas, myositis ossificans is not usually attached to the underlying osseous cortex.
- A well-known "Aunt Minnie" is the association between ossified pulmonary metastases and spontaneous pneumothorax.
- In relation to the knee, common routes of intra-articular extension include through the posterior capsule, along the cruciate ligaments, and into the suprapatellar recess anteriorly.

PITFALLS

- Skip metastases, seen in 1 to 25% of patients with conventional high-grade osteosarcoma, have a similar negative impact on prognosis as distant metastases: this feature reiterates one of the basic tenets of imaging bone lesions, which is the necessity of imaging the whole length of the affected bone.
- Osseous expansion is not a necessary feature, as high-grade intramedullary tumors often disrupt the overlying cortical bone without causing osseous expansion (reflecting their aggressive behavior).
- Joint invasion is usually best assessed on postcontrast T1-weighted images or standard T1-weighted images without fat suppression.
- Although the absence of a joint effusion has a high negative predictive value for tumor extension, the presence of an effusion does not necessarily imply or indicate tumor extension, as effusion may be sympathetic.

Suggested Readings

Murphey MD, Robbin MR, McRae GA, Flemming DJ, Temple HT, Kransdorf MJ. The many faces of osteosarcoma. Radiographics 1997;17:1205–1231

Nomikos GC, Murphey MD, Kransdorf MJ, Bancroft LW, Peterson JJ. Primary bone tumors of the lower extremities. Radiol Clin North Am 2002;40:971–990

Resnick D, Kyriakos M, Greenway G. Tumors and tumor-like lesions of bone: imaging and pathology of specific lesions. In: Resnick D, ed. Diagnosis of Bone and Joint Disorders. Philadelphia, PA: WB Saunders; 2002:3763–4128

White LM, Kandel R. Osteoid-producing tumors of bone. Semin Musculoskelet Radiol 2000;4:25–43

CASE 42

George Nomikos, Anthony G. Ryan, Peter L. Munk, and
Mark Murphey

Clinical Presentation

A 53-year-old man presented with pain in the proximal humerus for 3 months.

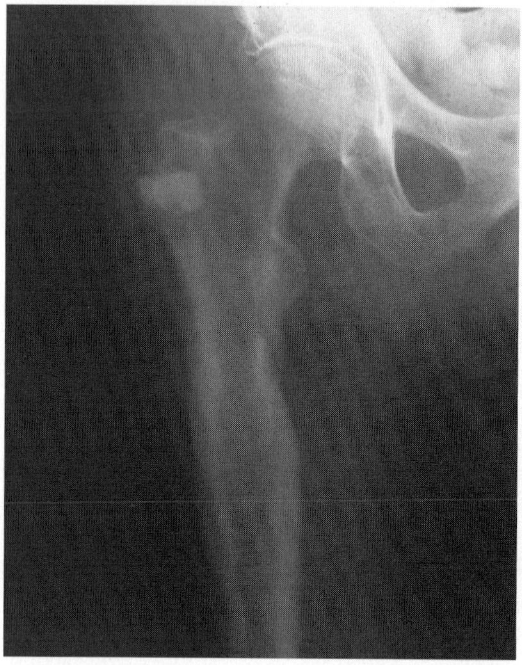

Figure 42A

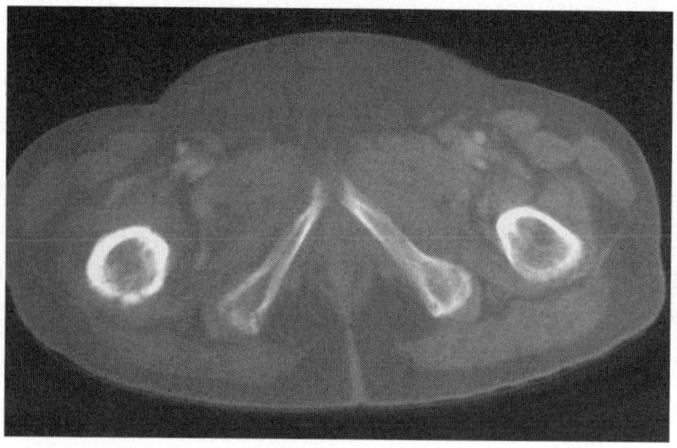

Figure 42B

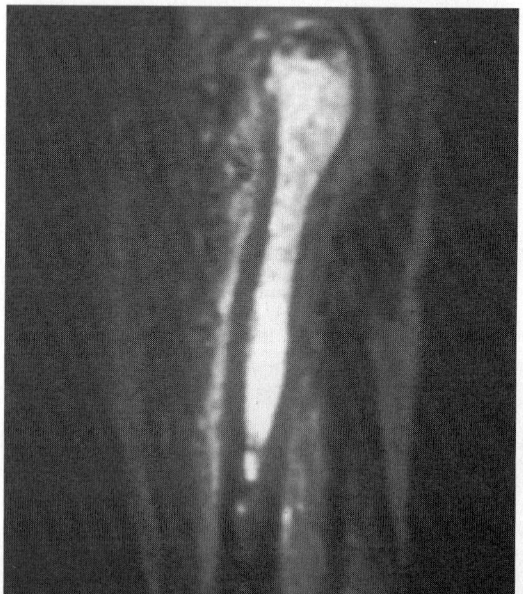

Figure 42C

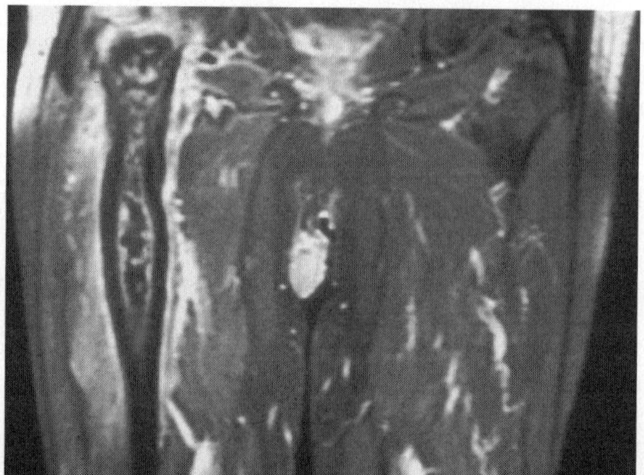

Figure 42D

Radiologic Findings

A radiograph (**Fig. 42A**) shows a lytic destructive lesion in the proximal femur. There is associated cortical thickening and periosteal reaction, as well as expansile remodeling and lobular endosteal scalloping. The density in the greater trochanter represents a methylmethacrylate plug from a prior biopsy. The CT (**Fig. 42B**) shows cortical destruction, faint internal mineralization, and soft-tissue thickening around the femur. The sagittal inversion recovery MRI (**Fig. 42C**) shows the extent of the lesion. The lesion is predominantly high signal intensity. The lower signal intensity foci within the lesion represent areas of mineralization. The postcontrast image (**Fig. 42D**) shows peripheral and septal enhancement, a characteristic pattern seen in hyaline cartilage lesions. There is also enhancement within the periosteal reaction around the femur.

Diagnosis

Chondrosarcoma.

Differential Diagnosis

- Bone infarction with secondary malignancy (malignant fibrous histiocytoma/fibrosarcoma)
- Enchondroma (effectively excluded in this case because of the presence of cortical destruction)

Discussion

Background

Chondrosarcomas account for ~8 to 17% of biopsied primary bone tumors. They may arise in the medullary canal (central type) or on the surface of the bone (peripheral type). Chondrosarcomas represent malignant cartilage lesions. They may arise de novo or from a preexisting cartilage lesion, such as an enchondroma or osteochondroma. Common locations include the pelvis, femur, humerus, ribs, tibia, scapula, and spine.

Clinical Findings

Most patients are in the fourth or fifth decade of life at the time of presentation and usually have a history of pain, often worse at night, and swelling. Patients reveal a palpable soft-tissue mass in ~28% of cases, and 27% show a pathological fracture at the time of diagnosis. Symptoms may be present for long periods (up to several years) prior to diagnosis.

Imaging Findings

RADIOGRAPHY

- Lesions usually demonstrate a geographic pattern of lysis with a wide zone of transition and lobulated margin.

- Mineralized matrix in a ring and arc pattern typical of hyaline cartilage lesions is seen in ~75% of cases.

COMPUTED TOMOGRAPHY

- Lesions are typically slightly lower in attenuation than skeletal muscle.
- Cortical scalloping and cortical penetration, as well as the presence of a soft-tissue mass, are well demonstrated.
- Matrix mineralization is seen in ~92% of cases on CT.

MAGNETIC RESONANCE IMAGING

- Histologically, higher grade lesions often demonstrate less prominent mineralization than lower grade lesions but larger soft-tissue masses.
- MRI delineates the degree of marrow replacement and the presence of a soft-tissue mass to better advantage than CT.
- Nonmineralized portions of the lesion are typically very high signal on T2-weighted images due to the high water content in the hyaline cartilage matrix.
- Postcontrast enhancement in a peripheral and septal enhancement pattern characteristic of hyaline cartilage lesions is typical; however, this pattern may also be seen in benign hyaline cartilage lesions, such as enchondromas, and is therefore not helpful in distinguishing benign from malignant lesions.

Variants

In addition to the relatively more common intramedullary and peripheral chondrosarcomas described above, several less common variants exist. Of special interest is the clear cell variant, which accounts for only 2% of chondrosarcomas but has an unusual predilection for the epiphyses of the proximal femur or humerus. This type of chondrosarcoma is seen in patients slightly younger than those affected with the traditional chondrosarcoma. It is usually predominantly lytic and may demonstrate a peripheral rim of sclerosis. Mineralization is seen in only approximately one third of cases, and formation of a soft-tissue mass is uncommon.

ENCHONDROMA VERSUS CHONDROSARCOMA

Differentiation of enchondroma and chondrosarcoma in long bones may be difficult both radiologically and histologically. Findings that are suggestive of chondrosarcoma rather than enchondroma in long bones include the following: cortical scalloping greater than two thirds of the cortical depth in any single location; uptake on scintigraphy greater than the anterior superior iliac spine; cortical destruction and soft-tissue mass (CT or MRI); periosteal reaction on radiography; pain directly attributable to the lesion; size > 5 to 6 cm; epiphyseal location (very uncommon site for enchondroma). Neither pattern nor degree of enhancement is helpful in distinguishing enchondroma from chondrosarcoma.

Treatment

- Treatment is surgical excision.
- Chemotherapy and radiotherapy have virtually no role in treatment.

Prognosis

- As expected, prognosis is much better for lower grade lesions than for higher grade lesions.

- The 10-year survival for grade 1 lesions is ~85%, but for grade 3 lesions, it is only 28%.
- Lesions are known to recur as long as 10 years after the initial treatment.

PEARLS

- Enhancement within the periosteal reaction around the affected bone is typical.
- Findings that are suggestive of chondrosarcoma rather than enchondroma in long bones include the following: cortical scalloping greater than two thirds of the cortical depth in any single location; uptake on scintigraphy greater than the anterior superior iliac spine; cortical destruction and soft-tissue mass (CT or MRI); periosteal reaction on radiography; pain directly attributable to the lesion; size > 5 to 6 cm; epiphyseal location (very uncommon site for enchondroma).
- Uncomplicated enchondroma is excluded if cortical destruction is present.

PITFALLS

- Histologically, higher grade lesions often demonstrate less prominent mineralization than lower grade lesions but larger soft-tissue masses.
- Postcontrast enhancement in a peripheral and septal enhancement pattern characteristic of hyaline cartilage lesions is typical; however, this pattern may also be seen in benign hyaline cartilage lesions, such as enchondromas, and is therefore not helpful in distinguishing benign from malignant lesions. Thus, neither pattern nor degree of enhancement is helpful in distinguishing enchondroma from chondrosarcoma.
- The clear cell variant (2% of chondrosarcomas) has an unusual predilection for the epiphyses of the proximal femur or humerus. This type of chondrosarcoma is seen in patients slightly younger than those affected with the traditional chondrosarcoma. It is usually predominantly lytic and may demonstrate a peripheral rim of sclerosis. The latter feature should not be mistaken as evidence that the lesion is benign.

Suggested Readings

Flemming DJ, Murphey MD. Enchondroma and chondrosarcoma. Semin Musculoskelet Radiol 2000;4:59–71

Giudici MA, Moser RP Jr, Kransdorf MJ. Cartilagenous bone tumors. Radiol Clin North Am 1993;31:237–259

Murphey MD, Flemming DJ, Boyea SR, Bojescul JA, Sweet DE, Temple HT. Enchondroma versus chondrosarcoma in the appendicular skeleton: differentiating features. Radiographics 1998;18:1213–1237

CASE 43

George Nomikos, Anthony G. Ryan, Peter L. Munk, and Mark Murphey

Clinical Presentation

A skeletally immature patient presented with a rapidly enlarging calf mass.

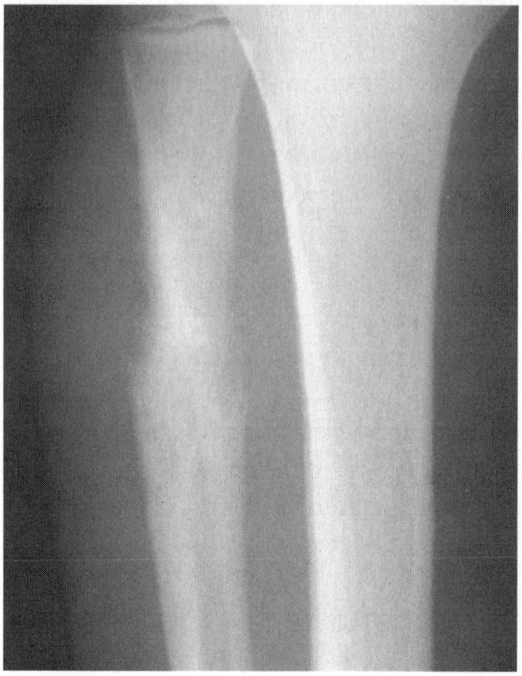

Figure 43A

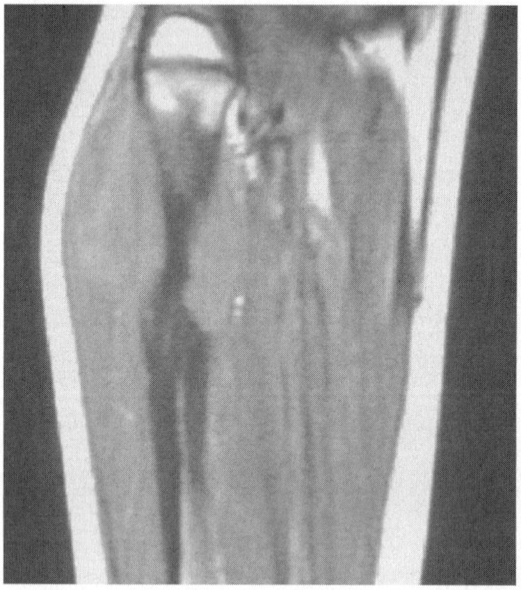

Figure 43B

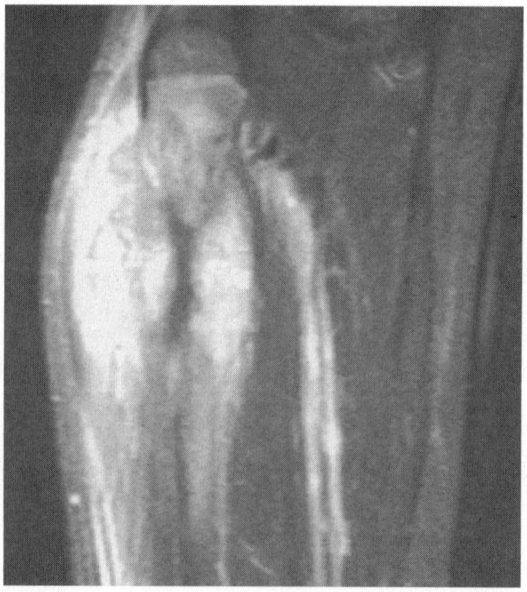

Figure 43C

Radiologic Findings

An anteroposterior radiograph (**Fig. 43A**) of the proximal lower leg shows a poorly marginated area of permeative bone destruction as well as mild sclerosis involving the proximal fibular diaphysis. Note the marked cortical destruction. No mineralized matrix is identified. Also note the aggressive periosteal reaction along the diaphysis adjacent to the area of cortical destruction.

A T1-weighted MRI (**Fig. 43B**) shows a large destructive mass arising from the proximal fibular diaphysis with formation of a large soft-tissue component. There is marrow replacement in the fibular shaft extending into the metaphysis. There is no evidence of extension across the physis. There is diffuse and heterogeneous enhancement of the mass after intravenous contrast administration (**Fig. 43C**).

Diagnosis

Ewing's sarcoma.

Differential Diagnosis

- Primitive neuroectodermal tumor (PNET)
- Lymphoma
- Leukemia
- Langerhans' cell histiocytosis
- Osteomyelitis (acute, bacterial)

Discussion

Background

Ewing's sarcoma and the closely related PNET represent the second most common primary bone malignancy occurring in children and adolescents, after osteosarcoma. Most patients present with pain and swelling and a palpable mass. Systemic symptoms simulating an infectious process, including fever and malaise, are also seen and imply diffuse disease.

Pathology

Pathologically, both lesions represent small, round blue cell tumors that often demonstrate a genetic translocation, most commonly at t(11;22).

Imaging Findings

RADIOGRAPHY

- May demonstrate permeative lysis (long bone lesions), sclerosis (flat bone lesions), and expansion (the sclerosis has been shown to correspond to areas of osteonecrosis and reactive osteoid histologically)

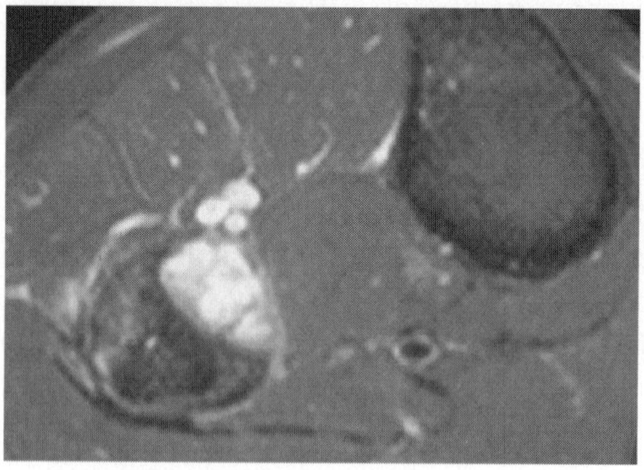

Figure 43D Transaxial T2-weighted image with fat saturation of the same lesion in **Figs. 34A** to **34C**, demonstrating high signal intensity throughout.

- Typically diaphyseal or metadiaphyseal in location
- Mineralized matrix is absent, but multilayered periosteal reaction may be seen.
- Soft-tissue involvement is very common (80%) and may be seen without focal cortical destruction, likely due to growth of tumor through the haversian canals into the surrounding soft tissues prior to gross cortical destruction (a feature common to all small, round blue cell tumors).

COMPUTED TOMOGRAPHY/MAGNETIC RESONANCE IMAGING

- Although CT reveals the soft-tissue mass, this is seen to better advantage on MRI.
- These lesions are usually nonspecific in appearance on MRI: heterogeneously low to intermediate signal intensity on T1-weighted images and intermediate to high signal on T2-weighted images (**Fig. 43D**).

Treatment

- Treatment consists of neoadjuvant chemotherapy combined with radiation therapy and wide or radical en bloc resection and reconstruction.

Prognosis

- Long-term survival has been improved significantly by the addition of neoadjuvant chemotherapy and radiation therapy to the treatment regimen (74% 5-year survival vs 34% previously).
- Poor prognostic indicators include size > 8 cm, pelvic location, elevated erythrocyte sedimentation rate, age > 17 years, gross soft-tissue mass, and metastatic disease at presentation.

PEARLS

- The classic presentation is that of a poorly marginated area of permeative bone destruction, marked cortical destruction, and aggressive periosteal reaction, but no mineralized matrix.
- Lesions typically do not cross the physis.
- Poor prognostic indicators include size > 8 cm, pelvic location, elevated erythrocyte sedimentation rate, age > 17 years, gross soft-tissue mass, and metastatic disease at presentation.

PITFALLS

- The variability in appearances (permeative lysis [long bone lesions], sclerosis [flat bone lesions], and expansion) occasionally may give rise to diagnostic confusion.
- Soft-tissue involvement is very common (80%) and may be seen without focal cortical destruction, likely due to growth of tumor through the haversian canals into the surrounding soft tissues prior to gross cortical destruction (a feature common to all small, round blue cell tumors). Thus, when radiographs only are reviewed, if one does not appreciate the soft-tissue mass, the cortical destruction may be subtle, leading to a missed diagnosis.
- These lesions are usually nonspecific in appearance on MRI: heterogeneously low to intermediate signal intensity on T1-weighted images and intermediate to high signal on T2-weighted images.

Suggested Readings

Frouge C, Vanel D, Coffre C, Couanet D, Contesso G, Sarrazin D. The role of magnetic resonance imaging in the evaluation of Ewing sarcoma: a report of 27 cases. Skeletal Radiol 1988;17:387–392

Kransdorf MJ, Smith SE. Lesions of unknown histogenesis: Langerhans cell histiocytosis and Ewing sarcoma. Semin Musculoskelet Radiol 2000;4:113–125

Resnick D, Kyriakos M, Greenway G. Tumors and tumor-like lesions of bone: imaging and pathology of specific lesions. In: Resnick D, ed. Diagnosis of Bone and Joint Disorders. Philadelphia, PA: WB Saunders; 2002:3763–4128

CASE 44

George Nomikos, Anthony G. Ryan, Peter L. Munk, and Mark Murphey

Clinical Presentation

A 40-year-old man presented with an 8-month history of a painless thigh mass.

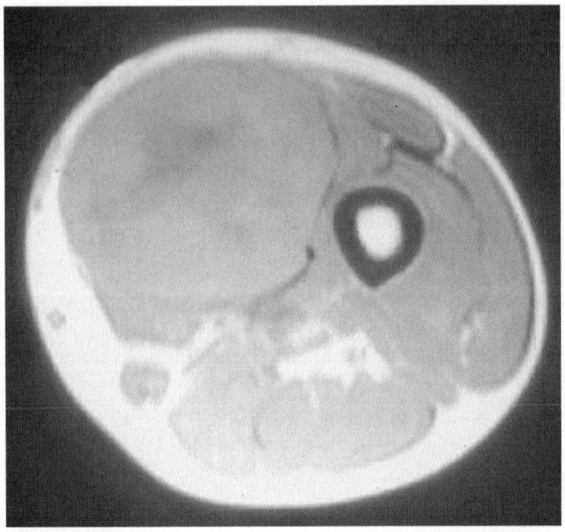

Figure 44A

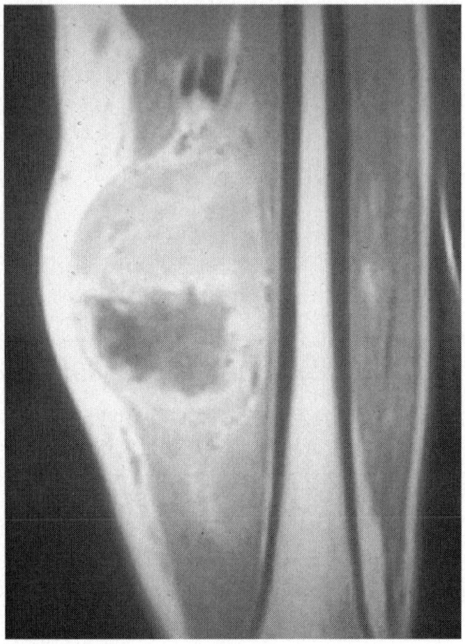

Figure 44B

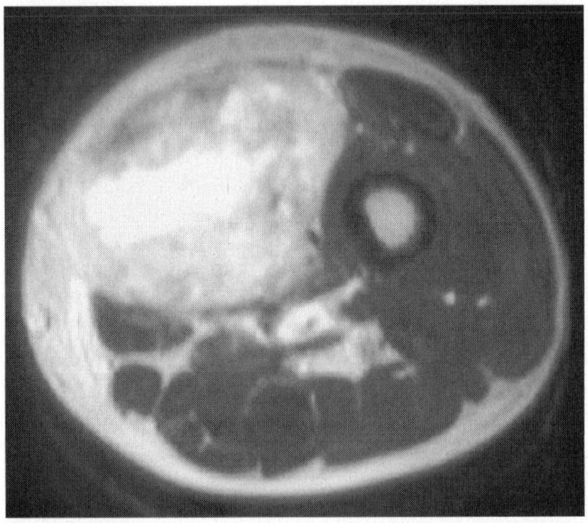

Figure 44C

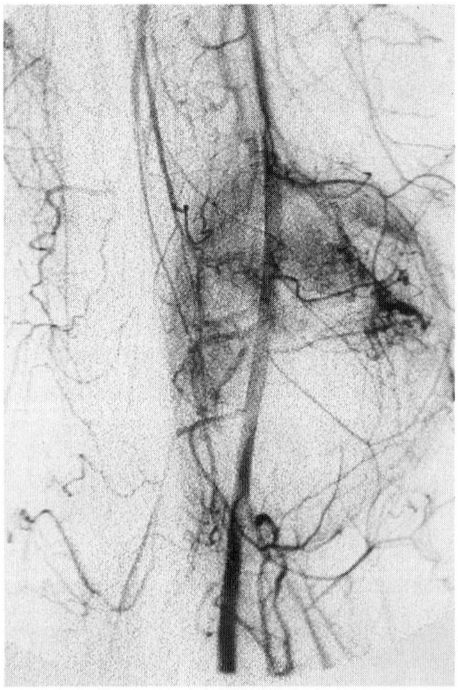

Figure 44D

Radiologic Findings

Axial T1- (**Fig. 44A**), postcontrast coronal T1- (**Fig. 44B**), and axial T2- (**Fig. 44C**) weighted images show a large intramuscular mass arising in the vastus medialis muscle. The lesion has a nonenhancing central area that is low signal on the T1-weighted image and high signal on the T2-weighted image, compatible with a region of central necrosis. The peripheral solid portion of the lesion is moderately heterogeneous on the T2-weighted image and shows diffuse enhancement. No fat is seen in the mass. No mineralization was identified in the mass on CT (not shown). The angiogram (**Fig. 44D**) shows marked tumor blush and neovascularity in the arterial phase of perfusion. There is also slight narrowing of the femoral artery, compatible with tumor encasement.

Diagnosis

Primary soft-tissue malignant fibrous histiocytoma (MFH).

Differential Diagnosis

- Fibrosarcoma
- Leiomyosarcoma
- Liposarcoma (usually intermuscular; some fat is usually identifiable in the lesion)

Discussion

Background

MFH, a malignant tumor of fibrohistiocytic origin, accounts for 20 to 30% of all soft-tissue sarcomas and is the most common soft-tissue sarcoma in the later adult years. It arises in a deep intramuscular location in two thirds of cases, and 70 to 75% occur in the extremities. Approximately 5 to 10% of lesions are subcutaneous, and these lesions have a better prognosis. The retroperitoneum accounts for 15% of cases, and the head and neck account for 5% of cases; half of all cases occur in the lower extremities. Although most lesions arise spontaneously, there is a well-known association between MFH and prior radiation therapy. There is also reported association between MFH and retained shrapnel, orthopedic hardware, and osteonecrosis.

Clinical Findings

Most patients present with an enlarging, painless soft-tissue mass. Internally, the lesions may bleed spontaneously, causing rapid enlargement. It is important to note that an occult MFH is the diagnosis of exclusion in any patient who presents with a "spontaneous hematoma" in the deep soft tissues. In addition, most true soft-tissue hematomas demonstrate marked surrounding edema and inflammatory change. Intratumoral hemorrhage often lacks this edema/inflammatory change because the blood products are contained within the tumor pseudocapsule and have not spread into the surrounding muscle, where they would cause inflammatory changes.

Pathology

There are multiple pathological subtypes of MFH. The majority of tumors are of the storiform/pleomorphic variety, which accounts for 50 to 60% of lesions. The myxoid variety, which accounts for ~25% of cases, contains prominent mucoid material that has large amounts of extracellular mucopolysaccharide and hyaluronic acid. The other subtypes are considerably less common. The inflammatory subtype (5 to 10%) deserves special mention as patients with this variety of tumor may present with signs of systemic infection (fever and leukocytosis). Pathologically, this variety of tumor demonstrates acute and chronic inflammatory cells. According to the 2002 World Health Organization terminology, MFH is properly referred to as *undifferentiated pleomorphic sarcoma*.

Imaging Findings

RADIOGRAPHY

- Nonspecific soft-tissue mass
- Calcification or ossification may be seen in 5 to 20% of cases, usually peripherally; mineralization may simulate the zonal phenomenon of myositis ossificans and represents metaplastic, not tumor, new bone formation.
- Cortical erosion or bone destruction may be seen. (This latter finding is highly suggestive of MFH. The only other soft-tissue sarcoma with a propensity for osseous invasion is synovial sarcoma.)

COMPUTED TOMOGRAPHY

- Large, lobular, well-defined, (usually) intramuscular mass with central low attenuation representing hemorrhage, necrosis, or myxoid areas
- Often adjacent to a long bone diaphysis
- Better defines mineralization, if present
- Demonstrates cortical erosion and bone invasion to better advantage than radiography
- Solid portions enhance, often in a peripheral and nodular pattern, and hemorrhagic/necrotic/myxoid areas do not enhance.

MAGNETIC RESONANCE IMAGING

- Intermediate signal on T1-weighted images
- Heterogeneously high signal on T2-weighted images. The myxoid variant is of diffusely high signal.
- Relatively well-defined margins owing to the pseudocapsule
- Enhancement pattern similar to CT
- Imaging features of MFH and fibrosarcoma are virtually identical.

Treatment and Prognosis

- Treatment by means of preoperative chemotherapy followed by wide resection
- Radiation commonly employed as well
- Osseous invasion by tumor may necessitate limb salvage procedure.
- The most common site of metastatic disease is the lungs (90%).
- Survival ranges from 82% at 5 years for lesions < 5 cm to 51% for lesions > 10 cm.
- Histologic variant has only a mild influence on survival, as most tumors are high-grade lesions.

PEARLS

- MFH is a vascular tumor, demonstrating marked tumor blush and neovascularity in the arterial phase of perfusion. Tumor encasement of adjacent arteries is not uncommon.
- Differentiating MFH from liposarcoma is often straightforward, as the latter is usually intermuscular and some fat is usually identifiable in the lesion.
- Most true soft-tissue hematomas demonstrate marked surrounding edema and inflammatory change. Intratumoral hemorrhage often lacks this edema/inflammatory change because the blood products are contained within the tumor pseudocapsule and have not spread into the surrounding muscle, where they would cause inflammatory changes.

PITFALLS

- It is important to note that an occult MFH is the diagnosis of exclusion in any patient who presents with a "spontaneous hematoma" in the deep soft tissues.
- The inflammatory subtype (5 to 10%) deserves special mention, as patients with this variety of tumor may present with signs of systemic infection (fever and leukocytosis).
- Imaging features of MFH and fibrosarcoma are virtually identical; differentiation is not possible on the basis of imaging alone.

Suggested Readings

Kransdorf M, Murphey M. Imaging of Soft Tissue Tumors. Philadelphia, PA: WB Saunders; 1997

Munk PL, Sallomi DF, Janzen DL, et al. Malignant fibrous histiocytoma of soft tissue: imaging with emphasis on MRI. J Comput Assist Tomogr 1998;22:819–826

Murphey MD, Gross TM, Rosenthal HG. Musculoskeletal malignant fibrous histiocytoma: radiologic-pathologic correlation. Radiographics 1994;14:807–826

CASE 45

Anthony G. Ryan and Peter L. Munk

Clinical Presentation

A 25-year-old woman presented with a large palpable swelling behind her knee. This case was referred to us to rule out a deep venous thrombosis (DVT).

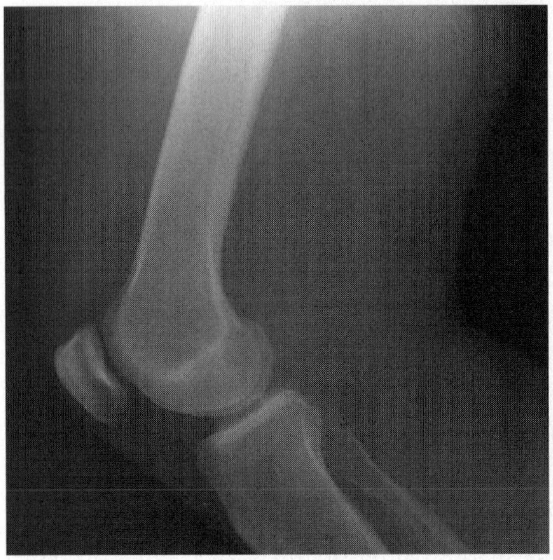

Figure 45A

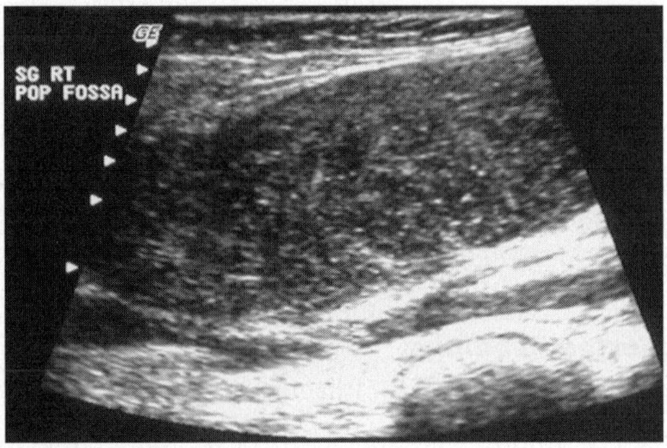

Figure 45B

Radiologic Findings

A lateral radiograph of the distal thigh (**Fig. 45A**) shows a lucent soft-tissue swelling posterior to the distal femur. Because of the clinical suspicion of DVT, an ultrasound (**Fig. 45B**) was performed. It revealed a mixed hyperechoic and hypoechoic lesion superficial to the popliteal neurovascular bundle, thought initially to be cystic, specifically a Baker's cyst, especially given the presence of posterior acoustic enhancement. No communication with the joint was demonstrable, however, and the patient was subsequently referred for MRI. An axial T2-weighted image (**Fig. 45C**) seems to confirm the suspicion of a cystic lesion, returning very high signal. However, coronal (**Fig. 45D**) and sagittal (**Fig. 45E**) T1-weighted images demonstrate the lesion returns intermediate signal intensity hyperintense to skeletal muscle, which is inconsistent with simple fluid, and several low signal intensity foci consistent with flow voids. Sagittal T1-weighted postintravenous gadolinium (**Fig. 45F**) and coronal T1-weighted postintravenous gadolinium with fat-saturated (**Fig. 45G**) images confirm that the lesion is solid, demonstrating intense enhancement throughout.

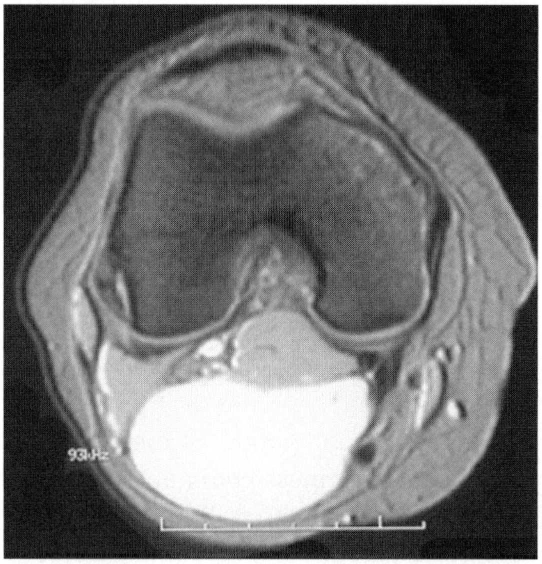

Figure 45C

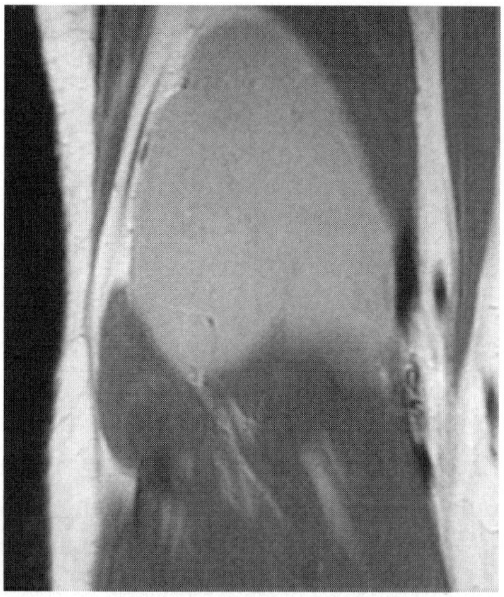

Figure 45D

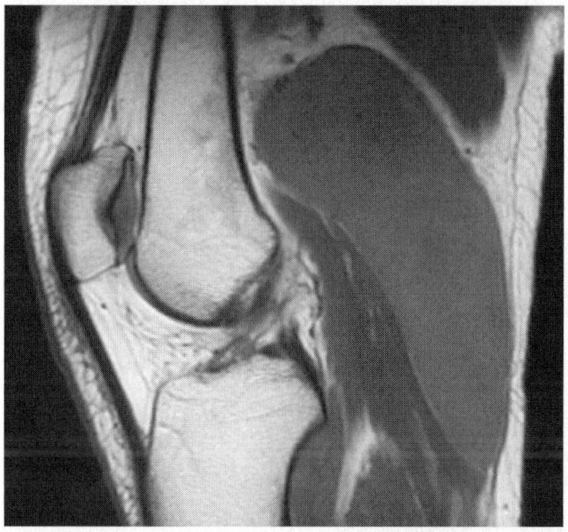

Figure 45E

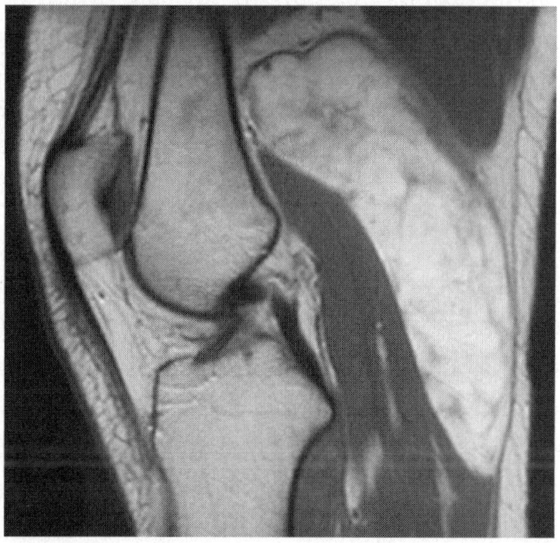

Figure 45F

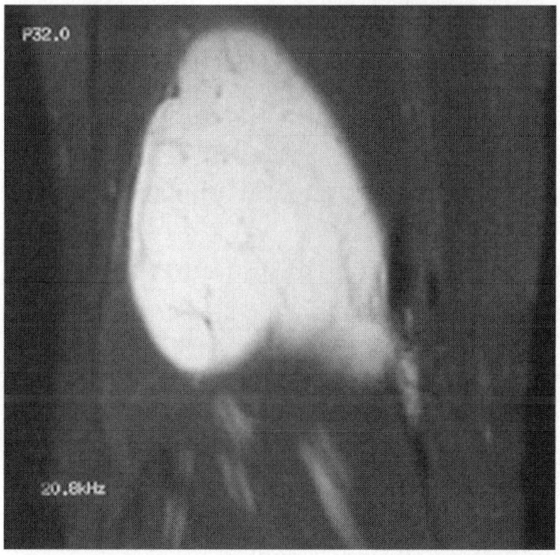

Figure 45G

Diagnosis

Liposarcoma: myxoid subtype.

Differential Diagnosis

- Dedifferentiated liposarcoma
- Malignant fibrous histiocytoma

Discussion

Background

Liposarcomas are a heterogeneous group of lesions comprising malignant tumors of mesenchymal origin containing variable adipose components. They are the second most common soft-tissue sarcoma in adults after malignant fibrous histiocytoma, comprising 12 to 18% of all malignant soft-tissue sarcomas. They occur most frequently in the fifth and sixth decades and are almost unheard of in the pediatric population.

The crucial decisions on imaging are the differentiation of a lipomatous or myxomatous lesion with malignant potential from benign lipomatous or myxomatous lesions, and to stratify those lesions with malignant potential into low-grade (e.g., nonmetastasizing), well-differentiated liposarcoma and high-grade lesions (e.g., the pleomorphic variant), although the final arbiter of this decision is invariably histological.

Etiology

All liposarcomas demonstrate a genetic clonal abnormality resulting in amplification of the 12q13–15 region. Lipomas do not share this genetic lesion, making this one of the criteria used by pathologists to differentiate these entities.

Dedifferentiation is thought to occur in roughly 10% of well-differentiated liposarcomas, occurring three times as often in retroperitoneal lesions (15% risk of differentiation) than in extremity lesions (5% risk). This difference is thought to be a result of the longer "time to discovery" for retroperitoneal lesions.

Pathophysiology

As with other sarcomas, hematogenous metastasis to the lungs followed by the visceral organs is the expected pattern.

Myxoid liposarcomas have a predilection for metastases to scerosal and pleural surfaces, subcutaneous tissues, and bone.

A concomitant mass in the retroperitoneum or thigh may be present in up to 10% of myxoid liposarcomas, presenting as either a multicentric lesion or a primary lesion with a secondary deposit at initial diagnosis.

Clinical Findings

WELL-DIFFERENTIATED LIPOSARCOMA

- The most common liposarcoma, accounting for roughly half of all liposarcomas
- Equal sex distribution, most prevalent in the sixth to seventh decades of life
- Slow-growing, intramuscular soft-tissue mass

- Usually painless, but may be painful in 10 to 15% of cases
- Half occur in the extremities (half of which occur in the thigh), half are retroperitoneal.
- Extremity lesions tend to present at an earlier age than retroperitoneal or mediastinal lesions, given the "hidden" nature of the latter, where they can grow to a considerable size (> 20 cm) before producing symptoms.

MYXOID LIPOSARCOMA

- The second most common type of liposarcoma
- Equal sex incidence, with peak prevalence in the fourth to fifth decades of life
- Painless soft-tissue mass reaching a large size (> 15 cm) before presentation
- 70 to 80% of cases are intermuscular, and 75 to 80% of cases affect the lower extremity.
- This is the most common type of liposarcoma to affect children, accounting for almost 80% of liposarcomatous lesions in patients ages 10 to 16 years.

PLEOMORPHIC LIPOSARCOMA

- Least common subtype, accounting for 5 to 15% of all liposarcomas
- Equal sex distribution, most arising in patients older than 50 years
- The lower extremity is most commonly affected (56%), the upper extremity is affected in 20% of cases, and the retroperitoneum in 9% of cases.
- A firm, painless soft-tissue mass that demonstrates rapid enlargement
- Most frequently intramuscular

DEDIFFERENTIATED LIPOSARCOMA

- Dedifferentiated liposarcoma comprises two distinct histological populations: well-differentiated liposarcoma and nonadipose cellular sarcoma, such as malignant fibrous histiocytoma.
- Equal sex distribution, with peak prevalence in the seventh decade
- Presents as a painless, slow-growing mass
- The clinical history of a rapid increase in size in an apparently well-differentiated liposarcoma suggests possible dedifferentiation.

MIXED LIPOSARCOMA

- Five to 12% of all liposarcomas
- Usually affects older patients and is most commonly found in the retroperitoneum and the abdominal cavity

Stages of Disease

Liposarcomas are subclassified by the World Health Organization into four major subtypes and a fifth subtype comprising a mixture of elements of the other subtypes:

1. Well-differentiated
2. Myxoid
3. Pleomorphic
4. Dedifferentiated
5. Mixed

Well-differentiated liposarcoma represents the lowest, and dedifferentiated liposarcoma the highest, grades of tumor.

Complications

- Low-grade lesions may dedifferentiate to a higher grade, for example, well-differentiated to dedifferentiated.

- Dedifferentiation to a different histological sarcoma may occur (e.g., osteosarcomatous change).
- Metastases occur to the lungs and viscera.
- Recurrence after treatment is common in retroperitoneal and abdominal lesions, and multiple recurrences may give rise to significant morbidity and mortality.
- Death

Pathology

WELL-DIFFERENTIATED LIPOSARCOMA

Gross

- Clearly marginated, large, pale, lobular mass

Microscopic

- Low-grade neoplasm with five described histologic variants, of which lipoma-like is the most common, containing abundant mature adipose tissue that may appear identical to classic lipoma
- The adipose tissue is studded by scattered lipoblasts or cells with enlarged hyperchromatic nuclei representing lipocytic atypia, a sine qua non of the lesion.
- The fibrous interlobular septae are seen to contain increased cellularity, including skeletal muscle fibers (particularly at the margin with adjacent muscle), in comparison to lipoma, where the septae remain fibrous.

MYXOID LIPOSARCOMA

Gross

- Well-circumscribed, multinodular mass
- Lesions consisting mostly of myxoid material are gelatinous with opaque white nodules representing focal cellular aggregates.
- Lesions consisting mostly of round cells have a white, fleshy appearance.

Microscopic

- 40 to 50% (most common): well-delineated lobules of myxoid matrix; plexiform capillary pattern; primitive proliferating fibroblasts with variable numbers of usually mono- and sometimes bivacuolated lipoblasts
- Overall, these tumors typically consist of less than 10% fat.
- Myxoid liposarcomas are generally considered intermediate-grade lesions if predominantly myxoid, but high-grade lesions if they contain a substantial round cell component.
- 90% of myxoid liposarcomas express a reciprocal translocation of t(12;16)(q13;p11), which is thus a very specific and sensitive marker for this lesion.

PLEOMORPHIC LIPOSARCOMA

Gross

- High-grade sarcoma comprising a large multinodular, pale mass
- Myxoid and necrotic areas may be present.

Microscopic

There are two distinguishable histologic types sharing cellular pleomorphism:

1. Malignant fibrous histiocytoma-like spindle cell tumor containing bizarre lipoblasts; frank adipose regions are sparse
2. Epithelioid pleomorphic liposarcoma
   - Solid sheets of epithelioid-appearing cells
   - Regions of fatty differentiation with bizarre lipoblasts

DEDIFFERENTIATED LIPOSARCOMA

Gross

- Multinodular mass with yellow well-differentiated regions
- Dedifferentiated foci often appear as distinct admixed tan-gray regions, with an abrupt transition between the two components.

Microscopic

- The dedifferentiated regions of the tumor consist of high-grade fibrosarcoma or malignant fibrous histiocytoma in 90% of cases.
- There may be a mixture of high- and low-grade components in the region of dedifferentiation; 10% of cases contain only low-grade components.

Imaging Findings

RADIOGRAPHY

There may be an inhomogeneous mass with clear soft-tissue and fatty components, or, in non–well-differentiated subtypes, a nonspecific soft-tissue mass; the latter is less likely to contain grossly visible lucent components.

Well-differentiated liposarcoma

- Soft-tissue mass with occasional calcific foci
- Fat is frequently seen in extremity lesions.

Myxoid liposarcoma

- Nonspecific soft-tissue mass
- The soft-tissue swelling may appear lucent (**Fig. 45A**).
- Calcification occurs much less frequently than with well-differentiated liposarcoma.

Pleomorphic liposarcoma

- Nonspecific soft-tissue mass

Dedifferentiated liposarcoma

- Metaplastic mineralization may be evident (e.g., well-defined bone, amorphous or punctuate calcification).

ULTRASOUND

General

- Nonspecific soft-tissue mass with variable/no fat content
- The apparent advantage of ultrasound in examining superficial lesions is often paradoxically lost, as fatty lesions may blend in imperceptibly with subcutaneous fat.
- Intramuscular lesions are easier to see due to tissue contrast.

Well-differentiated liposarcoma

- Well-defined multilobulated, heterogeneous mass
- Hyperechoic foci suggest fat, but this is neither a sensitive nor a specific finding, seen in other lipomatous lesions.
- Hyperechogenicity is often variable, similar to the situation.

Myxoid liposarcoma

- Complex, well-defined, hypoechoic (but not anechoic) mass with posterior acoustic enhancement (**Fig. 45B**)
- A popliteal location of myxoid liposarcomas is common, and such lesions may simulate a Baker's cyst.

- The more cellular areas of the lesion demonstrate nonspecific features of solid tissue with intermediate echogenicity on sonograms.

Pleomorphic liposarcoma

- Relatively well-defined mass, although infiltrative margins may be present

Dedifferentiated liposarcoma

- Areas of metaplastic mineralization may be seen as hyperechoic foci with posterior shadowing.

COMPUTED TOMOGRAPHY

Well-differentiated liposarcoma

- Largely lipomatous mass (> 75% of the lesion) with nonlipomatous components in thick septae or focal nodules (**Fig. 45H**)
- The fat may have altered characteristics (i.e., be of higher attenuation than normal, e.g., –20 Hounsfield units).
- Calcification or metaplastic ossification is seen in 10 to 32% of lesions.

Myxoid liposarcoma

- The high water content of the lesion is reflected as predominant low attenuation.
- Frequently, little or no fat is demonstrable.
- The more cellular areas of the lesion may have nonspecific features of solid tissue with attenuation similar to that of muscle.

Pleomorphic liposarcoma

- Little or no fat
- Relatively well-defined mass ± infiltrative margins
- Nonlipomatous areas have attenuation similar to muscle.

Dedifferentiated liposarcoma

- A well-defined fatty component is typically evident with an associated closely apposed, nonfatty region.
- The finding of a nodular focus > 1 cm in size of nonfatty tissue in a well-differentiated liposarcoma suggests dedifferentiation, the nonfat foci having attenuation similar to or slightly lower than that of skeletal muscle.
- Areas of metaplastic mineralization may be evident.

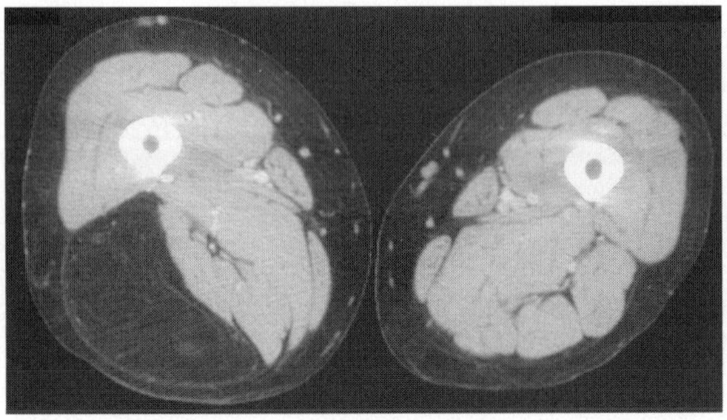

Figure 45H Transaxial CT of "giant" intermuscular lipoma with features suggestive of well-differentiated liposarcoma: size > 10 cm (coronal) and foci of high attenuation in an otherwise uniform fatty attenuation mass.

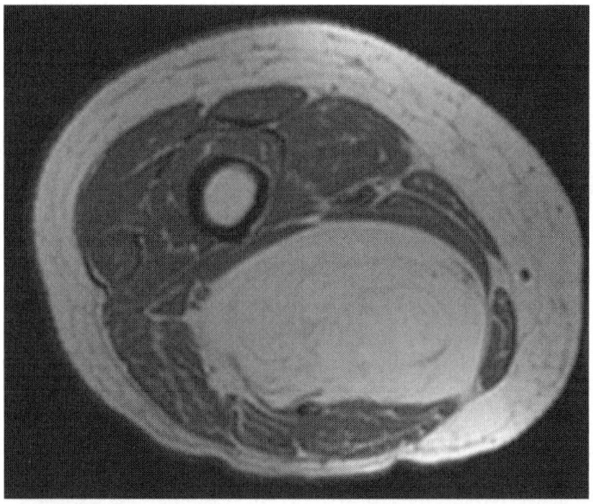

I

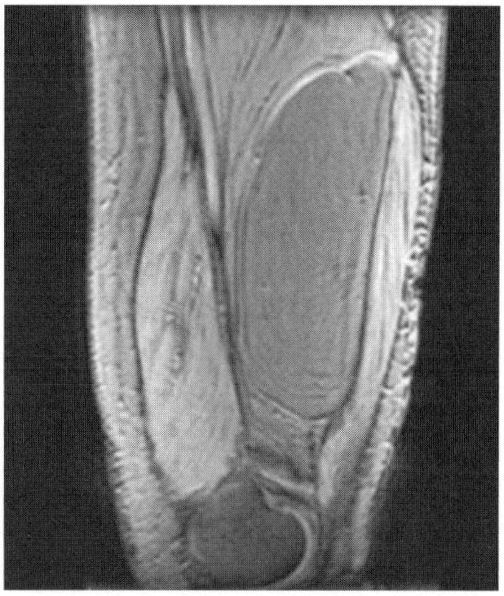

J

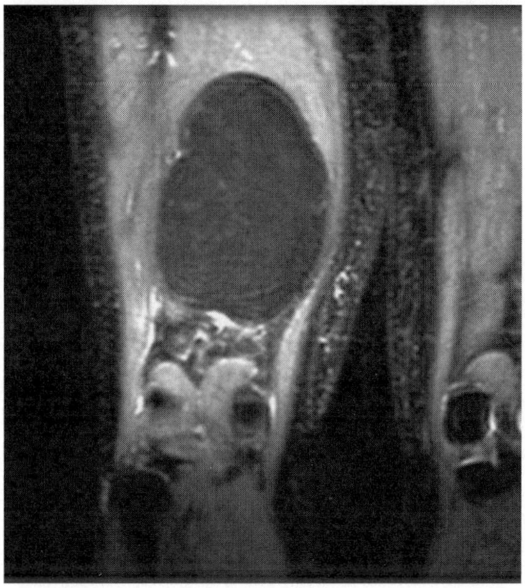

K

Figures 45I–45K Transaxial T1-weighted (**45I**), sagittal MPGR (**45J**), and coronal T2 fat-saturated (**45K**) images of a large intermuscular lipoma. There is uniform fat intensity return from all areas of the lesion, with uniform suppression on the fat-suppression sequence (**45K**). The only feature raising the suspicion of well-differentiated liposarcoma is the large size (> 10 cm in its coronal dimension).

MAGNETIC RESONANCE IMAGING

Lipomas

- Numerous studies have shown that tumors demonstrating homogeneous fat signal with no areas of nonfat signal (suppressing completely on fat suppression sequences) are benign lipomas ($p < .05$) (**Figs. 45I–K**).
- Although most lipomas (48 to 71%) are entirely composed of homogeneous fat (11 to 22% of cases) or are largely adipose with only thin (< 2 mm) septae, 30% of lipomas are not composed of homogeneous fat and can have a more complex appearance, simulating that of a well-differentiated liposarcoma.

Liposarcoma

- As the degree of malignancy increases, the fatty component is less apparent.
- There is a variable reactive pseudocapsule similar to that seen in malignant fibrous histiocytoma.

Well-differentiated liposarcoma

- More than 75% of the lesion is fatty and demonstrates classic fatty signal return, that is, high on both T1- and T2-weighted images (less intense on T2- than T1-weighted).
- 96% of lesions with thick (> 2 mm) nonfat septae and 83% of lesions with nodular or globular nonfat foci (usually < 2 cm in size) will be well-differentiated liposarcomas (versus lipomas).

- Well-differentiated liposarcomas reveal moderate (25%) to marked (75%) enhancement of the septae with gadolinium, reflecting the increased vascularity in the septae of well-differentiated liposarcoma.
- Fifty-eight percent of lipomas show no enhancement, and 37% show mild septal enhancement.
- Targeting the areas of signal enhancement when biopsying these lesions is most likely to provide a definitive result.

Statistically significant factors favoring the diagnosis of well-differentiated liposarcoma over lipoma include the following:

- Male sex (increases the risk of malignancy 13-fold)
- Age > 66 years
- A lower percentage of fat (< 75% of the lesion, $p < .001$)
- The presence of calcification
- Lesion size > 10 cm ($p < .001$)
- Thick (> 2 mm) nonfat septae ($p = .001$), increasing the risk of malignancy 9-fold
- Nonfatty nodular or patchy globular foci ($p = .003$) increase the risk of malignancy 32-fold. The latter were present more frequently in deep and retroperitoneal lesions than in the subcutaneous lesions ($p < .01$).

Intramuscular lipomas

- Intramuscular lipomas vary in size from < 3 cm to > 10 cm.
- Approximately 40% of intramuscular lipomas demonstrate intermingled muscle fibers within the mass.
- Although the majority of intramuscular lipomas are well defined, ~20% will have infiltrative margins.
- When the lesions are multinodular/multilobular, liposarcoma should be suspected (**Figs. 45L–45N**).

Myxoid liposarcoma

- The classic appearance of a myxoid liposarcoma on MRI is that of a large, well-defined, multilobulated, intermuscular lesion of apparent high water content that contains foci of fat within the septae or small nodular fatty foci. This appearance occurs between 42 and 78% of the time.
- Between 90 and 95% of myxoid liposarcomas demonstrate fat on MRI in a lacy or linear, amorphous pattern. Fat-suppression techniques increase the sensitivity in the demonstration of fat. Of those lesions in which fat is visible, it usually composes a minority of the bulk of the lesion (less than one quarter of the lesion).
- The myxoid component (which may predominate) is hypointense on T1 (**Figs. 45D,45E**) and hyperintense on T2 (**Fig. 45C**). The tumor may appear grossly cystic in 20%, especially on CT or ultrasound, but less frequently on MRI (5 to 10%), especially when gadolinium is employed when the solid component will enhance, unlike a cyst (**Figs. 45F,45G**).

Enhancement patterns described in myxoid liposarcoma include

- Peripheral nodular (61%)
- Central nodular (44%)
- Diffuse (17%) (**Figs. 45F,45G**)

The appearances in each case will depend on the relative composition of myxoid and cellular components, and the associated vascularity of each necrotic areas will not enhance.

- Components with a greater percentage of round cells are more heterogeneous and more solid, demonstrating intermediate signal intensity on T1- and T2-weighted MRI.

L M

N

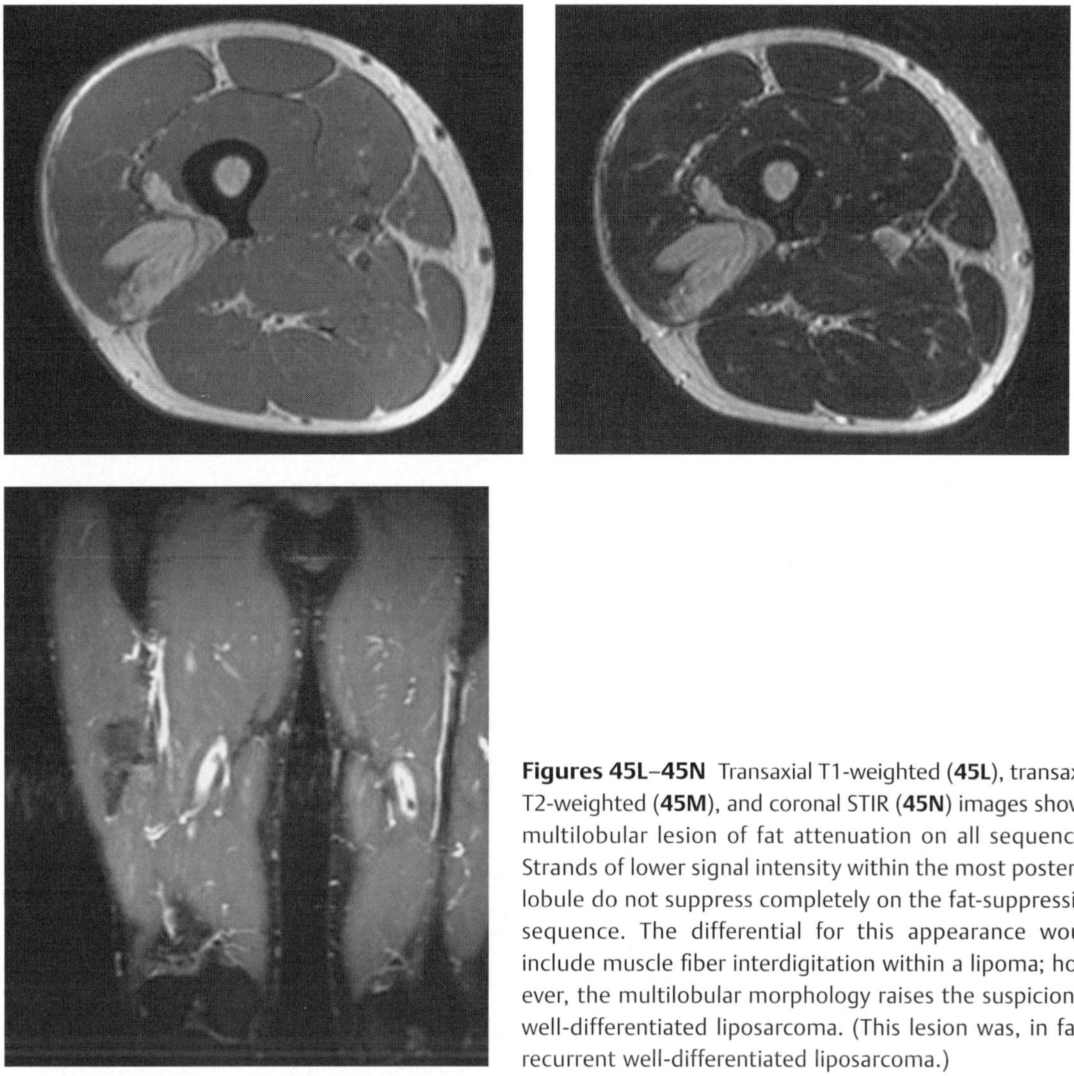

Figures 45L–45N Transaxial T1-weighted (**45L**), transaxial T2-weighted (**45M**), and coronal STIR (**45N**) images show a multilobular lesion of fat attenuation on all sequences. Strands of lower signal intensity within the most posterior lobule do not suppress completely on the fat-suppression sequence. The differential for this appearance would include muscle fiber interdigitation within a lipoma; however, the multilobular morphology raises the suspicion of well-differentiated liposarcoma. (This lesion was, in fact, recurrent well-differentiated liposarcoma.)

- The absence of thin septae or a capsule and prominent contrast enhancement (reflecting the hypervascularity that accompanies this subtype) suggest a more prominent round cell component with a consequently worse prognosis.

Benign intramuscular myxomas

- Myxomas are generally intramuscular lesions, in contrast to myxoid liposarcomas, which are typically intermuscular.
- Myxomas are typically associated with atrophy and edema of surrounding musculature, neither of which is usually seen in myxoid liposarcoma.

In addition, MR signs favoring a benign myxoma include the following:

- The lesion is very well circumscribed.
- T1-weighted images demonstrate uniform decreased signal intensity.
- T2-weighted images demonstrate uniform increased signal intensity.
- Gadolinium-enhanced images exhibit an inhomogeneous increase in signal intensity.

If any of these conditions are not met, then a myxoid-containing malignancy should be suspected.

Pleomorphic liposarcoma

- High-grade sarcomatous lesions demonstrated as a well-defined mass with occasional infiltrative margins (**Figs. 45O–45Q**)
- Usually more heterogeneous than other liposarcomas secondary to hemorrhage and necrosis
- Fewer than 50% of pleomorphic liposarcomas show macroscopic fat, although small amounts of fat are seen on MRI in 62 to 75% of cases.
- Because of tissue admixture, the fat may have a less-intense signal on T1-weighted images than is usually expected from fat.
- Of those lesions in which fat is visible, it usually composes less than a quarter of the bulk of the lesion.
- The nonfatty components have nonspecific features on MRI, having intermediate signal intensity with T1 and intermediate to high signal intensity with T2 sequences.
- Hemorrhage may mimic fat on T1-weighted images. as each can return high signal intensity; this is usually resolved on fat-suppressed T2-weighted images, as fat will have low signal intensity, whereas blood will return high signal intensity.

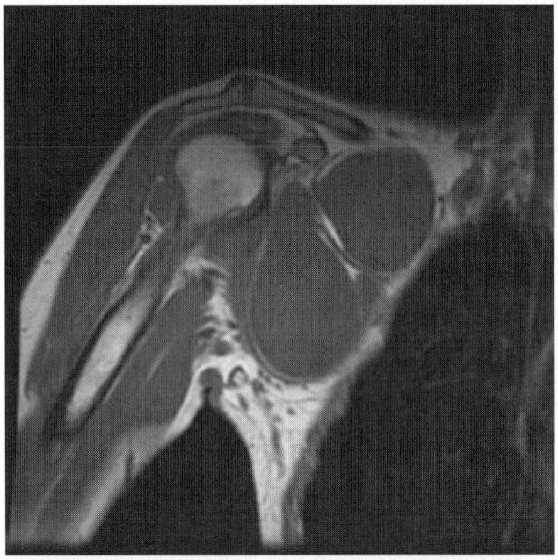

O

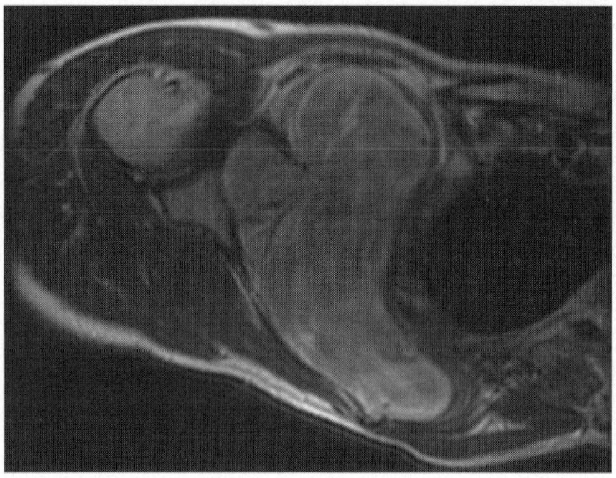

P

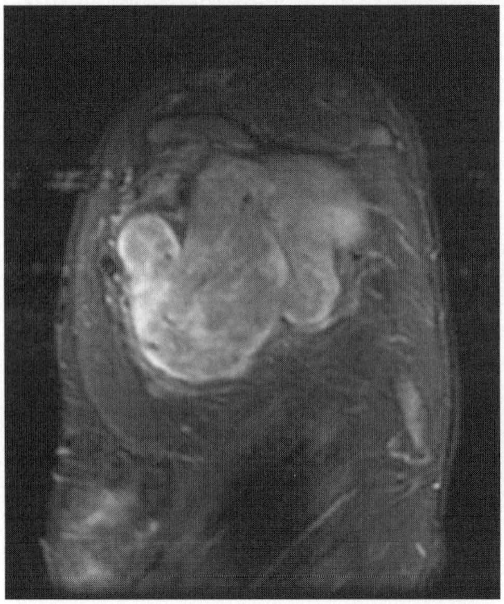

Q

Figures 45O–45Q Coronal T1-weighted (**45O**), transaxial T1-weighted postintravenous gadolinium (**45P**), and sagittal STIR (**45Q**) images show a large well-defined, multilobular pleomorphic liposarcoma in the region of the subscapularis, anterior and caudad to the scapula. The lesion, although subtly heterogeneous, is predominantly of intermediate intensity, isointense to skeletal muscle on the coronal T1-weighted image. The postcontrast images show diffuse enhancement, more prominent on the STIR image, confirming the solid nature of the tumor. No definite fat tissue is identifiable on any of the sequences. This lesion is a histologically confirmed pleomorphic liposarcoma.

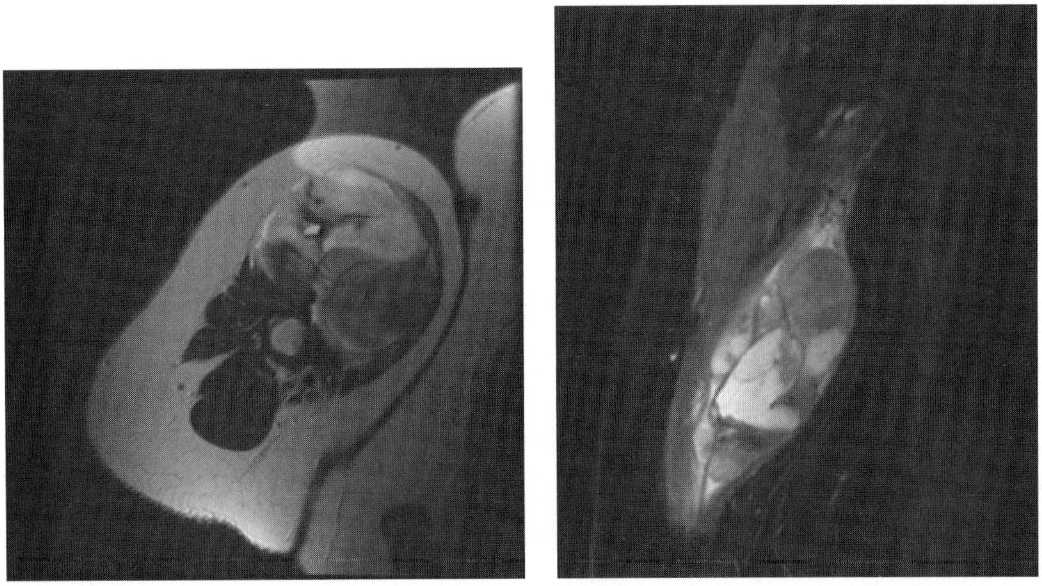

R S

Figures 45R and **45S** Transaxial T1-weighted postcontrast (**45R**) and coronal STIR postintravenous contrast (**45S**) images show a partly fatty lesion based in the medial head of the triceps muscle with multiple large enhancing nonfat nodules. The large nonenhancing nodules reflect either hemorrhage or necrosis. There is evidence of extension into the adjacent lateral head of the triceps and extramuscular extension to the deep fascia of the posterior compartment. This lesion is a dedifferentiated liposarcoma.

Dedifferentiated liposarcoma

Dedifferentiated liposarcoma occurs especially in the mediastinum, the retroperitoneum, and the inguinal/paratesticular regions.

Dedifferentiated liposarcoma is typically a large (mean maximum size of 24 cm) fatty mass (well-differentiated liposarcoma) with a closely apposed large nonfatty component (high-grade nonlipomatous sarcoma), which is described pathologically as a "biphasic tumor," that is, having two distinct cell populations.

The appearances overlap considerably with well-differentiated liposarcoma from which dedifferentiated liposarcomas arise. A nodular focus ($>$ 1 and usually $>$ 3 cm) of nonfat tissue in a well-differentiated liposarcoma suggests dedifferentiation.

It is more common for the fatty component to be larger than the nonfatty component. The nonfat component shows low to intermediate signal intensity on T1-weighted MRI and intermediate to high signal intensity on T2-weighted MRI, depending on the relative proportions of myxoid and fibrous tissue in the dedifferentiated mass (**Figs. 45R,S**).

Biopsies should be taken of both fatty and nonfat components.

Treatment

WELL-DIFFERENTIATED LIPOSARCOMA

- *Surgery* Wide local excision
- *Radiotherapy* Adjunctive utilized to avoid local recurrence where the tumor extent and its proximity to vital structures preclude a free surgical margin

MYXOID LIPOSARCOMA

- *Surgery* Wide local excision
- *Radiotherapy* Often used to reduce local recurrence if incomplete or marginal resection
- *Chemotherapy* Occasionally used as an adjunctive treatment

PLEOMORPHIC LIPOSARCOMA

- Multimodal therapeutic regimes, using a combination of surgery, radiotherapy, and ifosfamide-based chemotherapy, are suggested, given the marked propensity for local recurrence and metastases.
- Wide local excision or amputation and postoperative radiation therapy have been shown to reduce local recurrence.

DEDIFFERENTIATED LIPOSARCOMA

- *Surgery* Wide local excision, frequently with combined radiotherapy
- *Chemotherapy* Occasionally used as an adjunctive treatment

Prognosis

Histologic grading is the single most important prognostic factor for soft-tissue sarcomas.

WELL-DIFFERENTIATED LIPOSARCOMA

- These lesions do not metastasize (unless dedifferentiated); however, where complete excision is difficult or impossible, local recurrence is likely.
- Local recurrence of subcutaneous well-differentiated liposarcomas is rare; however, the rate of recurrence increases when the lesions are deep-seated, even in an extremity. For example, the rate of local recurrence is 43% for extremity lesions, 70% for groin lesions, and 91% for retroperitoneal lesions.
- The complications of multiple local recurrences and the consequent multiple disfiguring surgeries and associated radiotherapy are significant, giving rise to disease-related mortality; groin and retroperitoneal well-differentiated liposarcomas are associated with mortality rates of 14% and 33%, respectively.

MYXOID LIPOSARCOMA

Myxoid lesions have a strong predilection for extrapulmonary metastases.

- 94% of patients with metastatic myxoid liposarcoma develop lesions in extrapulmonary soft-tissue sites, such as the retroperitoneum, chest wall, pericardium, pleura, and within the pelvis.
- The metastatic deposits frequently appear typically myxoid.
- The overall 5-year survival rate for patients with myxoid liposarcoma ranges from 47 to 77%.

A worse prognosis is present in patients who

- Are older than 45 years at diagnosis
- Demonstrate evidence of spontaneous necrosis on histology

A greater proportion of round cells has also been shown to correlate closely with a worse prognosis, metastases occurring in

- 23% of patients with 0 to 5% round cell component
- 35% of patients with 5 to 10% round cell component
- 56% of patients with $>$ 25% round cell component

PLEOMORPHIC LIPOSARCOMA

The lungs are the site of predilection for pleomorphic liposarcoma metastases.

It has been shown that ifosfamide-based chemotherapy in patients with large, high-grade extremity liposarcomas is associated with an improved survival rate.

- 5-year survival rate: 63%
- Local recurrence-free: 58%
- Metastasis-free: 58%

- Disease-free survival rate: 39%

A poor prognosis is associated with

- Patients older than 60 years of age
- Nonextremity lesions
- Deep-seated tumor
- Tumor > 5 cm

DEDIFFERENTIATED LIPOSARCOMA

- The predominant morbidity associated with these lesions is secondary to the local tumor effects, such as on neighboring viscerae and bowel by retroperitoneal lesions, before metastases occur.
- Dedifferentiated liposarcomas recur locally more rapidly (41%) than well-differentiated lesions.
- Retroperitoneal lesions have essentially a 100% local recurrence rate and thus almost invariably lead to death.
- Metastases to the lungs, liver, and bone occur in 15 to 20% of cases.
- Overall, dedifferentiated liposarcomas have a mortality rate of 28 to 30%.

PEARLS

- Lipomatous lesions composed solely of fat or containing thin (< 2 mm) septae, without prominent contrast enhancement on MRI, are considered lipomas.
- Lipomas are very rare in the mediastinum or retroperitoneum, and any lipomatous mass should be considered a well-differentiated liposarcoma until proven otherwise.
- Liposarcomas are expected to demonstrate moderate to high enhancement postintravenous contrast, which helps to distinguish them from simple lipomas, which enhance only minimally.
- Although such signal enhancement can be seen in some types of benign lipomatous tumors with increased numbers of blood vessels, this technique is helpful in selection of a biopsy site, especially in a clinical setting of multiple fatty masses.
- Fat-suppressed T2-weighted images help to differentiate the fatty elements in pleomorphic liposarcoma from hemorrhage (both may have high intensity on T1-weighted images), as the fat has low signal intensity compared with the high signal intensity of blood products.
- Dedifferentiated liposarcomas recur locally more rapidly (41%) than well-differentiated lesions.

PITFALLS

- On ultrasound examination, hyperechogenicity is often difficult and variable in well-differentiated liposarcoma, as is frequently the case with lipoma.
- Hyperechoic foci suggest fat, but this is neither a sensitive nor a specific finding, as it is seen in other lipomatous lesions.
- Positron emission tomography cannot distinguish well-differentiated liposarcoma from lipoma because of the low metabolic rate of the former.
- Myxoid liposarcoma may be incorrectly identified initially on MRI due to the high water content of myxoid and the relative lack of fat, giving rise to a false diagnosis of a cystic lesion. A popliteal location of myxoid liposarcomas is common, and such lesions may simulate a Baker's cyst.
- Hemorrhage may mimic fat on T1 images, as each can return high signal intensity; this is usually resolved on fat-suppressed T2-weighted images, as fat will have low signal intensity, whereas blood will have high signal intensity.

Suggested Readings

Hosono M, Kobayashi H, Fujimoto R, et al. Septum-like structures in lipoma and liposarcoma: MR imaging and pathologic correlation. Skeletal Radiol 1997;26:150–154

Kransdorf MJ, Bancroft LW, Peterson JJ, Murphey MD, Foster WC, Temple HT. Imaging of fatty tumors: distinction of lipoma and well-differentiated liposarcoma. Radiology 2002;224:99–104

Logan PM, Janzen DL, O'Connell JX, Munk PL, Connell DG. Chondroid lipoma: MRI appearances with clinical and histologic correlation. Skeletal Radiol 1996;25:592–595

Munk PL, Lee MJ, Janzen DL, et al. Lipoma and liposarcoma: evaluation using CT and MR imaging. Am J Roentgenol 1997;169:589–594

Murphey MD, Arcara LK, Fanburg-Smith J. Imaging of musculoskeletal liposarcoma with radiologic-pathologic correlation. Radiographics 2005;25:1371–1395

Ohguri T, Aoki T, Hisaoka M, et al. Differential diagnosis of benign peripheral lipoma from well-differentiated liposarcoma on MR imaging: is comparison of margins and internal characteristics useful? Am J Roentgenol 2003;180:1689–1694

CASE 46

George Nomikos, Anthony G. Ryan, Peter L. Munk, and Mark Murphey

Clinical Presentation

A 55-year-old patient presented with left shoulder pain.

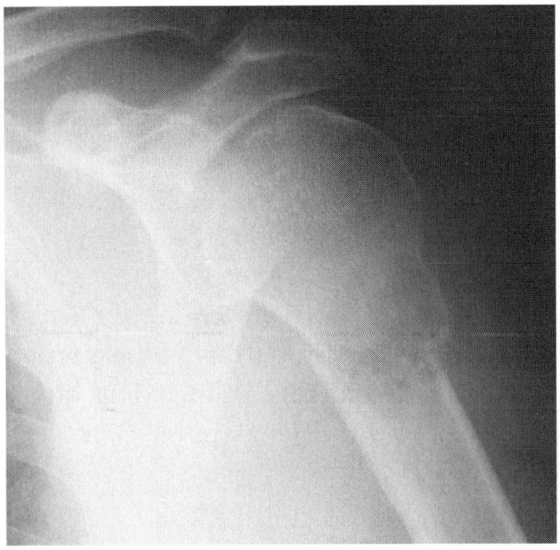

Figure 46A

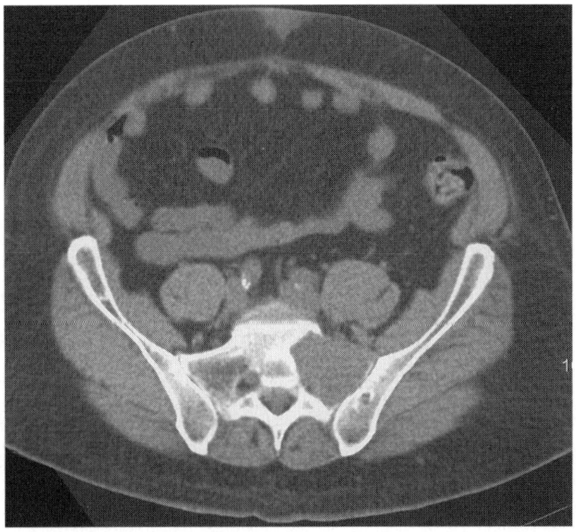

Figure 46B

Radiologic Findings

A single view of the shoulder (**Fig. 46A**) shows a pathologic fracture through a lytic destructive lesion of the left proximal humerus. The lesion involves the epiphysis, metaphysis, and diaphysis of the left proximal humerus. The lesion shows a relatively wide zone of transition. There is extensive bone destruction. No mineralized matrix is identified in the lesion. A single image from a CT scan through the pelvis in the same patient is shown in **Fig. 46B,** demonstrating a soft-tissue mass within the left sacral ala with extensive medullary replacement and cortical breakthrough anteriorly.

Diagnosis

Metastatic renal cell carcinoma.

Differential Diagnosis

- Multiple myeloma
- Lymphoma

Discussion

Background

After the lung and liver, bone is the third most common site of metastatic disease. Approximately 30% of patients with a primary carcinoma develop bone metastases, and ~70% of these patients suffer from pain related to the osseous disease.

Etiology

The most common malignancies to give rise to osseous metastases are in the kidney, prostate, breast, lung, and thyroid.

Pathophysiology

Most osseous metastases occur in the axial skeleton (80%), with the spine representing the single most common site. This is likely related to the large amount of hematopoietic marrow in this portion of the skeleton. Malignancies may spread to bone via several different routes, including direct extension, lymphatic spread, hematogenous dissemination, and intraspinal spread via the cerebrospinal fluid.

Clinical Findings

Although these lesions may be asymptomatic and only discovered incidentally, pain at the site of metastasis (which may be due to pathologic fracture) and neurologic compromise secondary to spinal involvement are the most common presentations.

Complications

- Pathologic fracture
- Neurologic compromise in the spine

Pathology

Histology reflects the primary malignancy.

Imaging Findings

RADIOGRAPHY

Skeletal metastases may be osteolytic, osteosclerotic, or mixed. **Tables 46–1** to **46–3** summarize the most common osteolytic (**Table 46–1**), mixed (**Table 46–2**), and osteosclerotic (**Table 46–3**) metastatic lesions.

Lesions are often multiple; however, solitary osseous metastases may occur. Periosteal reaction is less commonly seen in the setting of metastatic disease to bone than in the case of primary bone tumors.

Certain tumors have a predilection to cause prominent osseous expansion, particularly renal, thyroid, and liver carcinomas.

Large osteoblastic lesions may be identified in patients with metastatic prostate cancer.

Table 46–1 Common Osteolytic Metastases

Thyroid cancer
Renal cancer
Adrenal cancer
Uterine cancer
Gastrointestinal cancers
Melanoma
Hepatoma
Squamous cell carcinoma of the skin
Certain head and neck cancers
Ewing's sarcoma
Wilms' tumor
Pheochromocytoma

Table 46–2 Common Mixed Lytic and Sclerotic Metastases

Lung cancer
Breast cancer
Cervical cancer
Ovarian cancer
Testicular cancer

Table 46–3 Common Osteosclerotic Metastases

Prostate cancer
Bronchial carcinoid
Transitional cell cancer of the bladder
Mucinous gastrointestinal tumors
Some nasopharyngeal cancers
Medulloblastoma
Neuroblastoma

Soft-tissue masses in association with bone lesions are generally more common in the setting of primary bone tumors than in the setting of osseous metastatic disease; however, metastatic colon carcinoma is known to produce soft-tissue masses with areas of calcification on occasion (**Fig. 46C**).

Pathologic fracture is a serious potential complication of osseous metastases, with breast carcinoma the most common histology implicated. Common sites of pathologic fractures include the spine and proximal femora. Factors suggestive of an impending pathologic fracture include destruction of more than 50% of the cortical bone, increasing pain, and pain after radiation.

COMPUTED TOMOGRAPHY

Evaluation of the degree of cortical destruction is much better performed by CT than by routine radiography (**Figs. 46D,46E**).

- The presence of subtle calcifications, as in a mucinous metastasis, is best identified on CT.
- A prominent desmoplastic response may be evident in soft tissues adjacent to metastases, for example, sacral metastases secondary to colonic carcinoma.
- Although MRI has superior soft-tissue contrast, CT is moderately sensitive in the demonstration of muscle and subcutaneous metastases (**Fig. 46F**).
- CT angiography may be helpful in planning an embolization procedure.

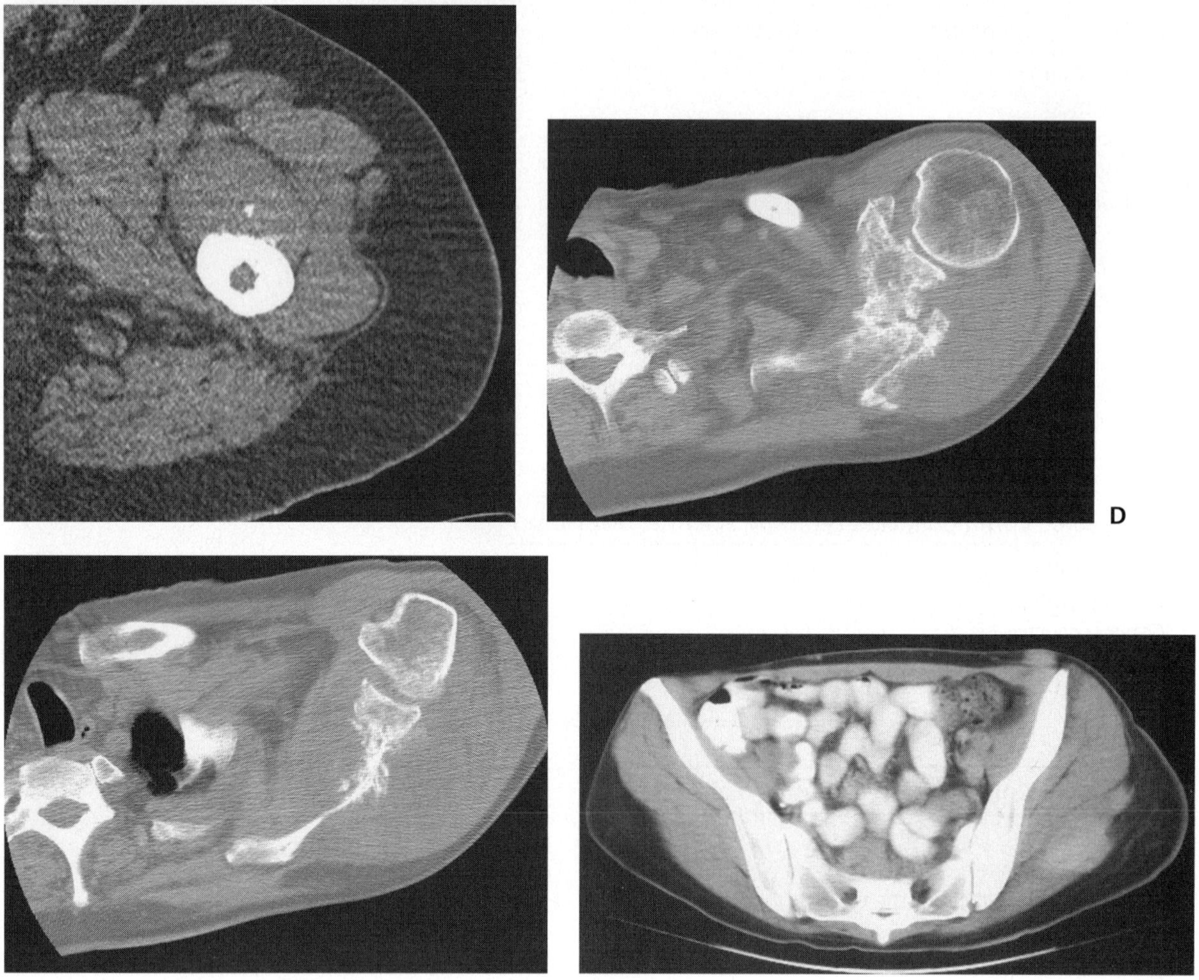

C D E F

Figures 46C A transaxial image from CT of the left femur shows a soft-tissue mass based on the surface of the femur with periosteal reaction and early saucerization. A focus of calcification is evident centrally within the lesion. The lesion is seen to displace the adjacent musculature. **46D** and **46E** Transaxial images of the left scapula in a patient with metastatic adenocarcinoma of the bronchus show florid destruction, pathologic fracture, and marked periosteal reaction centered within a large soft-tissue mass. Partly because of overlying ribs, the lesion was not immediately appreciated on a chest radiograph. **46F** Transaxial CT of the pelvis performed as a routine follow-up of a patient with melanoma shows multiple subcutaneous (adjacent to the anterior superior iliac crest) and intramuscular (left gluteus maximus) nodules: biopsy-proven melanoma metastases.

MAGNETIC RESONANCE IMAGING

Typical pathologic signal return is seen, that is, low T1 and high T2 signal, primarily secondary to high water content. Sclerotic metastases are low signal on both T1- and T2-weighted sequences.

MRI is the ideal modality to demonstrate the medullary extent and to characterize associated soft-tissue masses when present (**Figs. 46G,46H**).

Treatment and Prognosis

Treatment and prognosis are entirely dependent on the tissue of origin.

The World Health Organization has recommended a regime of therapy of escalating aggressiveness in the treatment of bone pain related to metastases.

The initial phase of treatment in all cases involves pharmacotherapy, starting with nonsteroidal anti-inflammatories and rapidly including opioids if the former are not effective. Nonsteroidal anti-inflammatories are frequently associated with gastritis/duodenitis in the elderly population, and

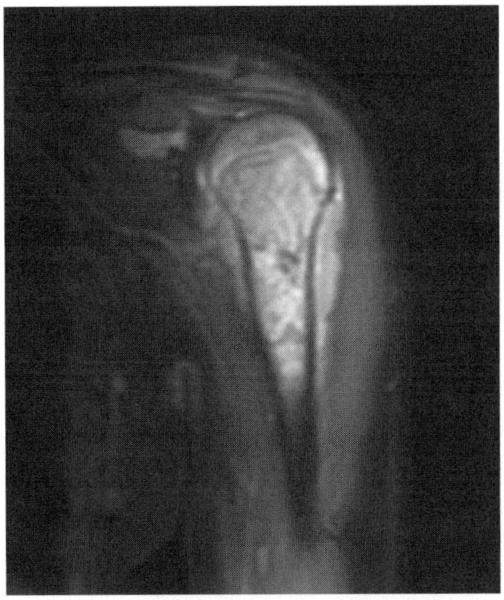
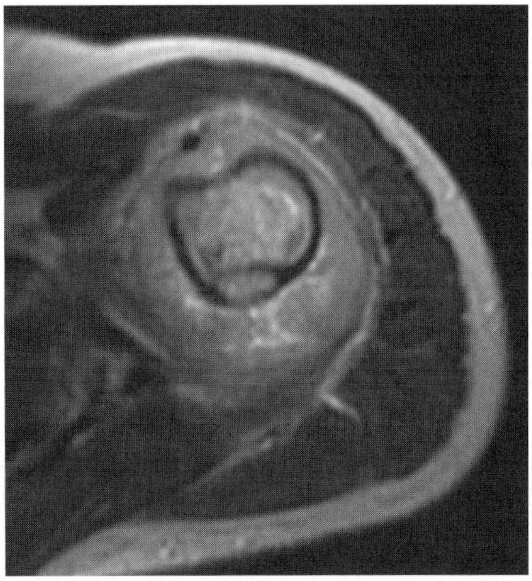

G H

Figures 46G and **46H** Coronal STIR and axial T2-weighted images show a large melanoma metastasis centered on the left proximal humeral diametaphysis with an associated encircling soft-tissue mass. Cortical breakthrough is evident anteriorly.

opioids may render a patient increasingly obtunded as tolerance develops and increasingly higher doses are required for analgesia.

Ongoing pain despite opiates has traditionally been treated with external beam radiotherapy. The latter is also used when the risk of pathologic fracture is high, frequently in association with internal rod fixation in the long bones or prosthesis insertion in the region of a joint (**Figs. 46I–46L**).

Radiotherapy is associated with several drawbacks, however, foremost of which is the lag time to maximal effectiveness, which can be as long as 12 weeks in some cases.

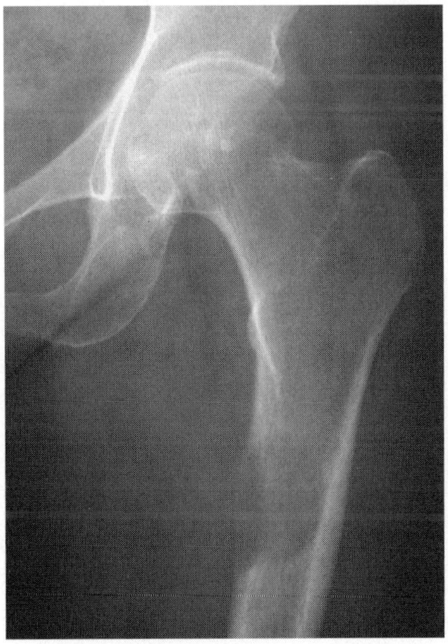
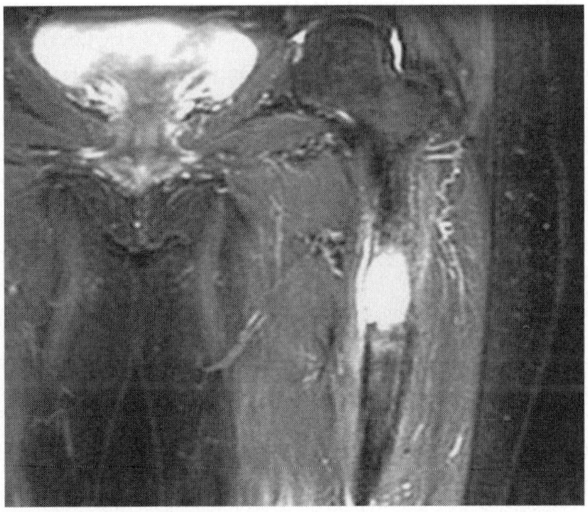

I J

Figures 46I A conventional radiograph of the left femur shows a focal lytic lesion in the proximal diaphysis in a patient with known renal cell carcinoma but with no other site of metastasis. **46J** A coronal T2-weighted image with fat saturation shows that the lesion returns an intensely high signal.

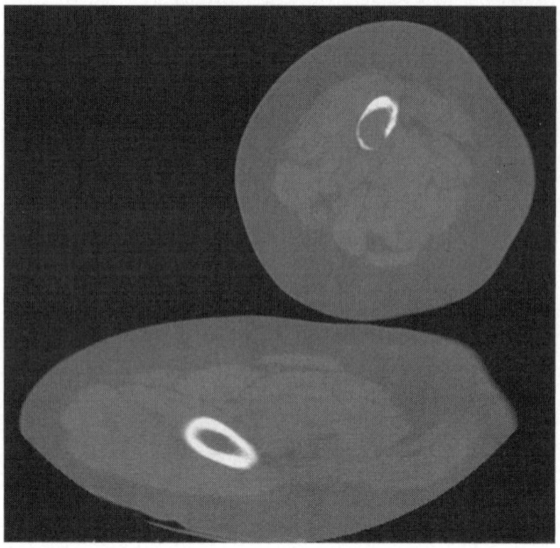

K

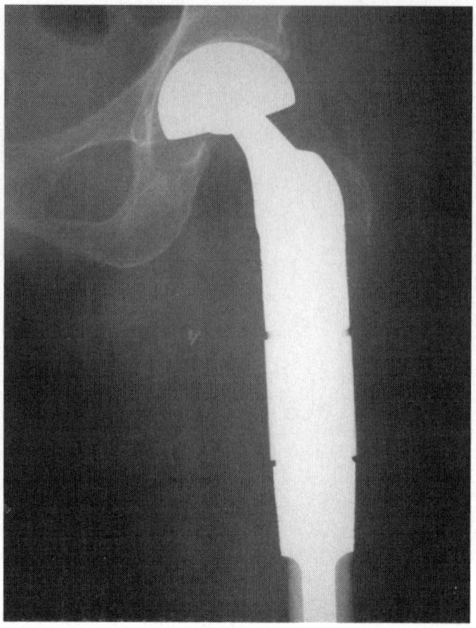

L

Figures 46K A single transaxial image from CT performed as part of a CT-guided biopsy procedure shows focal destruction of the posteromedial aspect of the diaphysis with endosteal scalloping of the remaining cortex. **46L** A postoperative radiograph shows arthroplasty left hip hemiarthroplasty with replacement of the proximal third of the femur.

In light of the disadvantages of the above therapies, interventional radiology has developed several palliative local treatments that are very efficacious in relieving the pain associated with bone metastases, particularly in those cases where other therapies are unsuccessful.

Radiofrequency ablation, osteoplasty, and cryotherapy have all shown very promising results in these cases. Occasionally, in the presence of hypervascular metastases, bland embolization may result in some relief of symptoms and render procedures such as internal stabilization less prone to hemorrhage.

PEARLS

- Soft-tissue masses in association with bone lesions are generally more common in the setting of primary bone tumors than in the setting of osseous metastatic disease.
- Factors suggestive of an impending pathologic fracture include destruction of more than 50% of the cortical bone, increasing pain, and pain after radiation.
- Periosteal reaction is less commonly seen in the setting of metastatic disease to bone than in the case of primary bone tumors.

PITFALLS

- Conventional radiographs are frequently insensitive in the detection of bone metastases until a considerable amount of cortical destruction has occurred. Unexplained pain should be investigated further with more sensitive modalities.
- Although soft-tissue masses are more common in association with bone lesions in the presence of primary bone tumors, certain malignancies, such as melanoma and renal cell carcinoma, have a predilection for producing soft-tissue masses, not only in bone but also in muscle and the subcutaneous soft tissues.

- In the presence of a known malignancy, discovery of a bone lesion is almost invariably diagnosed as metastatic; however, alternative diagnoses must always be considered, particularly in the case of a solitary bone lesion. Benign, no touch lesions should be recognized as such, and the possibility of infection should be considered, especially if the patient is immunocompromised.

Suggested Readings

Resnick D. Skeletal metastases. In: Resnick D, ed. Diagnosis of Bone and Joint Disorders. Philadelphia, PA: WB Saunders; 2002:4274–4351

Welber A, Rafii M. MR imaging of osseous metastatic disease. Contem Diagn Rad 2002;25:1–6

CASE 47

George Nomikos, Anthony G. Ryan, Peter L. Munk, and Mark Murphey

Clinical Presentation

A 49-year-old man was admitted to the hospital who was unconscious and had a fever.

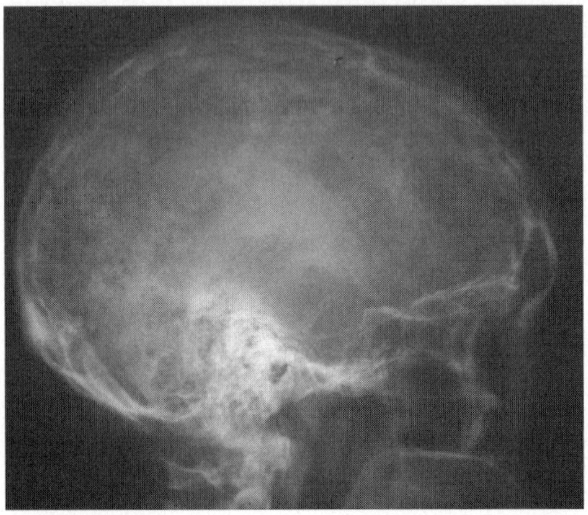

Figure 47A

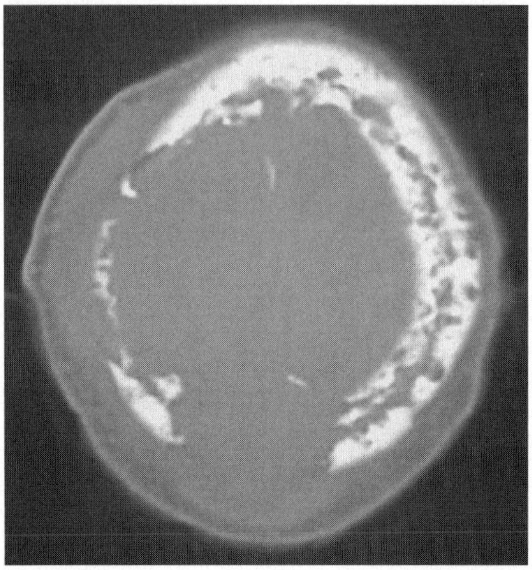

Figure 47B

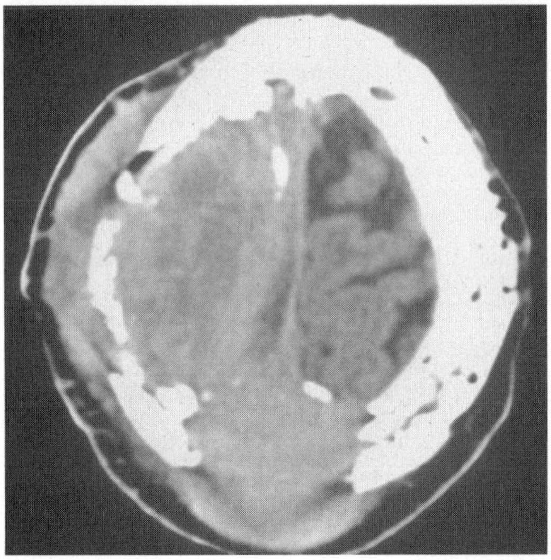

Figure 47C

Radiologic Findings

A lateral radiograph (**Fig. 47A**) shows diffuse osseous destruction throughout the skull in a moth-eaten/permeative pattern. The axial unenhanced CT image (**Fig. 47B**) also demonstrates this diffuse osseous infiltration and destruction throughout the skull. Several larger lytic areas with associated soft-tissue masses are also identified. No mineralized matrix is seen. The contrast-enhanced CT (**Fig. 47C**) obtained at a higher level shows two enhancing soft-tissue masses arising from the skull and causing compression of the underlying brain parenchyma.

Diagnosis

Multiple myeloma.

Differential Diagnosis

- Metastatic disease
- Lymphoma
- Leukemia
- Atypical infection, such as tuberculosis or fungal infection (e.g., coccidiomycosis)
- Waldenström's macroglobulinemia
- Histiocytosis
- Gaucher's disease
- Vascular tumors

Discussion

Background

Myeloma, a lymphoproliferative malignancy of monoclonal plasma cells, is the most common primary malignancy of bone, with an incidence of ~50 cases/100,000 people per year who have reached an age of 80 years. The majority of patients (55 to 60%) have multiple myeloma, which is characterized by multiple sites of involvement. The solitary form of the disease (solitary plasmacytoma) accounts for ~25% of patients, although these patients usually go on to develop multiple lesions within 3 to 5 years. Because areas of hematopoietic marrow are predominantly affected, lesions primarily affect the axial skeleton. Although lesions are most commonly lytic, a sclerotic form of myeloma does exist. This sclerotic form of myeloma (**Fig. 47D**) is often, although not invariably, associated with POEMS syndrome: polyneuropathy, organomegaly, endocrinopathy, monoclonal gammopathy (usually immunoglobulin A or G [IgA or IgG]), and skin changes.

Clinical Findings

Myeloma, which has a median patient age of 64 years, is most commonly a disease of older individuals. It is relatively common, with an incidence of ~3 cases/100,000 every year. Patients most commonly present with the chief complaint of bone pain. Fever, weight loss, bleeding, and

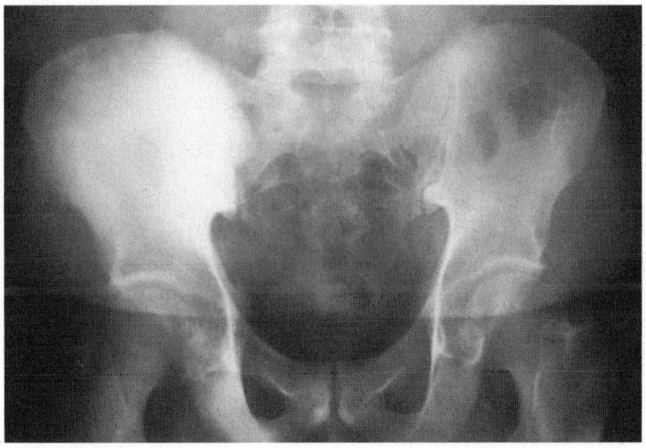

Figure 47D An anteroposterior radiograph of the pelvis in a patient with POEMS syndrome (polyneuropathy, organomegaly, endocrinopathy, monoclonal gammopathy, and skin changes) demonstrating profound sclerosis of the right ilium adjacent to the sacroiliac joint and a further less-intense focus in the right ischium.

neurologic symptoms are also commonly reported. Dissemination of disease has usually occurred by the time of diagnosis in most patients. Myeloma is also known to develop more frequently in Black patients.

Pathology

The lesions contain tightly packed plasma cells that replace the normal bone marrow. Myeloma lesions tend to be most common in regions of hematopoietic marrow, especially in the spine, although they can affect in any bone. The hematopoietic marrow infiltration can appear diffuse or as solid tumor nodules of marrow replacement. Amyloid deposition (which may calcify) is seen in association with myeloma in 10% of cases either in association with the tumor cells or in other areas, such as the joint capsule, tongue, or kidneys. The replacement of normal marrow elements, such as platelets and polymorphonuclear leukocytes, is responsible for common complications such as bleeding and infection.

Imaging Findings

RADIOGRAPHY

- Radiographs typically demonstrate multiple punched out lytic lesions throughout the skeleton, with a predilection for the axial skeleton.
- A skeletal survey is more reliable for detection of lesions than scintigraphy because of the substantial false-negative rate of the latter modality (~30%).
- The sclerotic form of myeloma is very uncommon (< 3%).
- Vertebral compression fractures are commonly encountered.
- Diffuse osteopenia may be the sole finding on radiographs.

COMPUTED TOMOGRAPHY

- CT demonstrates areas of marrow replacement by tumor cells.
- Multidetector CT (MDCT) may recognize areas of osseous lysis that can be missed on radiographs or MRI.
- Better assessment of trabecular and cortical destruction is available with MDCT than with MRI, which may aid in the prediction of unstable areas at risk for fracture.

MAGNETIC RESONANCE IMAGING

- MRI may demonstrate focal areas of marrow replacement or diffuse marrow infiltration.
- Typically, focal lesions are low signal intensity on T1-weighted images and high signal intensity on T2-weighted images.
- Focal lesions may demonstrate intermediate to low signal intensity on T2-weighted images after treatment.
- Lack of enhancement of nodules on post-therapy MRI is suggestive of a good response to the treatment.
- Diffusely infiltrated marrow may appear as intermediate, not low, signal intensity on T1-weighted images, which may make recognition of marrow replacement much more difficult.
- Diffuse infiltration on T2-weighted images has a speckled high signal intensity pattern.
- T2-weighted images are probably more sensitive for detection of focal lesions than T1-weighted images.
- MRI is excellent for evaluation of soft-tissue extension of lesions.
- Occult disease is often identified on MRI (especially in the lumbar spine) in patients with no or only one lesion seen on radiographs (stage 1 disease).

Treatment

- Chemotherapy and radiation
- The bone pain associated with myeloma has been shown to respond favorably to osteoplasty when other therapies (e.g., radiotherapy) have failed.

Prognosis

- Myeloma cell mass is determined by the staging system of Durie and Salmon.
- Median survival: 18 to 36 months
- Less than 3% 10-year survival

PEARLS

- Better assessment of trabecular and cortical destruction is available with MDCT than with MRI, which may aid in the prediction of unstable areas at risk for fracture.
- Diffuse infiltration on T2-weighted images has a speckled high signal intensity pattern.
- Lack of enhancement of nodules on post-therapy MRI is suggestive of a good response to the treatment.

PITFALLS

- Scintigraphy has a substantial false-negative rate (~30%) in the detection of myelomatous deposits; the latter are visualized more reliably with a radiographic skeletal survey.
- The pattern of destruction seen in the skull affected by myeloma has been described as a "raindrop," demonstrating multiple lytic lesions of different sizes, but usually intermediate to large. This should not be mistaken for the "pepper pot" or "salt and pepper" pattern seen in hyperparathyroidism, where the lucent lesions tend to be innumerable uniform small foci on a background of normally mineralized skull.
- Diffusely infiltrated marrow may appear as intermediate, not low, signal intensity on T1-weighted images, which may make recognition of marrow replacement much more difficult.

Suggested Readings

Durie BG. The role of anatomic and functional staging in myeloma: description of Durie/Salmon plus staging system. Eur J Cancer 2006;42:1539–1543

Libshitz HI, Malthouse SR, Cunningham D, MacVicar AD, Husband JE. Multiple myeloma: appearance at MR imaging. Radiology 1992;182:833–837

Mahnken AH, Wildberger JE, Gehbauer G, et al. Multidetector CT of the spine in multiple myeloma: comparison with MR imaging and radiography. Am J Roentgenol 2002;178:1429–1436

Mulligan ME. Myeloma and lymphoma. Semin Musculoskelet Radiol 2000;4:127–135

Rahmouni A, Divine M, Mathieu D, et al. MR appearance of multiple myeloma of the spine before and after treatment. Am J Roentgenol 1993;160:1053–1057

Resnick D. Plasma cell dyscrasias and dysgammaglobulinemias. In: Resnick D, ed. Diagnosis of Bone and Joint Disorders. Philadelphia, PA: WB Saunders; 2002:2188–2232

Shah BK, Saifuddin A, Price GJ. Magnetic resonance imaging of spinal plasmacytoma. Clin Radiol 2000;55:439–445

CASE 48

George Nomikos, Anthony G. Ryan, Peter L. Munk, and Mark Murphey

Clinical Presentation

A 23-year-old man presented with intermittent aching in the left shoulder following a sports injury $1^1/_2$ years prior to his visit to the hospital.

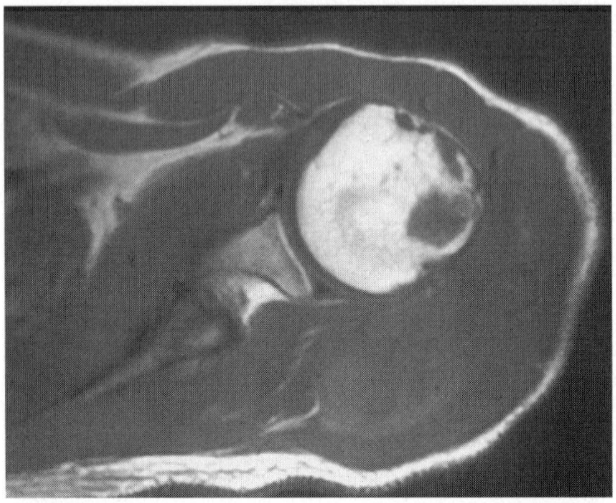

Figure 48A

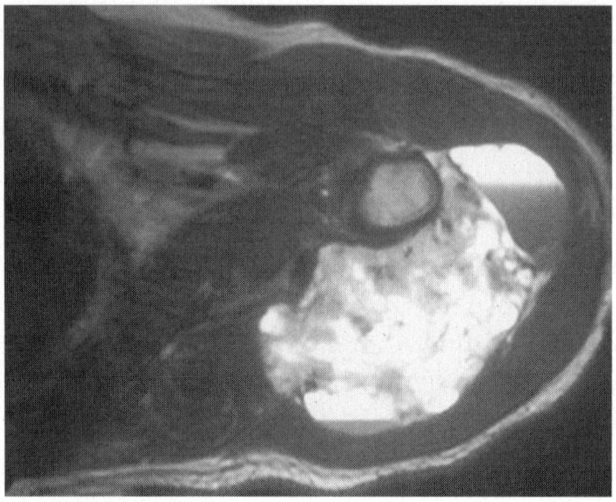

Figure 48B

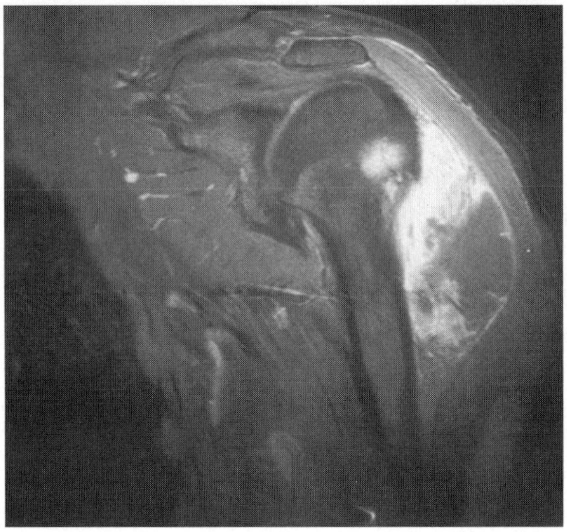

Figure 48C

Radiographic Findings

The axial T1-weighted image (**Fig. 48A**) shows a soft-tissue mass around the proximal humerus. The mass is isointense to muscle. Note the focal area of marrow replacement in the humeral head compatible with osseous invasion. The mass is heterogeneously high signal intensity on the axial T2-weighted image (**Fig. 48B**) with no significant surrounding edema. Also note the fluid levels in the mass resulting from internal hemorrhage. The postcontrast T1-weighted image (**Fig. 48C**) demonstrates diffuse enhancement of the solid portion of the mass and peripheral enhancement of the cystic/hemorrhagic portion. The focal area of osseous invasion is also well illustrated on this coronal image.

Diagnosis

Synovial sarcoma.

Differential Diagnosis

- Malignant fibrous histiocytoma/fibrosarcoma
- Malignant peripheral nerve sheath tumor (MPNST)
- Leiomyosarcoma
- Atypical infection

Discussion

Background

The majority of synovial sarcomas, which account for 5 to 10% of all sarcomas, arise in the extremities (80 to 95%). These lesions most commonly arise in a deep intermuscular location near a large joint. Despite their name, they do not arise from synovial tissue, and very few are thought to have a primary intra-articular origin. Like malignant fibrous histiocytoma, synovial sarcoma has a propensity for osseous invasion, as demonstrated in this case.

Clinical Findings

Most lesions occur in patients between the ages of 15 and 35, although lesions have been seen in children as well, including neonates. Most patients present with a painful or painless mass that has demonstrated slow growth over time. It is not uncommon for symptoms to have been present for many years prior to diagnosis. Neurologic deficits distal to the mass have been reported in association with these lesions.

Pathology

These tumors arise from primitive mesenchymal cells (not synovial tissue) and display a genetic translocation between the X chromosome and chromosome 18t (X,18). Lesions may be monophasic (contain spindle cell components only) or biphasic (contain both spindle cell and epithelial components).

Imaging Findings

RADIOGRAPHY

- Calcification (often peripheral) may be seen in these lesions in up to 30% of cases.
- Cortical erosion, osseous remodeling, periosteal reaction, or osseous invasion is often encountered (11 to 20%).

COMPUTED TOMOGRAPHY

- Lesional calcification is better demonstrated on CT than on radiographs.
- Osseous remodeling, periosteal reaction, and invasion are also well demonstrated.
- Low-attenuation regions represent cystic, hemorrhagic, or necrotic areas.
- Best for evaluation of pulmonary metastases (which may demonstrate internal mineralization)

MAGNETIC RESONANCE IMAGING

- Usually a well-defined lobular mass with internal septations
- Isointense to muscle on T1-weighted images
- Often heterogeneously high signal on T2-weighted images

- A triple signal intensity pattern is described on T2-weighted images: areas that are hypointense, isointense, and hyperintense to subcutaneous fat on standard spin-echo T2-weighted images secondary to the presence of cystic, hemorrhagic, fibrous, and other solid-tissue areas.
- Cystic areas and fluid levels (compatible with internal hemorrhage) are common.
- Best modality for demonstrating extracompartmental spread and neurovascular involvement

Treatment

- Treatment is wide excision and postoperative radiation.
- Adjuvant chemotherapy is controversial but may be useful in cases with more aggressive biological behavior.

Prognosis

- Poor prognostic indicators include tumor size > 5 cm (most important), nonextremity lesion location, and older age.
- Metastases or local recurrence is seen in 80% of patients.
- Metastases may be seen several decades after the primary treatment.
- Five-year survival rate: 27 to 55%

PEARLS

- These lesions most commonly arise in a deep intermuscular location near a large joint.
- Cortical erosion, osseous remodeling, periosteal reaction, or osseous invasion is often encountered (11 to 20%).
- Triple signal intensity pattern is described on T2-weighted images: areas that are hypointense, isointense, and hyperintense to subcutaneous fat on standard spin-echo T2-weighted images secondary to the presence of cystic, hemorrhagic, fibrous, and other solid-tissue areas.

PITFALLS

- Despite their name, synovial sarcomas do not arise from synovial tissue, and very few are thought to have a primary intra-articular origin.
- Peripheral calcification may be seen in these lesions in up to 30%, thus potentially raising confusion with myositis ossificans.
- Pulmonary metastases may demonstrate internal mineralization on CT, raising the differential of osteosarcoma metastases, although the latter are usually ossified.
- Metastases may be seen several decades after the primary treatment.

Suggested Readings

Jones BC, Sundaram M, Kransdorf MJ. Synovial sarcoma: MR findings in 34 patients. Am J Roentgenol 1993;161:827–830

Kransdorf M, Murphey M. Imaging of Soft Tissue Tumors. Philadelphia, PA: WB Saunders; 1997

McCarville MB, Spunt SL, Skapek SX, Pappo AS. Synovial sarcoma in pediatric patients. Am J Roentgenol 2002;179:797–801

Morton MJ, Berquist TH, McLeod RA, Unni KK, Sim FH. MR imaging of synovial sarcoma. Am J Roentgenol 1991;156:337–340

CASE 49

George Nomikos, Anthony G. Ryan, Peter L. Munk, and Mark Murphey

Clinical Presentation

A 16-year-old boy presented with pain in the lower leg.

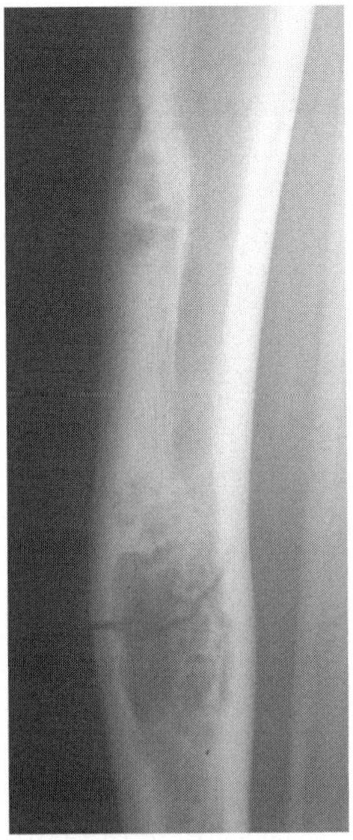

Figure 49A

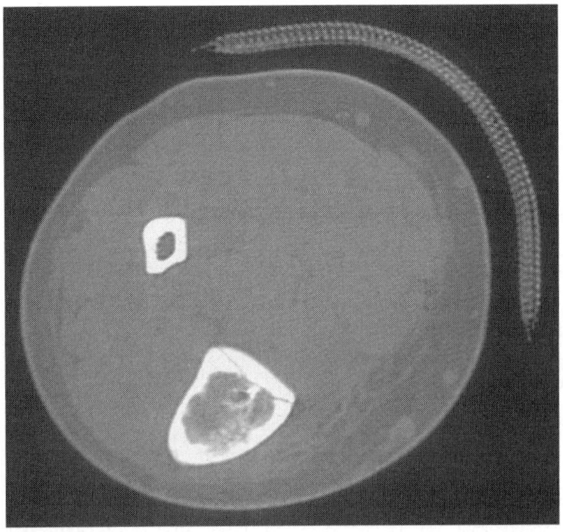

Figure 49B

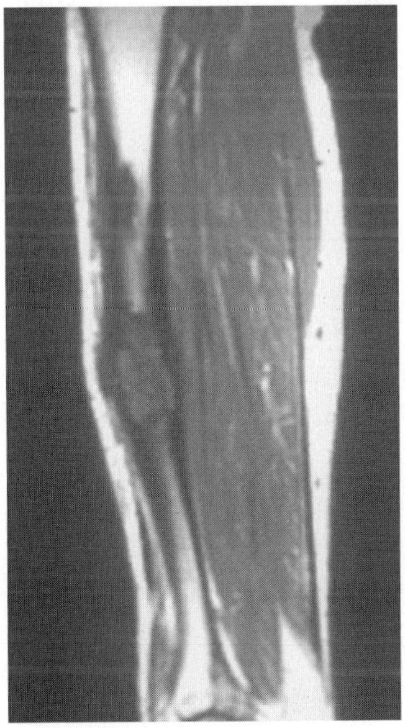

Figure 49C

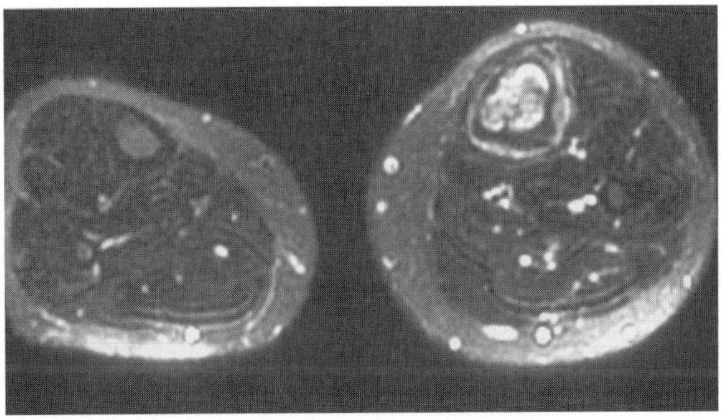

Figure 49D

Radiologic Findings

The lateral radiograph of the tibia (**Fig. 49A**) shows a bubbly, mildly expansile, lytic lesion of the midtibia with surrounding sclerosis. The dominant lesion appears to involve the cortex and medullary canal. A smaller satellite lesion is identified proximally that appears to involve the cortical bone alone. The axial CT image (**Fig. 49B**) through the lesion demonstrates the cortical and medullary involvement of the dominant lesion, as well as the internal trabeculation. The sagittal T1-weighted image (**Fig. 49C**) shows the multifocal nature of this lesion, with the superior focus of involvement isolated to the cortex. The lesion is predominantly high signal on the T2-weighted image (**Fig. 49D**), with low signal intensity septations internally. Note the rim of high signal periosteal reaction surrounding the tibial cortex.

Diagnosis

Adamantinoma.

Differential Diagnosis

- Osteofibrous dysplasia (OFD)
- Fibrous dysplasia (FD)
- Hemangioma
- Angiosarcoma or other vascular malignancy

Discussion

Background

Adamantinoma, generally considered to represent a low-grade malignancy, is a rare neoplasm, representing less than 1% of all primary bone neoplasms. The vast majority of lesions, between 80 and 90%, occur in the tibia, usually in the anterior midshaft of the diaphysis. This tumor is a distinct entity from adamantinoma of the jaw. Satellite lesions in the same bone are not uncommonly encountered, as in this case.

Clinical Findings

The age distribution for adamantinoma is wide; however, the majority of patients are in their second through fifth decades of life. Presenting symptoms most commonly include pain and/or swelling, as well as pathologic fracture. Symptoms are often present for many years prior to diagnosis, and a significant number of patients relate a history of trauma or other prior pathology, such as osteomyelitis, in the involved area. The biologic behavior of the tumor appears to be slightly more aggressive in males than in females, and metastatic disease and local recurrence may occur many years after initial treatment.

Pathology

The cell of origin is uncertain, but it does appear to be of an epithelial lineage. There is speculation that adamantinoma may be histologically related to OFD, such that the former represents a malignant degeneration of the latter, via an intermediate lesion of OFD-like adamantinoma.

Imaging Findings

RADIOGRAPHY

- Lesions are typically lytic, appearing as "soap bubble" tumors involving both the cortex and medullary canal of the tibia or fibula; occasionally a "moth-eaten" pattern of destruction is observed.
- Areas of internal density or internal septations may be present.
- Multilayered periosteal reaction is not uncommon.
- The presence of internal ground glass opacity, anterior tibial bowing, and a younger patient age all suggest the diagnosis of FD over adamantinoma.
- Exclusive or predominant cortical involvement is seen in ~10% of lesions.
- Lesions arise in an intracortical location; however, medullary involvement is common, as opposed to osteofibrous dysplasia, which also arises in the cortex but only uncommonly (10%) extends into the medullary canal.
- The presence of infantile/congenital pseudoarthrosis eliminates the possibility of adamantinoma.

COMPUTED TOMOGRAPHY

- CT demonstrates the intracortical and intramedullary components of the tumor well.
- Internal trabeculations are often seen.

MAGNETIC RESONANCE IMAGING

- Findings on MRI are nonspecific, including low signal intensity on T1-weighted images and high signal intensity on T2-weighted images.
- MRI often shows areas of marked contrast enhancement.

Treatment

- Limb salvage with en bloc resection of the tumor and reconstruction with an intercalary allograft or autograft is the preferred treatment.
- Complication rate related to the reconstructive procedure is relatively high (48% in a recent study), especially from nonunion and fracture of the graft.
- Metastatic rate (~15%) and recurrence rate are higher in patients treated with curettage.

Prognosis

- A recent study reported an 87.2% 10-year survival rate.

PEARLS

- Satellite lesions in the same bone are not uncommonly encountered, as in the reference case above.
- The presence of internal ground glass opacity, anterior tibial bowing, and a younger patient age all suggest the diagnosis of FD over adamantinoma.
- The presence of infantile/congenital pseudoarthrosis eliminates the possibility of adamantinoma.

PITFALLS

- This tumor is a distinct entity from adamantinoma of the jaw.
- Lesions arise in an intracortical location; however, medullary involvement is common (as opposed to osteofibrous dysplasia, which also arises in the cortex but only extends into the medullary canal in 10% of cases).
- The metastatic rate (~15%) and recurrence rate are higher in patients treated with curettage; however, the complication rate related to reconstructive procedures is relatively high (48% in a recent study), especially from nonunion and fracture of the graft.

Suggested Readings

Bloem JL, van der Heul RO, Schuttevaer HM, Kuipers D. Fibrous dysplasia vs. adamantinoma of the tibia: differentiation based on discriminant analysis of clinical and plain film findings. Am J Roentgenol 1991;156:1017–1023

Hazelbag HM, Taminiau AH, Fleuren GJ, Hogendoorn PC. Adamantinoma of the long bones. J Bone Joint Surg Am 1994;76:1482–1499

Qureshi AA, Shott SS, Mallin BA, Gitelis S. Current trends in the management of adamantinoma of long bones: an international study. J Bone Joint Surg Am 2000;82-A:1122–1131

Springfield DS, Rosenberg AE, Mankin HJ, Mindell ER. Relationship between osteofibrous dysplasia and adamantinoma. Clin Orthop Relat Res 1994;309:234–244

Sweet DE, Vinh TN, Devaney K. Cortical osteofibrous dysplasia of long bone and its relationship to adamantinoma: a clinicopathologic study of 30 cases. Am J Surg Pathol 1992;16:282–290

Zehr RJ, Recht MP, Bauer TW. Adamantinoma. Skeletal Radiol 1995;24:553–555

CASE 50

George Nomikos, Anthony G. Ryan, Peter L. Munk, and Mark Murphey

Clinical Presentation

A 38-year-old man presented with left hip pain.

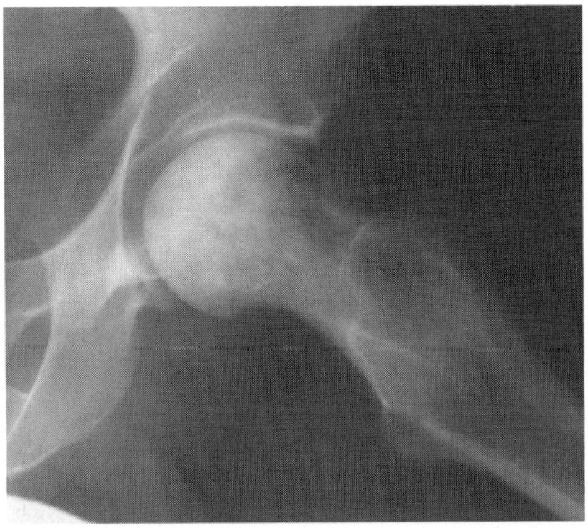

Figure 50A

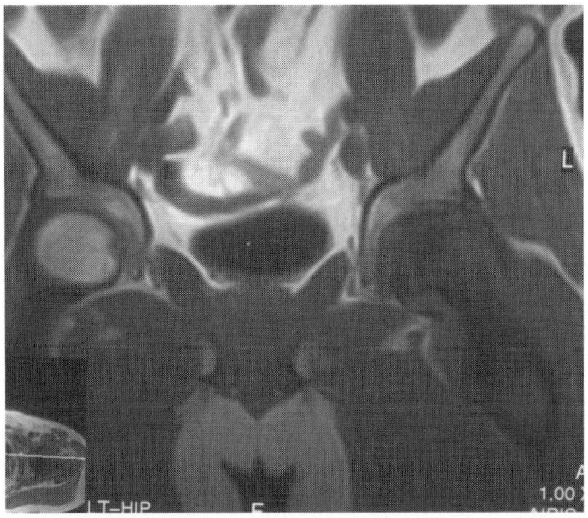

Figure 50B

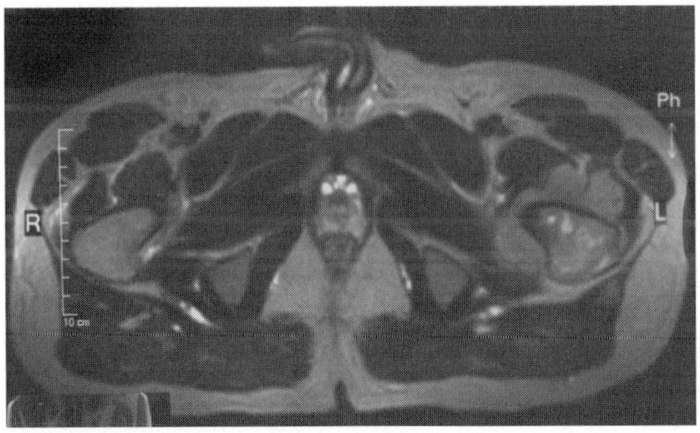

Figure 50C

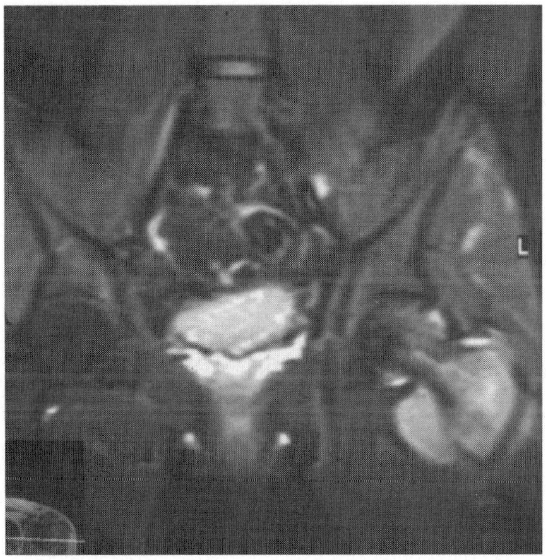

Figure 50D

Radiologic Findings

The frog-leg view of the left hip (**Fig. 50A**) shows sclerosis with some intermixed areas of lucency within the left femoral head and neck. The T1-weighted image (**Fig. 50B**) from the MRI examination shows marrow replacement in the femoral head and neck, as well as a large soft-tissue mass. On the T2-weighted image (**Fig. 50C**), marrow replacement is again seen in the proximal femur. The lesion is intermediate in signal intensity on the T2-weighted image. Also note the lack of obvious cortical destruction, despite the presence of a large soft-tissue mass. The large soft-tissue component with relative preservation of the cortex is also demonstrated on the STIR image (**Fig. 50D**).

Diagnosis

Primary lymphoma of bone.

Differential Diagnosis

- Metastatic disease
- Ewing's sarcoma/primitive neuroectodermal tumors (PNETs)
- Myeloma
- Leukemia
- Langerhans' cell histiocytosis
- Osteosarcoma
- Malignant fibrous histiocytoma or fibrosarcoma of bone
- Infection

Discussion

Background

Primary lymphoma of bone (PLB) is an uncommon primary osseous malignancy, accounting for ~3% of all primary bone tumors. Virtually all cases represent the non-Hodgkin's form of the disease, although there are rare reports of the Hodgkin's type. The presence of a primary soft-tissue site of origin with metastatic disease to the bone must be excluded before making the diagnosis of PLB. Although usually solitary, PLB can be multifocal (defined as involving more than one bone without involvement of lymph nodes or viscera for at least 6 months after presentation). This may represent between 11 and 31% of all PLB. Lesions are most commonly located in the metaphysis or diametaphysis of long bones, with the femur, tibia, and humerus the most frequently involved sites. Lesions are occasionally noted to be centered in the epiphysis. Flat bones are affected in ~25% of cases, most commonly the pelvis, scapula, and ribs.

Clinical Findings

Patients may present with pain, a palpable mass, or constitutional symptoms such as fever, weight loss, and night sweats. There is a male predominance of ~1.8:1 and a wide age distribution (2–88 years age range, with a mean of 42 years in one recent series).

Pathology

The vast majority of cases are the non-Hodgkin's form, and the most common subtype is the diffuse large cell variant. Reticulin staining is useful to demonstrate a typical meshwork of fibrous tissue around the lymphoma cells. Percutaneous biopsy of these lesions may result in crush artifact owing to the discohesive cells and require immunohistochemical staining for diagnosis.

Imaging Findings

RADIOGRAPHY

- Most cases show a lytic pattern of destruction (70%), usually in a "moth-eaten" or permeative pattern.
- A mixed pattern of lysis and sclerosis is seen in ~28% of cases.
- Periosteal reaction is also common, often in an aggressive pattern (single interrupted layer or multiple layers).
- Nonaggressive-appearing periosteal reaction (solid single layer) is seen in ~30% of cases.
- Pathologic fractures are not uncommon.
- Sequestra formation has been reported in 11 to 16% of cases; other processes that may demonstrate sequestra or sequestra-like appearance include Langerhans' cell histiocytosis, metastases, chronic osteomyelitis, fibrosarcoma, malignant fibrous histiocytoma, and desmoplastic fibroma.
- Transarticular spread may occur; other tumors that are reported to demonstrate this include chordoma, metastases, and chondrosarcoma.

SCINTIGRAPHY

- Increased activity is present in the vast majority of cases on bone scintigraphy, usually markedly.
- A combination of markedly increased activity on scintigraphy and normal-appearing radiographs is highly suggestive of the diagnosis of lymphoma (also seen with other small blue cell tumors such as Ewing's sarcoma, leukemia, and myeloma).
- A pattern of multifocal abnormal uptake in the skull, distal femur, and proximal tibia has been reported as suggestive of multifocal PLB.

COMPUTED TOMOGRAPHY

- Demonstrates marrow replacement, cortical destruction, and soft-tissue mass
- Also demonstrates sequestra formation, pathologic fracture, and transarticular spread to better advantage than radiographs

MAGNETIC RESONANCE IMAGING

- Variable signal intensity is seen on both T1- and T2-weighted images.
- Lesions may be hypo-, iso-, or hyperintense to muscle on T1-weighted images.
- Lesions may be hypo-, iso-, or hyperintense to fat on T2-weighted images.
- The variability of signal intensity on T2-weighted images is of uncertain etiology; intralesional collagen content or a high degree of cellularity may be responsible for the lower signal intensity seen in some lesions.
- Soft-tissue masses are very common.
- Primary lymphoma of the bone may present as an area of marrow replacement and large associated soft-tissue mass without significant associated focal cortical destruction. The lack of cortical destruction is due to tumor extension into the soft tissues from the medullary space through the small vascular channels in the cortical bone (as can also be seen in Ewing's sarcoma and other small round blue cell tumors).

Treatment

- Multidrug chemotherapy

Prognosis

- Average 5-year survival rate: up to 64%

PEARLS

- Most cases show a lytic pattern of destruction (70%), usually in a "moth-eaten" or permeative pattern. Alternatively, the presence of a large soft-tissue mass in the absence of obvious cortical destruction is suggestive.
- A combination of markedly increased activity on scintigraphy and normal-appearing radiographs is highly suggestive of the diagnosis of lymphoma (also seen with other small blue cell tumors, such as Ewing's sarcoma, leukemia, and myeloma). A pattern of multifocal abnormal uptake in the skull, distal femur, and proximal tibia has been reported as suggestive of multifocal primary lymphoma of bone.
- Transarticular spread may occur; other tumors that are reported to demonstrate this include chordoma, metastases, and chondrosarcoma.

PITFALLS

- Sequestra formation has been reported in 11 to 16% of cases; however, other processes may demonstrate sequestra or sequestra-like appearance, including Langerhans' cell histiocytosis, metastases, chronic osteomyelitis, fibrosarcoma, malignant fibrous histiocytoma, and desmoplastic fibroma.
- Percutaneous biopsy of these lesions may result in crush artifact owing to the discohesive cells and consequently require immunohistochemical staining for diagnosis.
- Lesions may be hypo-, iso-, or hyperintense to muscle on T1-weighted images and may be hypo-, iso-, or hyperintense to fat on T2-weighted images.

Suggested Readings

Hermann G, Klein M, Abdelwahab I, Kenan S. MRI appearance of primary non-Hodgkin's lymphoma of bone. Skeletal Radiol 1997;26:629–632

Melamed JW, Martinez S, Hoffman CJ. Imaging of primary multifocal osseous lymphoma. Skeletal Radiol 1997;26:35–41

Mulligan ME. Myeloma and lymphoma. Semin Musculoskelet Radiol 2000;4:127–135

Mulligan ME, Kransdorf MJ. Sequestra in primary lymphoma of bone: prevalence and radiologic features. Am J Roentgenol 1993;160:1245–1248

Mulligan ME, McRae GA, Murphey MD. Imaging features of primary lymphoma of bone. AJR Am J Roentgenol 1999;173:1691–1697

White LM, Schweitzer ME, Khalili K, Howarth DJ, Wunder JS, Bell RS. MR imaging of primary lymphoma of bone: variability of T2-weighted signal intensity. Am J Roentgenol 1998;170:1243–1247

CASE 51

George Nomikos, Anthony G. Ryan, Peter L. Munk, and Mark Murphey

Clinical Presentation

A 45-year-old woman with rheumatoid arthritis was incidentally noted to have a lesion in the left fibular head.

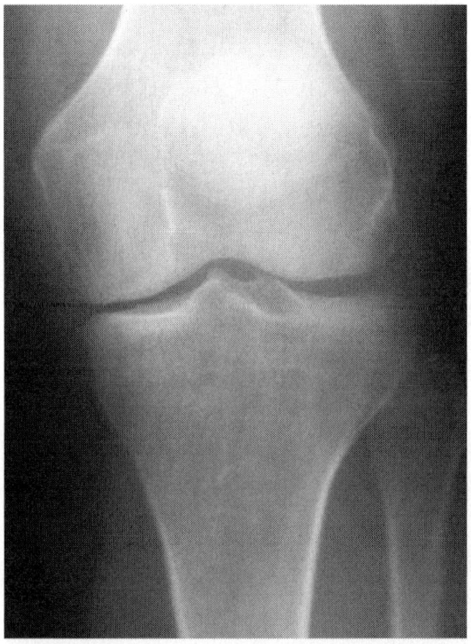

Figure 51A

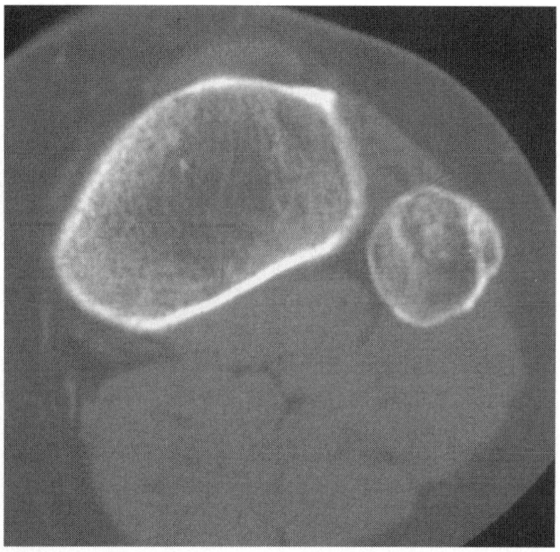

Figure 51B

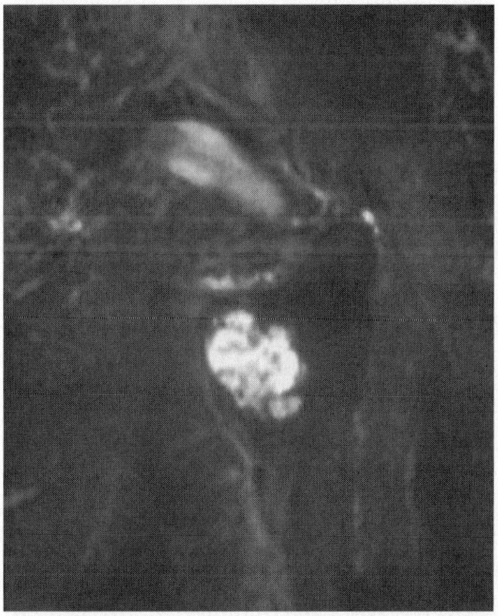

Figure 51C

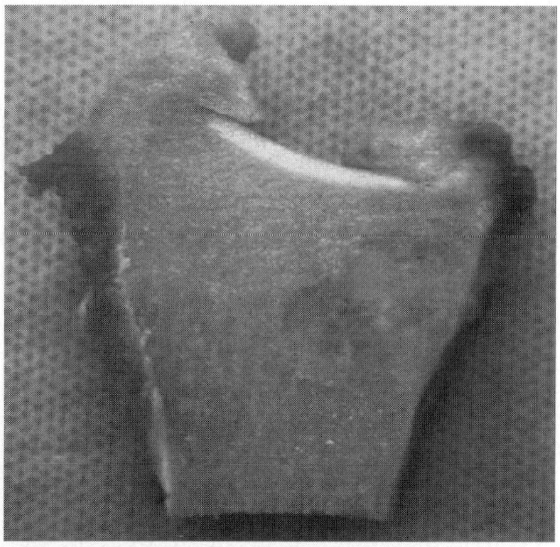

Figure 51D (See **Figure 51D** in color insert.)

Radiologic Findings

An anteroposterior radiograph of the knee (**Fig. 51A**) shows a vague area of radiolucency in the proximal fibular head with punctuate internal mineralization. There is no evidence of cortical destruction. A CT scan at the level of the fibular head (**Fig. 51B**) shows a well-defined lytic lesion with a narrow zone of transition. The lesion margin is partially sclerotic and partially nonsclerotic. There is internal matrix mineralization in a ring and arc pattern, compatible with a hyaline cartilage lesion. The lesion is predominantly very high signal intensity on the sagittal fat-suppressed T2-weighted image (**Fig. 51C**), similar to the signal intensity of fluid. The areas of low signal intensity on the T2-weighted image correspond to areas of mineralization on radiography and CT, and the lesion shows lobulated margins. Corresponding sagittally sectioned gross specimen of the fibular head (**Fig. 51D**) shows the glistening blue-white lobular lesion in the medullary canal. There is no evidence of destruction of the overlying cortex.

Diagnosis

Enchondroma.

Differential Diagnosis

- Low-grade chondrosarcoma
- Osteoblastoma
- Chondromyxoid fibroma
- Chondroblastoma
- Osteocartilaginous fibrous dysplasia

Discussion

Background

Enchondromas account for ~20% of all chondroid lesions of bone, are second in prevalence to osteochondromas (30%), and are the most common tumor of the hands. Lesions in the small bones of the hand account for ~40 to 65% of lesions and most commonly affect the proximal phalanges (40 to 50%) or metacarpals (15 to 30%). Long tubular bone lesions account for ~25% of enchondromas, and most commonly involve the femur, humerus, and tibia. Isolated flat bone or carpal bone involvement is very uncommon, and the possibility of chondrosarcoma should be excluded in the case of lesions in this location. Lesions arise when a fragment of hyaline cartilage from the growth plate becomes entrapped in the medullary canal metaphysis of a growing long bone. Instead of becoming ossified, it continues to grow and enlarge until skeletal maturity. As growth of the bone proceeds, the lesion may migrate into the diaphysis, which is more likely the earlier the lesion develops.

Clinical Findings

Lesions are frequently discovered incidentally in asymptomatic patients in the third to fourth decades of life. Enchondromas also often present because of pathologic fracture, particularly in the case of

Table 51–1 Findings Suggestive of Chondrosarcoma in Long Bone

Cortical scalloping > two thirds of the cortical depth in any one location
Uptake on scintigraphy greater than that seen in the anterior superior iliac spine
Cortical destruction
Soft-tissue mass
Pain directly referable to the lesion
Size > 5 to 6 cm
Epiphyseal location
Periosteal reaction or cortical thickening on radiography

hand lesions. Hand lesions may also cause mild surrounding soft-tissue swelling. Pain that is directly referable to a long bone enchondroma is worrisome for malignant transformation to chondrosarcoma (see **Table 51–1**).

Pathology

Lesions may appear as benign islands of cartilage with normal marrow fat interposed between the cartilaginous lobules, or they may be surrounded by lamellar bone. There should be no permeation or invasion of the surrounding marrow fat or entrapment of trabecular bone by the cartilage lesion. Differentiation between benign enchondroma and low-grade chondrosarcoma can be difficult pathologically because these lesions may demonstrate overlap in degrees of polynuclearity, mitoses, and cellularity. The radiologic appearance of lesions is therefore often very important in the distinction between benign and malignant cartilage lesions (see Case 42). It is also important to note that lesions arising in the hands or feet, lesions identified during pregnancy, lesions arising on the surface of bone (juxtacortical chondroma), and lesions arising in the setting of multiple enchondromatosis may all demonstrate a more "active-appearing" histology than typical enchondromas and yet still be benign.

Imaging Findings

RADIOGRAPHY

- Lesions are lytic, with a narrow zone of transition without surrounding sclerosis.
- Epiphyseal lesions (2 to 5% of enchondromas) often demonstrate a rim of sclerosis and may be confused with chondroblastoma.
- Lesions in the hand are usually lobular, well marginated, and within the diaphysis of the bone centrally.
- Metaphyseal lesions are less common and may extend to the end of the bone.
- Deep endosteal scalloping is often seen in hand lesions; however, periosteal reaction and cortical thickening should be absent unless there is a pathologic fracture.
- Chondroid mineralization (punctate or rings and arcs) is usually present but may be subtle, particularly in hand lesions or in anatomically complex areas.
- Long bone lesions may be central or eccentric and may be located in the metaphysis (epiphyseal extension is uncommon) or diaphysis.
- Long bone lesions are usually < 6 cm in size and may show mild cortical scalloping (depth < two thirds of the cortical thickness), mild expansion, and mild cortical thickening; chondroid calcification is very common (95%) but variable in degree.
- Eccentric expansion may be seen in rib or fibular lesions, producing a more worrisome radiographic appearance (enchondroma protuberans).

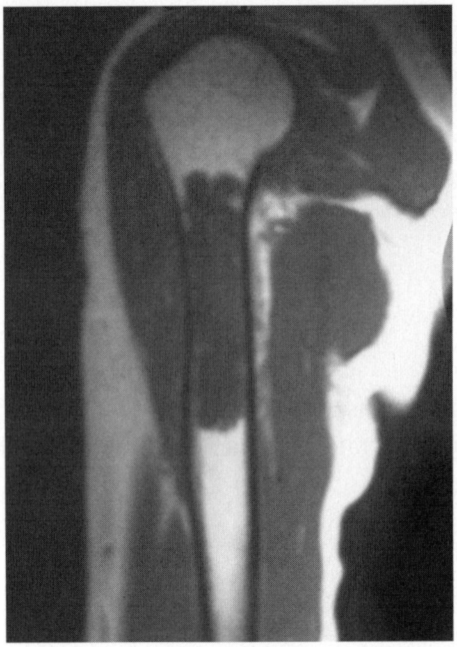

E

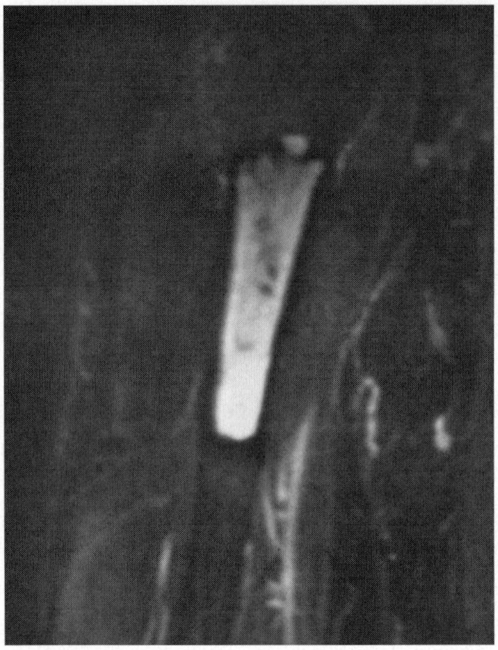

F

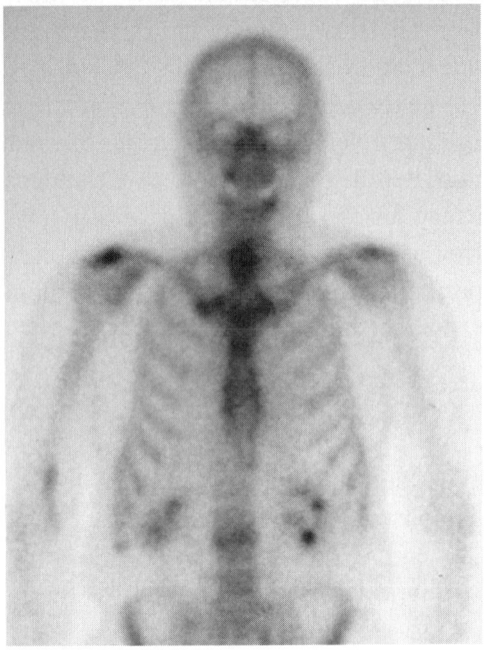

G

Figures 51E–51G A coronal T1-weighted image (**51E**) shows an intra-axial uniform intermediate signal intensity lesion in the proximal humerus with no evidence of cortical breach. A T2-weighted image (**51F**) shows the lesion to have high signal intensity. A radionuclide bone scan (**51G**) demonstrates mild to moderate homogeneous uptake in the location of the lesion.

SCINTIGRAPHY

- Mild to moderate homogeneous uptake is typical (**Fig. 51E**).
- Uptake greater than that in the anterior superior iliac crest is very suggestive of malignant degeneration to chondrosarcoma (**Fig. 51H,51I**).

COMPUTED TOMOGRAPHY

- Best modality for determining the extent and type of mineralization, as well as degree of endosteal scalloping
- Also good for detection of subtle pathologic fracture

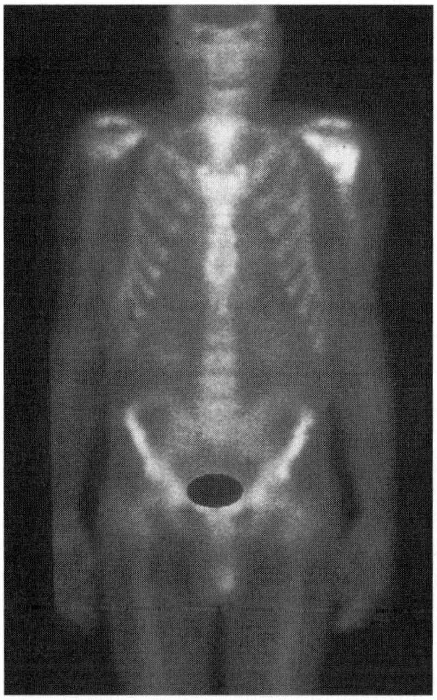

H

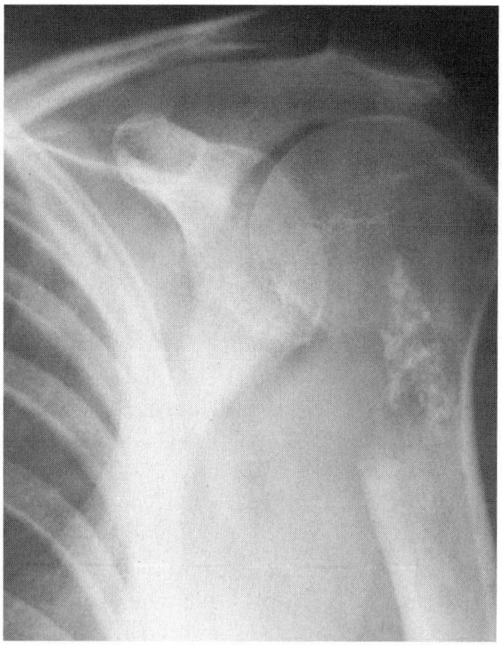

I

Figures 51H,51I Marked uptake (greater than in the anterior superior iliac crest) is demonstrated on scintigraphy (**51H**) at the location of the left proximal humeral lesion. Corresponding radiograph (**51I**) shows cortical destruction medially. This combination of findings is diagnostic of malignant degeneration to chondrosarcoma.

MAGNETIC RESONANCE IMAGING

- Predominant signal intensity similar to skeletal muscle on T1-weighted images
- Foci of high signal may be seen on T1-weighted images corresponding to fat in the intervening normal yellow marrow.
- High signal intensity on T2-weighted images because of the high water content of hyaline cartilage
- Lobular margins are best appreciated on T2-weighted images.
- Areas of mineralization or septations are low signal intensity on all pulse sequences.
- Evaluation for soft-tissue mass (diagnostic of malignant transformation) is best performed by MRI.
- Peripheral and septal enhancement after gadolinium administration

Variants

1. Ollier's disease (**Fig. 51J**) is a nonheritable dyschondroplasia in which multiple enchondromas are present throughout the skeleton. Lesions are often predominantly or completely localized to one side of the body. Patients usually present at an early age because of the high prevalence of pathologic fractures, masses, and skeletal deformities. Radiographs in young patients demonstrate multiple radiolucent enchondromas that are often connected to the physeal plate by multiple radiolucent columns of metaphyseal cartilage, which produce a fan-like appearance in the metaphysis. This columnar appearance is diagnostic of enchondromatosis. The risk of malignant degeneration of the enchondromatosis is 5 to 30%. There is also increased risk of development of other malignancies, such as ovarian carcinoma, pancreatic carcinoma, and gliomas.
2. Maffucci's syndrome (**Fig. 51K,51L**) is the association of multiple enchondromata with multiple soft-tissue hemangiomas or lymphangiomas. Like Ollier's disease, and unlike hereditary

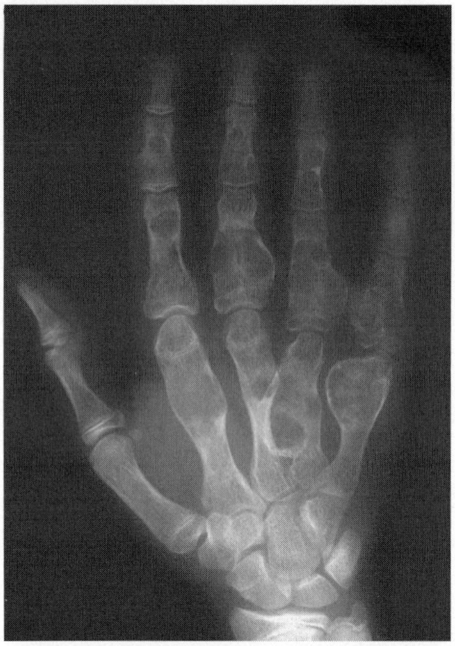

J

Figures 51J An anteroposterior radiograph of the hand in a patient with Ollier's disease shows multiple radiolucent enchondromas throughout the small bones of the hand. **51K,51L** Radiographs of the hands in a patient with Maffucci's syndrome show the combination of multiple enchondromata and multiple soft-tissue hemangiomas, the latter evinced by the presence of phleboliths.

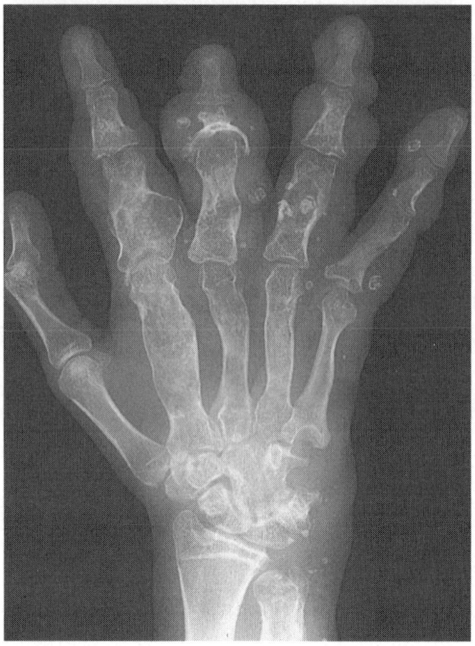

K

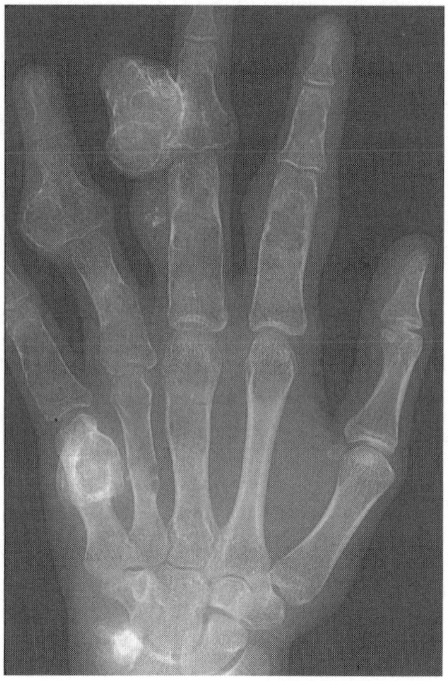

L

multiple enchondromatosis (HME), Maffucci's syndrome is nonheritable and often favors one side of the body. Maffucci's syndrome is diagnosed at birth in ~25% of cases, and 78% are diagnosed by puberty. The associated hemangiomas are often subcutaneous, although deep hemangiomas may occur. Enchondromas most commonly affect the tubular bones, particularly the small tubular bones of the hands and feet. The soft-tissue hemangiomas can be recognized radiographically by the presence of phleboliths. Malignant transformation of the enchondromas to chondrosarcoma (most common) or fibrosarcoma occurs at a rate similar to that seen in Ollier's disease. However, the rate of development of nonmusculoskeletal malignancies is much higher in Maffucci's syndrome (vascular tumors, carcinoma of the gastrointestinal (GI) tract, pancreas, and ovaries, as well as gliomas). Overall, the reported rate of development of malignancy in Maffucci's syndrome varies widely (23 to 100%).

3. Metachondromatosis is a condition in which multiple osteochondromas and enchondromas both develop. There is a familial predisposition.

Treatment and Prognosis

- Treatment of solitary enchondromas is not required unless they are symptomatic or there is concern for malignant degeneration.
- When treatment is required, curettage and bone grafting are usually adequate.
- Recurrence is uncommon.
- Malignant transformation of a solitary enchondroma occurs with less frequency than in the setting of multiple enchondromas, at a reported rate ranging from 2 to 5%.
- Malignant transformation is usually to chondrosarcoma, but transformation to fibrosarcoma, malignant fibrous histiocytoma, and osteosarcoma has been reported.

PEARLS

- In the presence of a radiographically suspicious lesion, radiotracer uptake greater than in the anterior superior iliac crest on scintigraphy is suggestive of malignant degeneration.
- Radiographs in young patients demonstrate multiple radiolucent enchondromas that are often connected to the physeal plate by multiple radiolucent columns of metaphyseal cartilage, which produce a fanlike appearance in the metaphysis. This columnar appearance is diagnostic of enchondromatosis.
- CT is the best modality for determining the extent and type of mineralization and the degree of endosteal scalloping, as well as for detecting any subtle pathologic fracture.

PITFALLS

- Although increased radiotracer uptake may suggest malignant degeneration, it is important to exclude pathologic fracture as a cause of the increase.
- The risk of malignant degeneration in the enchondromas encountered in Ollier's disease is 5 to 30%; however, there is an additional risk of extraosseous malignancies, such as ovarian carcinoma, pancreatic carcinoma, and gliomas.
- Malignant transformation of the enchondromas to chondrosarcoma (most common) or fibrosarcoma in Maffucci's syndrome occurs at a rate similar to that seen in Ollier's disease; however, the rate of development of nonmusculoskeletal malignancies is much higher in Maffucci's syndrome (vascular tumors; carcinoma of the GI tract, pancreas, and ovaries; and gliomas).

Suggested Readings

Brien EW, Mirra JM, Kerr R. Benign and malignant cartilage tumors of bone and joint: their anatomic and theoretical basis with an emphasis on radiology, pathology and clinical biology. I. The intramedullary tumors. Skeletal Radiol 1997;26:325–353

Flemming DJ, Murphey MD. Enchondroma and chondrosarcoma. Semin Musculoskelet Radiol 2000;4:59–71

Giudici MA, Moser RP Jr, Kransdorf MJ. Cartilagenous bone tumors. Radiol Clin North Am 1993;31:237–259

Murphey MD, Flemming DJ, Boyea SR, Bojescul JA, Sweet DE, Temple HT. Enchondroma versus chondrosarcoma in the appendicular skeleton: differentiating features. Radiographics 1998;18:1213–1237

Zwenneke Flach H, Ginai AZ, Wolter Oosterhuis J. Best cases from the AFIP: Maffucci syndrome: radiologic and pathologic findings. Armed Forces Institutes of Pathology. Radiographics 2001;21:1311–1316

CASE 52

George Nomikos, Anthony G. Ryan, Peter L. Munk, and Mark Murphey

Clinical Presentation

A 31-year-old woman presented with increasing left elbow pain that began 3 to 4 years ago, now persisting at rest.

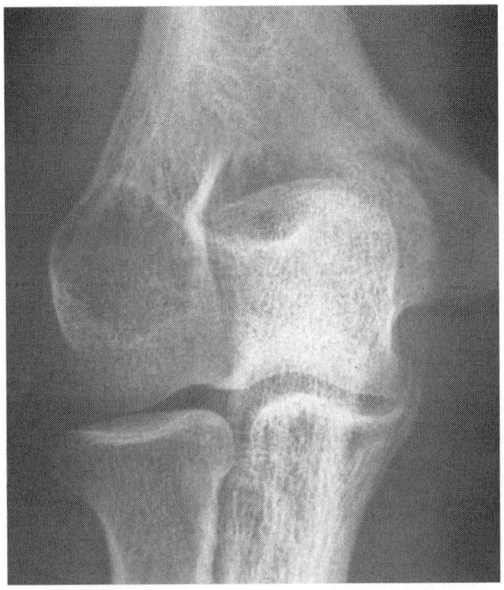

Figure 52A

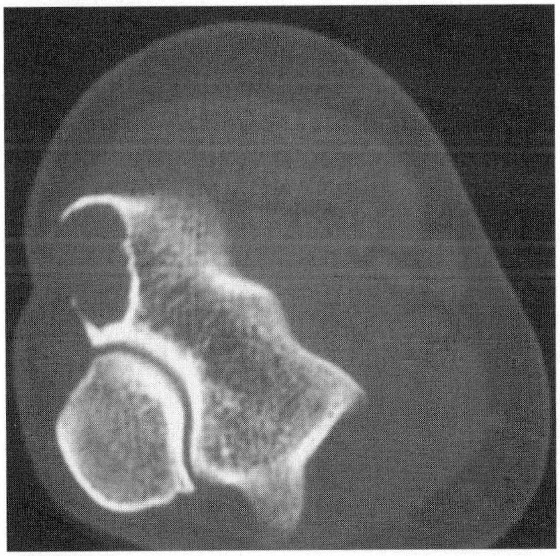

Figure 52B

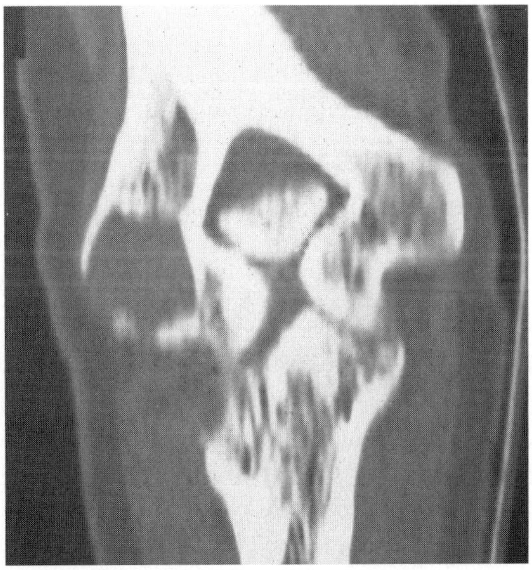

Figure 52C

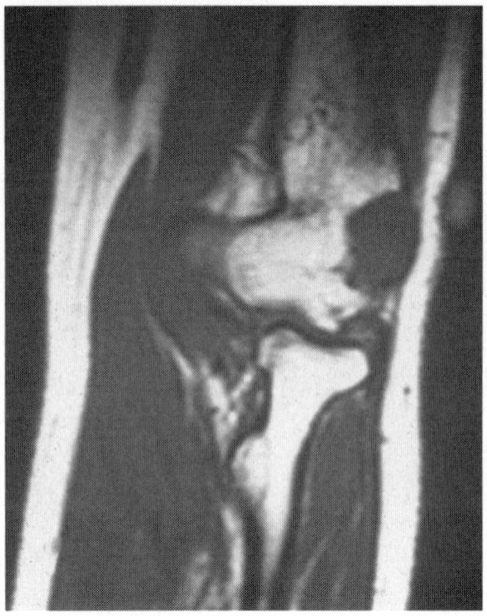

Figure 52D

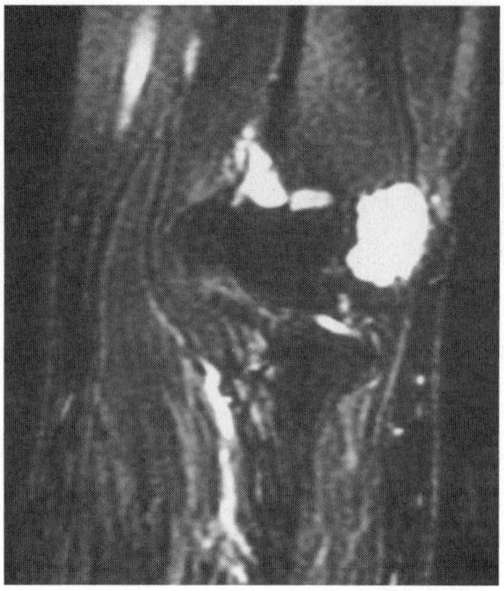

Figure 52E

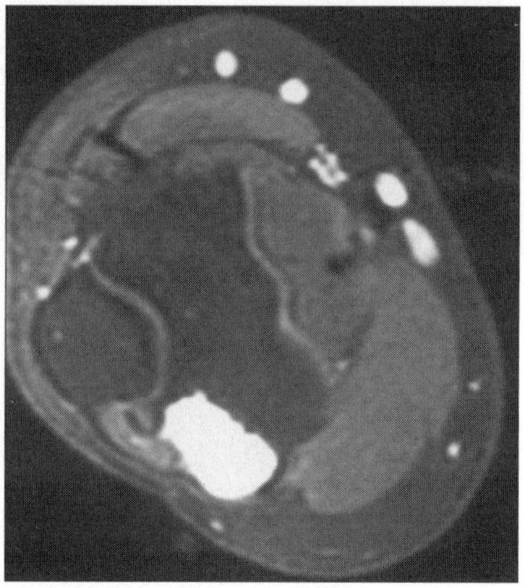

Figure 52F

Radiologic Findings

An anteroposterior radiograph of the left elbow shows a mildly expansile lytic lesion arising in the lateral epicondyle of the humerus. The lesion demonstrates a narrow zone of transition with a partially sclerotic rim and no mineralized matrix (**Fig. 52A**). An axial CT scan and a coronal reformatted image (**Figs. 52B,52C**) through the lesion show expansion and marked thinning of the overlying cortical bone. The inner border of the lesion is more indolent in appearance and reveals a thin sclerotic rim. The lesion is similar to skeletal muscle in attenuation and does not demonstrate matrix mineralization. The lesion is also similar to skeletal muscle in signal intensity on the T1-weighted MRI (**Fig. 52D**) and demonstrates very high signal, similar to fluid, on the fat-suppressed T2-weighted image (**Fig. 52E**). It demonstrates marked diffuse enhancement on the fat-suppressed T1-weighted image (**Fig. 52F**) after intravenous gadolinium administration.

Diagnosis

Chondromyxoid fibroma (CMF) of bone.

Differential Diagnosis

- Aneurysmal bone cyst (ABC)
- Giant cell tumor (should extend to subchondral bone)
- Chondroblastoma

- Periosteal chondroma
- Enchondroma
- Fibroxanthoma
- Monostotic fibrous dysplasia
- Langerhans' cell histiocytosis

Discussion

Background

CMF is a rare primary benign cartilaginous tumor of bone that accounts for less than 1% of all primary bone tumors.

Clinical Findings

Although these tumors have been reported over a wide age range (6 to 87 years, with an average of 31.1 years in one large study), most patients are in their second or third decade of life (50% of cases). Lesions in the small bones of the hands or feet, recurrent tumors, and tumors with histological atypia tend to be seen in younger patients. Lesions most frequently affect the lower extremity, particularly around the knee, and are most commonly located in long bones (47%), particularly the tibia, femur, and fibula. The humerus accounts for ~6% of all long bone lesions. Other common locations include flat bones (30%), most commonly the ilium and ribs, and the small bones of the hands and feet (17%). Lesions show a mild male predilection. Most patients have a nonspecific clinical presentation, including pain, swelling, and a palpable soft-tissue mass.

Pathology

Histologically, these lesions may demonstrate variable patterns. Lesions are characterized by spindle-shaped or stellate tumor cells, usually arranged in a lobular pattern, set in a myxoid background. Mature hyaline cartilage, giant cells, chondroblastoma-like regions, mitotic figures, and bizarre cytological features are commonly seen. Calcification was seen histologically in ~35% of lesions in a recent review. Soft-tissue extension is also common at pathologic examination, especially in lesions involving the small bones of the hands and feet (44%). Secondary ABC formation is uncommon (9%).

Imaging Findings

RADIOGRAPHY

- Lesions are typically lytic and metaphyseal, often with lobular margins, and demonstrate a geographic pattern of lysis, commonly with a rim of sclerosis. Internal trabeculation is frequent.
- Matrix mineralization is identified in fewer than 10% of lesions on radiographs.
- Long bone lesions are usually eccentric or intracortical in location, whereas lesions in the small bones of the feet are often central in location.
- Expansile remodeling is common, particularly along the outer margin of lesions.
- The outer margin is often markedly expanded or even absent-appearing on radiographs (simulating an aneurysmal bone cyst), whereas the inner margin of the lesion has an intact and indolent appearance.
- Although epiphyseal extension is common, extension to the subchondral bone plate is infrequent.
- Expansile remodeling and trabeculation are often very prominent in lesions located in the small bones of the feet.

COMPUTED TOMOGRAPHY

- Lesions are lower attenuation compared with muscle on CT and may demonstrate minimal calcification to better advantage than radiography.
- Although the expanded outer margin of CMF may appear absent on radiography, CT typically demonstrates an intact outer margin composed of thickened and expanded periosteum.

MAGNETIC RESONANCE IMAGING

- Signal intensity may be heterogeneous, due to the diverse pathologic components of these lesions.
- Lesions demonstrate low signal intensity on T1-weighted images and very high signal intensity on T2-weighted images, reflecting the high water (myxoid) content of the lesions.
- As on CT, an intact outer margin is often identifiable on MRI, even when it appears absent on radiographs.
- Cystic or secondary ABC components are rare.

Treatment and Prognosis

- Curettage or excision and bone grafting
- Recurrence rate of 26% in one large study from the Mayo Clinic
- Malignant transformation to chondrosarcoma very uncommon

PEARLS

- Lesions are lower attenuation compared with muscle on CT.
- Although similar in both appearance and location, giant cell tumor of bone may be differentiated from CMF, as the latter does not extend to subchondral bone.
- Secondary ABC formation is an uncommon (9%) occurrence.

PITFALLS

- Although the expanded outer margin of CMF may appear absent on radiography, CT typically demonstrates an intact outer margin composed of thickened and expanded periosteum.
- Despite treatment with curettage and bone grafting, there is a very high recurrence rate of 26%.
- Malignant transformation to chondrosarcoma, although uncommon, is possible, and an index of suspicion should be present in the presence of a growing, painful lesion.

Suggested Readings

Giudici MA, Moser RP Jr, Kransdorf MJ. Cartilaginous bone tumors. Radiol Clin North Am 1993;31:237–259

O'Connor PJ, Gibbon WW, Hardy G, Butt WP. Chondromyxoid fibroma of the foot. Skeletal Radiol 1996;25:143–148

Robbin MR, Murphey MD. Benign chondroid neoplasms of bone. Semin Musculoskelet Radiol 2000;4:45–58

Schajowicz F, Gallardo H. Chondromyxoid fibroma (fibromyxoid chondroma) of bone: a clinico-pathologic study of thirty-two cases. J Bone Joint Surg Br 1971;53:198–216

Wu CT, Inwards CY, O'Laughlin SS, Rock MG, Beabout JW, Unni KK. Chondromyxoid fibroma of bone: a clinicopathologic review of 278 cases. Hum Pathol 1998;29:438–446

CASE 53

George Nomikos, Mark Murphey, Anthony G. Ryan, and Peter L. Munk

Clinical Presentation

A 32-year-old man presented with foot pain.

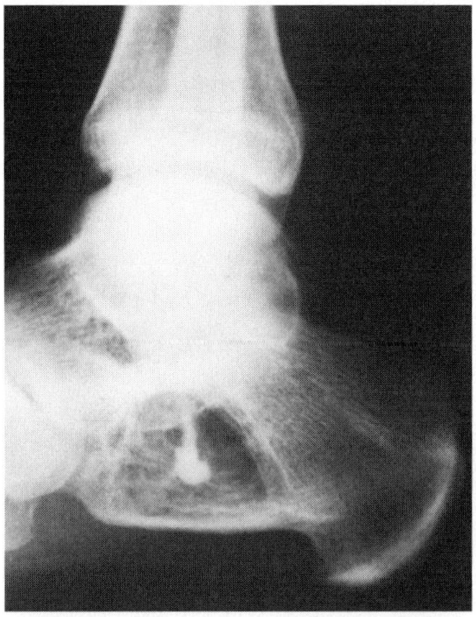

Figure 53A

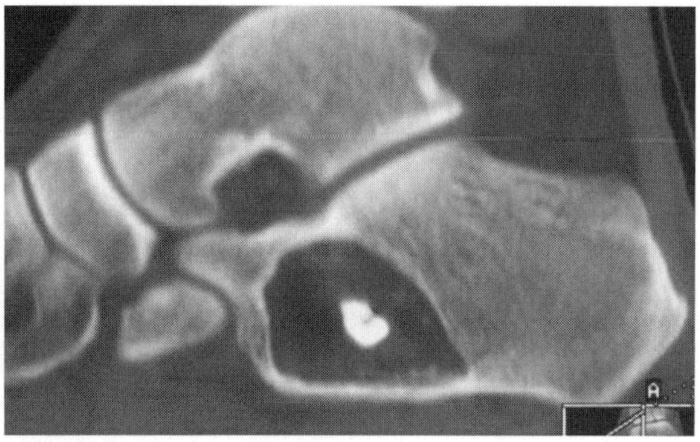

Figure 53B

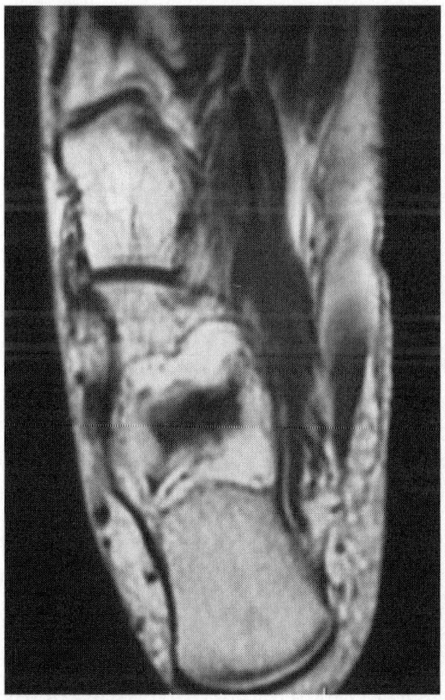

Figure 53C

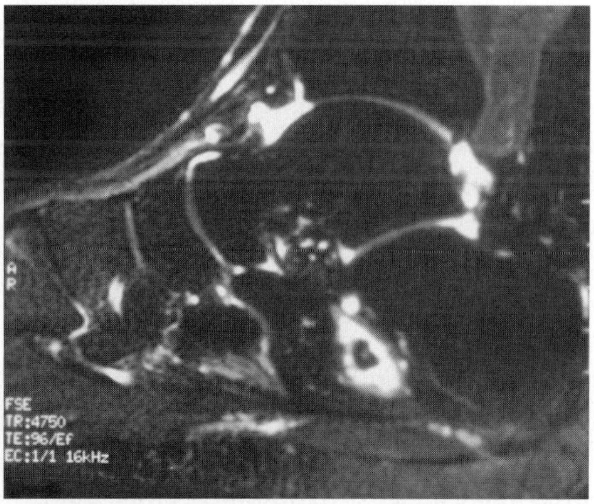

Figure 53D

Radiologic Findings

The lateral radiograph of the ankle (**Fig. 53A**) shows a geographic lytic lesion in the anterior calcaneus with a narrow zone of transition and significant surrounding sclerosis. There is a central area of dense mineralization in the lesion. There is no evidence of pathologic fracture or aggressive bone destruction. CT (**Fig. 53B**) shows a well-marginated lesion arising in the anterior calcaneus. Note the sclerotic margin and central dense focus of mineralization. The predominant internal attenuation of the lesion is identical to subcutaneous fat. Axial T1- and sagittal fat-suppressed T2-weighted images demonstrate that the majority of the lesion follows fat signal intensity on the T1- and T2-weighted images (**Figs. 53C,53D**); however, there is central fluid signal intensity in the lesion, around the area of mineralization.

Diagnosis

Involuting intraosseous lipoma.

Differential Diagnosis

- Involuting infarction
- Simple bone cyst
- Fibrous dysplasia
- Aneurysmal bone cyst
- Cartilaginous lesions
- Liposclerosing myxofibrous tumor (LSMFT)

Discussion

Background

Intraosseous lipomas are uncommon benign bone tumors, accounting for ~0.1% of bone tumors. However, in our opinion and experience, they are much more frequent. Although the radiographic appearance of lesions in the calcaneus is often diagnostic, lesions in other locations may have a more variable appearance (see differential diagnosis list above). Three stages have been described: lesions composed virtually entirely of mature fat cells; lesions composed of mature fat cells, fat necrosis, and mineralization; and lesions demonstrating cyst formation, myxoid degeneration, and reactive woven bone production.

Clinical Findings

Lesions have been reported in patients ranging in age from 14 to 75 years. Most patients are asymptomatic, and most lesions are incidentally discovered. However, some patients report mild pain, and symptoms may result from associated pathologic fracture. The single most commonly reported location is the proximal femur (intertrochanteric/subtrochanteric region). Other common locations include the calcaneus, ilium (near the sacroiliac joint), and fibula. Spinal lesions are uncommon.

Pathology

According to Milgram, stage 1 lesions are composed of mature fat cells. Stage 2 lesions demonstrate partial fat necrosis and mineralization intermixed with areas of mature fat cells. Stage 3 lesions contain areas in which the fat cells have died and there has been subsequent cyst formation, mineralization, and new bone formation. Advancement from one stage to the next is due to progressive ischemia and infarction, which in turn may be due to expansion of the lesion in the rigid surrounding bone.

Imaging

RADIOGRAPHY

- Lesions are most commonly metadiaphyseal in location.
- Lesions typically have a narrow zone of transition, often with a sclerotic rim.

Stage 1

- Purely lytic lesion demonstrating osseous resorption and expansile remodeling (the latter is a distinguishing feature from infarctions that do not show evidence of expansion)

Stage 2

- Similar to stage 1, but demonstrates areas of increased density secondary to fat necrosis and subsequent dystrophic calcification

Stage 3

- There is no residual trabecular bone; the overall density of the lesion is greater than stage 1 or 2 lesions because of extensive fat necrosis and mineralization in the lesion; a thick rim of sclerosis is often present, also likely related to the involutional changes.

COMPUTED TOMOGRAPHY

Stage 1

- Lesions demonstrate homogeneous internal attenuation equivalent to subcutaneous fat.

Stage 2

- Lesions have areas of mineralization due to fat necrosis in the fatty lesion.

Stage 3

- Lesions demonstrate extensive fat necrosis leading to widespread ossification and calcification as well as cyst formation.
- The presence of central calcification and a peripheral rind of fat is diagnostic of an intraosseous lipoma because mineralization does not occur in this area of osteonecrosis.

MAGNETIC RESONANCE IMAGING

Stage 1

- Lesions are similar to subcutaneous fat on all pulse sequences and demonstrate a low signal intensity rim corresponding to surrounding reactive sclerosis.

Stage 2

- Lesions are predominantly fat signal intensity on all pulse sequences but also demonstrate regions that are low signal intensity on all pulse sequences, corresponding to areas of mineralization.

Stage 3

- Lesions demonstrate extensive internal mineralization that is often central, a thick margin of low signal intensity corresponding to reactive sclerosis, as well as a peripheral rind of fat signal intensity within the outer sclerosis and surrounding the mineralization.
- Lesions may also demonstrate areas of fat necrosis and cyst formation that are high signal intensity on T2-weighted images and variable in intensity on T1-weighted images.

Treatment and Prognosis

- No treatment or simple curettage is adequate for most lesions.
- Rare cases of malignant transformation are reported.

Variants

Parosteal lipoma represents an uncommon lipoma variant that arises on or adjacent to the surface of bone, most frequently a long tubular bone. Common locations include the thigh adjacent to the femur and the upper extremity adjacent to the radius. Compression of adjacent motor or sensory nerves by the mass is not infrequent. Periosteal reaction and cortical thickening of the adjacent bone are common. In addition, an osseous excrescence simulating an osteochondroma, but which does not show cortical or medullary continuity with the underlying bone, may extend from the surface of the involved bone into the fatty mass (**Figs. 53E,53F**).

PEARLS

- The presence of central calcification and a peripheral rind of fat is diagnostic of an intraosseous lipoma.
- The single most common location of intraosseous lipomas is the intertrochanteric/subtrochanteric region of the proximal femur.
- The osseous resorption and expansile remodeling demonstrated by purely lytic stage 1 lesions differentiate them from infarctions, which do not show evidence of expansion.

PITFALLS

- Parosteal lipoma may give rise to an osseous excrescence simulating an osteochondroma; however, a parosteal lipoma does not show cortical or medullary continuity with the underlying bone and may extend from the surface of the involved bone into a fatty mass.

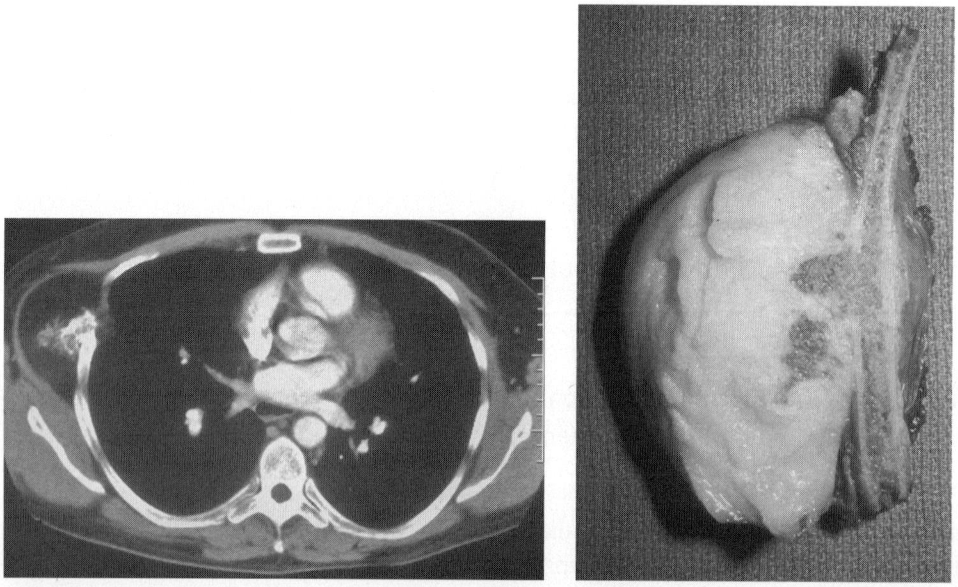

E F

Figures 53E and **53F** Transaxial CT thorax (**53E**) and corresponding gross specimen (**53F**) demonstrating an osseous excrescence arising from the lateral aspect of a rib with no corticomedullary continuity surrounded by a fatty mass. Biopsy confirmed a diagnosis of parosteal lipoma. (See also **Figure 53F** in color insert.)

- Although quoted as accounting for only 0.1% of bone tumors, in practice intraosseous lipomas appear to be more common, and so consideration should be given to the diagnosis in the appropriate circumstances.

Suggested Readings

Blacksin MF, Ende N, Benevenia J. Magnetic resonance imaging of intraosseous lipomas: a radiologic-pathologic correlation. Skeletal Radiol 1995;24:37–41

Milgram JW. Intraosseous lipomas: a clinicopathologic study of 66 cases. Clin Orthop Relat Res 1988;231:277–302

Murphey MD, Carroll JF, Flemming DJ, Pope TL, Gannon FH, Kransdorf MJ. From the archives of the AFIP: benign musculoskeletal lipomatous lesions. Radiographics 2004;24:1433–1466

Propeck T, Bullard MA, Lin J, Doi K, Martel W. Radiologic-pathologic correlation of intraosseous lipomas. Am J Roentgenol 2000;175:673–678

Williams CE, Close PJ, Meaney J, Ritchie M, Cogley D, Carty AT. Intraosseous lipomas. Clin Radiol 1993;47:348–350

CASE 54

George Nomikos, Anthony G. Ryan, Peter L. Munk, and Mark Murphey

Clinical Presentation

A 15-year-old girl presented with ankle pain.

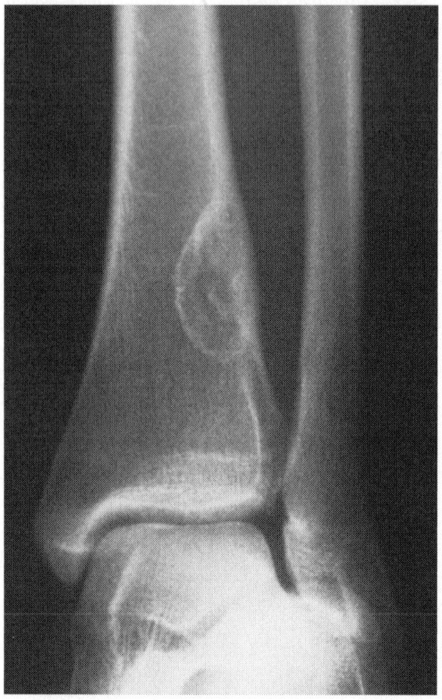

Figure 54A

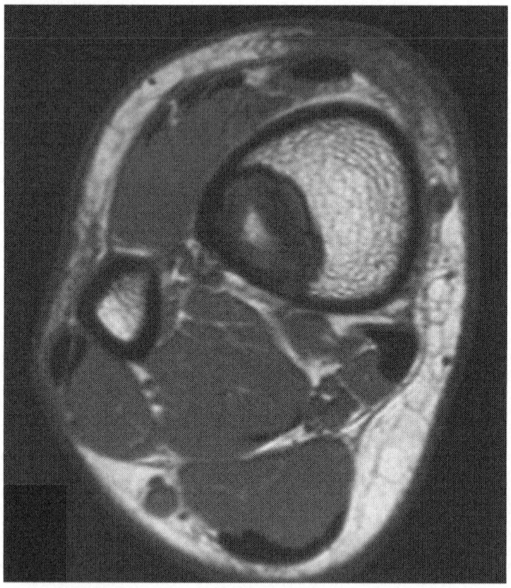

Figure 54B

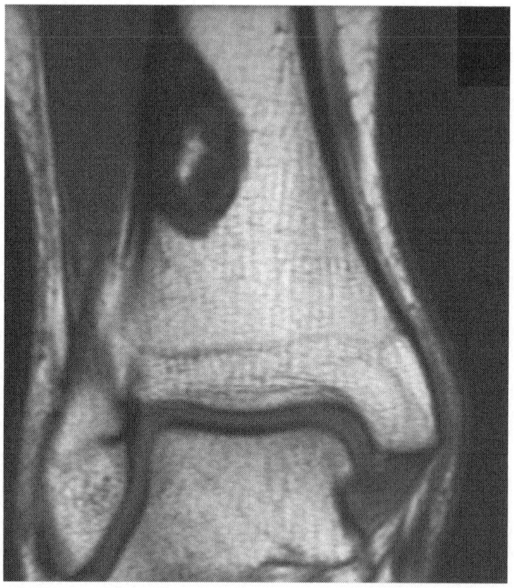

Figure 54C

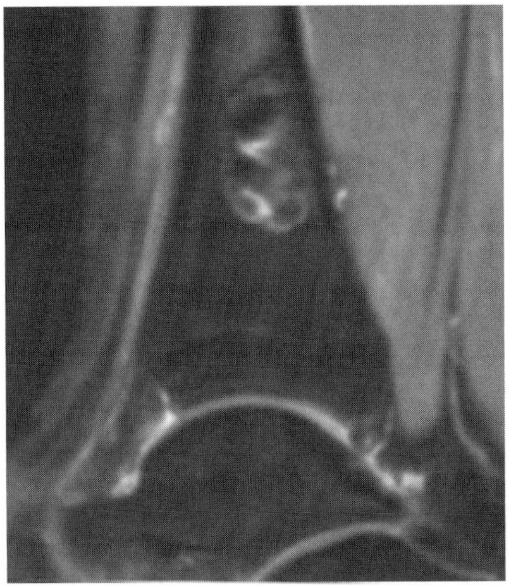

Figure 54D

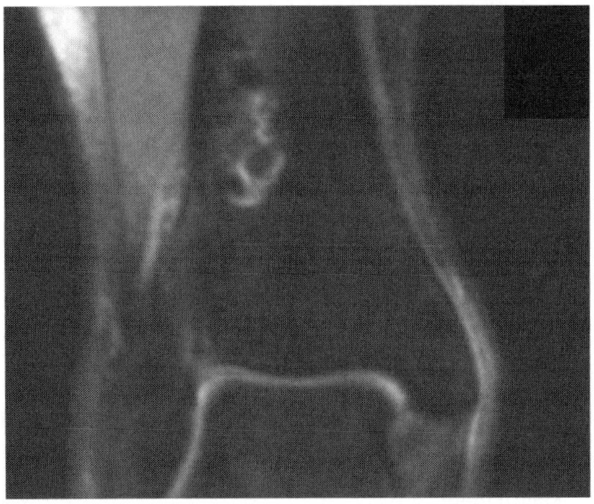

Figure 54E

Radiologic Findings

The oblique radiograph of the ankle (**Fig. 54A**) shows an expansile lytic lesion centered in the cortex of the distal tibia. The lesion has a narrow zone of transition and a sclerotic rim. There is no aggressive-appearing periosteal reaction. The lesion is predominantly low signal intensity on T1-weighted images (**Figs. 54B,54C**) but demonstrates a central area of high signal intensity that represents a residual island of normal fatty marrow entrapped in the lesion. The lesion is predominantly low signal intensity on the fat-saturated T2-weighted image (**Figs. 54D,54E**) but does contain small regions of high signal intensity.

Diagnosis

Fibroxanthoma (nonossifying fibroma/fibrous cortical defect).

Differential Diagnosis

- Fibrous dysplasia
- Chondromyxoid fibroma
- Aneurysmal bone cyst
- Periosteal chondroma
- Desmoplastic fibroma

Discussion

Background

The terms *fibrous cortical defect, nonossifying fibroma,* and *fibroxanthoma* are often used interchangeably to describe a related group of benign fibrous lesions of bone. The term *fibrous cortical defect* is best reserved for small lesions isolated to the cortical bone that commonly resolve spontaneously. The term *nonossifying fibroma* is typically used to refer to larger lesions that extend from the cortical into the medullary bone and may persist into adulthood. These lesions are perhaps best referred to by the term *fibroxanthoma,* as this name best describes the underlying histology of these lesions. Multiple fibroxanthomas have been reported in association with neurofibromatosis type 1

(5% of cases). The presence of multiple fibroxanthomas in association with multiple café-au-lait spots but without the other findings of neurofibromatosis is referred to as Jaffe-Campanacci syndrome. These patients also demonstrate mental retardation, hypogonadism, or cryptorchidism, as well as ophthalmologic and cardiovascular abnormalities. The term *benign fibrous histiocytoma* has been used to describe fibroxanthoma-like lesions occurring in patients over 25 years old. The latter lesions frequently show medullary extension and are more often symptomatic than typical fibroxanthomas.

Clinical Findings

Fibroxanthomas are common lesions, particularly in adolescents, who account for ~70% of all lesions. Lesions are approximately twice as common in men as in women, and most (90%) occur in long bones. Lesions are most commonly located around the knee (55% of cases). The femur and tibia account for ~80% of all lesions. A fibular location accounts for ~8 to 10% of lesions, and interestingly, these lesions are usually located in the medullary canal. The upper extremity accounts for only ~8% of all lesions. Smaller lesions are often asymptomatic. Larger lesions may cause pain and may be associated with pathologic fracture.

Pathology

Lesions are predominantly composed of fibroblasts arranged in a storiform pattern. Giant cells and xanthomatous elements are commonly intermixed with the fibrous tissue. Although hemosiderin may be prominent, collagen is not a major component of these lesions.

Imaging Findings

RADIOGRAPHY

- The radiographic appearance of these lesions is usually diagnostic.
- Lesions are eccentric, oval, and either metaphyseal or diametaphyseal in location.
- Lesions arise near the growth plate but may migrate toward or into a diaphyseal location with continued skeletal growth.
- Epiphyseal location is rare.
- Typically, these are lytic tumors with a narrow zone of transition and a sclerotic rim.
- Smaller lesions tend to be isolated to the cortex.
- Larger lesions and lesions in thin bones (e.g., the fibula) often extend into the medullary canal.
- Larger lesions often demonstrate a multilocular, "soap bubble" appearance and expansile remodeling.
- Periosteal reaction is seen only if there is a pathologic fracture.

COMPUTED TOMOGRAPHY

- Not usually required
- Appearance on CT is similar to radiographic appearance.
- Internal attenuation is usually soft-tissue attenuation.
- Useful to identify small pathologic fractures in painful lesions.

MAGNETIC RESONANCE IMAGING

- Low signal intensity on T1-weighted images
- Usually low signal intensity on T2-weighted images (80% of cases) due to the hypercellular fibrous tissue and/or hemosiderin in these lesions
- Diffuse (80%) or peripheral and septal (20%) enhancement after intravenous gadolinium administration

Treatment and Prognosis

- Most lesions will involute and gradually heal with sclerotic bone.
- Treatment is required only if the diagnosis is unsure or if there is risk for a pathologic fracture.
- Lesions at risk for pathologic fracture (> 3 cm or involving > 50% of the diameter of a weight-bearing bone) should be treated with curettage and bone grafting.

PEARLS

- Histologically, nonossifying fibroma and fibrous cortical defect are the same lesion, differing only by size, with a fibrous cortical defect generally < 2 cm and a nonossifying fibroma > 2 cm.
- 8% of patients have multiple lesions, most commonly in the lower extremities, in one of four patterns: (1) clustered (usually around the knee), (2) nonclustered (opposite ends of long bones), (3) coalescent (several lesions coalescing over time), and (4) emergent (appearing in previously unaffected bone).
- When found in the midshaft of the tibia, adamantinoma should be considered in the differential.

PITFALLS

- Because lesions in the fibula often involve the entire medullary canal and may have an unusual appearance, biopsy is often required.
- Chondromyxoid fibroma may be mistaken for a fibrous cortical defect, but the former should demonstrate a more prominent cortical bulge.
- Concurrent osteomalacia in the presence of a fibrous cortical defect should not be ascribed solely to dietary deficiencies, as hypophosphotemic vitamin D-resistant rickets may be caused secondary to a substance secreted by the tumor that increases renal tubular resorption of phosphorus.

Suggested Readings

Jee WH, Choe BY, Kang HS, et al. Nonossifying fibroma: characteristics at MR imaging with pathologic correlation. Radiology 1998;209:197–202

Kransdorf MJ, Utz J, Gilkey F, Berry B. MR appearance of fibroxanthoma. J Comput Assist Tomogr 1988;12:612–615

Resnick D, Kyriakos M, Greenway G. Tumors and tumor-like lesions of bone: imaging and pathology of specific lesions. In: Resnick D, ed. Diagnosis of Bone and Joint Disorders. Philadelphia, PA: WB Saunders; 2002:3763–4128

Smith SE, Kransdorf MJ. Primary musculoskeletal tumors of fibrous origin. Semin Musculoskelet Radiol 2000;4:73–88

CASE 55

George Nomikos, Anthony G. Ryan, Peter L. Munk, and Mark Murphey

Clinical Presentation

A 12-year-old boy presented with a complaint of sudden onset of arm pain while playing. A radiograph was taken of the area (**Fig. 55A**). The next image (**Fig. 55B**) was obtained 3 years later.

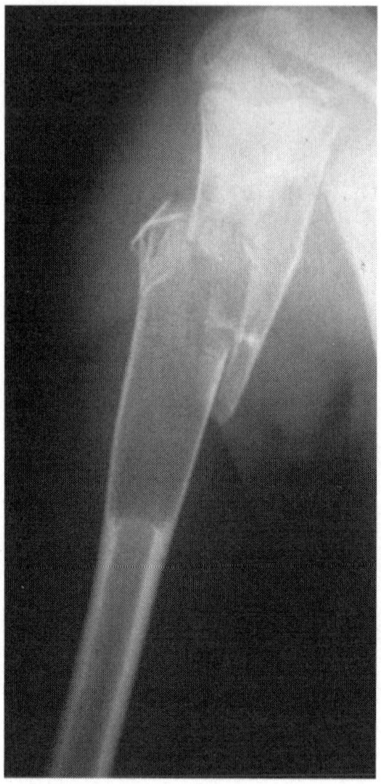

Figure 55A

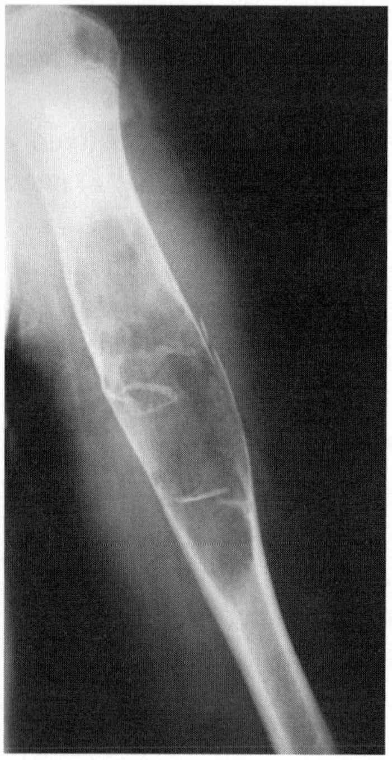

Figure 55B

Radiologic Findings

A single view of the left humerus (**Fig. 55A**) shows a pathologic fracture through a lytic lesion in the central medullary canal of the proximal humeral diaphysis. The lesion is mildly expansile and has a narrow zone of transition with mild surrounding sclerosis. There is no mineralized matrix in the lesion. The second image obtained 3 years later (**Fig. 55B**) shows a new pathologic fracture through the lesion. Both the humerus and the lesion had grown since the prior study. The lesion appears slightly more expansile on the current study than previously. Note the fragment of bone that has been displaced from the fracture site and has fallen into a dependent location of the lesion (fallen fragment).

Diagnosis

Simple (unicameral) bone cyst (SBC) with pathologic fracture.

Differential Diagnosis

- Aneurysmal bone cyst
- Fibrous dysplasia
- Telangiectatic osteosarcoma
- Osteoblastoma

Discussion

Background

SBCs are nonneoplastic and represent the only true cystic lesion of bone. These lesions are benign and have an extremely low incidence of malignant transformation (there are rare reports of malignant transformation in the wall to osteosarcoma). SBCs are purely lytic lesions consisting of a fluid-filled cavity lined by a single layer of mesothelial-like cells. The etiology of these lesions is unknown, but various theories have been postulated, including (1) a defect of enchondral bone formation, (2) increased venous pressure, and (3) biochemical factors.

Clinical Findings

Lesions most commonly occur in patients between 5 and 15 years old, and only 15% of lesions are seen in patients over 20 years old. There is a 2.5:1 male-to-female predominance. Lesions are usually asymptomatic unless a pathologic fracture occurs. They are usually located centrally in the metaphysis adjacent to the open physis, which acts as a barrier to epiphyseal extension. With continued growth of the long bone and no further growth of the SBC, the lesion migrates into the diaphysis and is often referred to as a latent SBC. If both the SBC and long bone continue to grow, the lesion remains in the metaphysis abutting the physeal plate (active SBC). In young patients, the proximal humerus is the single most common site (60%), followed by the proximal femur (30%). Lesions in adults have a propensity to involve the distal calcaneus and ileum adjacent to the sacroiliac joints.

Pathology

Nontraumatized SBCs are composed of clear serous fluid surrounded by a single layer of mesothelial cells. Fibroblasts, collagen, osteoclast-like giant cells, areas of hemorrhage, lymphocytes, and osteoid may all be identified deep to the mesothelial lining. The lesion should not contain hemorrhage or reparative tissue unless there has been a pathologic fracture or mechanical stress.

Imaging Findings

RADIOGRAPHY

- Purely lytic central metaphyseal or diaphyseal lesion with a narrow zone of transition with or without a thin rim of sclerosis (geographic 1A or 1B margin)
- No mineralized matrix
- No periosteal reaction in the absence of fracture
- Causes mild expansile remodeling as well as thinning of the overlying cortical bone
- Internal trabeculation may be seen, creating a multilocular appearance.

- The fallen fragment sign (5% of cases) (**Fig. 55B**) is pathognomonic of an SBC and represents displacement of a fracture fragment from the fracture site into the dependent portion of the lesion (which occurs because the purely fluid lesion does not obstruct the movement of the fragment).

SCINTIGRAPHY

- Mild peripherally increased uptake and central photopenia ("doughnut" sign)
- Healing fracture may demonstrate intense uptake.

COMPUTED TOMOGRAPHY AND MAGNETIC RESONANCE IMAGING

- Internal characteristics should be similar to simple fluid on CT and MRI.
- SBC may be mildly higher in signal intensity than water on T1-weighted images because of the elevated protein content of the fluid.
- Fluid levels, multiloculation, surrounding edema, and solid areas of reparative tissue may be seen in lesions that have undergone previous fracture.
- Subtle fracture may be more easily detected with CT/MRI than with radiography.

Treatment and Prognosis

- Traditional treatment consists of curettage and bone grafting.
- Recurrence rate with this treatment is 40 to 45%.
- Injection of methylprednisolone acetate is as effective as if not more effective than surgery and is less invasive.
- Injection of sclerosis-inducing embolization agents has also shown promising results.
- Each loculation of a multilocular lesion must be injected to completely treat the lesion (communication between loculations can be assessed with contrast injection to help in planning therapeutic injections).

PEARLS

- With continued growth of the long bone and no further growth of the SBC, the lesion migrates into the diaphysis and is often referred to as a latent SBC. If both the SBC and long bone continue to grow, the lesion remains in the metaphysis abutting the physeal plate (active SBC).
- Lesions in adults have a propensity to involve the distal calcaneus and ileum adjacent to the sacroiliac joints.
- The fallen fragment sign (5% of cases) (**Fig. 55B**) is pathognomonic of an SBC and represents displacement of a fracture fragment from the fracture site into the dependent portion of the lesion (which occurs because the purely fluid lesion does not obstruct the movement of the fragment).

PITFALLS

- If hemorrhage or reparative tissue is seen in the absence of a pathologic fracture or mechanical stress, these features should be considered suspicious, and an alternative diagnosis to SBC should be considered.
- Healing fracture may demonstrate intense uptake, masking the typical "doughnut" sign (mild peripherally increased uptake and central photopenia).
- Radiography may miss subtle fractures (more easily detected with CT/MRI).

Suggested Readings

Burr BA, Resnick D, Syklawer R, Haghighi P. Fluid-fluid levels in a unicameral bone cyst: CT and MR findings. J Comput Assist Tomogr 1993;17:134–136

Capanna R, Campanacci D, Manfrini M. Unicameral and aneurysmal bone cysts. Orthop Clin North Am 1996;27:605–614

Parman LM, Murphey MD. Alphabet soup: cystic lesions of bone. Semin Musculoskelet Radiol 2000;4:89–101

CASE 56

George Nomikos, Anthony G. Ryan, Peter L. Munk, and Mark Murphey

Clinical Presentation

A 13 year-old-boy presented with a history of 2 months of back pain. He reported that the pain radiated down his right lateral thigh and worsened with activity.

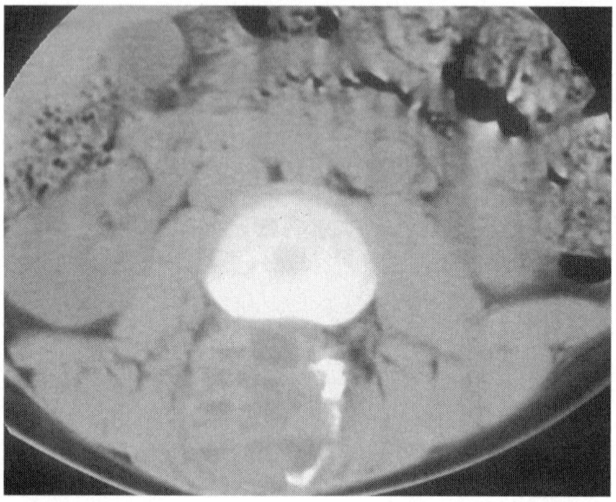

Figure 56A

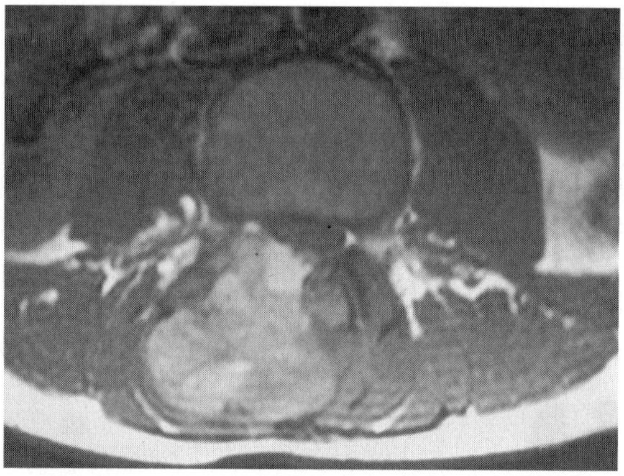

Figure 56B

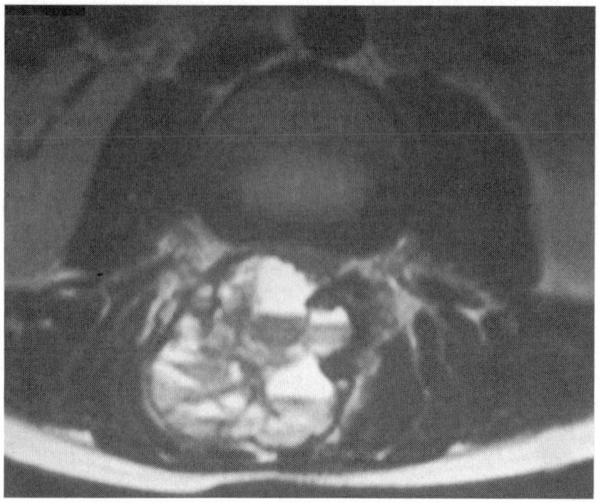

Figure 56C

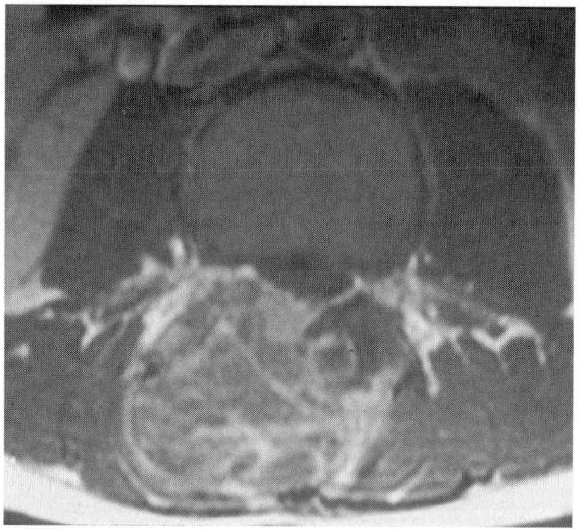

Figure 56D

Radiologic Findings

The CT scan (**Fig. 56A**) shows a markedly expansile lesion arising in the posterior elements of the spine at the L2 level. Multiple fluid levels are identified in the lesion on CT and no mineralized matrix is seen. The lesion causes mild compression of the thecal sac. The axial T1- and T2-weighted images (**Figs. 56B,56C**) demonstrate multiple fluid levels in all areas of the lesion with no identifiable solid component. Despite its marked expansion, the mass appears well circumscribed. The postcontrast MRI (**Fig. 56D**) shows peripheral and septal enhancement of the lesion. No solid enhancing nodular component is identified.

Diagnosis

Primary aneurysmal bone cyst (ABC).

Differential Diagnosis

- Osteoblastoma
- Giant cell tumor
- Telangiectatic osteosarcoma
- Chondroblastoma
- Chondromyxoid fibroma (long bone lesions)

Discussion

Background

ABCs are reactive, not neoplastic, lesions composed of multiple blood-filled spaces. Primary ABCs represent lesions not associated with an underlying tumor, and secondary ABCs represent lesions associated with an antecedent tumor (**Table 56–1**). ABCs are considered secondary in from 1 to 30% of cases. An ABC is thought to arise when there is disruption in the normal vascular system of the host bone, which often occurs secondary to trauma or tumor. There is often a history of trauma to the affected area in cases of primary ABC, particularly in subperiosteal or intracortical lesions. This alteration in the normal hemodynamics leads to rapid enlargement of multiple blood-filled vascular spaces as well as proliferation of the osseous mesenchymal tissue. The patient in **Fig. 56E** presented initially

Table 56–1 Primary Bone Tumors that Commonly Demonstrate Secondary ABC Components

Giant cell tumor of bone
Osteoblastoma
Chondroblastoma
Telangiectatic osteosarcoma

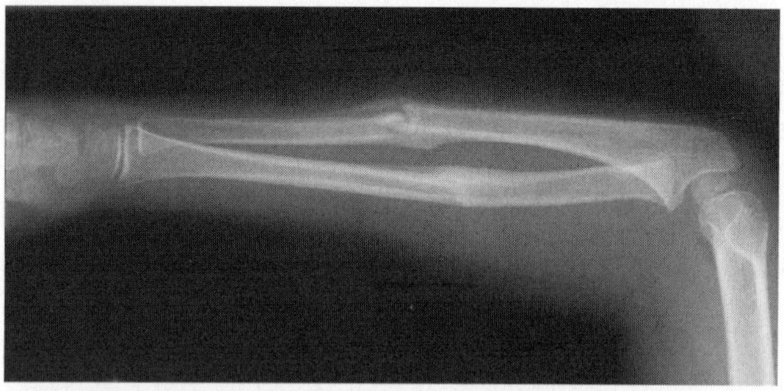

E

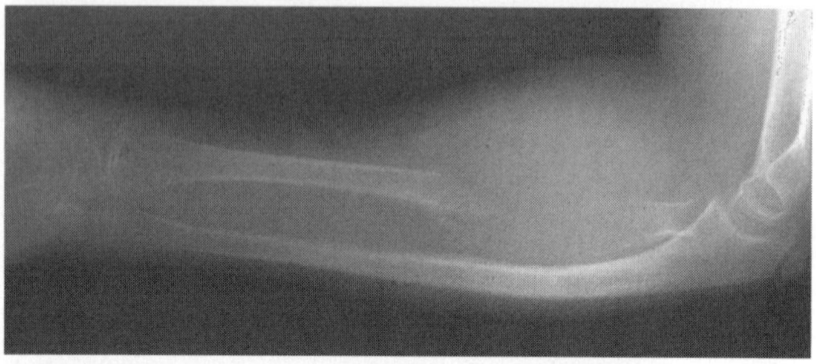

F

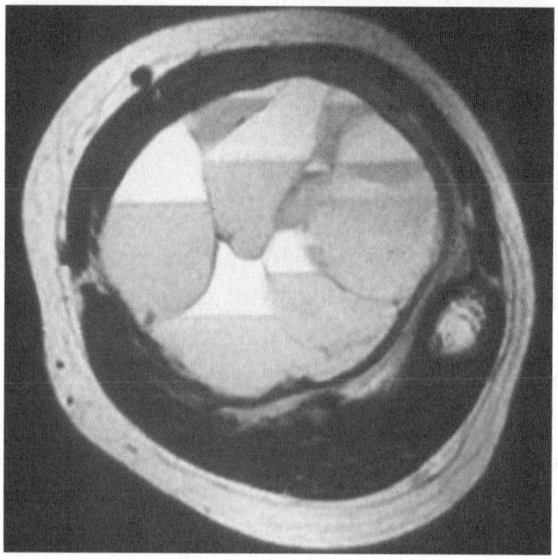

G

Figures 56E–56G A lateral radiograph of the forearm (**56E**) shows healing fractures of the midshafts of the radius and ulna. Six years later, the same patient presented with swelling in the left arm. A lateral radiograph (**56F**) shows a markedly expansile lytic lesion arising in the radius at the site of the prior fracture, representing a primary ABC. A transaxial T2-weighted image (**56G**) through the area of maximal swelling elegantly shows multiple fluid levels within the ABC.

with uncomplicated fractures of the radius and ulna. Six years later, the patient presented with swelling in the left arm. The radiograph at that time showed a markedly expansile lytic lesion arising in the radius at the site of the prior fracture (**Fig. 56F**), representing a primary ABC. The multiple fluid levels within the ABC are well demonstrated on the MRI (**Fig. 56G**).

Clinical Findings

Most patients (approximately 80%) are younger than 20 years at the time of diagnosis, although ABC is uncommon in patients under 5 years. Lesions are commonly seen in the metadiaphysis of long tubular bones (50%) and in the posterior elements of the spine (20%). Long bone lesions are more frequently encountered in the lower extremity than in the upper extremity. ABCs are more commonly eccentric than central in long tubular bones, as opposed to simple bone cysts. The pelvis accounts for 50% of all flat bone lesions. ABCs do not usually extend across the open physis. Involvement of contiguous bones has rarely been reported. Patients usually present with nonspecific pain and swelling. Neurologic symptoms are particularly common with spinal lesions. Pathologic fracture is seen in up to 20% of cases and is particularly common in spine lesions.

Pathology

Primary ABCs consist of interconnecting blood-filled cystic spaces encapsulated by a thin fibrous periosteal membrane. The blood-filled spaces are lined by fibrous septations. Lesions contain reticulated chondroid-like material that is highly suggestive of a reparative process in approximately 30% of primary ABCs. There is a solid variant of ABC (also known as giant cell reparative granuloma of long bone) that contains the same solid elements as typical ABCs, including the chondroid-like material, but it does not contain the usual blood-filled cavities. These lesions may be easily confused with low-grade osteosarcoma and are seen especially in the spine.

Imaging Findings

RADIOGRAPHY

- Initially, the lesions usually demonstrate an eccentric metadiaphyseal osteolytic lesion without significant expansion.
- Patients usually present during the active phase, which is characterized by rapid osseous expansion and bone destruction, at which time the lesion may appear central in location (**Fig. 56F**).
- During the active phase, the osseous shell or surrounding periosteal membrane may not be demonstrable on radiographs.
- The osseous expansion is usually most prominent along the outer border of the lesion, whereas the inner margin is often less aggressive in appearance and may even demonstrate a thin rim of sclerosis (dichotomous border).
- Alternatively, all borders may be markedly expansile and aggressive in appearance ("finger in the balloon" appearance).
- Periosteal reaction, even in the form of a Codman's triangle, may be seen.
- Periosteal extension of new bone may arise from the Codman's triangle and envelop the lesion, a finding that is highly suggestive of ABC.
- As the lesion stabilizes and heals, there is progressive ossification of the periosteal shell.
- In the spine, ABCs are most commonly expansile lesions centered in the posterior elements, often with extension into the vertebral body.
- Spinal lesions often grow to involve adjacent vertebral bodies, disks, posterior ribs, and the surrounding soft tissues.

COMPUTED TOMOGRAPHY AND MAGNETIC RESONANCE IMAGING

- CT and MRI demonstrate the thin surrounding osseous shell (CT) or periosteal membrane better than radiographs (lesions tend to appear less aggressive on advanced imaging).
- Thin calcification may occasionally be seen in the rim and septae due to the presence of chondroid-like material.
- Fluid levels are seen in up to 35% of cases on CT.
- MRI is much more sensitive for the detection of fluid levels than CT.
- Primary ABCs demonstrate no soft-tissue mass.
- Thin peripheral and septal enhancement of the lesion can be seen after contrast administration without foci of solid tissue in primary ABC.
- In the case of secondary ABC, there will be regions of enhancing solid tissue that represent the primary lesion, separate from the ABC component.
- In the case of secondary ABC, biopsy must be directed to the solid portion of the lesion, which harbors the diagnostic tissue, not toward the secondary ABC component.

SCINTIGRAPHY

- Peripherally increased activity with central photopenia ("doughnut" sign) is seen in 70% of cases.

Treatment and Prognosis

- Curettage and bone grafting with intraoperative extension of resection, with cryosurgery or phenol often employed
- Wide resection for lesion in expendable bones
- Preoperative embolization may be employed to reduce intraoperative hemorrhage or in unresectable lesions.
- Radiation therapy may also be used for unresectable lesions.
- In the case of secondary ABC, treatment must be directed at the underlying tumor.
- Recurrence rate: 20 to 25%
- Malignant degeneration has not been reported.

PEARLS

- Lesions are commonly seen in the metadiaphysis of long tubular bones (50%) and in the posterior elements of the spine (20%).
- Long bone lesions are more frequently encountered in the lower extremity than in the upper extremity. The pelvis accounts for 50% of all flat bone lesions.
- ABCs are more commonly eccentric than central in long tubular bones, as opposed to unicameral bone cysts.
- Periosteal extension of new bone may arise from the Codman's triangle and envelop the lesion, a finding that is highly suggestive of ABC.

PITFALLS

- Lesions thought to be very aggressive on conventional radiography tend to appear less aggressive on advanced imaging (CT and MRI), as the thin surrounding osseous shell or periosteal membrane is clearly demonstrated.
- Involvement of contiguous bones occurs rarely.
- In the case of secondary ABC, biopsy must be directed to the solid portion of the lesion, which harbors the diagnostic tissue, not toward the secondary ABC component.

Suggested Readings

Capanna R, Campanacci D, Manfrini M. Unicameral and aneurysmal bone cysts. Orthop Clin North Am 1996;27:605–614

Kransdorf MJ, Sweet DE. Aneurysmal bone cyst: concept, controversy, clinical presentation, and imaging. Am J Roentgenol 1995;164:573–580

Munk PL, Helms CA, Johnson J, Steinbach L, Neumann C. MR imaging of aneurysmal bone cyst. AGR 1989;153:99–101

Murphey MD, Andrews CL, Flemming DJ, Temple HT, Smith WS, Smirniotopoulos JG. From the archives of the AFIP. Primary tumors of the spine: radiologic-pathologic correlation. Radiographics 1996;16:1131–1158

Parman LM, Murphey MD. Alphabet soup: cystic lesions of bone. Semin Musculoskelet Radiol 2000;4:89–101

CASE 57

George Nomikos, Anthony G. Ryan, Peter L. Munk, and Mark Murphey

Clinical Presentation

A 25-year-old woman presented with a chief complaint of knee pain.

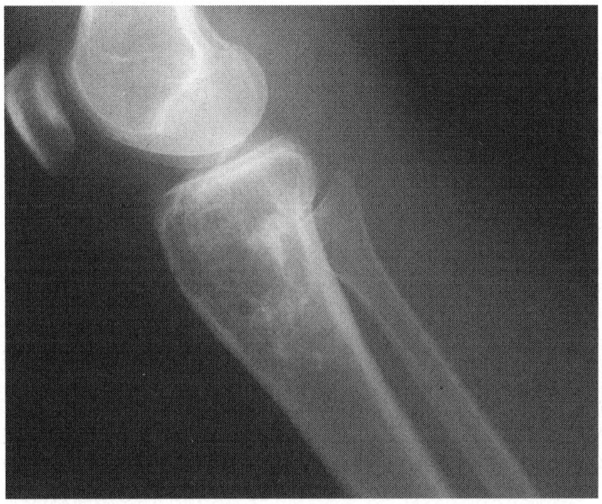

Figure 57A

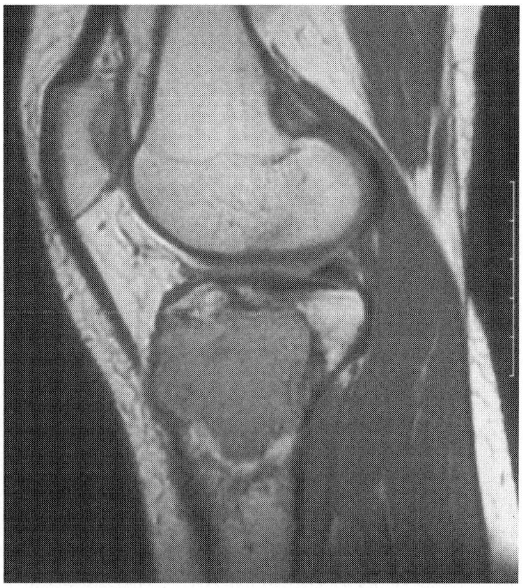

Figure 57B

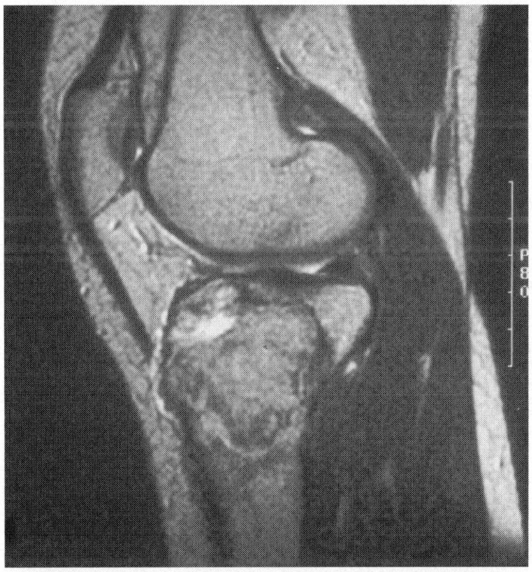

Figure 57C

Radiologic Findings

The lateral radiograph of the knee (**Fig. 57A**) shows a lytic lesion in the proximal tibia. The center of the lesion appears to be in the proximal metaphysis of the tibia; however, the lesion extends to the subchondral bone plate. The lesion demonstrates a narrow zone of transition, with adjacent patchy sclerosis in the surrounding bone. No mineralized matrix is identified in the lesion. The lesion is mildly heterogeneous on the sagittal T1-weighted image (**Fig. 57B**), with intensity slightly greater than that of skeletal muscle. On the sagittal T2-weighted image (**Fig. 57C**), the lesion remains predominantly intermediate in signal intensity. There is focal high signal intensity in the lesion that likely represents an area of cyst formation. Note the low signal intensity rim visible around portions of the lesion on both the T1- and T2-weighted images, representing a fibrous pseudocapsule.

Diagnosis

Giant cell tumor (GCT) of bone.

Differential Diagnosis

- Aneurysmal bone cyst
- Chondroblastoma
- Chondromyxoid fibroma
- Brown tumor
- Telangiectatic osteosarcoma

Discussion

Background

GCT of bone is a relatively common osseous neoplasm, accounting for 18 to 23% of benign primary bone tumors and 4 to 9.5% of all bone neoplasms. It is now generally agreed that these lesions arise in the metaphysis adjacent to the growth plate and rapidly extend to the subchondral bone plate, as seen in this lesion. Approximately 84 to 99% of lesions extend to within 1 cm of the subchondral bone plate. Secondary cystic or aneurysmal bone cyst (ABC) areas are commonly seen. Over half of all cases occur about the knee, with the distal femur accounting for 23 to 30% of cases and the proximal tibia accounting for 20 to 25%. The distal radius is the third most common site (10–12%), followed by the sacrum (4–9%). When lesions occur in the spine (3–6%), they usually originate in the vertebral body, and from there they may extend into the posterior elements. Lesions are usually solitary. Multifocal lesions are rare (< 1% of all cases). However, there is a known association between Paget's disease and multifocal GCT (predilection for skull, facial bones, and spine). In any case of multifocal GCT (**Fig. 57D**—the same patient as above, with a second lesion in the patella 6 years later), the possibility of hyperparathyroidism with multiple brown tumors must be excluded by laboratory analysis, as GCTs can be indistinguishable from brown tumors of hyperparathyroidism both radiologically and pathologically.

Clinical Findings

Patients are most commonly between the ages of 20 and 50 years, and there is a mild female predilection. Only 1 to 3% of GCTs occur in skeletally immature patients. Symptoms most frequently include pain, swelling, and decreased range of motion. Neurologic symptoms are commonly seen in patients with spine lesions. Pathologic fracture is relatively common.

Pathology

GCTs are composed of diffusely scattered giant cells in a background mononuclear stroma. The nuclei of the giant cells should be identical to those of the mononuclear cells. Secondary cystic or ABC areas are common. The majority of GCTs are benign; however, up to 5 to 10% are malignant (either primarily malig-

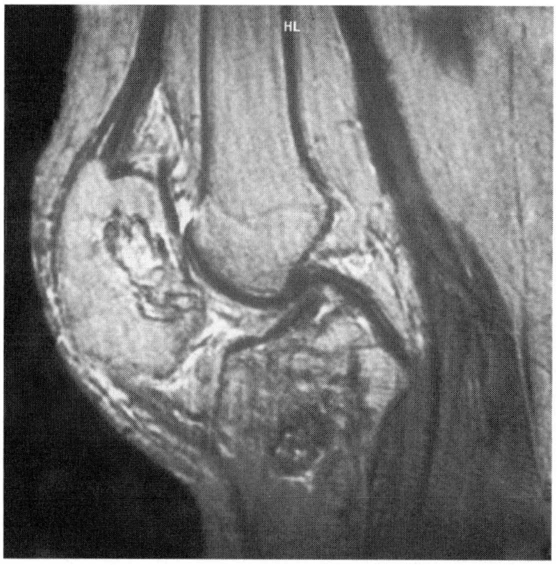

Figure 57D A sagittal T2-weighted image in the same case as above shows a further giant cell tumor within the patella (multifocal giant cell tumor), six years after treatment of the tibial lesion.

nant or secondarily malignant after previous therapy, particularly related to prior radiation therapy) and may demonstrate pulmonary metastases. A "benign metastasizing" form of GCT has also been reported.

Imaging Findings

RADIOGRAPHY

- Eccentric lytic lesion with a geographic pattern of bone destruction (although large lesions may appear centrally located)
- Metaphyseal center but extends to the subchondral bone plate
- Most commonly demonstrate a narrow zone of transition and lack of a surrounding rim sclerosis; patchy peripheral sclerosis is not uncommon, particularly on CT (as in this case).
- 10 to 15% of cases demonstrate a wide zone of transition.
- No mineralized matrix (with the exception that recurrent GCT in the soft tissues may demonstrate a peripheral rim of ossification simulating myositis ossificans)
- Periosteal reaction is uncommon (10 to 30%) and when present suggests the presence of a pathologic fracture.
- Trabeculation or pseudotrabeculation (created by the formation of osseous ridges as a result of endosteal scalloping) is common.

COMPUTED TOMOGRAPHY

- No internal mineralization
- Predominant attenuation similar to muscle
- Cystic areas or fluid levels (secondary ABC component) may be seen.
- Cortical destruction and the presence of soft-tissue mass is better evaluated on CT than on radiographs.

MAGNETIC RESONANCE IMAGING

- Better delineation of soft-tissue component, if present
- Cystic areas are common.
- Areas of internal hemorrhage (high signal on both T1- and T2-weighted images or multiple fluid levels) owing to secondary ABC are common and may be prominent.
- Solid areas are similar to muscle in signal intensity on T1-weighted images.

- GCTs remain low to intermediate signal intensity on standard T2-weighted images (likely as a result of high cellularity or collagen deposition).
- The presence of peritumoral edema suggests pathologic fracture.
- Diffuse enhancement of the solid portions of the lesion

Treatment

- Curettage and bone grafting have been the traditional method of treatment, although this has been associated with a relatively high rate of recurrence (40 to 60%).
- Addition of high-speed burring and chemical agents (e.g., phenol) or cryosurgery (liquid nitrogen) to the treatment protocol has significantly reduced the recurrence rate (2 to 20%)
- Polymethylmethacrylate is often used in place of bone graft material to fill the surgical defect, as it provides more mechanical support than graft material.
- Larger lesions require more radical resection and reconstruction.
- Because of the risk of inducing malignant transformation, radiation is contraindicated except in nonoperable tumors.

Prognosis

- The recurrence rate varies, but efforts to extend the surgical margins, as described above, have significantly improved the recurrence rate (2 to 20%).
- Most, but not all, recurrences occur in the first 3 years after therapy.

PEARLS

- 84 to 99% of lesions extend to within 1 cm of the subchondral bone plate.
- When lesions occur in the spine (3 to 6%), they usually originate in the vertebral body and extend into the posterior elements.
- Periosteal reaction is uncommon (10 to 30%) and when present suggests the presence of a pathologic fracture, in which case peritumoral edema is likely to be visible on MRI.

PITFALLS

- In any case of multifocal GCT, the possibility of hyperparathyroidism with multiple brown tumors must be excluded, as GCTs can be indistinguishable from brown tumors of hyperparathyroidism both radiologically and pathologically.
- GCTs are rare (1 to 3%) in skeletally immature patients, and the diagnosis should thus be reserved in this population.
- Unlike the primary lesion, where no mineralized matrix occurs, recurrent GCT in the soft tissues may demonstrate a peripheral rim of ossification simulating myositis ossificans.

Suggested Readings

Manaster BJ, Doyle AJ. Giant cell tumors of bone. Radiol Clin North Am 1993;31:299–323

Murphey MD, Nomikos G, Flemming D, Gannon F, Temple T, Kransdorf M. Imaging of giant cell tumor and giant cell reparative granuloma of bone: radiologic-pathologic correlation. Radiographics 2001;21:1283–1309

Parman LM, Murphey MD. Alphabet soup: cystic lesions of bone. Semin Musculoskelet Radiol 2000;4:89–101

CASE 58

Anthony G. Ryan and Peter L. Munk

Clinical Presentation

A 53-year-old woman presented with unremitting pain in her foot, exacerbated by walking, with occasional shooting pain into her toes.

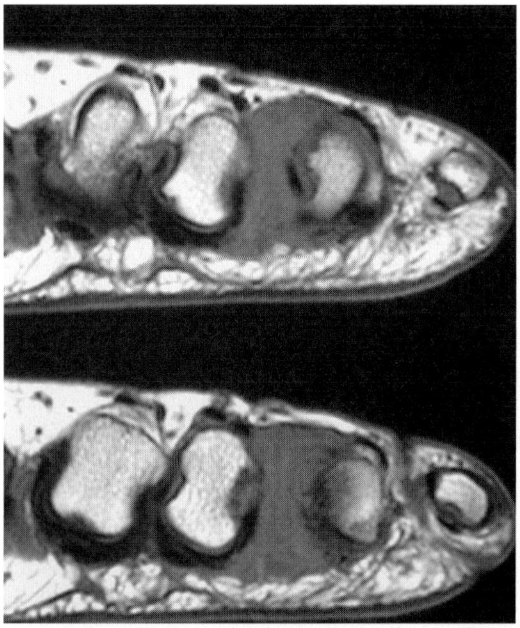

Figure 58A

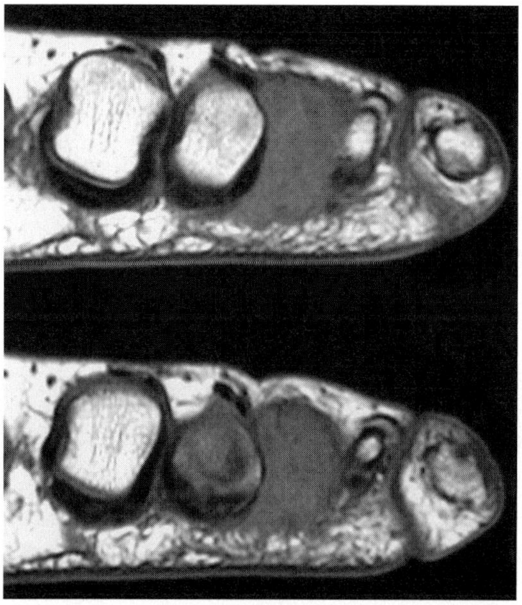

Figure 58B

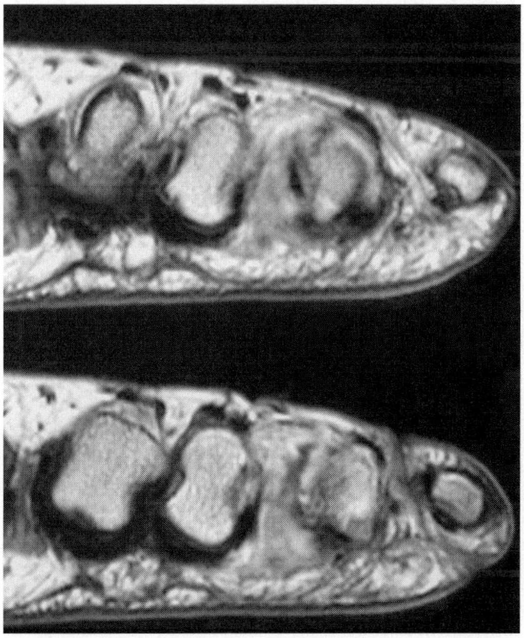

Figure 58C

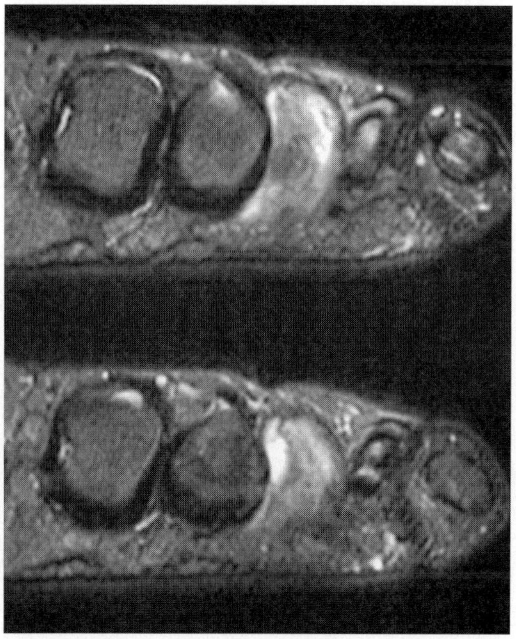

Figure 58D

Radiologic Findings

Consecutive coronal slices from a T1-weighted sequence (**Figs. 58A,58B**) demonstrate a large, well-defined, dumbbell-shaped intermediate signal intensity lesion splaying the heads of the third and fourth metatarsals. The lesion shows intense enhancement on both T1-weighted postintravenous gadolinium (**Fig. 58C**) and STIR postintravenous gadolinium (**Fig. 58D**) images.

Diagnosis

Giant Morton's neuroma.

Differential Diagnosis

- Infected intermetatarsal bursa
- Foreign body reaction
- Tendon sheath ganglion cyst
- Synovial cyst with infarcted tissue
- Giant cell tumor of tendon sheath

Discussion

Background

Foot pain is an increasingly common clinical complaint, especially in an aging population engaged in physical exercise programs. The referral of a patient with forefoot pain where Morton's neuroma is the working clinical diagnosis is an increasing source of referrals, particularly from podiatrists.

Etiology

This lesion is not a true neoplasm, but a fibrotic overgrowth, the cause of which is unknown, although repetitive biomechanical trauma (e.g., secondary to wearing high-heeled shoes) has been implicated.

Pathophysiology

It is thought that dorsiflexion of the toes produces friction of the affected nerve against the edge of the intermetatarsal ligament, resulting in fibrosis and consequent enlargement of the nerve sheath, predisposing to further friction.

The lesion (bilateral in ~10% and multiple in as many as 28%) is most commonly found between the second and third metatarsal heads. Compression of the neuroma on walking irritates the associated interdigital nerve, giving rise to the characteristic neuralgia.

Clinical Findings

Eighty percent of patients are middle-aged women. The presenting complaint is either pain in the foot localized to the affected web space or adjacent metatarsal phalangeal (MTP) joint and/or paresthesia on walking. The pain may progress over time. Critically, the pain secondary to a neuroma is constant and not relieved by rest. Clinical examination usually reproduces the typical pain with exquisite tenderness on compression of the affected web space and circumferential compression of the metatarsal heads.

Pathology

GROSS

A mass of pale fibrous tissue is demonstrable wrapped around the normal nerve.

MICROSCOPIC

The mass is seen to be composed of benign perineural fibrosis surrounding a plantar interdigital nerve.

Imaging Findings

RADIOGRAPHY

Radiographs are rarely contributory, although widening of the web space may be demonstrable when the lesion is large.

ULTRASOUND

- Normal nerves appear as linear, fibrillar structures, hyperechoic relative to muscle but slightly hypoechoic to tendon ~2 mm in diameter.
- The vessels of the neurovascular bundle are usually easily seen in close proximity; therefore, if one is having difficulty finding the nerve, one should find the associated interdigital artery alongside which the nerve will invariably run.
- Morton's neuromas typically appear as hypoechoic, well-defined ovoid masses between 5 and 7 mm in diameter, usually found at the bifurcation of the interdigital nerve, at or proximal to the metatarsal head. Fifty percent of neuromas are located dorsal to the plantar aspect of the metatarsal heads, and 50% are both dorsal and plantar.
- The sensitivity and specificity of ultrasound are increased when the mass is equal to or greater than 5 mm. It has been estimated that the use of sonography correctly identifies neuromas in 85% of cases, with variable echogenicities identified:
    - Hypoechoic compared with muscle: 79.2%
    - Mixed echotexture: 12.5%
    - Anechoic: 8.3%
- The mass may be hourglass-shaped, secondary to compression by the transverse metatarsal ligament deep to which the interdigital nerve runs.
- Visualizing the nerve coursing in and out of a suspected neuroma increases the diagnostic confidence. The associated nerve may demonstrate secondary signs of irritation, such as edema and fusiform swelling. In more severe cases, the neuroma may become adherent to the adjacent bursa, which may then give rise to a large hypoechoic mass.
- Pressing the transducer on the neuroma may reproduce the characteristic pain.
- The finding of an interdigital mass > 20 mm in length should raise suspicion of an abnormality other than a Morton's neuroma because statistically, nonneuromatous lesions are longer than neuromas.
- True tumors of the nerve are typically fusiform and hypoechoic.
- Although a bursa may appear as hyperechoic as a neuroma, a bursa should be compressible, whereas a neuroma is not.

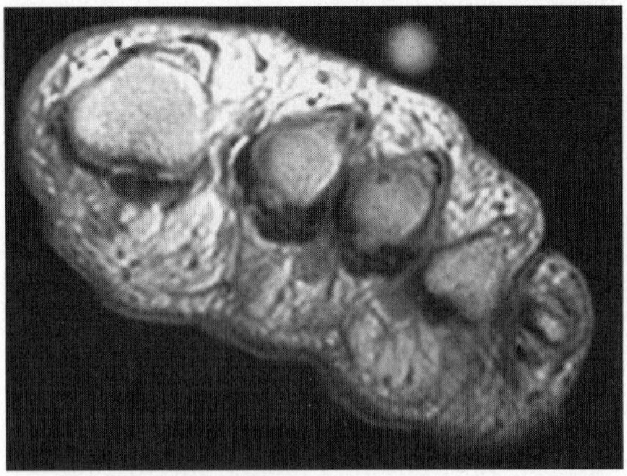

E

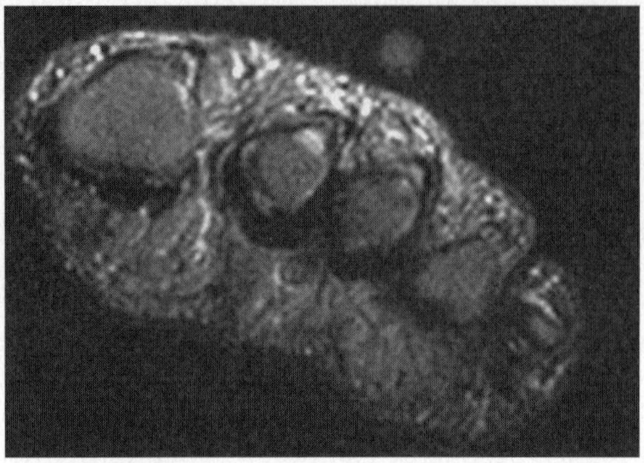

F

Figures 58E and **58F** A coronal T1-weighted image (**58E**) shows two small round Morton's neuromas (plantar to the second and third interspaces), that are of intermediate signal intensity and hypointense compared to surrounding fat, and consequently, more conspicuous than on the corresponding unenhanced fat-saturated image (**58F**). On the latter, although the larger second interspace lesion remains visible, the smaller, third interspace lesion is essentially invisible.

MAGNETIC RESONANCE IMAGING

- Morton neuromas demonstrate with intermediate to low signal intensity on both T1- (**Figs. 58A,58B**) and T2-weighted images.
- T1 sequences render Morton's neuromas more conspicuous as the fibrous tissue within the lesion is hypointense compared to the surrounding high-signal intensity fat secondary to (**Figs. 58E,58F**).
- The lesions appear as a dumbbell-shaped mass secondary to compression by the transverse metatarsal ligament (**Figs. 58A–58D**).
- Morton's neuromas typically display mild to moderate enhancement with intravenous gadolinium enhancement (**Figs. 58C,58D**).
- Unless intravenous gadolinium is employed, a neuroma is likely to be rendered less conspicuous with the application of fat suppression (**Figs. 58E,58F**).
- A lesion in the typical location of a Morton's neuroma but which is homogeneously hyperintense on T2 is almost certainly an intermetatarsal bursa as opposed to a Morton's neuroma. Where doubt remains between these entities, gadolinium can help distinguish the solid neuromas from the more cystic bursa, by virtue of the diffuse enhancement of the former and rim pattern of enhancement of the latter.
- It should be noted that the MRI diagnosis of Morton's neuroma does not imply symptomatology, as the prevalence of Morton's neuroma in patients with no symptoms or physical findings suggestive of this condition is as high as 33%. In one study, slightly larger lesions were observed in symptomatic patients; the mean transverse diameter of symptomatic neuromas was 5.3 mm (standard deviation, 2.14) compared with 4.1 mm (standard deviation, 1.75) for asymptomatic neuromas. Although examination of the above standard deviations reveals considerable overlap between the symptomatic and asymptomatic groups, this difference reached statistical significance ($p = .05$).

Treatment

The clinical differential for intermetatarsal space pain includes metatarsalgia; however, the latter is usually relieved by rest and appropriate orthotics, whereas the pain from a Morton's neuroma is unremitting and is relieved by neither rest nor orthotics.

Prior to imaging, the majority of patients will have already failed a trial of foot pads or orthotics. Surgical excision is then indicated through a longitudinal incision over the dorsal interspace, proximal to the intermetarsal ligament.

Prognosis

Division of the interdigital nerve to excise the neuroma results in sensory denervation of the involved digits.

Adequate excision results in dramatic relief of symptoms in the vast majority of patients; however, occasionally, if the initial incision is made too close to the intermetatarsal ligament, the cut end of the nerve may adhere to the ligament and result in a recurrence of pain.

PEARLS

- On ultrasound, the vessels of the neurovascular bundle are usually easily seen in close proximity to the nerve; thus, if one is having difficulty finding the nerve, locating the associated interdigital artery will almost invariably reveal the location of the nerve.
- Although a bursa may be hyperechoic like a neuroma, it should be compressible, whereas a neuroma is not.
- Although gadolinium enhancement does not contribute to the differential diagnosis or patient management in the vast majority of patients (estimated at 89%), it may at times be helpful in the initial assessment. Examples of this include differentiating between synovitis, Morton's neuroma, and intramuscular myxoma.

PITFALLS

- The finding of an interdigital mass > 20 mm in length should raise suspicion of an abnormality other than a neuroma.
- Unless intravenous gadolinium is used, a neuroma is likely to be rendered less conspicuous by the application of fat suppression (**Figs. 58E,58F**).
- If a lesion is seen in the typical location of a Morton's neuroma but appears homogeneously hyperintense on a T-2 weighted image, it is almost certainly an intermetatarsal bursa.
- The MRI diagnosis of Morton's neuroma does not imply symptomatology, as the prevalence of Morton's neuroma in patients with no clinical evidence of this condition is as high as 33%.

Suggested Readings

Bencardino J, Rosenberg ZS, Beltran J, Liu X, Marty-Delfaut E. Morton's neuroma: is it always symptomatic? Am J Roentgenol 2000;175:649–653

Erickson SJ, Canale PB, Carrera GF, et al. Interdigital (Morton) neuroma: high-resolution MR imaging with a solenoid coil. Radiology 1991;181:833–836

Keogh C, Torreggiani WC, Al-Ismail K, Munk PL. Musculoskeletal case 25. Morton's neuroma. Can J Surg 2002;45:448, 467–468

May DA, Good RB, Smith DK, Parsons TW. MR imaging of musculoskeletal tumors and tumor mimickers with intravenous gadolinium: experience with 242 patients. Skeletal Radiol 1997;26:2–15

Pollak RA, Bellacosa RA, Dornbluth NC, et al. Sonographic analysis of Morton's neuroma. J Foot Surg 1992;31:534–537

Quinn TJ, Jacobson JA, Craig JG, van Holsbeeck MT. Sonography of Morton's neuromas. Am J Roentgenol 2000;174:1723–1728

Terk MR, Kwong PK, Suthar M, Horvath BC, Colletti PM. Morton neuroma: evaluation with MR imaging performed with contrast enhancement at fat suppression. Radiology 1993;189:239–241

Zanetti M, Ledermann T, Zollinger H, Hodler J. Efficacy of MR imaging in patients suspected of having Morton's neuroma. Am J Roentgenol 1997;168:529–532

CASE 59

George Nomikos, Anthony G. Ryan, Peter L. Munk, and Mark Murphey

Clinical Presentation

A 15-year-old boy presented with deformity of the right, slowly progressive over a period of several years.

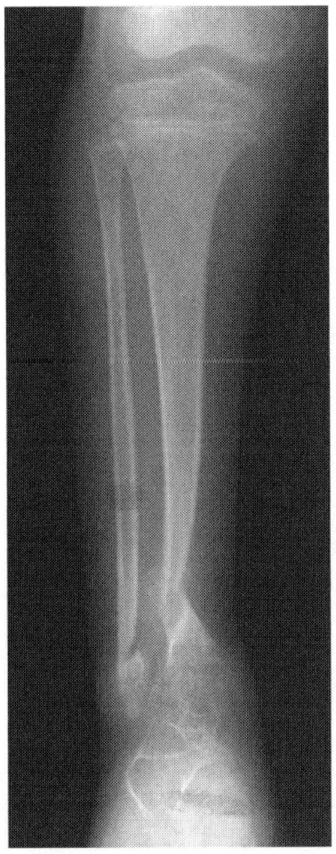

Figure 59A

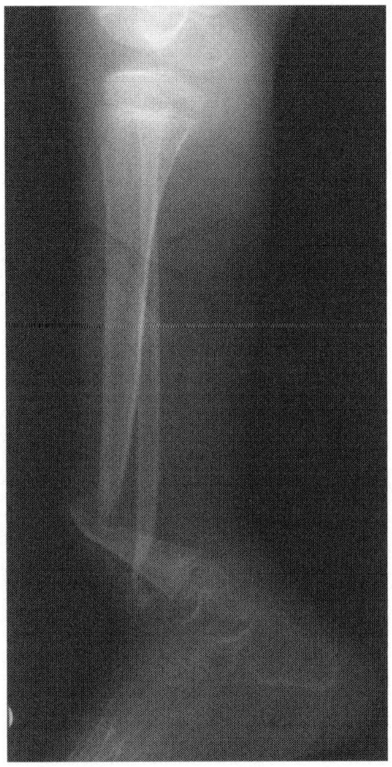

Figure 59B

Radiologic Findings

Anteroposterior (**Fig. 59A**) and lateral (**Fig. 59B**) radiographs of the lower leg in this skeletally immature patient demonstrate chronic pseudarthroses of the distal tibial and fibular shafts. The visualized bones are gracile and osteopenic.

Diagnosis

Neurofibromatosis Type 1 (von Recklinghausen's disease).

Differential Diagnosis

Congenital or infantile pseudarthrosis of the tibia may be seen sporadically in the general population and may also been seen in association with osteofibrous dysplasia. However, ~50% of all cases of congenital or infantile pseudarthrosis occur in the setting of neurofibromatosis type 1 (NF1).

Discussion

Background

NF1 is a common genetic disease, with a frequency of 1 case in every 2500 to 3000 births, and is the most common of the phakomatoses. It is inherited in an autosomal dominant pattern; however,

Table 59–1 Criteria for Diagnosis of Neurofibromatosis Type 1

Six or more café-au-lait spots > 5 mm in diameter in children or > 15 mm in diameter in adults
Two or more neurofibromas or one plexiform neurofibroma
Optic glioma
Two or more iris hamartomas (Lisch nodules)
Axillary or inguinal freckling
Distinctive osseous lesions (sphenoid dysplasia, pseudarthrosis, vertebral scalloping, dystrophic scoliosis)
A first-degree relative with neurofibromatosis type 1 as diagnosed by these criteria

up to 50% of new cases are thought to arise from spontaneous mutations. It is a mesodermal dysplasia that affects multiple organ systems. Advanced paternal age is thought to be one potential predisposing factor. An abnormality in the pericentromeric region of chromosome 17, which is responsible for coding for the protein neurofibromin, is the underlying genetic abnormality.

Clinical Findings

The clinical criteria for establishing a diagnosis of NF1 are summarized in **Table 59–1**. The diagnosis can be established when two or more of these criteria are present. The classic triad of NF1 consists of cutaneous lesions, skeletal deformity, and mental deficiency. Café-au-lait spots not only are seen in patients with NF1 but also may be seen in the setting of fibrous dysplasia and tuberous sclerosis.

The orthopedic abnormalities seen with NF1 are the following:

- Dystrophic scoliosis
  - Sharply angulated curve (most commonly a thoracic curvature involving four to six vertebrae with sharp angulation and severe rotation)
  - Posterior vertebral body scalloping
  - Extreme rotation
  - Severe deformity in the sagittal plane
  - Vertebral wedging
  - Neural foraminal enlargement
  - Spinal canal widening
  - Abnormal pedicles
  - Thin (ribbon) ribs
- Nondystrophic scoliosis (more common than the dystrophic type)
- Congenital or infantile pseudarthrosis of the tibia (**Fig. 59A,59B**) or less commonly of other bones such as the clavicle, radius, ulna, and femur
- Anterior tibial bowing may be identified before formation of a pseudarthrosis (**Fig. 59C**).
- Disproportionate overgrowth of part of an extremity (e.g., macrodactyly)
- Multiple nonossifying fibromas or fibroxanthomas
- Marked subperiosteal bone formation
- Facial or orbital dysplasia
- Lamboid suture defects (left-sided)
- Coxa valga
- Acetabuli protrusio

Imaging Findings

RADIOGRAPHY

Plain films may demonstrate any of the above osseus abnormalities.

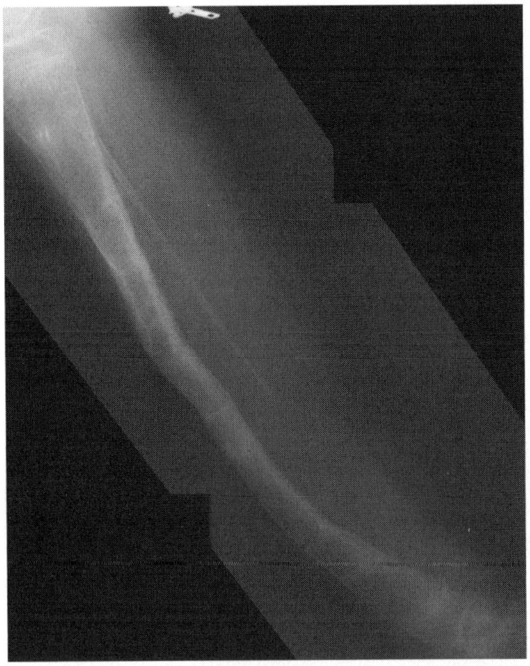

Figure 59C Anterior tibial bowing, cortical irregularity, fracture, and periosteal reaction. Note, in addition, the abnormal tapered fibula.

MAGNETIC RESONANCE IMAGING

Localized neurofibromas are most commonly seen in the setting of NF1. In patients with NF1, localized neurofibromas often involve deep large nerves (e.g., sciatic nerve and brachial plexus). On MRI, typically they are low signal intensity on T1-weighted images, and variable high signal but with heterogeneity on T2-weighted images; occasionally, they are described as having a "salt and pepper" or "target" appearance (**Figs. 59D–59G**). In common with other neurogenic tumors, they arise in the line of an existing nerve and consequently have a "neural tail." They are usually large and multiple (**Fig. 59H**). They may also involve the subcutaneous tissues and dermis as well produce nodules under the skin.

The plexiform neurofibroma is virtually pathognomonic of NF1. These neurofibromas involve long segments of nerves and their branches (**Figs. 59I–59L**). The involved nerves will be markedly expanded and may resemble a "bag of worms." These large lesions extend into the surrounding soft tissues and may cause marked enlargement and deformity of an extremity (elephantiasis neuromatosa). Associated osseous overgrowth may occur due to hyperemia of the affected extremity.

The most worrisome complication in these patients is malignant transformation into a malignant peripheral nerve sheath tumor (MPNST). A sudden increase in pain or in the size of a known neurofibroma is suggestive of malignant transformation into an MPNST (**Figs. 59M–59O**). The estimated overall lifetime risk of malignant transformation is ~5%.

PEARLS

- The presence of one plexiform neurofibroma is adequate for the diagnosis of NF1.
- The scoliosis associated with neurofibromatosis is characteristic, having most commonly an upper thoracic curvature involving four to six vertebrae with sharp angulation and severe rotation.
- Neurofibromas tend to cause concentric expansion of the involved nerve, whereas schwannomas cause eccentric growth.

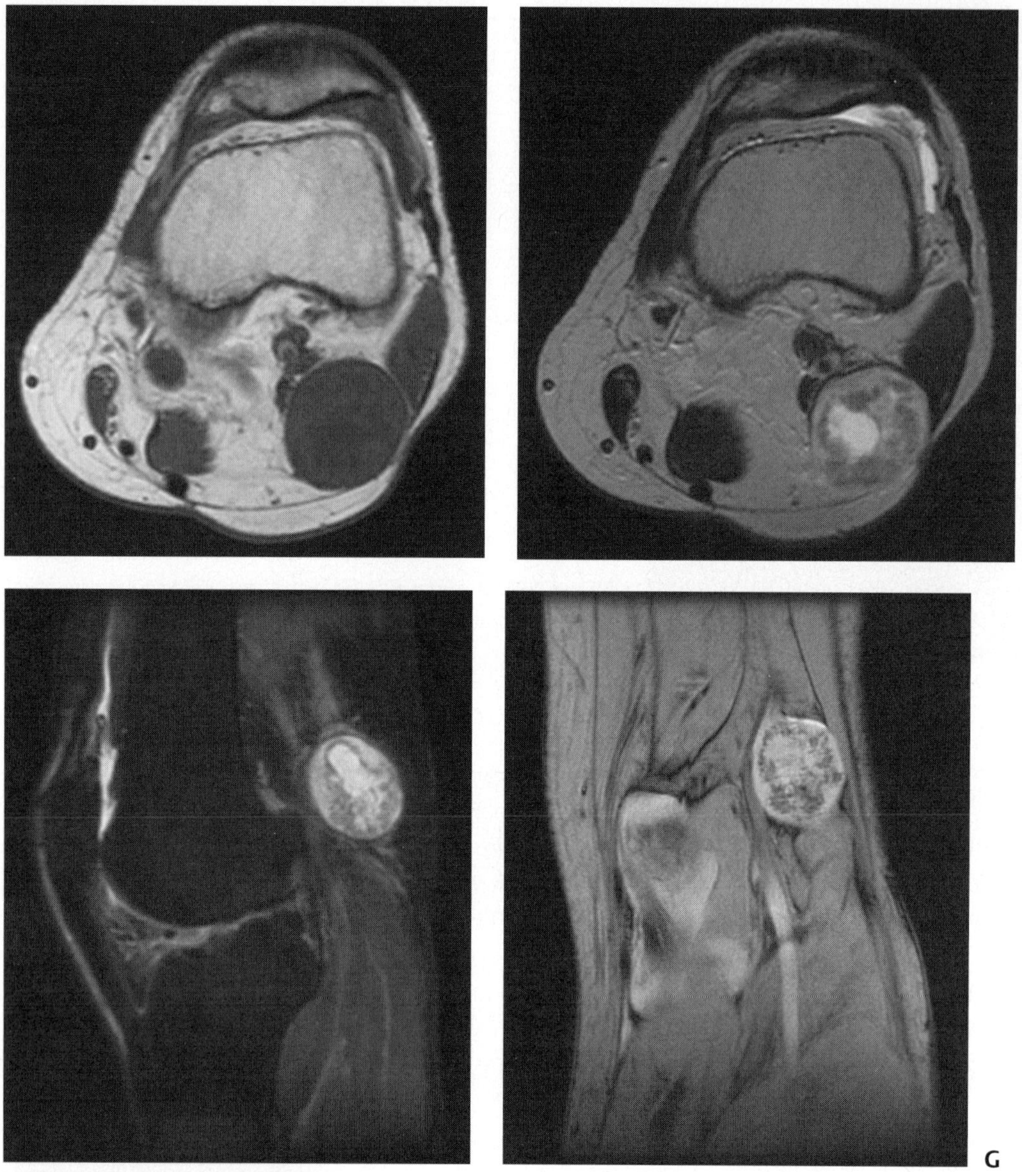

D E F G

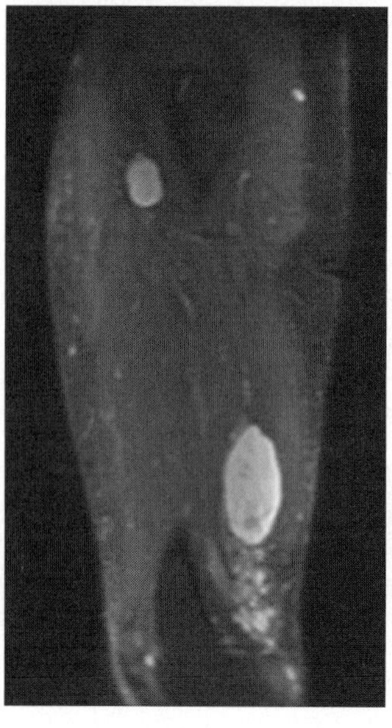

H

Figures 59D–59H Transaxial T1-weighted (**59D**), transaxial T2-weighted (**59E**), sagittal T2-weighted fat-saturated (**59F**), and coronal MPGR (**59G**) images show a large neurofibroma of the distal sciatic nerve that demonstrates intermediate low signal intensity on T1, heterogeneous but predominantly high-signal intensity on T2 (the latter becoming more marked with fat saturation), and a prominent "salt and pepper" sign on the MPGR image. **59H** Patient with neurofibromatosis type 1 demonstrating multiple large neurofibromas of the sciatic nerve on a sagittal T2 fat-saturated image.

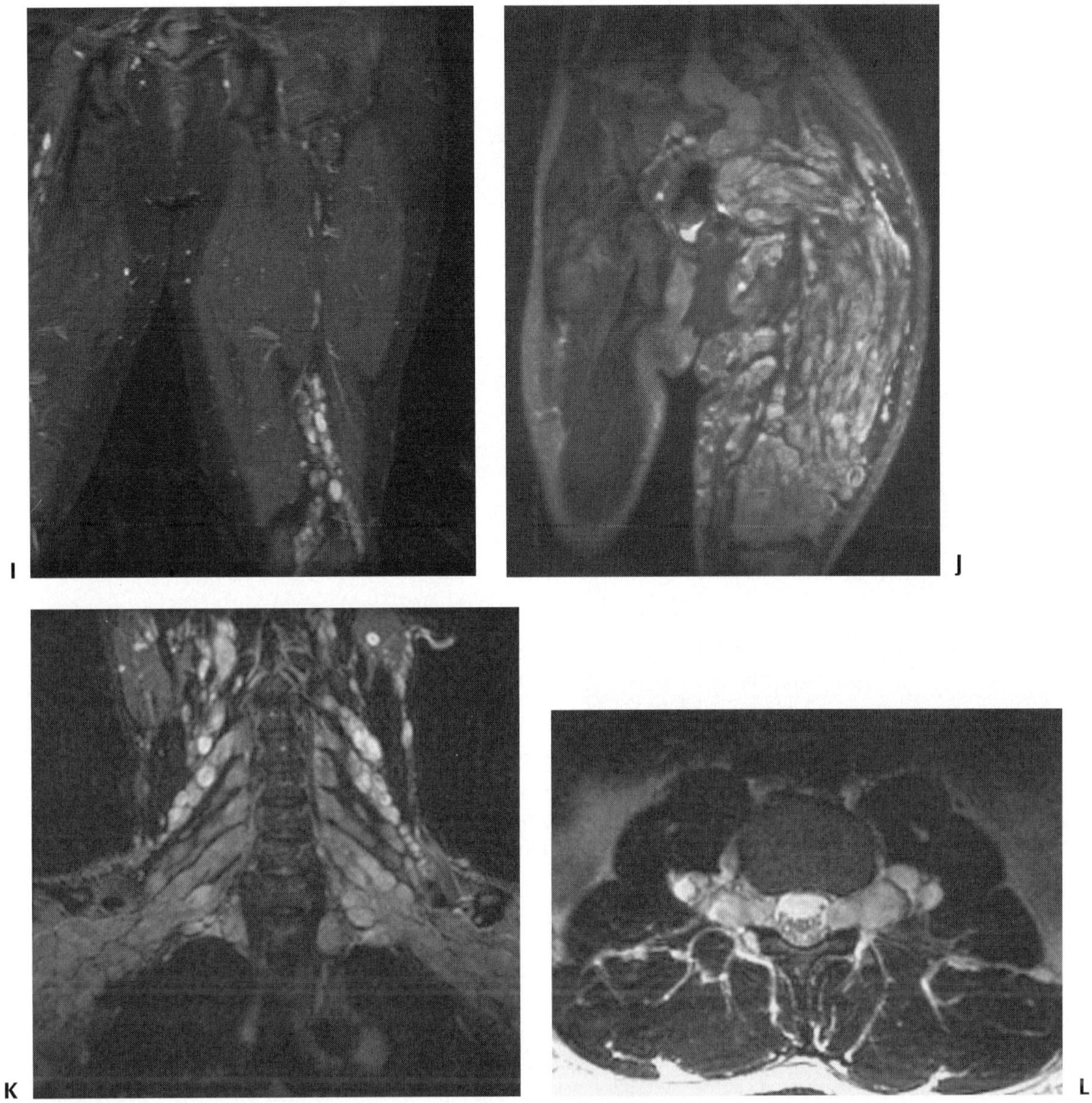

Figures 59I–59L Plexiform neurofibromata of the distal sciatic (**59I,** coronal T2-weighted fat-saturated image), proximal thigh (**59J**, coronal T2-weighted fat-saturated image, demonstrating a "bag of worms" configuration), and the cervical nerves as they exit the neural foramina (**59K**, coronal T2-weighted fat-saturated image). **59L** A transaxial T2-weighted image shows the typical expansion of the foramen caused by the plexiform neurofibroma, particularly on the left.

PITFALLS

- Neurofibromatosis is inherited in an autosomal dominant pattern; however, up to 50% of new cases are thought to arise from spontaneous mutations.
- Café-au-lait spots not only are seen in patients with NF1 but also may be seen in the setting of fibrous dysplasia and tuberous sclerosis.
- A sudden increase in pain or in the size of a known neurofibroma should not be ignored, as it usually heralds the development of malignant transformation into an MPNST, estimated overall lifetime risk of which is ~5%.

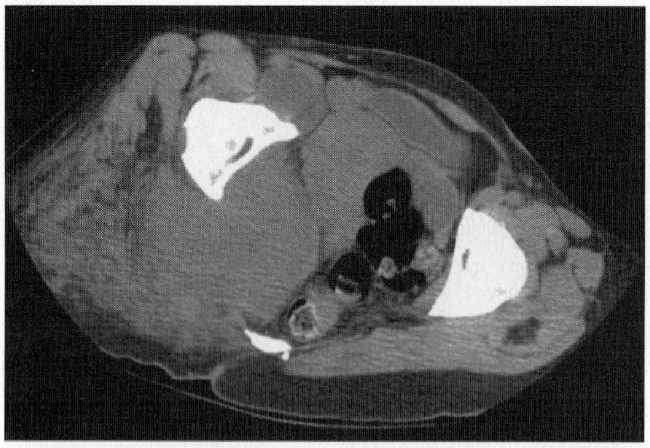

M

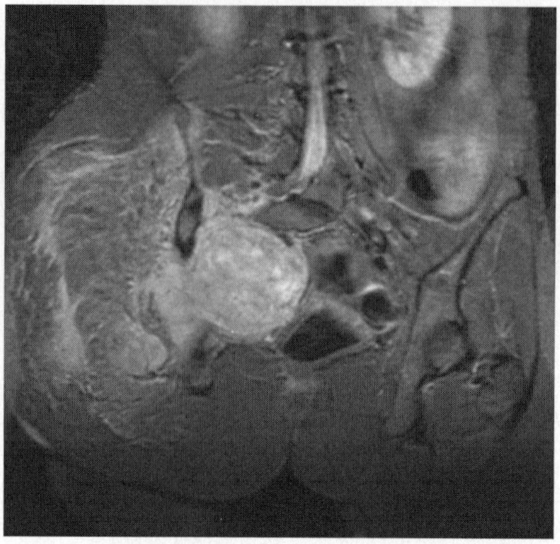

N

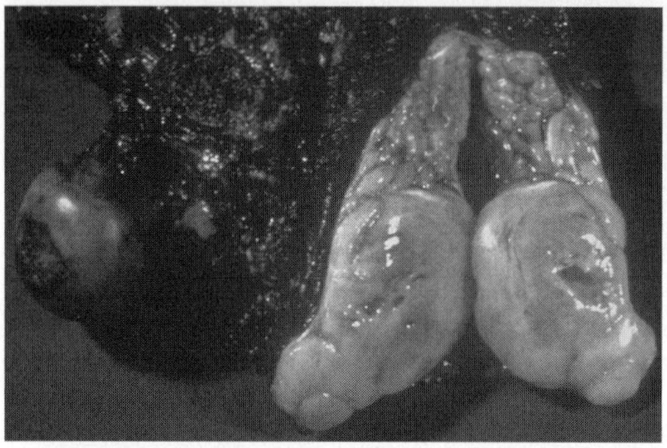

O

Figures 59M–59O Transaxial image from CT of the pelvis at the level of the sciatic notch shows a massive expansion of the sciatic nerve on the region of a previously identified neurofibroma in a patient with neurofibromatosis 1 (**59M**). Coronal T2 fat-saturated image (**59N**) shows a large intrapelvic component and a smaller more distal extrapelvic component. (**59O**) The cut surgical specimen is depicted. (See also **Figure 59O**, page 318.)

Suggested Readings

Fortman BJ, Kuszyk BS, Urban BA, Fishman EK. Neurofibromatosis type 1: a diagnostic mimicker at CT. Radiographics 2001;21:601–612

Khong PL, Goh WH, Wong VC, Fung CW, Ooi GC. MR imaging of spinal tumors in children with neurofibromatosis 1. Am J Roentgenol 2003;180:413–417

Lim R, Jaramillo D, Poussaint T, Chang Y, Korf B. Superficial neurofibroma: a lesion with unique MRI characteristics in patients with neurofibromatosis type 1. Am J Roentgenol 2005;184:962–968

Murphey MD, Smith WS, Smith SE, Kransdorf MJ, Temple HT. Imaging of musculoskeletal neurogenic tumors: radiologic-pathologic correlation. Radiographics 1999;19:1253–1280

Vitale MG, Guha A, Skaggs DL. Orthopaedic manifestations of neurofibromatosis in children: an update. Clin Orthop Relat Res 2002;401:107–118

CASE 60

Anthony G. Ryan and Peter L. Munk

Clinical Presentation

A 51-year-old woman presented complaining of a slightly painful lump at the base of her index finger. No bone or joint abnormality was seen on plain film.

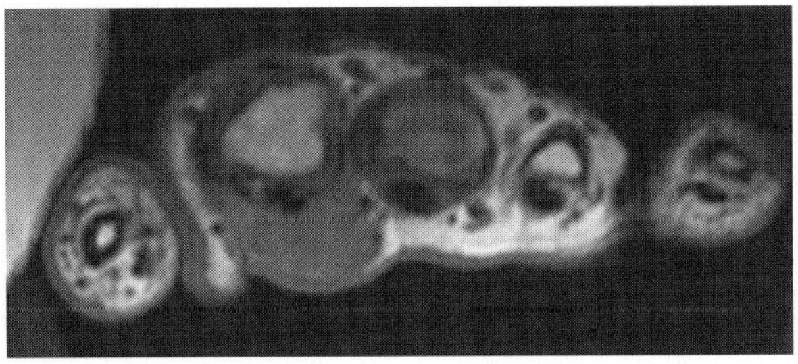

Figure 60A

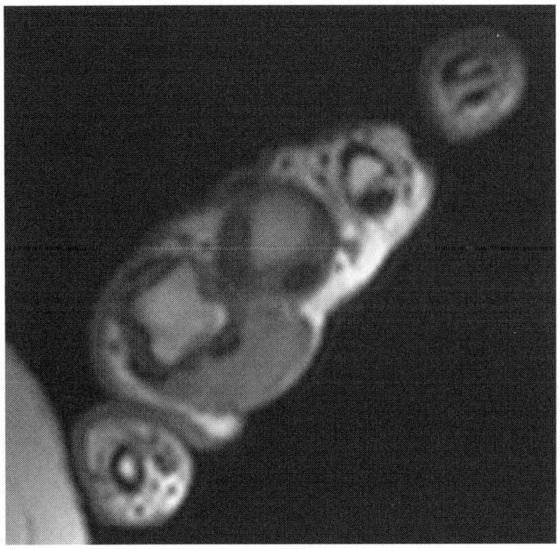

Figure 60B

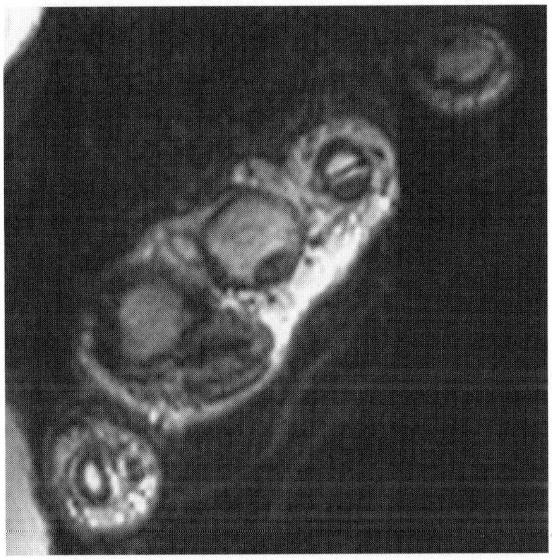

Figure 60C

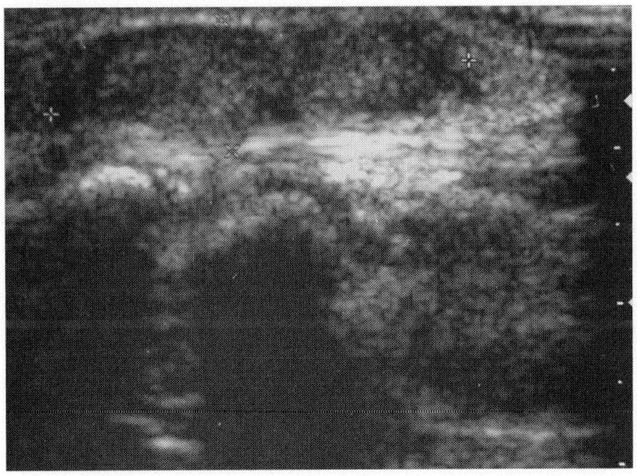

Figure 60D

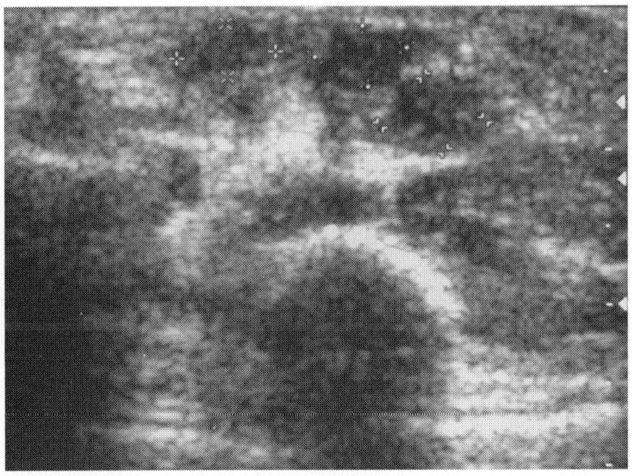

Figure 60E

Radiologic Findings

Transaxial T1-weighted (**Fig. 60A**) and T2-weighted (**Fig. 60B**) images of the hand at the level of the metacarpophalangeal joints show an intermediate signal intensity mass on the volar aspect of the flexor tendons palmar to the head of the second metacarpal. The mass is seen to extend dorsally on either side of the tendons. The lesion extends from just deep to the dermis to the metacarpal periosteum, but without osseous invasion. A transaxial gradient image (**Fig. 60C**) demonstrates linear, very low signal intensity within the lesion with minimal associated "blooming."

Images taken at the time of ultrasound-guided biopsy, sagittal (**Fig. 60D**) and transverse (**Fig. 60E**), show a lobulated heterogeneous hypoechoic mass anterior to the tendon, which is seen deep to the mass as a typical hyperechoic fibrillar structure. The tendon sheath is draped over the top of the mass from which it is inseparable.

Diagnosis

Giant cell tumor of the tendon sheath (GCTTS).

Differential Diagnosis

- Ganglion
- Tenosynovitis
- Amyloid
- Synovial fibroma
- Synovial sarcoma
- Synovial chondromatosis

Discussion

Background

GCTTS is a proliferative disorder of tendon sheaths that is the second most common cause of a mass of the hand and wrist. Previously known as nodular synovitis, GCTTS is now recognized as pathologically indistinguishable from pigmented villonodular synovitis (PVNS), occurring as a localized form of the latter, of which it accounts for 75 to 85% of all PVNS lesions (diffuse lesions accounting for 15 to 25%).

Etiology

Unknown. Inflammatory, neoplastic, and traumatic etiologies have all been proposed.

Pathophysiology

The lesion gives rise to symptoms primarily secondary to local mass effects, for example, impingement on digital nerves, pressure erosion on adjacent bone, and hindering flexion of the affected digit.

Clinical Findings

GCTTS has a maximum incidence between ages 40 and 60, with a wide range from 14 to 77 years reported. There is a slight female preponderance (6:4). The lesions are most common in the fingers (80%), followed by the knee, hand and wrist, feet, and hip. Lesions are found twice as often on the palmar aspect on the hand than on the dorsum, usually opposite a distal interphalangeal (DIP) or metacarpal phalangeal (MCP) joint.

These lesions typically present as a small lobulated, firm, and laterally mobile swelling measuring between 5 mm and 3 cm. They are typically covered by normal skin but are frequently fixed on the deep aspect. They are usually painless but may give rise to pain as a result of pressure on local nerves. They usually have been present for several months before presentation and typically demonstrate steady, progressive growth that eventually interferes with joint excursion.

Bony erosion is uncommon, occurring in only 10 to 15% (compared with the diffuse form of PVNS, in which erosion occurs, on average, in 50% of affected knees).

Complications

- Pain secondary to neural impingement
- Diminished range of motion in adjacent joint
- Osseous erosion
- Locally aggressive

Pathology

GROSS

Seen on examination is a brownish yellow, lobulated, incompletely encapsulated lesion inseparable from the synovium of the tendon sheath, with well-defined, firm, fibrous nodules, each measuring up to 4 cm (though usually less than 2 cm) in size. Thin septations arising from the capsule are demonstrated throughout the internal architecture of the lesion.

Similar to the diffuse form of PVNS, pigmentation secondary to hemosiderin deposition may be evident.

MICROSCOPIC

This is a very cellular tumor divided into lobules by the capsular septations. The septations are composed of bands of fibrous connective tissue compressed around the cellular tumor, which in combination with the surrounding, incomplete capsule, constitute the complete pseudocapsule.

There is a mixed cellular population, namely

- Giant cells resembling osteoclasts
- Histiocyte-derived mononucleated foam cells/xanthoma cells, from which comes the tumor's alternative name: xanthoma
- Hemosiderin-containing macrophages

Within the lesion, there is an extracellular component containing deposits of hemosiderin and fat.

HISTOLOGICAL DIFFERENTIAL

The lesion may be mistaken for rheumatoid tenosynovitis and synovial sarcoma.

Imaging Findings

RADIOGRAPHY

- Soft-tissue mass that rarely calcifies (**Fig. 60F**)
- With or without erosion of the underlying bone (**Fig. 60F**)

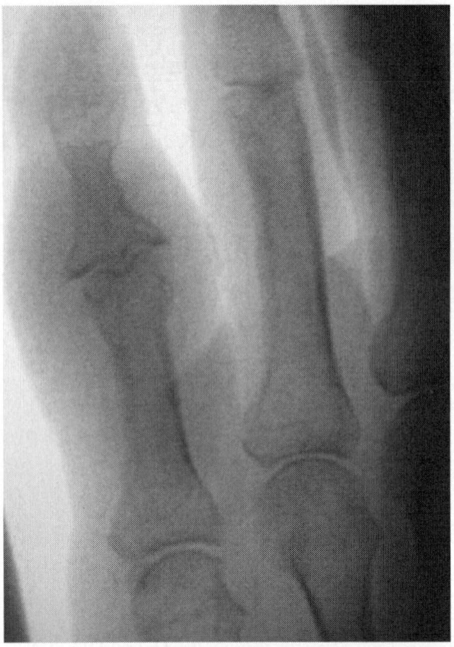

F

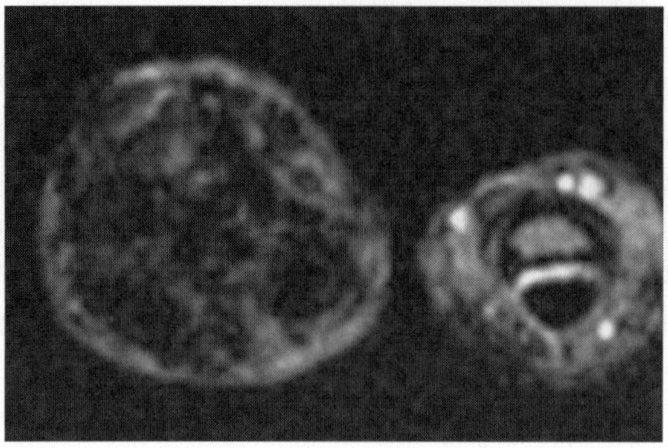

G

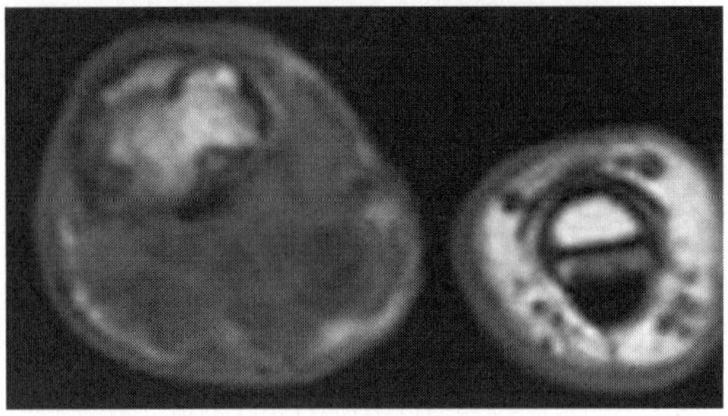

H

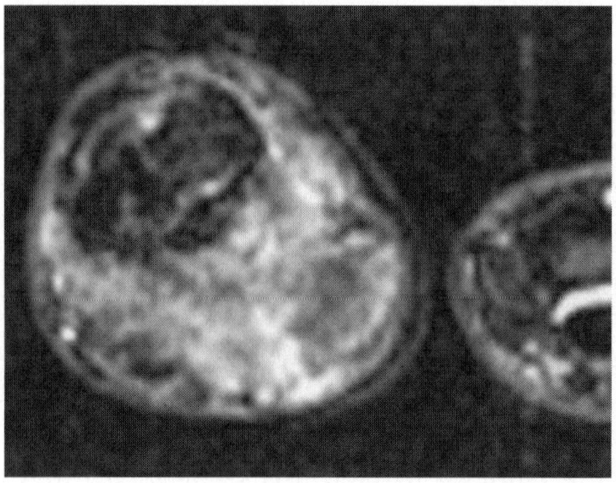

I

Figures 60F–60I (**Figs. 60F–60L** are of the same case.) **60F** Control film from angiography of the left upper limb in a 54-year-old woman complaining of a painful soft-tissue swelling affecting the entirety of the fifth digit shows pronounced soft-tissue swelling apparently centered on the proximal interphalangeal (PIP) joint of the fifth digit, at which joint space narrowing and irregular osteophyte formation is evident. The head of the middle phalanx is expanded and lucent compared with the remainder of the bone. **60G** A transaxial gradient image at the level of the soft-tissue swelling in which no normal anatomy is discernible secondary to the presence of pronounced blooming as a result of magnetic susceptibility artifact due to the high hemosiderin content of the lesion. **60H** A transaxial T2-weighted image shows a large lobular mass returning heterogeneous but predominantly intermediate signal intensity. The lesion extends from the periosteum to the dermis, which is variably involved. The digital tendons are seen abutting the metacarpal, almost completely surrounded by the lesion. The neurovascular bundles are clearly involved. **60I** A transaxial T1-weighted image with fat saturation after intravenous gadolinium at the level of the phalangeal head shows not only intense enhancement but also destruction and invasion of the underlying bone at the level of the bony changes seen on the plain film.

- When osseous erosion is present, it is usually a surface pressure phenomenon; however, true intraosseous invasion occurs rarely (**Figs. 60F–60L**).
- Degeneration of the subjacent joints is common.
- Periostitis

ULTRASOUND

In transverse scanning, the tumor is seen to be a typically hypoechoic or inhomogeneous irregular swelling within the tendon sheath (**Figs. 60D,60E**). The lesion has a broad base along the tendon sheath, eccentric in relation to the tendon (which is usually normal), and demonstrates prominent vascularity on ultrasound.

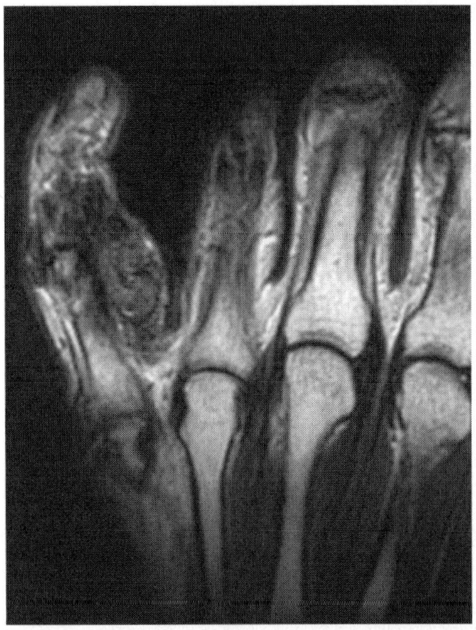

J

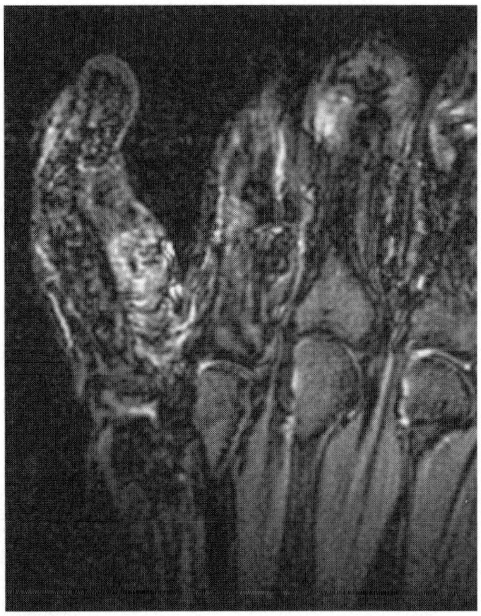

K

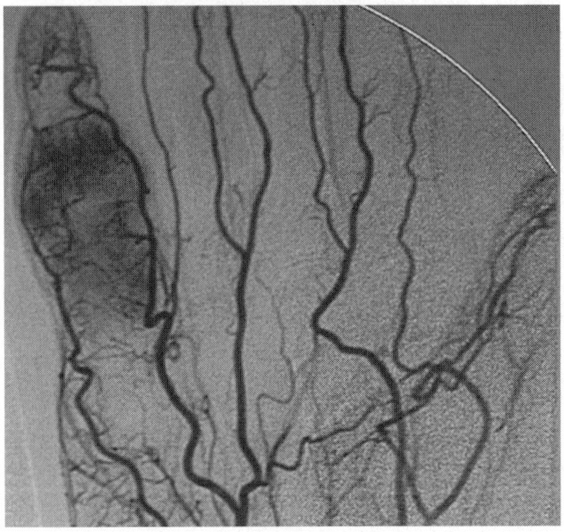

L

Figures 60J A sagittal T1-weighted image shows the longitudinal extent of the lesion, the internal signal heterogeneity, and the profound low signal intensity at the level of the invaded phalanx. Extension onto the dorsum of the finger is also clearly seen. **60K** A sagittal T1-weighted image with fat saturation after intravenous gadolinium again shows intense enhancement in the main tumor bulk. **60L** Preoperative selective digital angiography demonstrating the prominent vascularity and dense vascular blush associated with the tumor, the latter most dense in the region of intraosseous invasion. Abnormal spiral neovessels are seen at the level of the dense blush.

These appearances on ultrasound raise a differential including:

- *Synovial fibromas* A fibroma of the tendon sheath would be hypoechoic (but does not demonstrate enhanced through-transmission) and displace the tendon. Fibromas are typically very firm and have internal echoes.
- *Synovial chondromatosis* Multiple echogenic nodules
- *Tenosynovitis* The presence of a (usually) normal tendon and the definite irregular masslike characteristics of the findings in GCTTS permit its distinction from tenosynovitis.
- *Ganglion* Demonstrates enhanced through-transmission

COMPUTED TOMOGRAPHY

- Soft-tissue mass of increased attenuation. Multidector CT elegantly demonstrates the lesion, its vascularity, and its relationship to the adjacent tendon.

MAGNETIC RESONANCE IMAGING

The classic description is of marked low signal intensity on T1- and T2-weighted images in the synovial lining and the tendons secondary to the presence of hemosiderin, similar to that frequently described in relation to PVNS.

Hemosiderin, when present, gives rise to prominent “blooming” on gradient sequences (**Fig. 60G**).

Not all lesions contain hemosiderin, however, in which case the majority of lesions demonstrate hypointense or intermediate signal, approximately equal to that of skeletal muscle on both T1- and T2-weighted images (**Figs. 60A,60B**).

T2-weighted images reveal a more variable pattern, ranging from hypointense, isointense, and slightly hyperintense relative to skeletal muscle but hypointense relative to fat, or frank heterogeneity (**Fig. 60H**). Despite this variability, prominent low-intensity foci are usually seen on T2-weighted images.

Moderate to pronounced enhancement after intravenous gadolinium is typical (**Figs. 60I–60K**).

ANGIOGRAPHY

Angiography is occasionally requested preoperatively, at which time the lesions are almost invariably hypervascular (**Fig. 60L**) and demonstrate neovascularity.

Treatment

Although surgical resection is the proposed treatment, these tumors are difficult to treat because they may wrap around the associated tendon(s) and extend into subjacent joints.

Prognosis

The recurrence rate after resection is 10 to 20%.

PEARLS

- Low signal intensity on both T1- and T2-weighted images is an uncommon appearance of extra-articular soft-tissue masses, in particular when they occur in the hands or feet, and should thus suggest the diagnosis of GCTTS.
- The ultrasound appearances raise a differential, as follows:
  - *Synovial fibromas* A fibroma of the tendon sheath would be hypoechoic (but does not demonstrate enhanced through-transmission) and displace the tendon. Fibromas are typically very firm and contain internal echoes.
  - *Ganglion* Demonstrates enhanced through-transmission

PITFALLS

- Tenosynovitis is unlikely to be mistaken for a GCTTS, given the usually very painful nature of the former. Similarly, the presence of a (usually) normal tendon and the definite irregular masslike characteristics of the findings in GCTTS permit its distinction from tenosynovitis.
- Because these tumors are difficult to excise completely, it is important to visualize the full extent of the lesion before surgery is planned. Ideally, this should include at least the whole of the ray involved by the tumor.
- Not all CGTTS demonstrate hemosiderin deposition and consequent “blooming”; thus, the absence of the latter does not exclude the diagnosis.

Suggested Readings

Fogelson MH, Dao KD, Shin AY. Intraosseous metacarpal involvement of giant cell tumor of the tendon sheath: report of 2 cases. Am J Orthop 2003;32:32–34

Jelinek JS, Kransdorf MJ, Shmookler BM, Aboulafia AA, Malawer MM. Giant cell tumor of the tendon sheath: MR findings in nine cases. Am J Roentgenol 1994;162:919–922

Karasick D, Karasick S. Giant cell tumor of tendon sheath: spectrum of radiologic findings. Skeletal Radiol 1992;21:219–224

CASE 61

George Nomikos, Anthony G. Ryan, Peter L. Munk, and Mark Murphey

Clinical Presentation

A 28-year-old woman presented with elbow pain.

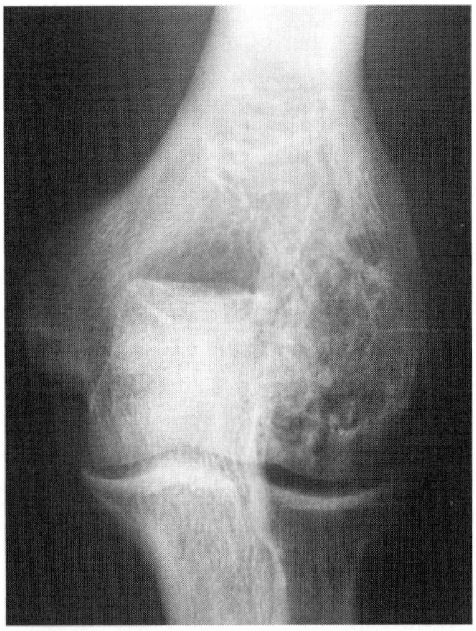

Figure 61A

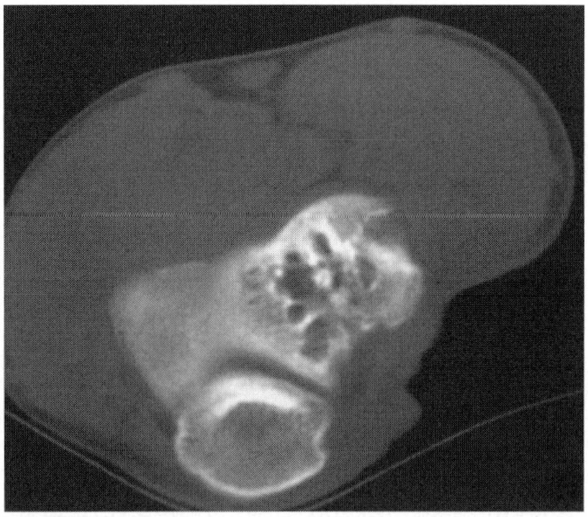

Figure 61B

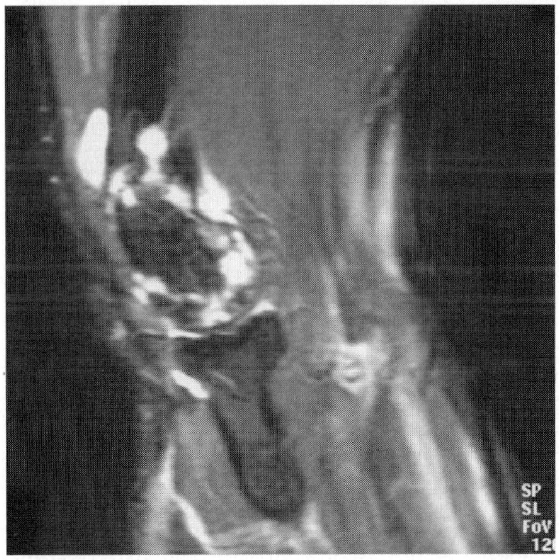

Figure 61C

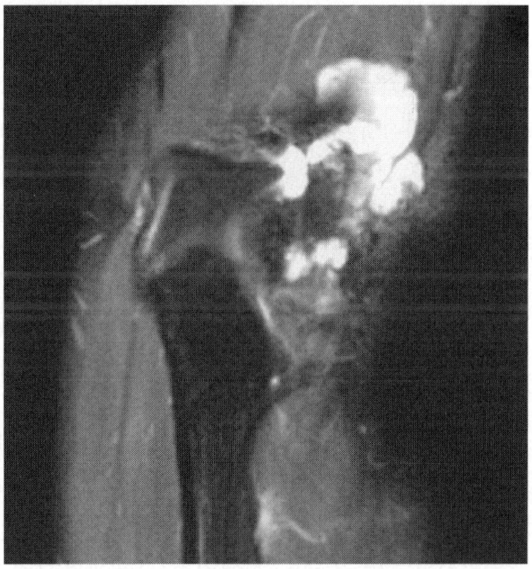

Figure 61D

Radiologic Findings

An anteroposterior radiograph of the elbow (**Fig. 61A**) shows multiple round lucencies in the lateral humeral condyle with intervening trabeculae (reticular pattern). There is associated sclerosis around the areas of lucency. There is no associated periosteal reaction. The CT (**Fig. 61B**) demonstrates similar findings. The lucencies have a tubular appearance. No mineralized matrix is identified. Sagittal T2-weighted (**Fig. 61C**) and coronal inversion recovery (**Fig. 61D**) images show multiple high signal intensity tubular structures in the lateral humeral condyle extending into the surrounding soft tissues and into the elbow joint. The entire lesion is composed of these serpentine tubular structures.

Diagnosis

Osseous hemangioma.

Differential Diagnosis

- Paget's disease
- Fluorosis

Discussion

Background

Angiomatous lesions, particularly hemangiomas, are very common in the musculoskeletal system. Although capillary hemangiomas are the most common type in general, they are usually very superficial, usually involute by age 7, and thus rarely come to radiographic evaluation. Cavernous hemangiomas, which are composed of large blood-filled vascular channels, are the form most commonly encountered by radiologists, as they usually involve the deep tissues and do not usually involute with age. Arteriovenous hemangiomas represent a localized abnormal persistence of a portion of the fetal capillary circulation and may be superficial (frequently asymptomatic) or deep (frequently symptomatic). They are almost exclusively soft-tissue lesions found in young patients and may cause complications associated with shunt vascularity. Venous hemangiomas are most commonly seen in the deep soft tissues of the retroperitoneum, mesentery, or lower extremity muscles and are composed of thick-walled vessels.

Clinical Findings

Osseous hemangiomas are most commonly encountered in the vertebrae (thoracic or lumbar segments usually) or skull, accounting for 23% and 20% of all skeletal hemangiomas, respectively. Lesions in the vertebrae and skull are usually asymptomatic. In the vertebrae, hemangiomas usually originate in the vertebral body, but they may extend to involve the posterior elements or surrounding soft tissues, potentially causing neurologic compromise. Pathologic fracture may occur, but it is unlikely in lesions demonstrating significant trabecular thickening and reinforcement. Lesions that contain greater amounts of fat tend to be asymptomatic (quiescent hemangioma). Unlike spinal and skull hemangiomas, extremity lesions are symptomatic in $>$ 90% of cases (pain, swelling, or mass). Appendicular lesions most commonly occur in the lower extremities (73%), particularly the tibia and femur. These lesions are most commonly medullary and are diaphyseal or metadiaphyseal, although periosteal and intracortical lesions also occur.

Imaging Findings

RADIOGRAPHY

- Vertebral hemangiomas typically demonstrate trabecular coarsening and thickening between channel-like areas of radiolucency, representing vascular channels, producing the classic "corduroy" appearance (**Fig. 61E**).
- Skull lesions typically begin in the diploic space, cause osseous expansion (particularly of the outer table), and demonstrate osteolysis with a central spoke-wheel or sunburst area of radiating trabeculae.
- Extremity lesions do not usually demonstrate the classic patterns seen in the vertebrae and skull.
- Extremity lesions may demonstrate multilocular areas of lucency with thin surrounding osseous trabeculae (reticular pattern), larger lucencies with more coarse osseous trabeculae (soap-bubble appearance), multiple well-defined areas of radiolucency without trabeculation, or (rarely) a pseudopermeative pattern resembling myeloma or metastatic disease.
- Extremity lesions in the medullary canal may demonstrate osseous expansion and endosteal scalloping.
- Intracortical lesions may appear as a radiolucent central area with surrounding sclerosis, much like an osteoid osteoma, adamantinoma, or osteofibrous dysplasia.

COMPUTED TOMOGRAPHY

- CT demonstrates the trabecular thickening and coarsening of spinal and skull lesions well.
- In cross section, the thickened trabeculae produce a "polka dot" appearance (**Fig. 61F**).

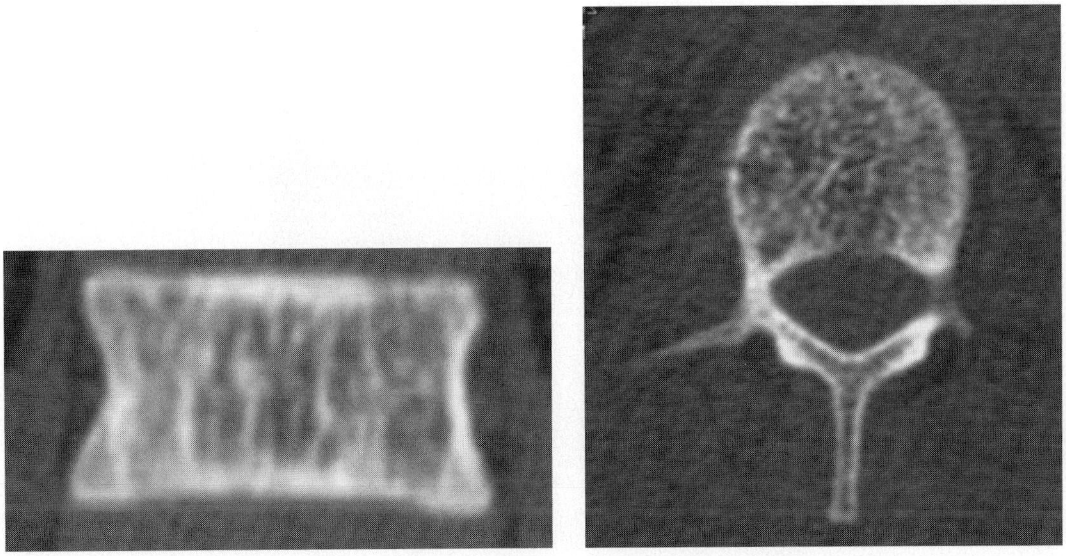

E F

Figures 61E Coronal reconstruction of transaxially acquired CT of a vertebral hemangioma demonstrating the classic "corduroy" appearance, that is, trabecular coarsening and thickening between linear radiolucencies, the latter representing vascular channels. **61F** Same vertebra as **61E** showing the "polka dot" appearance of the thickened trabeculae in cross section.

- May demonstrate fat overgrowth in the lesion, which is characteristic of asymptomatic hemangiomas
- Enhancement after contrast administration
- Soft-tissue mass may be present secondary to extraosseous spread (particularly with symptomatic lesions).

MAGNETIC RESONANCE IMAGING

- Variable signal intensity found on T1-weighted images, as lesions with larger amounts of fat are high signal intensity, and lesions with little internal fat are lower in signal intensity.
- Blood-filled spaces with slow flow, as seen in cavernous lesions, are high signal intensity on T2-weighted images.
- Lesions with high flow (arteriovenous hemangiomas) show signal voids on all sequences.
- Areas of trabecular thickening are low signal intensity on all sequences.
- A soft-tissue mass may be present.

Variants and Syndromes

1. Angiomatosis (**Figs. 61G,61H**) is a rare condition in which there is diffuse proliferation of hemangiomatous and/or lymphangiomatous elements in bone and soft tissue. Cases with predominantly osseous involvement carry a better prognosis than those with more soft tissue, and specifically visceral, involvement. Radiographically, osseous lesions appear as multiple lytic lesions, often with surrounding sclerosis, producing a honeycomb or lattice appearance in the involved bones. This is similar in appearance to a solitary lesion but with more extensive involvement. The thickened trabeculae seen in solitary lesions are not usually apparent. Bones on both sides of a joint are commonly involved. The femur, rib, spine, and pelvis are commonly involved.

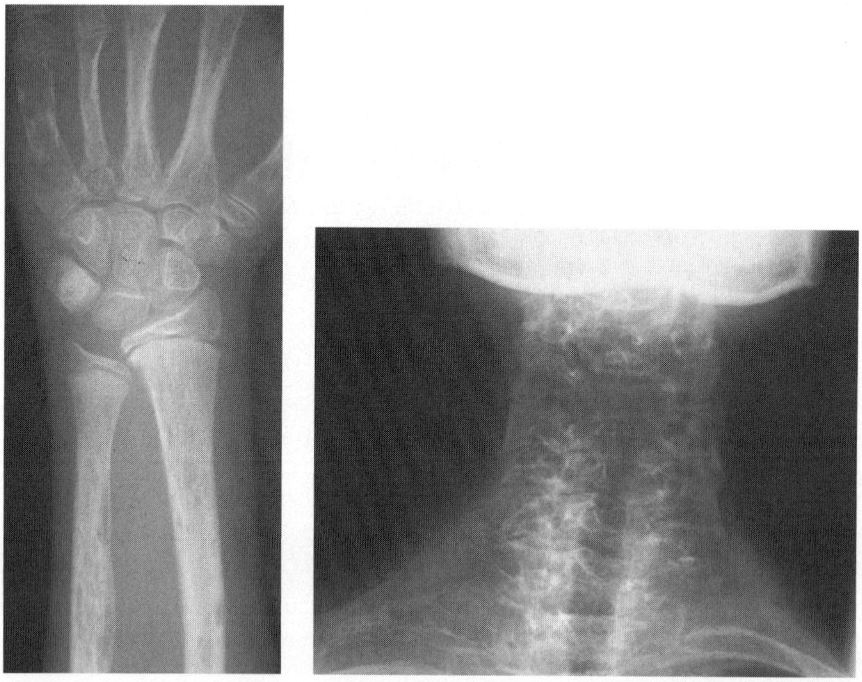

G H

Figures 61G and **61H** Radiographs of the left wrist and hand (**61G**) and cervical spine (**61H**) in a patient with angiomatosis show multiple lesions affecting radius, ulna, fifth metacarpal, and first and second ribs characterized by lysis with surrounding sclerosis, producing a honeycomb or lattice appearance in the involved bones.

2. Klippel-Trénaunay-Weber syndrome represents the association of cutaneous hemangiomas (usually capillary), bone and soft-tissue hypertrophy, and varicose veins. There is unilateral involvement of a single lower extremity with characteristic bone and soft-tissue overgrowth of all or a portion of the involved limb. When this triad of abnormalities is associated with a high flow component, it is called Parkes Weber syndrome.
3. Massive osteolysis of Gorham is a self-limited condition that results in rapid osteolysis and bone destruction. A single bone may be involved, or there may be involvement of multiple bones across a joint. Soft-tissue involvement is usually minimal, and tapering of osseous lesion margins is absent. The process begins as focal areas of bone resorption that progress to massive bone destruction and osteolysis. There is an association with trauma in 50% of patients. Common locations include the shoulder girdle/upper arm and mandible. These lesions are considered angiomatous because the tissue replacing bone has an appearance of vascularized granulation tissue.
4. Kasabach-Merritt syndrome is the association of a hemangioma or malignant vascular lesion with thrombocytopenia and purpura, owing to reduced platelets.
5. Hemangioendothelioma and hemangiopericytoma are vascular neoplasms with a behavior more aggressive than hemangiomas that may be benign or malignant. Both most commonly involve the soft tissues. Hemangioendotheliomas usually affect the deep soft tissues of the extremities and are often associated with a blood vessel. When in bone, they are often seen in the skull, spine, or lower extremity. Hemangiopericytomas often demonstrate large peripheral vessels and have a predilection for the soft tissues of the thigh, pelvis, and retroperitoneum.
6. Angiosarcoma is a malignant vascular neoplasm that usually displays aggressive behavior and demonstrates internal vascular channels. Local recurrence and metastatic disease are common. Commonly affected sites include the skin and soft tissue. Common osseous locations include the femur, tibia, humerus, and pelvis. There is an association with chronic lymphedema (of any cause), and this combination is referred to as Stewart-Treves syndrome.

Hemangioendothelioma, hemangiopericytoma, and angiosarcoma all demonstrate imaging features similar to hemangiomas; however, osseous lesions often demonstrate a more aggressive pattern of bone destruction and often produce a soft-tissue mass. Osseous lesions also often demonstrate multiple lytic areas in one or more bones (**Figs. 61I–61K**) separated by normal bone or by an intervening joint. Advanced imaging may demonstrate obvious areas of internal vessels with high flow as areas of signal voids and regions of nonspecific soft tissue. But unlike hemangiomas, fat overgrowth is not seen. Other sarcomas that may demonstrate prominent internal vascular channels include extraskeletal Ewing's sarcoma or primitive neuroectodermal tumor (PNET), alveolar soft part sarcoma, and rhabdomyosarcoma. Soft-tissue lesions frequently demonstrating prominent vascular channels are given in **Table 61–1**.

Treatment

- Surgical excision, laser therapy, and/or embolization for hemangiomas
- Radiation therapy is also used for unresectable hemangiomas that require therapy.
- Surgery for malignant lesions with adjuvant chemotherapy and radiation

Prognosis

- Recurrence rate for soft-tissue hemangiomas is 28%.
- Malignant vascular lesions have a poor prognosis, with high local recurrence and metastatic rates.

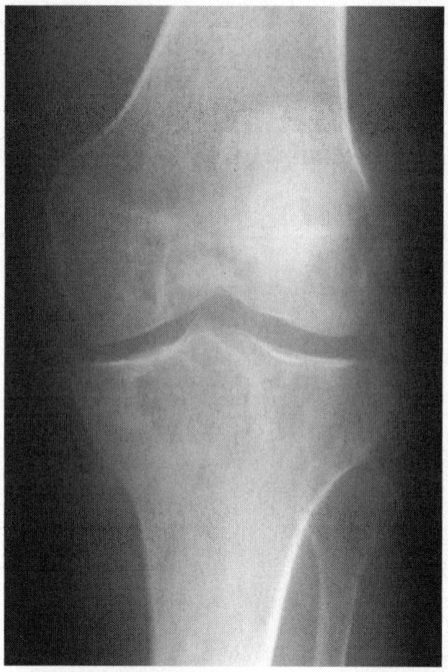

I

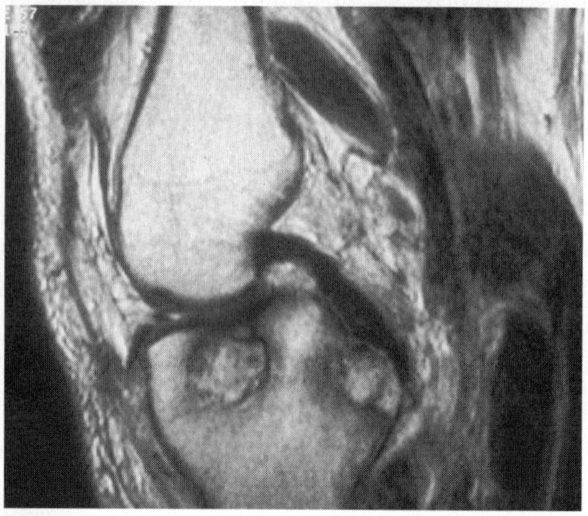

J

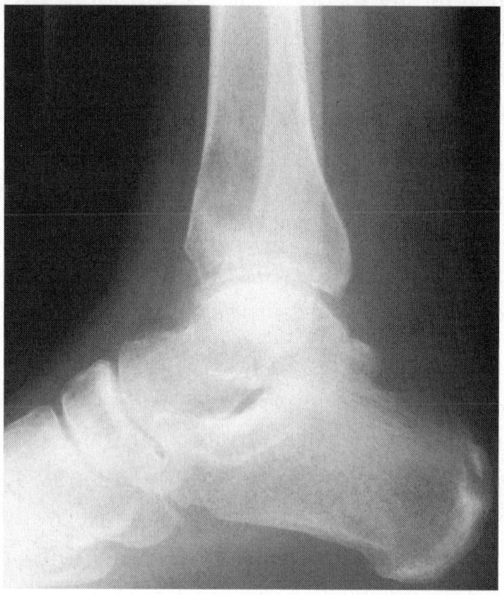

K

Figures 61I–61K Anteroposterior radiograph (**61I**) and sagittal T2-weighted image (**61J**) of a patient with multifocal hemangioendothelioma; the radiograph shows a reasonably well-defined lytic lesion underlying the medial tibial plateau and a less well-defined lesion laterally with a wide zone of transition. The MRI shows the medial plateau lesion and a further lesion posteriorly underlying the posterior cruciate ligament origin as patchily high signal intensity lesions with a sclerotic low signal margin. A lateral radiograph of the ankle (**61K**) in the same patient (same limb) shows a permeative-appearing lytic lesion in the anterior tibia with a wide zone of transition: a further focus of hemangioendothelioma.

Table 61–1 Soft-Tissue Lesions that Often Demonstrate Prominent Vascular Channels on Imaging

Hemangioma
Hemangioendothelioma
Hemangiopericytoma
Rhabdomyosarcoma
Synovial sarcoma
Alveolar soft part sarcoma (often demonstrates very large internal vessels)
Extraskeletal Ewing's sarcoma/primitive neuroectodermal tumor (PNET)
Angiosarcoma (often, however, do not see prominent internal vessels)

PEARLS

- Vertebral hemangiomas typically demonstrate trabecular coarsening and thickening between channel-like areas of radiolucency, representing vascular channels, producing the classic "corduroy" appearance (**Fig. 61E**); in cross section, the thickened trabeculae produce a "polka dot" appearance (**Fig. 61F**).
- Unlike spinal and skull hemangiomas, extremity lesions are symptomatic in > 90% of cases (pain, swelling, or mass).
- Hemangioendothelioma, hemangiopericytoma, and angiosarcoma all demonstrate imaging features similar to hemangiomas; however, fat overgrowth is not seen.

PITFALLS

- Extremity lesions do not usually demonstrate the classic patterns seen in the vertebrae and skull and may demonstrate multilocular areas of lucency with thin surrounding osseous trabeculae (reticular pattern), larger lucencies with more coarse osseous trabeculae (soap-bubble appearance), multiple well-defined areas of radiolucency without trabeculation, or (rarely) a pseudopermeative pattern resembling myeloma or metastatic disease.
- Extremity lesions in the medullary canal may demonstrate osseous expansion and endosteal scalloping.
- Blood-filled spaces with slow flow, as seen in cavernous lesions, are high signal intensity on T2-weighted images, whereas lesions with high flow (arteriovenous hemangiomas) show signal voids on all sequences.

Suggested Readings

Kaleem Z, Kyriakos M, Totty W. Solitary skeletal hemangioma of the extremities. Skeletal Radiol 2000;29:502–513

Murphey MD, Fairbairn K, Parman L, Baxter K, Parsa M, Smith S. Musculoskeletal angiomatous lesions: radiologic-pathologic correlation. Radiographics 1995;15:893–917

Wenger DE, Wold LE. Benign vascular lesions of bone: radiologic and pathologic features. Skeletal Radiol 2000;29:63–74

CASE 62

Anthony G. Ryan and Peter L. Munk

Clinical Presentation

A 29-year-old male snowboarder presented with an intermittent mass that "came and went" over a period of years, but that recently grew bigger and did not subside as usual. On examination, a large, minimally indentable firm swelling was palpable on the volar aspect of the wrist. The request read "suspected sarcoma."

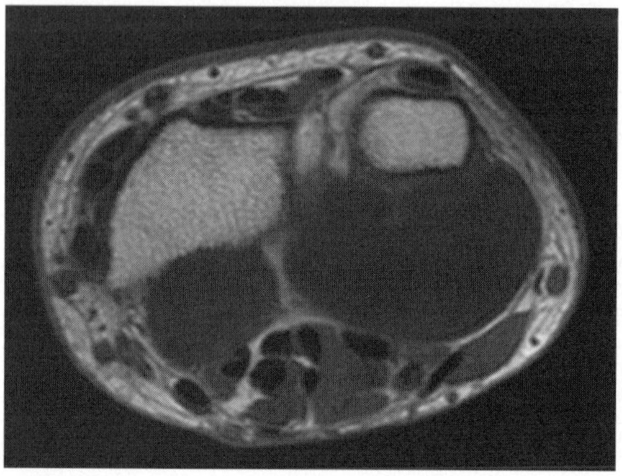

Figure 62A

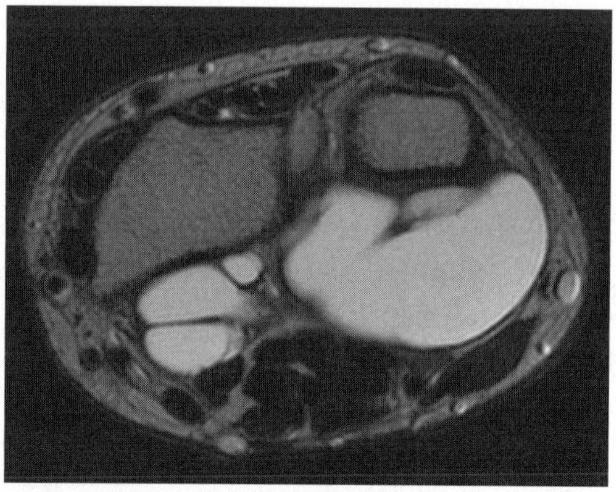

Figure 62B

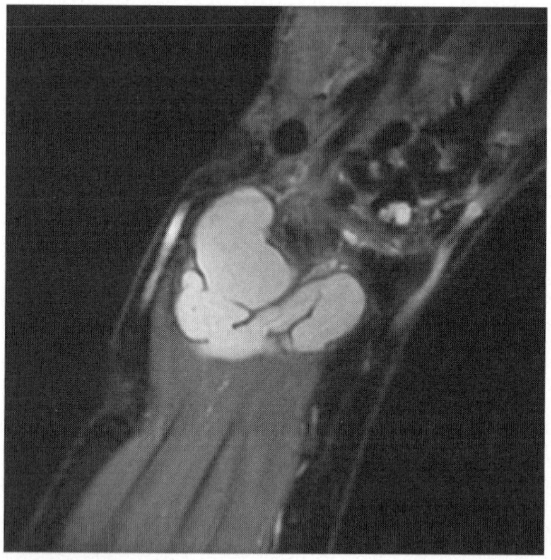

Figure 62C

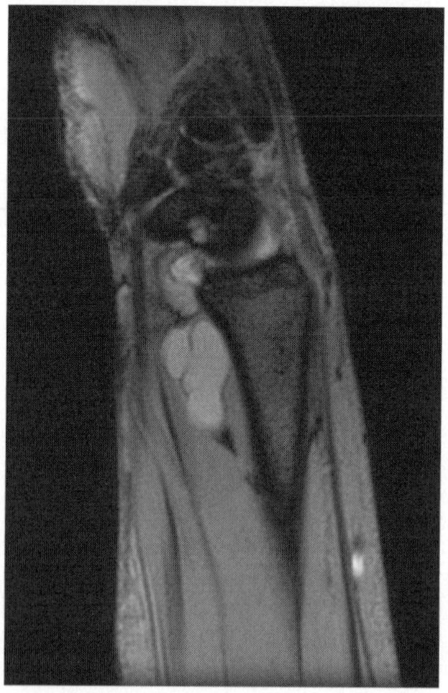

Figure 62D

Radiologic Findings

MRI examination of the wrist shows a large lobular septated lesion palmar to the distal radioulnar joint that returns low signal intensity on a transaxial T1-weighted image (**Fig. 62A**) and high signal intensity on a transaxial T2-weighted image (**Fig. 62B**) and a coronal T2-weighted image with fat saturation (**Fig. 62C**). Within the scaphoid is a further lesion demonstrating similar signal characteristics and which, on the sagittal MPGR image (**Fig. 62D**), appears to be in continuity with the larger lesion. Normal signal intensity is returned from the remainder of the scaphoid.

Diagnosis

Large soft-tissue ganglion in contiguity with a small intraosseous ganglion of the scaphoid.

Differential Diagnosis

None.

Discussion

Background

The most common tumor of the soft parts of the hand, soft-tissue ganglia are mucin-containing uni- or multilocular cysts lined by flat, spindle-shaped cells arising from a tendon sheath, a joint capsule, a bursa, or a subchondral bone. The term *synovial cyst* is used synonymously when the lesion arises from a herniated joint capsule with synovium in contiguity. Although some sources distinguish these lesions (ganglia and synovial cysts) on this basis, the imaging literature at large does not, and all lesions in this chapter are referred to as ganglia. Ganglia are most frequently found in relation to the hand, wrist (**Figs. 62E–62G**), or foot (**Figs. 62H–62K**).

An intraosseous ganglion is histologically identical to a soft-tissue ganglion but much less common, occurring in subchondral bone. Recognized as a potential source of mild pain, it occurs most frequently in the medial malleolus of the tibia, proximal tibia, femoral head, and acetabulum. Intraosseous ganglia have been described within the carpus and metacarpals. Of those occurring in the wrist, a scapholunate ganglion is relatively common, thought to be related to a tear of the dorsal scapholunate ligament.

Etiology

Both soft-tissue and intraosseous ganglia occur secondary to myxomatous degeneration of periarticular or intraosseous connective tissue, which is thought to happen as a result of repetitive trauma, possibly involving an ischemic element.

It is thought that, as a result of trauma, a focal defect in a joint capsule or ligament, combined with subsequent myxoid degeneration, gives rise to a synovial herniation. The latter theory is supported by studies demonstrating a significant association of ganglia with internal derangements

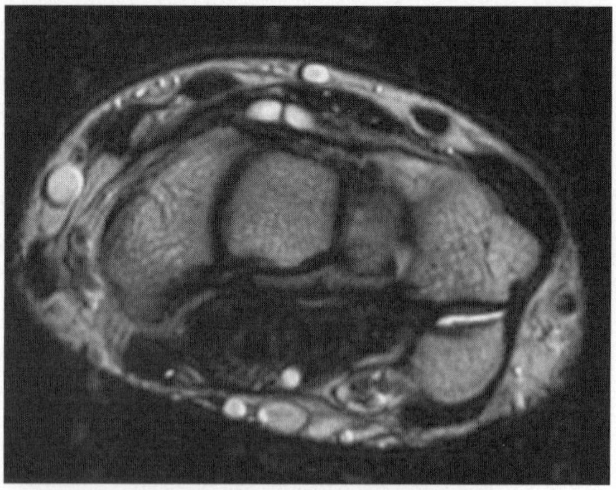

E

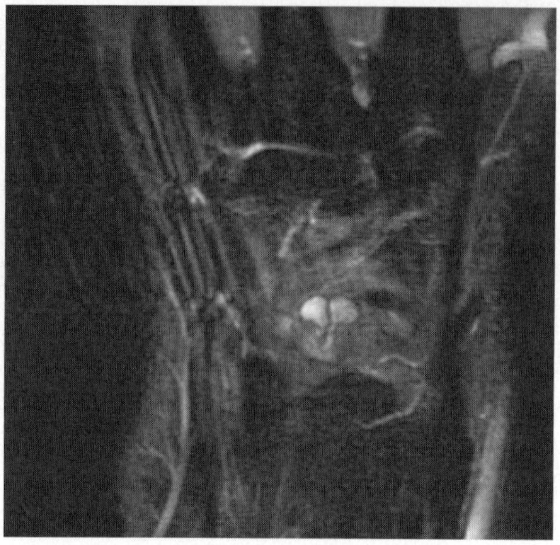

F

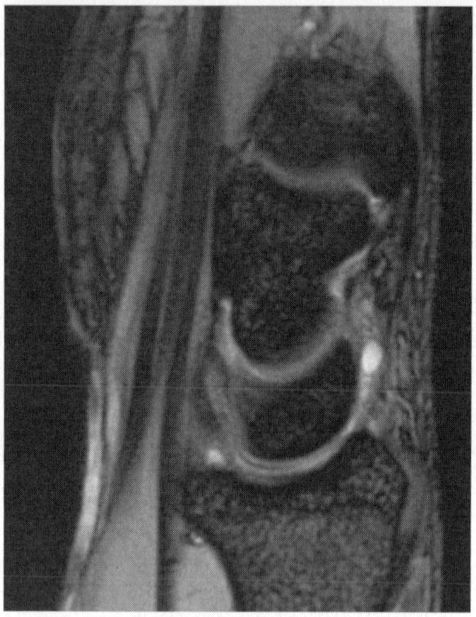

G

Figures 62E–62G Transaxial T2-weighted (**62E**), coronal STIR (**62F**), and sagittal MPGR (**62G**) images of the wrist show a very small bilobar ganglion arising from the dorsum of the carpus, which, despite its size, had been a cause of considerable discomfort for years. Subsequent arthrography (not shown) revealed a subtle tear of the dorsal scapholunate ligament.

of the wrist, where between 28 and 45% of ganglia are associated with tears of the triangular fibrocartilage complex, the scapholunate ligament, or the lunotriquetral ligament.

In the case of intraosseous ganglia, rather than an intrinsic osseous abnormality, it is thought that some arise secondary to erosion and penetration by an overlying soft-tissue ganglion, which may have been the etiology of the reference case (**Figs. 62A–62D**). This is not always the case, however, as intraosseous ganglia occur in the absence of associated soft-tissue ganglia.

Pathophysiology

When the fluid within the ganglion becomes tense, the lesion acts as a mass and can consequently give rise to considerable discomfort due to pressure effects on adjacent nerves or vessels. The mass may interfere with joint excursion and, as a result, interfere with a patient's occupation.

Clinical Findings

Ganglia are most common between the ages of 20 and 29. Although thought to be posttraumatic, many patients cannot remember an inciting incident. Ganglia tend to cause mild pain, usually after

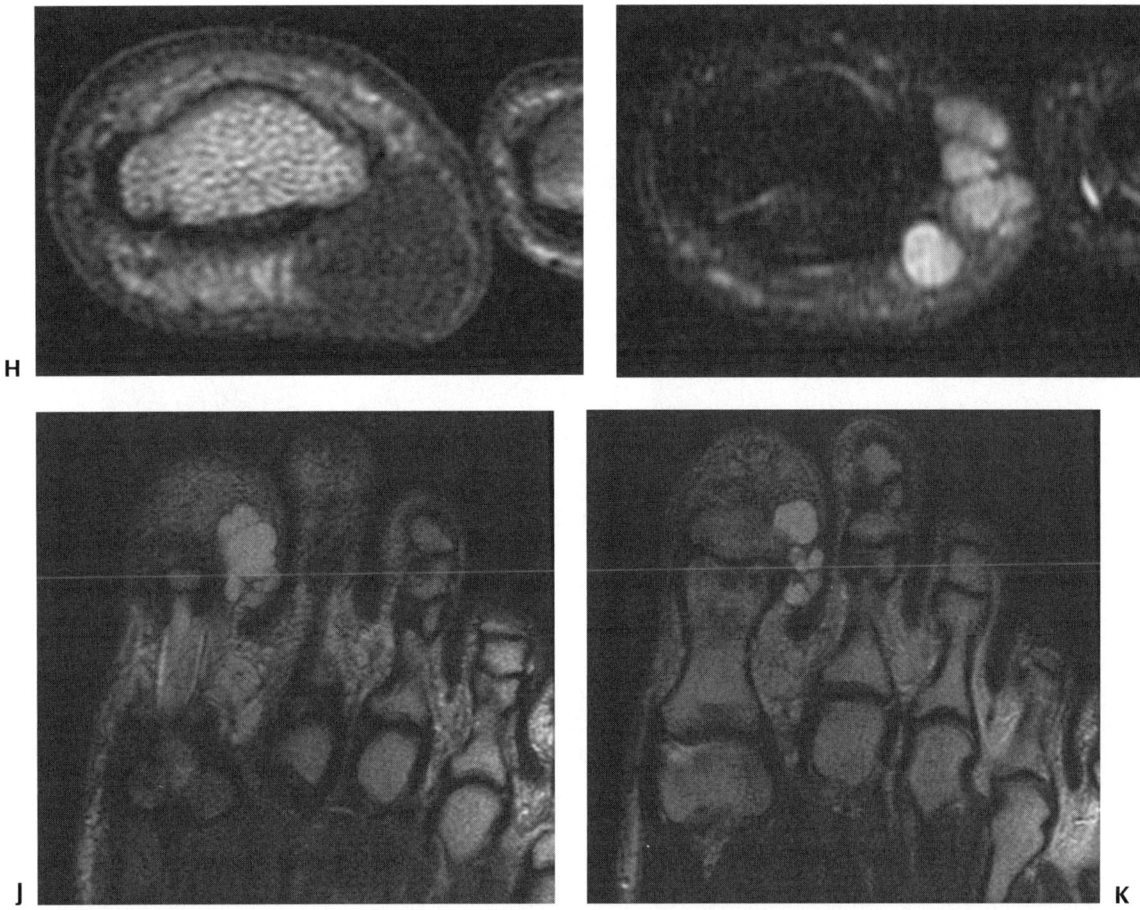

Figures 62H–62K Coronal T1-weighted fat-saturated (**62H**), coronal T2-weighted fat-saturated (**62I**), and transaxial T2-weighted (**62J** and **62K**) images of the great toe of the left foot in a 30-year-old woman complaining of chronic pain made worse by jogging, although the pain and swelling resolved with rest and elevation. The images show a moderate-sized multilocular ganglion arising from the interphalangeal joint. Although radiography had revealed no significant abnormality, the patient had been treated with orthotics as a result of a comment being made on the presence of a "Morton's foot" (second metatarsal projecting further distally than the first—a recognized cause of chronic foot pain in a jogger).

a period of repetitive motion of the adjacent joint. As above, the mass may be intermittent and resolve partly or completely over a period of time. On examination, the lesion may not be palpable or else may be grossly visible and be so hard on palpation as to be mistaken for a bony prominence (**Figs. 62L,62M**).

Transmitted pulsations from an underlying artery may be misleading and give rise to suspicion of a posttraumatic aneurysm.

Complications

Local pressure effects on adjacent bones, articulations, or neurovascular bundles may give rise to pain and/or paresthesias.

The latter is more likely to happen when a ganglion occurs in an anatomically restricted space, for example, in the carpal tunnel (producing carpal tunnel syndrome), the tarsal tunnel (producing tarsal tunnel syndrome), the Guyon's canal, or a spinoglenoid notch (**Fig. 62N).**

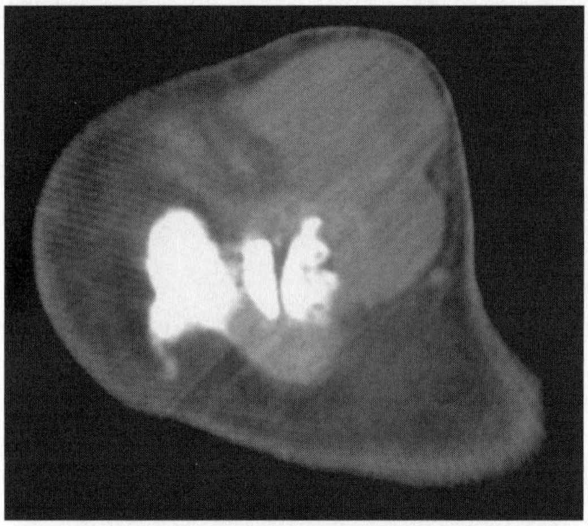
L

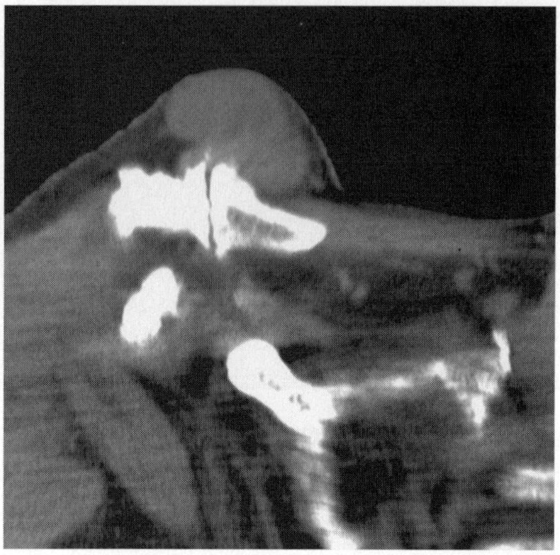
M

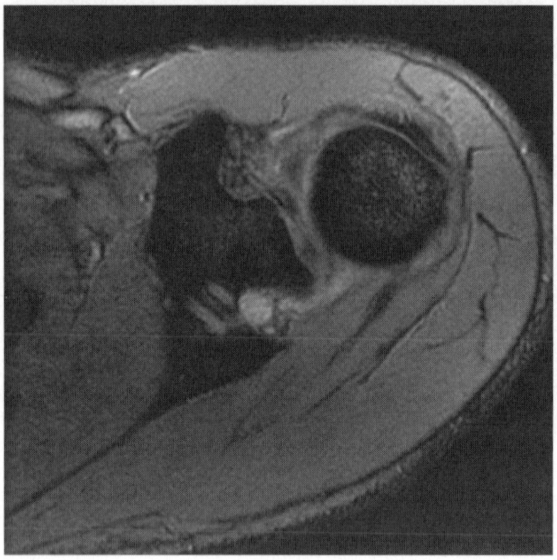
N

Figures 62L and **62M** Transaxial (**62L**) and coronal reformat (**62M**) of the right shoulder show a large multilocular ganglion arising from a clearly degenerate acromioclavicular joint. The hyperdensity in relation to the joint represents synovial hypertrophy. The lesion was thought to be a bony neoplasm, as it was so hard on examination. The patient experienced considerable relief from initial simple aspiration. **62N** Transaxial T2-weighted fat-saturated image shows a small spinoglenoid notch ganglion, giving rise to some weakness; however, no gross atrophy of the infraspinatus was evident.

Pathology

GROSS

These are uni- or multilocular cystic lesions surrounded by a thick fibrous wall usually attached to a joint or tendon sheath. They may contain internal septations. The fluid is not simple, having a consistency that is described variably as mucinous, gelatinous, or jelly-like. The communication to the underlying joint or tendon sheath is invariably tortuous and may be very difficult to track at excision.

MICROSCOPIC

Histologically, the cysts are lined by flat, spindle-shaped cells, frequently seen to be in contiguity with tendon sheath or joint capsule, and the contained fluid is composed predominantly of mucopolysaccharides.

The contained material of intraosseous ganglia differs slightly from the above in that the myxoid material becomes more fibrous, presumably because it is so much less mobile than that within soft-tissue ganglia.

Imaging Findings

RADIOGRAPHY

- Radiography is usually unremarkable.
- If the lesion is large enough, a soft-tissue mass may be demonstrable with surface resorption of adjacent bone, which may also demonstrate periosteal new bone formation.
- Rarely, calcification or ossification within the soft-tissue mass may be evident and may be florid, resembling myositis ossificans; however, this is atypical.
- Rarely, nitrogen gas may be evident within a ganglion secondary to communication with an underlying degenerate joint.
- Intraosseous ganglia tend to appear as solitary, subchondral juxta-articular lucent lesions with clear sclerotic margins.

ARTHROGRAPHY

- This modality may reveal communication with the joint or tendon sheath; however, additional delayed radiographs should be taken after the procedure, as circulation and adequate admixture of contrast may be inadequate or incomplete earlier, given the viscosity of the fluid within the ganglion. The patient is advised to exercise the joint in the interim.
- These delayed films are now rarely performed, as delayed CT is more sensitive and consequently preferred.

RADIONUCLIDE SCANNING

- 10% of intraosseous ganglia demonstrate increased uptake on technetium 99m–methylene diphosphonate scanning.

ULTRASOUND

- The cost-efficacy and real-time nature of ultrasound make it the ideal first line of investigation of suspected but clinically occult ganglia, where potential mimics of ganglia, for example, a compressible capsular recess, can be confidently distinguished.
- Given their fluid composition, superficial ganglia will be clearly demonstrated, and occasionally their communication to an underlying structure (tendon sheath or joint) may be identified.
- Although ganglia appear as focal hypoechoic, marginated collections, they are not as characteristically hypoechoic as the fluid around the tendon in tenosynovitis.
- Internal septations are frequently found.

COMPUTED TOMOGRAPHY

- CT arthrography with delayed acquisition 1 to 2 hours after arthrographic injection is a sensitive and reliable means of demonstrating communication of a ganglion with an underlying joint or tendon sheath.
- In patients who proceed directly to CT, even in the absence of intra-articular contrast, the communication with the underlying joint may be evident.
- The high protein content of the contained fluid can cause moderate internal hyperattenuation and heterogeneity (**Figs. 62L,62M**), as can the presence of septations, which enhance in keeping with the fibrous wall after intravenous contrast.

MAGNETIC RESONANCE IMAGING

- Given the fluid characteristics of the lesion and the soft-tissue resolution and multiplanar capacity of MRI, it is the investigation of choice in the identification of soft-tissue ganglia and their communication with underlying structures.

- In particular, ganglia in relation to complex joints, such as the wrist, and ganglia arising from unusual locations within large joints (e.g., the meniscofemoral ligament of Humphrey) are ideally suited to imaging assessment by MRI.
- Particular symptom complexes with ganglia as a potential cause, for example, carpal or tarsal tunnel symptom complexes, are ideally suited to investigation by MRI. In the latter, the presence of a ganglion within the tarsal tunnel arising from one of the many joints or tendon sheaths in the region (e.g., the flexor hallucis longus tendon) will be clearly evident, as will the site of its impingement on the posterior tibial nerve or its divisions (e.g., the medial calcaneal sensory branch(es) or the medial and lateral plantar nerves).
- It should be noted, however, that in small (0.5 mm or less) occult ganglia, ultrasound may have greater diagnostic confidence, especially when the examination is performed in real time.
- If the lesion has ruptured by the time of examination, considerable edema may be evident in the surrounding soft tissues, and the original lesion may be rendered inconspicuous.

Treatment

Because approximately one third of ganglia can be expected to resolve spontaneously, nonaggressive measures are usually pursued initially. Sudden force applied to the lesion, such as striking the visible lump with a heavy book in an attempt to cause rupture, was the classic treatment. Success is visible immediately, as the lesion should promptly disappear.

- The success is usually short-lived, as the lesions recur in 50 to 60% of cases.
- Aspiration has been utilized (e.g., of intra-articular ganglia of the knee) under both ultrasound and CT guidance, which provides temporary relief.
- At the time of aspiration, medications (e.g., steroids) have been injected, with variable success.
- Neither aspiration nor aspiration/injection is likely to provide lasting relief, as the lining of the lesion persists.

SURGICAL EXCISION

Surgical excision is the standard of care.

- The ideal procedure removes the whole cyst without rupture; however, the complex course of the track to the underlying joint makes this difficult, resulting in a recurrence rate of 5 to 20%.
- For this reason, more aggressive resections have been recommended, involving the excision of the ganglion in its entirety and its communication with adjacent synovium, along with pericystic tissue, including a wide rim of the joint capsule.
- It is reported that more aggressive resections give rise to a much-reduced recurrence rate without significantly increased joint instability.

Prognosis

- One third of ganglia are expected to resolve spontaneously.
- Although surgical excision is the standard of care, there remains a high recurrence rate of 5 to 20%.

PEARLS

- Although the contents of a ganglion tend to be anechoic, they are typically not as hypoechoic as the fluid seen around the tendon in tenosynovitis.
- Arthrography or CT arthrography with a view to establishing communication between a ganglion and the underlying joint or tendon sheath requires delayed imaging after contrast injection.
- An intraosseous ganglion is a rare cause of a fluid-fluid level in a periarticular lesion on MRI.

PITFALLS

- Posterior cruciate ligament (PCL) ganglion cysts may be simulated by pericruciate meniscal cysts. The latter will be suggested by the presence of an associated medial meniscal posterior horn horizontal tear. The site of communication between the cyst and the meniscal tear responsible will frequently be evident.
- The fluid within a ganglion may not return uniform low signal on T1-weighted images, as the high protein content may give rise to a variable intermediate signal. Similarly, multiple internal septations may return intermediate signal. These septations may enhance postintravenous gadolinium, in keeping with the surrounding wall.
- If the lesion has ruptured by the time of examination, considerable edema may be evident in the surrounding soft tissues, and the original lesion may be rendered inconspicuous.

Suggested Readings

Cardinal E, Buckwalter KA, Braunstein EM, Mih AD. Occult dorsal carpal ganglion: comparison of US and MR imaging. Radiology 1994;193:259–262

el-Noueam KI, Schweitzer ME, Blasbalg R, et al. Is a subset of wrist ganglia the sequela of internal derangements of the wrist joint? MR imaging findings. Radiology 1999;212:537–540

Erickson SJ, Quinn SF, Kneeland JB, et al. MR imaging of the tarsal tunnel and related spaces: normal and abnormal findings with anatomic correlation. Am J Roentgenol 1990;155:323–328

Malghem J, Vandeberg BC, Lebon C, Lecouvet FE, Maldague BE. Ganglion cysts of the knee: articular communication revealed by delayed radiography and CT after arthrography. Am J Roentgenol 1998;170:1579–1583

CASE 63

George Nomikos, Anthony G. Ryan, Peter L. Munk, and Mark Murphey

Clinical Presentation

A skeletally immature male presented with a knee pain complaint.

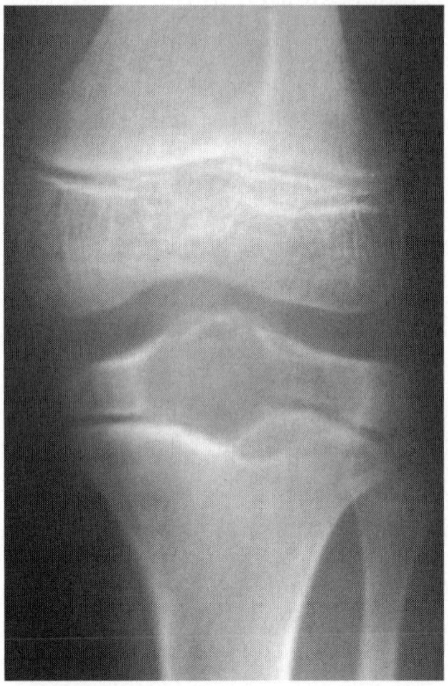

Figure 63A

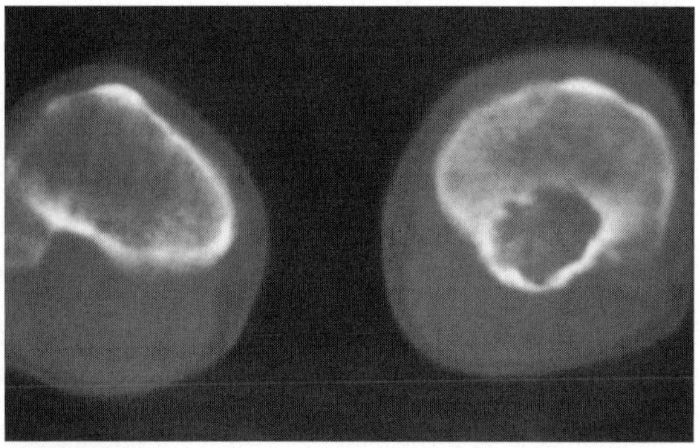

Figure 63B

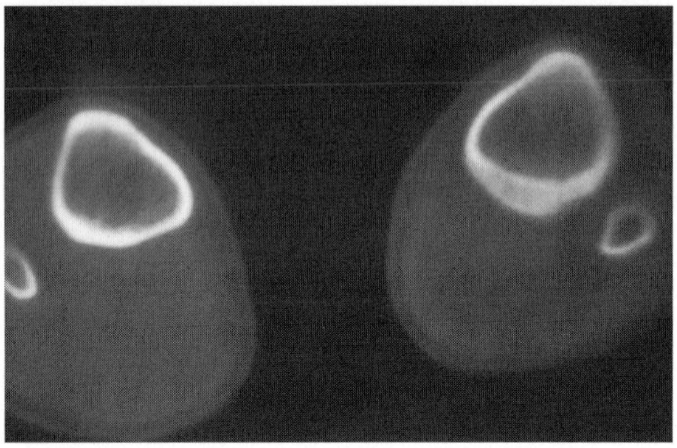

Figure 63C

Radiologic Findings

Radiologic work-up shows a lytic lesion in the proximal tibial epiphysis that has a narrow zone of transition with a mild rim of surrounding sclerosis (**Fig. 63A**). The lesion does not cross the physis. There is faint punctate mineralization in the lesion, better seen on the CT scan (**Fig. 63B**), with an appearance of chondroid matrix. There is also marked cortical thinning caused by the lesion posteriorly. There is no evidence of cortical penetration. CT scan obtained through the tibia more distally (**Fig. 63C**) shows smooth, thick, nonaggressive periosteal reaction along the tibial shaft distal to the lesion.

Diagnosis

Chondroblastoma.

Differential Diagnosis

- Clear cell chondrosarcoma
- Langerhans' cell histiocytosis
- Giant cell tumor
- Subchondral cyst/ganglion
- Brodie's abscess

Discussion

Background

Chondroblastoma is an uncommon benign primary neoplasm of bone, accounting for ~1% of all primary bone tumors. Most lesions arise in the epiphysis or apophysis of long tubular bones. The knee accounts for ~30 to 40% of cases. The femur is the most commonly involved bone (33% of all cases and equally divided between proximal and distal locations), followed by the humerus and tibia. The talus and calcaneus are common sites of involvement in the hindfoot. Equivalent epiphyseal and apophyseal locations such as the patella and greater trochanter of the femur are not uncommon. Isolated metaphyseal involvement is uncommon (10% in our experience). The hands and feet account for 10% of lesions.

Clinical Findings

Although the reported age range is broad, most patients are in their second decade of life at the time of diagnosis, and 90% of all lesions occur in patients between 5 and 25 years of age. Chondroblastoma is 1.4 to 2.0 times more common in men than in women. The most common presenting symptoms are pain, swelling, and limited range of motion. Muscle wasting may also be seen.

Pathology

The characteristic cell is the immature cartilage cell termed the chondroblast. Lesions typically consist of tightly packed mononuclear cells. The high degree of cellularity is different from many other cartilage lesions (except for chondromyxoid fibroma, which may also have similar high cellularity). The nuclei of the chondroblasts have a characteristic longitudinal cleft ("coffee bean" appearance). Areas of calcification, metaplastic bone, fibrosis, and necrosis may be seen, and areas of secondary aneurysmal bone cyst formation or serous cyst formation are common. Chondroblastoma demonstrates a typical "chicken wire" pattern of calcification when stained with sulfate.

Imaging Findings

RADIOGRAPHY

- Central or eccentric lytic lesion centered in the epiphysis or epiphyseal equivalent (apophysis or sesamoid) with a narrow zone of transition with or without surrounding sclerosis
- Lesions often show internal trabeculation and extend to the subchondral bone plate.
- Metaphyseal extension is seen in up to 55% of cases.

- Calcification is visible in 30 to 50% of cases.
- Mature-appearing, nonaggressive periosteal reaction is common and is often identified away from the lesion along the diametaphysis.
- The etiology of the periosteal reaction may be secondary to the marked inflammatory response often seen around these lesions.
- Pathologic fractures and soft-tissue masses are rare.

COMPUTED TOMOGRAPHY

- Cortical thinning caused by endosteal scalloping is often identified on CT.
- Calcification is very common (81 to 92%) but may be subtle.
- CT may demonstrate fluid levels or low attenuation regions if cystic (serous or secondary aneurysmal bone cyst) areas are present; however, solid components should also be identifiable.

MAGNETIC RESONANCE IMAGING

- Homogeneous and similar to muscle in signal intensity on T1-weighted images
- Heterogeneous on T2-weighted images
- The solid portion of the lesion remains low to intermediate signal intensity on T2-weighted images in the vast majority of cases (95% of cases in our experience) (**Fig. 63D**).
- Low to intermediate signal intensity on T2-weighted images may be due to hypercellularity or fibrosis in the tumor.
- Cyst formation and secondary aneurysmal bone cyst formation are very common.
- Secondary aneurysmal bone cyst areas are seen as fluid levels, regions of low or high signal on T1-weighted images, and marked high signal on T2-weighted images (**Fig. 63E**).
- Extensive inflammatory changes in the surrounding bone marrow (**Fig. 63F**) and soft tissues are commonly seen, as is adjacent joint effusion.
- The solid portions of the lesion enhance diffusely and homogeneously after contrast administration, whereas the cystic portions enhance peripherally and septally (**Fig. 63G**).

Treatment and Prognosis

- Treatment usually consists of curettage and placement of bone graft or methylmethacrylate.
- Cryosurgery or phenolization is also used to extend resection margins.
- Risk of recurrence is reportedly increased with lesions located in the proximal femur or pelvis.
- Metastatic disease is extremely rare, but when it occurs, it is most commonly in the lungs (benign metastasizing chondroblastoma).
- Redevelopment of bone marrow reaction/edema may herald tumor recurrence.

PEARLS

- Chondroblastoma is a central or eccentric lytic lesion centered in the epiphysis or epiphyseal equivalent (apophysis or sesamoid) with a narrow zone of transition, with or without surrounding sclerosis.
- These lesions are homogeneous and similar to muscle in signal intensity on T1-weighted images. They are heterogeneous on T2-weighted images. The solid portions of the lesion enhance diffusely and homogeneously after contrast administration, whereas the cystic portions enhance peripherally and septally.
- Redevelopment of bone marrow reaction/edema may herald tumor recurrence.

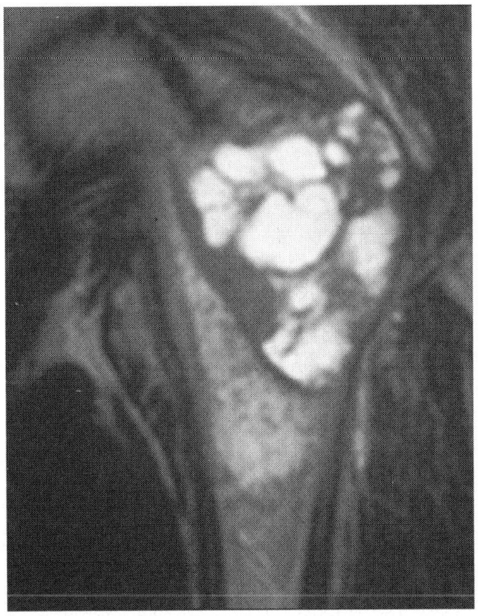

D

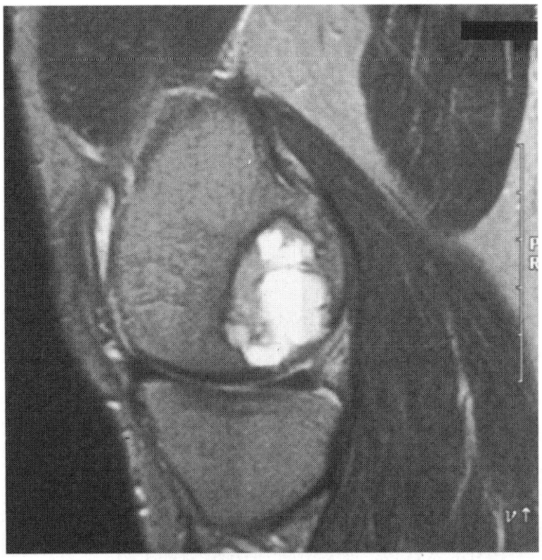

E

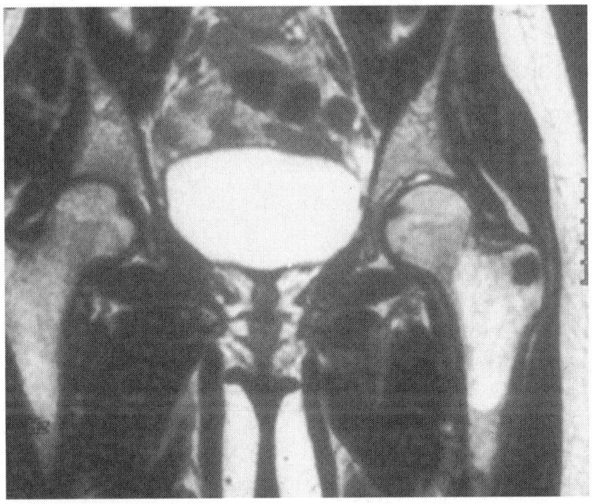

F

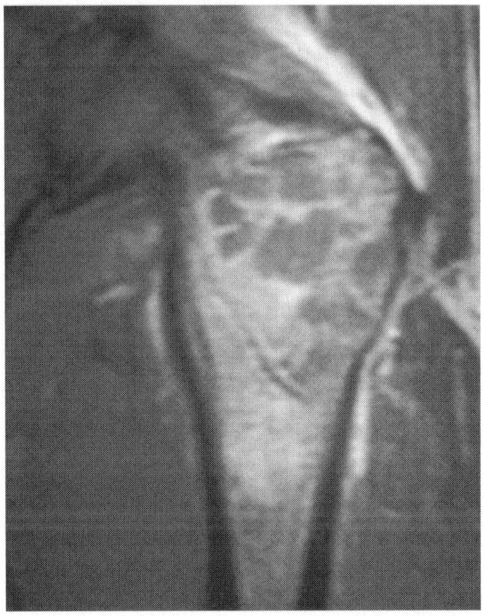

G

Figures 63D A coronal T2-weighted image of a chondroblastoma originating in the greater trochanter apophysis shows high signal change evincing cyst and secondary aneurysmal bone cyst formation, with the residual solid portion of the lesion visible medially as a focus of low to intermediate signal intensity. **63E** A sagittal T2-weighted image shows a further example of cyst and secondary aneurysmal bone cyst formation in a lesion arising in the distal femoral epiphysis. **63F** A coronal T2-weighted image shows the solid portion of a greater trochanteric chondroblastoma as a low-signal focus and extensive inflammatory changes in the bone marrow caudad to the lesion as diffuse high signal. No soft-tissue edema or joint effusion is present in this case; the latter is less common in apophyseal compared with epiphyseal lesions. **63G** A sagittal T1-weighted image of the hip in the same patient as in **63D** shows the diffuse and homogeneous enhancement of the solid portions of the lesion after contrast administration, whereas the cystic portions enhance peripherally and septally.

PITFALLS

- Although metaphyseal extension may be seen in up to 55% of cases, isolated involvement is seen in only 10%.
- Although periosteal reaction is common secondary to the marked inflammatory response, it is mature-appearing and nonaggressive.

- The solid portion of the lesion remains low to intermediate signal intensity on T2-weighted images in the vast majority of cases. This may represent either hypercellularity or fibrosis, the latter a potential pitfall when biopsying these lesions.

Suggested Readings

Brien EW, Mirra JM, Kerr R. Benign and malignant cartilage tumors of bone and joint: their anatomic and theoretical basis with an emphasis on radiology, pathology and clinical biology. I. The intramedullary tumors. Skeletal Radiol 1997;26:325–353

Brower AC, Moser RP, Kransdorf MJ. The frequency and diagnostic significance of periostitis in chondroblastoma. Am J Roentgenol 1990;154:309–314

Giudici MA, Moser RP Jr, Kransdorf MJ. Cartilagenous bone tumors. Radiol Clin North Am 1993;31:237–259

Jee WH, Park YK, McCauley TR, et al. Chondroblastoma: MR characteristics with pathologic correlation. J Comput Assist Tomogr 1999;23:721–726

Oxtoby JW, Davies AM. MRI characteristics of chondroblastoma. Clin Radiol 1996;51:22–26

Robbin MR, Murphey MD. Benign chondroid neoplasms of bone. Semin Musculoskelet Radiol 2000;4:45–58

Weatherall PT, Maale GE, Mendelsohn DB, Sherry CS, Erdman WE, Pascoe ER. Chondroblastoma: classic and confusing appearance at MR imaging. Radiology 1994;190:467–474

Yamamura S, Sato K, Sugiura H, Iwata H. Inflammatory reaction in chondroblastoma. Skeletal Radiol 1996;25:371–376

CASE 64

George Nomikos, Anthony G. Ryan, Peter L. Munk, and Mark Murphey

Clinical Presentation

A 21-year-old man presented with progressive inferior displacement of the right globe.

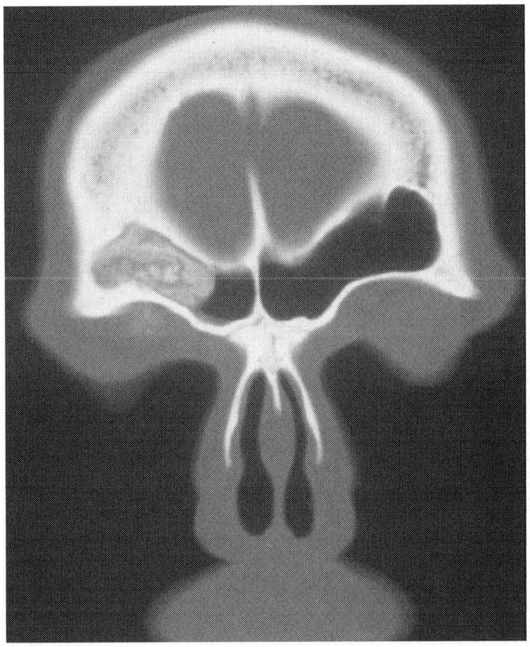

Figure 64A

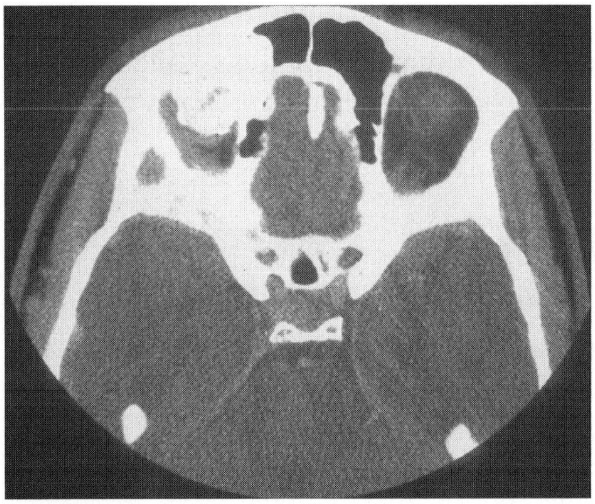

Figure 64B

Radiologic Findings

CT scans of the sinuses (**Fig. 64A**, coronal, and **Fig. 64B**, axial) reveal a dense, homogeneously mineralized mass in the right frontal sinus that is extending through the roof of the orbit and displacing the globe inferiorly. The overlying cortical bone remains intact. The mineralization has a cloudlike appearance, consistent with osteoid mineralization. The lesion has a nonaggressive appearance without associated periosteal reaction or soft-tissue mass.

Diagnosis

Osteoma.

Differential Diagnosis

- Parosteal osteosarcoma
- Osteochondroma

- Periosteal osteoblastoma
- Ossified parosteal lipoma
- Myositis ossificans
- Calcified meningioma (when on the inner table of the skull)

Discussion

Background

Osteomas are benign osteoid-producing tumors that arise on the surface of bone and are composed of mature lamellar bone. These lesions most commonly occur in the frontal or ethmoid sinuses (75%), skull, and jaw, although they occasionally occur in the appendicular skeleton. There is an association between multiple osteomas and Gardner's syndrome, which is an autosomal dominant condition characterized by multiple colonic polyps (with an increased propensity to malignant degeneration), soft-tissue desmoid tumors (both intra- and extra-abdominal), and multiple osteomas. There is also an association between tuberous sclerosis and the development of osteomas. There is no risk of malignant degeneration.

Clinical Findings

Lesions are often asymptomatic. Sinus lesions may block drainage and cause sinusitis, headache, pain, and even mucocele formation. They also occasionally extend into the orbit (as in this case) or cranium. Osteomas rarely compress the optic nerve, causing visual loss, and may be associated with loss of smell.

Pathology

These lesions are composed of mature lamellar-type bone (that may occasionally contain haversian systems) with a thin surrounding rim of spindle cells. The chief distinguishing feature of osteomas is the lack of densely collagenized stroma that is characteristic of parosteal osteosarcoma, along with the location in the skull and face.

Imaging Findings

RADIOGRAPHY

- Dense sclerotic mass arising on the surface of the involved bone
- Margins may be smooth or lobulated.

COMPUTED TOMOGRAPHY

- Homogeneously ossified surface lesion without internal lucencies
- Densely mineralized both peripherally and centrally
- Often demonstrates a mushroom shape with a stalk of connection to the underlying bone
- Lack of corticomedullary continuity with the underlying bone as seen in osteochondroma
- Lack of medullary backgrowth (medullary backgrowth is often seen with parosteal osteosarcoma)
- No contrast enhancement

MAGNETIC RESONANCE IMAGING

- Very low signal intensity on T1- and T2-weighted images, similar to cortical bone

Treatment and Prognosis

- Symptomatic lesions may be treated with local resection.
- Peripheral lesions should be adequately biopsied or completely excised because of the similarity in appearance to parosteal osteosarcoma.

PEARLS

- There is an association between multiple osteomas and Gardner's syndrome, which is an autosomal dominant condition characterized by multiple colonic polyps (with an increased propensity to malignant degeneration), soft-tissue desmoid tumors (both intra- and extra-abdominal), and multiple osteomas.
- There is also an association between tuberous sclerosis and the development of osteomas.
- The chief distinguishing feature of osteomas is the lack of densely collagenized stroma that is characteristic of parosteal osteosarcoma, along with the location in the skull and face.
- The lesion is densely mineralized both peripherally and centrally, differentiating it from myositis ossificans.

PITFALLS

- There is a lack of corticomedullary continuity with the underlying bone as seen in osteochondroma.
- There is a lack of medullary backgrowth as often seen with parosteal osteosarcoma.
- Despite the differentiating features, peripheral lesions should be adequately biopsied or completely excised because of the similarity in appearance to parosteal osteosarcoma.

Suggested Readings

Avrahami E, Even A. Osteoma of the inner table of the skull—CT diagnosis. Clin Radiol 2000;55:435–438

Greenspan A. Benign bone-forming lesions—osteoma, osteoid osteoma, and osteoblastoma: clinical, imaging, pathologic, and differential considerations. Skeletal Radiol 1993;22:485–500

Sundaram M, Falbo S, McDonald D, Janney C. Surface osteomas of the appendicular skeleton. Am J Roentgenol 1996;167:1529–1533

White LM, Kandel R. Osteoid-producing tumors of bone. Semin Musculoskelet Radiol 2000;4:25–43

CASE 65

George Nomikos, Anthony G. Ryan, Peter L. Munk, and Mark Murphey

Clinical Presentation

A 14-year-old boy presented with a several-month history of pain in the left thigh. He reported that the pain was worse at night and that it responded temporarily to ibuprofen.

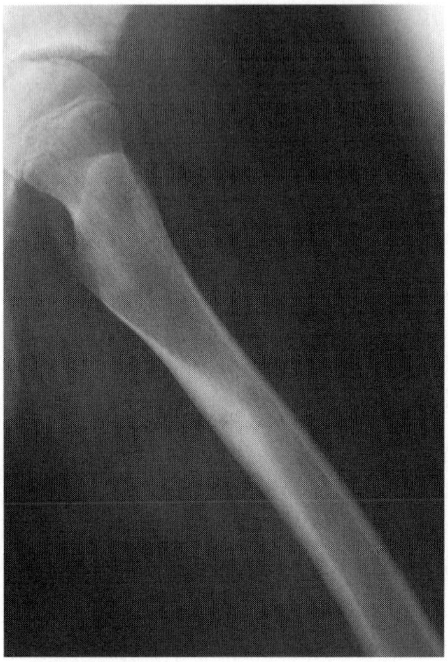

Figure 65A

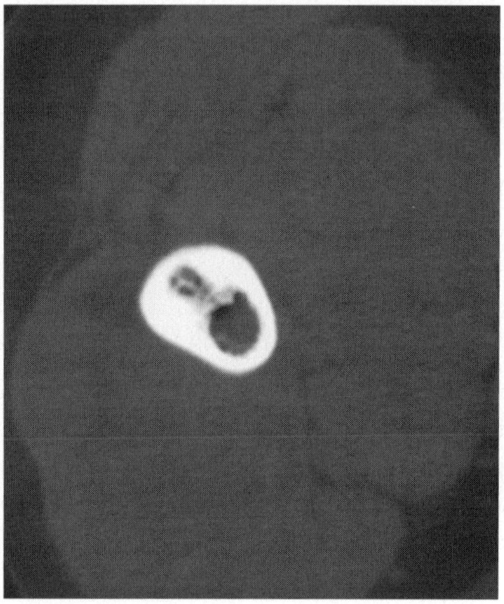

Figure 65B

Radiologic Findings

The radiograph demonstrates a long area of cortical thickening and mature-appearing periosteal reaction in the left proximal femoral cortex (**Fig. 65A**). In this area of dense new bone formation is a small central cortical lucency. A CT scan (**Fig. 65B**) shows the small radiolucent nidus surrounded by marked mature-appearing new bone formation. Note the central calcification in the radiolucent nidus.

Diagnosis

Osteoid osteoma.

Differential Diagnosis

- Infection (Brodie's abscess)
- Langerhans' cell histiocytosis
- Intracortical osteosarcoma

Discussion

Background

Osteoid osteoma represents the third most common bone tumor, after osteochondroma and nonossifying fibroma, and accounts for ~10 to 11% of all benign bone tumors. The majority of lesions are cortically based. Cortical lesions most commonly (70 to 80%) occur in the diaphysis of long tubular bones, particularly the femur (intertrochanteric region), tibia, and humerus. The posterior elements of the spine account for 10% of lesions. Lesions may also occur in an intramedullary, subperiosteal (most common along the femoral neck or talus), or intra-articular (intertrochanteric regions particularly) location.

Clinical Findings

The classical presentation is a several-month history of dull, aching pain, at its most severe at night, relieved by aspirin or other nonsteroidal anti-inflammatory medications. Children may also present with a limp. Bowing or varus/valgus deformities, as well as leg length discrepancies (with the affected limb being longer), are not uncommon. Intra-articular lesions (**Fig. 65C**) may cause synovitis, joint effusion, and joint pain, whereas spinal lesions classically produce painful scoliosis (concave to the side of the lesion). This scoliosis characteristically worsens in the supine position relative to the erect position, unlike patients with idiopathic scoliosis, in whom the scoliosis is worse when the patient is standing. Although there is a broad age range of reported cases, most lesions occur in the first three decades of life, and ~70% of patients are younger than age 20 at the time of diagnosis.

Pathology

The central nidus is composed of osteoid surrounded by extensive osteoblastic rimming, mineralized matrix, and prominent fibrovascular stroma. The surrounding bone demonstrates reactive changes

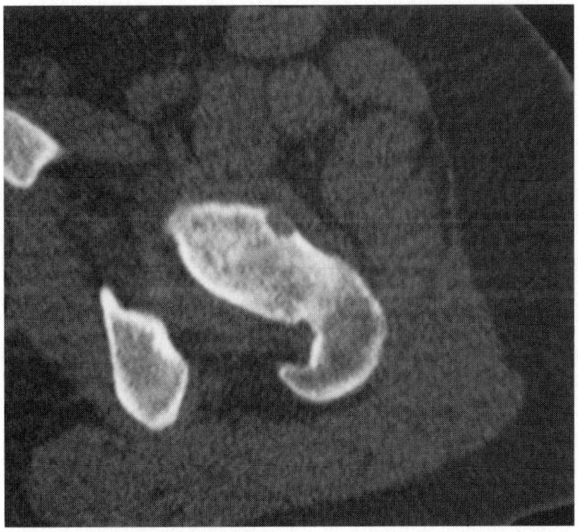

Figure 65C Transaxial CT in a young girl with severe hip pain on both motion and at rest demonstrating an anterior femoral cortical osteoid osteoma and a very small joint effusion (best seen posteriorly).

and new bone formation. Nerve fibers are also present in the nidus. These lesions release prostaglandins that increase vascular pressure in the surrounding tissue, which may in turn stimulate the nerves in the lesion and be the cause of severe pain. This theory is supported by the strong effect that nonsteroidal anti-inflammatory medications have on reducing pain in these patients.

Imaging Findings

RADIOGRAPHY

- Intracortical lesions typically appear as a small (< 1.0- to 1.5-cm), round or oval, radiolucent nidus surrounded by reactive sclerosis and cortical and periosteal thickening.
- Central calcification in the nidus is often very difficult to see on radiographs.
- Because of the lack of functional surrounding periosteum, intra-articular and intramedullary lesions are not associated with prominent cortical thickening or reactive bone formation, although joint effusion, synovitis, and periarticular osteopenia are common.
- Intramedullary lesions typically do not demonstrate significant surrounding sclerosis (except lesions located in the posterior elements of the spine).

COMPUTED TOMOGRAPHY

- The best modality for demonstrating the radiolucent nidus and central punctate mineralization in the nidus
- Large amount of surrounding sclerosis and new bone formation in typical intracortical lesions
- 1- to 1.5-mm scans should be performed through the region of reactive bone formation to localize the nidus.

MAGNETIC RESONANCE IMAGING

- Less useful in detection of lesion nidus than CT
- May demonstrate nonspecific surrounding inflammatory change, which may involve the surrounding bone and soft tissues, representing inflammatory cell infiltrate
- Intense surrounding inflammatory change on MRI (**Fig. 65D**), which is especially prominent in patients younger than age 15, may lead to a false impression of a more aggressive lesion (see **Table 65–1**).
- The nidus is typically low to intermediate on T1-weighted images and variable on T2-weighted images.
- Variability on T2-weighted images may be related to age, vascularity, and calcification of the nidus.

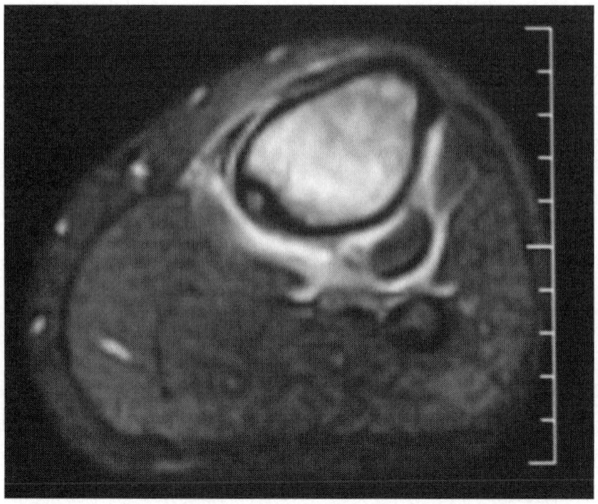

Figure 65D Transaxial T2-weighted image of the midcalf in a 9-year-old girl with a posteromedial tibial osteoid osteoma demonstrating intense surrounding inflammatory change within the underlying marrow edema and the surrounding soft tissues. The nidus is seen as an intermediate signal intensity lesion with surrounding low signal intensity sclerosis.

Table 65–1 Benign Lesions Commonly Demonstrating Intense Surrounding Inflammatory Change on MRI

Osteoid osteoma
Chondroblastoma
Osteoblastoma
Langerhans' cell histiocytosis
Brodie's abscess
Stress fracture

- Nonspecific joint effusion and synovitis are seen with intra-articular lesions.
- Dynamic gadolinium enhancement may improve the ability to identify the nidus, which shows enhancement that may be marked.

SCINTIGRAPHY

- Increased activity on all three phases of bone scan
- The delayed images may demonstrate very intense uptake in the nidus, with a surrounding area of less intense uptake in the region of reactive change (double-uptake sign).

Treatment and Prognosis

- Surgical excision of the nidus has been the standard treatment; however, the nidus can be difficult to localize at surgery.
- Preoperative CT localization, tetracycline labeling, and scintigraphic techniques have all been employed to improve lesion conspicuity at the time of surgery.
- CT-guided radiofrequency (RF) ablation is currently a popular alternative to surgery, with a success rate equal to or better than surgery, a minimal complication rate, and a rapid recovery period.
- RF ablation is accomplished by passing an RF probe into the nidus under CT guidance, then heating the lesion using RF energy (standard protocol is 90°C for 6 minutes) (**Fig. 65E**).

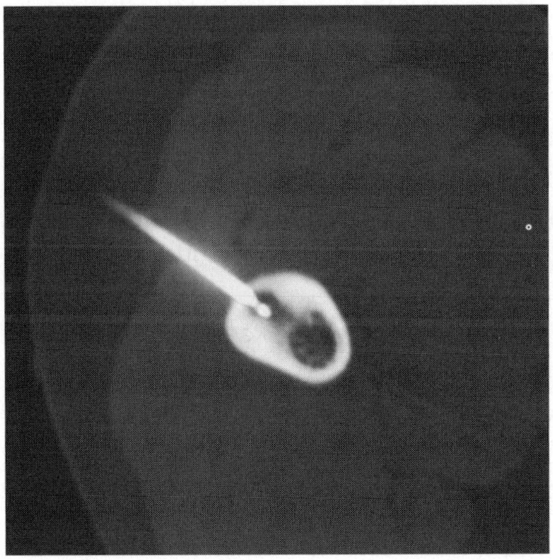

Figure 65E Intraprocedural transaxial CT image during a radiofrequency ablation procedure demonstrating the tip of a single fiber probe in the nidus during ablation.

- Untreated lesions may spontaneously regress; however, complications may include leg length discrepancies, deformities, premature arthritis (intra-articular lesions), personality disturbances, and side effects from long-term anti-inflammatory use.

PEARLS

- The scoliosis associated with a spinal osteoid osteoma characteristically worsens in the supine relative to the erect position, unlike patients with idiopathic scoliosis in whom the scoliosis is worse when the patient is standing.
- Dynamic gadolinium enhancement may improve the ability to identify the nidus, showing enhancement that may be marked.
- The delayed images of a radionuclide bone scan may demonstrate very intense uptake in the nidus, with a surrounding area of less intense uptake in the region of reactive change (double-uptake sign).

PITFALLS

- The central calcification in the nidus is often very difficult to see on radiographs.
- Because of the lack of functional surrounding periosteum, intra-articular and intramedullary lesions are not associated with prominent cortical thickening or reactive bone formation (**Fig. 65C**), although joint effusion, synovitis, and periarticular osteopenia are common.
- Intramedullary lesions typically do not demonstrate significant surrounding sclerosis (except lesions located in the posterior elements of the spine).
- Intense surrounding inflammatory change on MRI may lead to a false impression of a more aggressive lesion.

Suggested Readings

Assoun J, Richardi G, Railhac J, et al. Osteoid osteoma: MR imaging versus CT. Radiology 1994;191:217–223

Davies M, Cassar-Pullicino V, Davies A, McCall I, Tyrrell P. The diagnostic accuracy of MR imaging in osteoid osteoma. Skeletal Radiol 2002;31:559–569

Ehara S, Rosenthal D, Aoki J, et al. Peritumoral edema in osteoid osteoma on magnetic resonance imaging. Skeletal Radiol 1999;28:265–270

Frassica FJ, Waltrip RL, Sponseller PD, Ma LD, McCarthy EF Jr. Clinicopathologic features and treatment of osteoid osteoma and osteoblastoma in children and adolescents. Orthop Clin North Am 1996;27:559–574

Klein MH, Shankman S. Osteoid osteoma: radiologic and pathologic correlation. Skeletal Radiol 1992;21:23–31

Rosenthal D, Hornicek F, Wolfe M, Jennings L, Gebhart M, Mankin H. Percutaneous radiofrequency coagulation of osteoid osteoma compared with operative treatment. J Bone Joint Surg Am 1999;81:437–438

White LM, Kandel R. Osteoid-producing tumors of bone. Semin Musculoskelet Radiol 2000;4:25–43

Woertler K, Vestrig T, Boettner F, Winkelmann W, Heindel W, Lindner N. Osteoid osteoma: CT-guided percutaneous radiofrequency ablation and follow-up in 47 patients. J Vasc Interv Radiol 2001;12:717–722

CASE 66

George Nomikos, Anthony G. Ryan, Peter L. Munk, and Mark Murphey

Clinical Presentation

An 18-year-old man presented with a history of trauma to the knee 1 year previously. He had noticed progressive development of a painful soft-tissue mass posteriorly in the knee since that time.

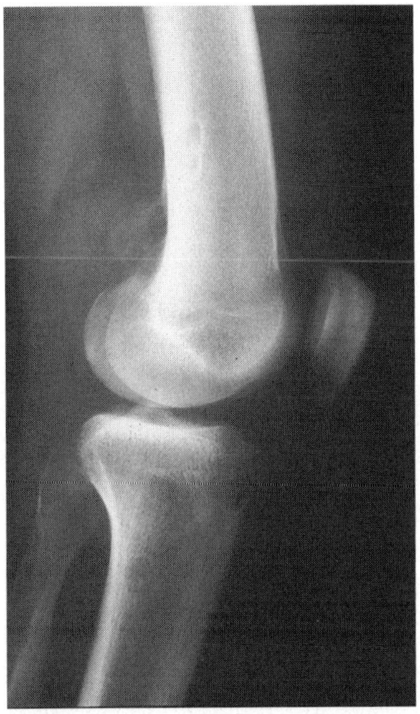

Figure 66A

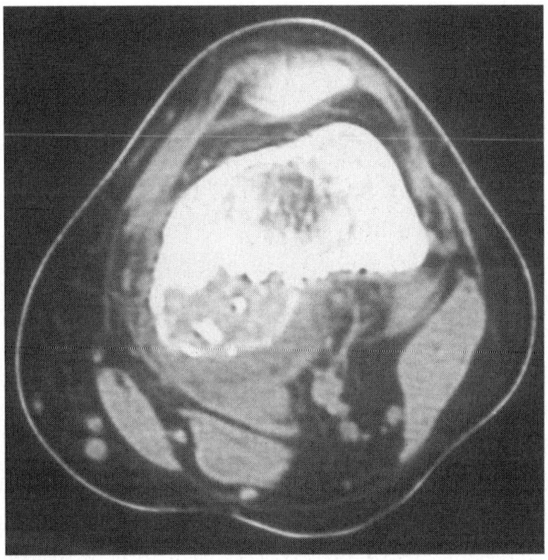

Figure 66B

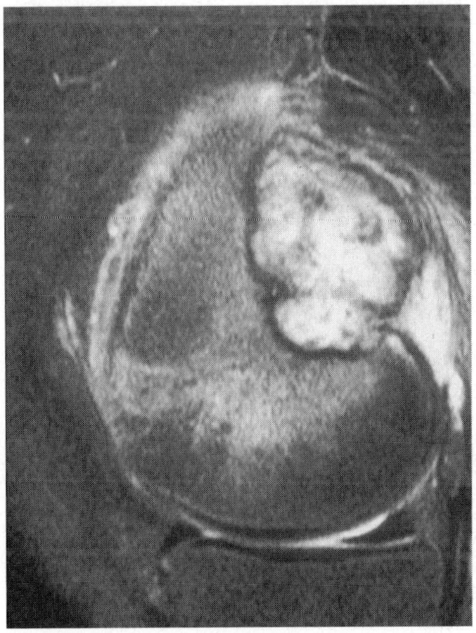

Figure 66C

Radiologic Findings

The lateral radiograph of the knee (**Fig. 66A**) shows a large expansile mass arising from the posterior surface of the distal femur. There is punctate mineralization in the mass as well as an intact surrounding rim of bone. The CT scan (**Fig. 66B**) confirms that the lesion is arising from the surface of the femur and demonstrates the internal mineralization. The nonmineralized portion of the mass has an attenuation similar to skeletal muscle. The lesion is predominantly high signal on the sagittal T2-weighted image (**Fig. 66C**). There is marked surrounding inflammatory reaction and edema, in both the soft tissues and bone. The low signal intensity areas correspond to regions of mineralization.

Diagnosis

Subperiosteal osteoblastoma.

Differential Diagnosis

- Periosteal chondroma
- Chondromyxoid fibroma
- Surface osteosarcoma
- Aneurysmal bone cyst (ABC)

Discussion

Background

Osteoblastomas are rare primary bone neoplasms, accounting for $< 1\%$ of all bone tumors and $\sim 3.5\%$ of all benign bone tumors. They are pathologically similar to osteoid osteomas but are larger. Lesions commonly occur in the long tubular bones (34%), spine and sacrum (30%), facial bones (especially the mandible) and skull (15%), small bones of the hands and feet (10%), and pelvis (5%). As with osteoid osteoma, pelvic osteoblastomas often arise in a periacetabular region. Spinal lesions most commonly involve the posterior elements alone (55%), with the remainder usually involving the posterior elements with extension into the vertebral body. Isolated vertebral body involvement is rare. Long bone lesions are diaphyseal (75%) or metaphyseal. The femur is the most commonly involved long bone. Lesions may be intramedullary, cortical, or subperiosteal in location.

Clinical Findings

Most patients present with complaints of a dull, aching pain and, depending on the location, a palpable mass. Symptoms similar to those of an osteoid osteoma are less common. Spinal lesions may cause scoliosis, muscle spasm, and neurologic symptoms. Gait disturbances are also reported. Although the reported age distribution is wide, most tumors occur in patients in their third decade of life. There is a 2:1 to 3:1 male-to-female ratio. Osteoblastoma is one of the tumors associated with oncogenic osteomalacia (see case 59). Toxic osteoblastoma is an uncommon variant in which patients experience severe systemic symptoms, including fever, leukocytosis, weight loss, anemia, cachexia, and generalized periosteal reaction, that remit when the tumor is removed.

Pathology

Lesions are typically composed of long, thick, interconnecting osteoid trabeculae that are lined by a single layer of osteoblasts. Although these osteoblasts are usually benign in appearance, some may appear atypical. Islands of chondroid matrix or hyaline can also be seen. Like osteoid osteoma, these lesions are highly vascular; however, the nidus of an osteoblastoma is much larger than that of an osteoid osteoma. There is often overlap between the histologic appearance of osteoblastoma and that of low-grade osteosarcoma. Approximately 10 to 15% of lesions contain areas of secondary aneurysmal bone cyst formation.

A controversial form of osteoblastoma, the aggressive osteoblastoma, has been described that demonstrates more aggressive histologic characteristics than traditional osteoblastomas. These characteristics include epithelioid osteoblasts, mitoses in the fibrovascular stroma, increased cellularity, osteoclast-like giant cells, spiculated tumor bone like that seen in conventional osteosarcoma, and disorganized matrix production. Unlike osteosarcoma, however, these lesions lack atypical mitoses and have a low mitotic rate. Aggressive osteoblastomas have been rarely reported to metastasize; however, they demonstrate a high local recurrence rate (up to 50%). Radiologically, as expected, they have a more aggressive appearance, including large, infiltrating soft-tissue components.

Imaging Findings

RADIOGRAPHY

- Three patterns: (1) central lytic area (with or without mineralization) and surrounding sclerosis (similar to, but larger than, an osteoid osteoma); (2) expansile lytic lesion with internal calcifications and a rim of sclerosis; and (3) more aggressive appearance with marked osseous expansion and destruction, soft-tissue invasion, and scattered calcification
- The character of mineralization may be similar to chondroid mineralization (rings and arcs or popcorn-like).
- The mineralization may have a variable appearance, including ground glass appearance, punctate mineralization, and trabecular bone.
- Mineralization is often multifocal throughout the lesion, as opposed to central, in an osteoid osteoma.
- The lesion may look like an osteoid osteoma, but it is larger (> 1.5 to 2.0 cm).
- Surrounding sclerosis is often present, although this is usually less prominent than that seen around osteoid osteomas.
- The adjacent cortical bone is often thinned and expanded (unlike an osteoid osteoma).
- Periosteal reaction may be present.
- Some lesions may have a more aggressive appearance, including cortical destruction and soft-tissue extension.
- Spinal lesions often extend into the paraspinal or epidural spaces.

COMPUTED TOMOGRAPHY

- Better detection and characterization of matrix mineralization and cortical destruction
- Best modality for evaluation of lesion extent
- Sclerosis in vertebral lesions may be multilevel.

MAGNETIC RESONANCE IMAGING

- Usually similar to muscle in signal intensity on T1-weighted images
- Usually low to intermediate signal intensity on T2-weighted images, likely due to nonmineralized osteoid or dense mineralization

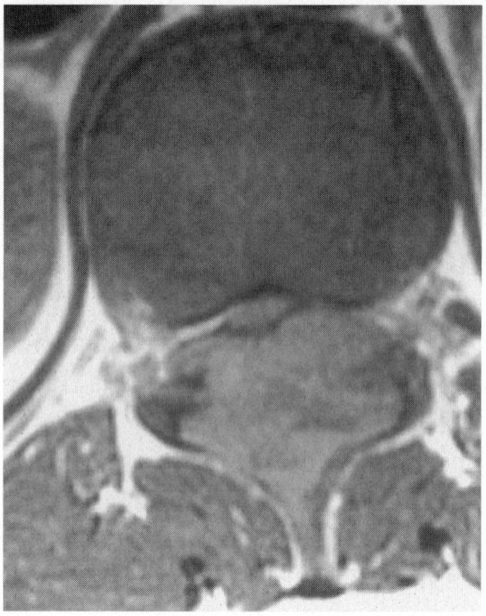

Figure 66D A transaxial T2-weighted image shows an extensive posterior element lesion causing severe spinal stenosis, complete effacement of the cerebrospinal fluid space, and flattening of the cord.

- Posterior element lesions elegantly demonstrated (**Fig. 66D**)
- May demonstrate extensive surrounding bone and soft-tissue edema that will enhance after intravenous contrast administration
- May overestimate extent of the lesion because of the extensive reactive and soft-tissue changes
- May see fluid levels consistent with secondary ABC formation

Treatment and Prognosis

- Local resection or curettage is performed for most tumors.
- Resection margin is extended by use of a high-speed burr or drill, chemical cautery (phenol), or cryosurgery (liquid nitrogen).
- Recurrence rate of 10 to 20% for conventional lesions
- Aggressive osteoblastoma requires wide local resection, similar to the treatment for low-grade osteosarcoma.

PEARLS

- Spinal lesions most commonly involve the posterior elements alone (55%), with the remainder usually involving the posterior elements with extension into the vertebral body.
- Toxic osteoblastoma is an uncommon variant in which patients experience severe systemic symptoms, including fever, leukocytosis, weight loss, anemia, cachexia, and generalized periosteal reaction, that remit when the tumor is removed.
- Mineralization is often multifocal throughout the lesion, as opposed to central as in an osteoid osteoma.
- The adjacent cortical bone is often thinned and expanded (unlike an osteoid osteoma).
- Spinal lesions often extend into the paraspinal or epidural spaces.

PITFALLS

- The character of mineralization may be similar to chondroid mineralization (rings and arcs or popcorn-like).

- The mineralization has an inconstant appearance, including ground glass appearance, punctate mineralization, and trabecular bone.
- Some lesions may have a more aggressive appearance, including cortical destruction and soft-tissue extension.
- MRI may overestimate the extent of the lesion because of the extensive reactive and soft-tissue changes.

Suggested Readings

Greenspan A. Benign bone-forming lesions: osteoma, osteoid osteoma, and osteoblastoma. Clinical, imaging, pathologic, and differential considerations. Skeletal Radiol 1993;22:485–500

Murphey MD, Andrews C, Flemming D, Temple H, Smith W, Smirniotopoulos J. Primary tumors of the spine: radiologic-pathologic correlation. Radiographics 1996;16:1131–1158

Ruggieri P, McLeod R, Unni K, Sim F. Osteoblastoma. Orthopedics 1996;19:621–624

Shaikh MI, Saifuddin A, Pringle J, Natali C, Sherazi Z. Spinal osteoblastoma: CT and MR imaging with pathologic correlation. Skeletal Radiol 1999;28:33–40

White LM, Kandel R. Osteoid-producing tumors of bone. Semin Musculoskelet Radiol 2000;4:25–43

CASE 67

Sam Y. Chun, Ali Islam, Alison Spouge, Anthony G. Ryan, and Peter L. Munk

Clinical Presentation

A 10-year-old girl presented with a 3-week history of thigh pain. Her blood work showed a mildly elevated erythrocyte sedimentation rate and normal white cell count.

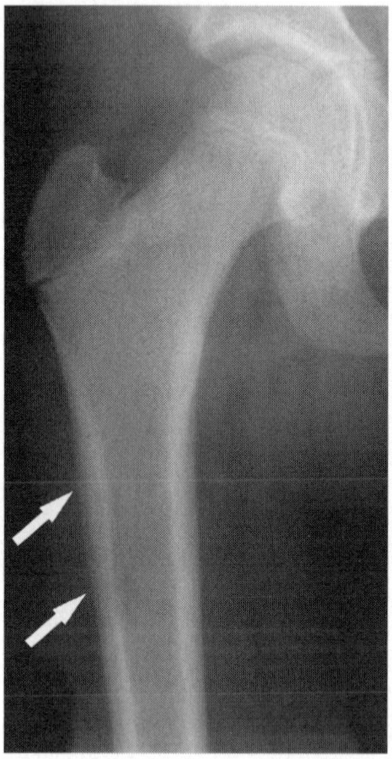

Figure 67A

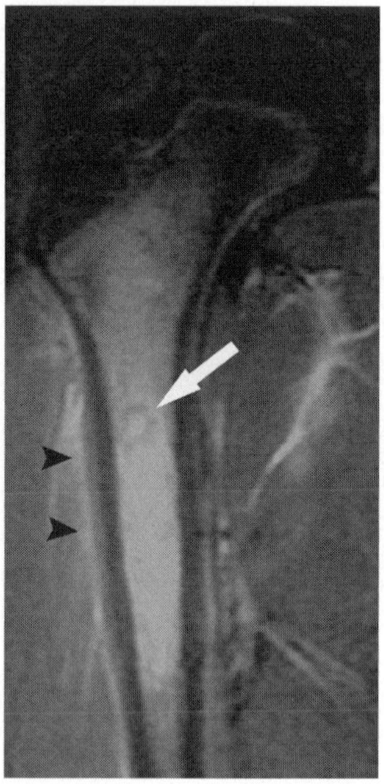

Figure 67B

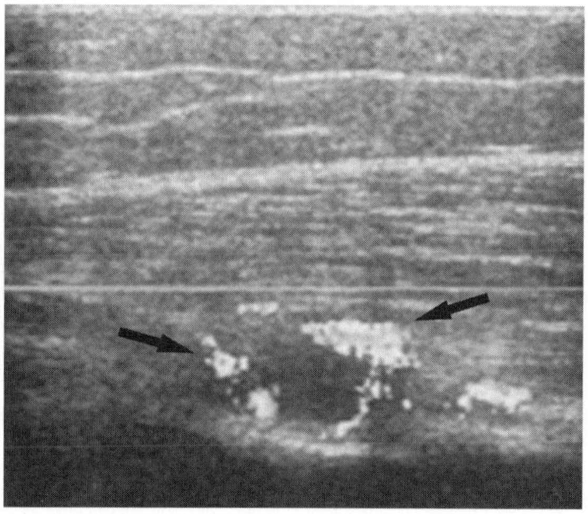

Figure 67C

Radiologic Findings

An anteroposterior radiograph of the femur (**Fig. 67A**) shows a subtle periosteal reaction (white arrows) along the lateral aspect of the diaphysis. Coronal fast inversion recovery (**Fig. 67B**) shows extensive high signal bone marrow edema in the proximal femoral metadiaphysis with a small spherical central ringlike low signal intensity consistent with very early abscess formation (arrow). A trace of fluid is also present in the periosseous soft tissues (arrowheads). Longitudinal sonogram (**Fig. 67C**) shows a small fluid collection (arrows) in the deep soft tissues adjacent to the proximal femur with a rim of hyperemia seen on color Doppler. The fluid collection was aspirated using ultrasound guidance, and subsequent cultures grew *Staphylococcus aureus*.

Diagnosis

Acute osteomyelitis.

Differential Diagnosis

- Eosinophilic granuloma
- Ewing's sarcoma
- Lymphoma or leukemia

Discussion

Background

Osteomyelitis is an infection of bone. The term *acute osteomyelitis* is reserved for recent onset of osseous infection characterized by a relatively abrupt clinical presentation. Relapse of a previously documented infection or persistence of symptoms for more than 6 weeks is generally classified as subacute or chronic. Osteomyelitis occurs via three routes of contamination: hematogenous, spread from a contiguous source of infection, or direct implantation. In many instances the source of contamination cannot be identified, and occasionally more than one route may contribute to the infection. In children and adult populations with osteomyelitis, males appear to be more frequently affected than females; however, in infants, both sexes are affected with equal frequency.

Although hematogenous osteomyelitis can affect patients of all ages, it is considered a disease of childhood (3 to 15 years). The primary site of infection in children is the metaphysis of the long bones, particularly those bones involved in rapid growth, such as around the knee, the wrist, and the proximal humerus. In adults, the pelvis, spine, and small bones are more commonly affected. The primary focus of infection is sometimes evident (ear, skin, throat), but more often than not, no source can be found. Hematogenous osteomyelitis can involve single or multiple bones; in infants, multiple sites of infection are often seen due to septicemia from infected umbilical catheters.

In adults, osteomyelitis of the appendicular skeleton is more commonly due to spread from a contiguous source of infection or direct implantation. Osteomyelitis from a contiguous source of infection includes spread from burns, soft-tissue infection, sinus disease, periodontal infection, and skin ulcers caused by peripheral vascular disease. Soft-tissue infections leading to bone contamination are often seen with bites (animal and human) and puncture wounds. Other common mechanisms of direct inoculation include penetrating wounds, compound fractures, and orthopedic instrumentation.

Etiology

The most common organism responsible for hematogenous osteomyelitis in childhood is *Staphylococcus aureus,* followed by β-hemolytic *Streptococcus*, the latter more frequently seen in neonates. In adults, the pathogens are *Staphylococcus aureus*, the enteric species, and *Streptococcus*. In addition, certain microbes are associated with specific disease conditions, including salmonella in sickle cell disease and *Pseudomonas* with intravenous drug abuse.

Osteomyelitis, due to spread from a contiguous source, is most often from *Staphylococcus*, *Streptococcus pneumoniae,* and *Haemophilus influenzae*. The microbes responsible for direct inoculation osteomyelitis vary depending on the scenario; however, *Pseudomonas* is often found following penetrating foot trauma. Infection from human bites often involves *Staphylococcus*, *Streptococcus,* and anaerobes. With regard to animal bites, dog bites are far more common than cat bites, but a far greater proportion of cat bites can lead to osteomyelitis resulting from *Pasteurella multocida* in addition to other organisms, including *Staphylococcus aureus, Staphylococcus epidermidis*, and the *Bacteroides* species.

Clinical Findings

In children, the typical clinical presentation of acute osteomyelitis is sudden onset of high fever and bone pain. Physical examination findings include localized tenderness, swelling, erythema, and warmth, as well as decreased range of motion of the affected limb, with or without a primary source of infection. In adults, the onset is more insidious, with a longer period between onset of symptoms and correct diagnosis.

Complications

- Chronic osteomyelitis
- Secondary septic arthritis
- Pathologic fracture

Pathogenesis

The pathophysiology of hematogenous osteomyelitis differs in the infant, child, and adult, mainly due to differences in vascular anatomy. In infants under 1 year of age and adults, the physis is traversed by vessels, allowing infections to spread into the epiphysis. In children, the growth plate is relatively avascular because the metaphyseal vessels terminate in the large venous sinuses of the distal metaphysis. The blood flow in these areas is slow, predisposing the metaphysis to bacterial seeding, resulting in septic thrombophlebitis and bone necrosis. Increasing intramedullary pressure from vascular engorgement, edema, and pus leads to spread of the infection along the haversian and Volkmann's canals, causing more widespread bone infarction (sequestra) and involvement of the cortex. As the inflammatory exudate reaches the cortex, periosteal elevation and new bone formation (involucrum) can occur, particularly in infants and children, where the periosteum is loosely attached to the underlying bone. The involucrum may ultimately surround the infection. In adults, the periosteum is more firmly attached to the cortex, and periosteal elevation is less common. However, sinus tract formation (cloaca) through the periosteum or involucrum to the adjacent soft tissues or skin surface is more common.

In nonhematogenous osteomyelitis, the infection extends from the soft tissues to the bone. As a result, the chronologic pathogenetic sequence is initiated with soft-tissue infection, followed by periosteal/cortical invasion and eventual spread of infection through the haversian and Volkmann's canals to the marrow.

Imaging Findings

RADIOGRAPHY

Conventional radiography remains the initial step in imaging osteomyelitis. The first sign is often soft-tissue swelling causing obliteration of the fat planes, which may be seen as early as 3 days following the onset of infection. Osseous involvement is characterized by regional osteopenia and focal bone resorption in the medullary space and occurs 10 to 21 days after onset of infection. Later findings include more extensive osteolysis, cortical lucencies, and involucrum formation. The sequestra usually appear dense due to osteolysis of the surrounding bone. Occasionally, a sinus (cloaca) may be seen through the cortex or involucrum, which may be accompanied by soft-tissue swelling and mass, suggesting a soft-tissue abscess. The classic radiographic appearance of permeative bone destruction is not specific and may be seen in a variety of other conditions, including round cell tumors and other malignancies. Because of these limitations, the sensitivity and specificity of conventional radiography for acute osteomyelitis are 43 to 75% and 76 to 83%, respectively.

SCINTIGRAPHY

Bone and labeled white cell scans are both sensitive and specific. The most commonly used bone scan agent is radioactive technetium, which is highly sensitive (up to 100%) in the detection of acute osteomyelitis and is positive within 24 to 48 hours after clinical onset of infection. Osteomyelitis appears as a focus of increased activity on the blood flow, blood pool, and delayed phases of the scan. Technetium scintigraphy is nonspecific in isolation, as other conditions, such as tumors, trauma, and neuropathic osteoarthropathy, can result in uptake of the radiotracer. When used in combination with indium 111–labeled leukocytes, increased specificity (90%) in the diagnosis is achieved. The labeled white cells accumulate in infected bone, which is interpreted as being positive for osteomyelitis when the white cell uptake is greater than the technetium uptake.

SONOGRAPHY

- Ultrasound facilitates the detection and aspiration of periosseous fluid collections.

COMPUTED TOMOGRAPHY

- CT is utilized in the detection of osseous changes that are frequently evident earlier than on plain films, including cortical destruction, periosteal proliferation, sequestra, intraosseous gas, and small foreign bodies.
- Soft-tissue changes are less conspicuous but may also be identified on CT. Intravenous contrast may be administered to help characterize abnormalities such as cloacae, abscesses, and necrotic tissue that do not enhance from the surrounding enhancing tissues.

MAGNETIC RESONANCE IMAGING

The high inherent tissue contrast provided by MRI results in high sensitivity (up to 100%) in diagnosis of all stages of osteomyelitis. In the early phases of infection, the marrow edema seen on MRI is relatively nonspecific, but as the disease progresses, additional findings of extensive soft-tissue edema and developing soft-tissue and intraosseous abscess strongly suggest the diagnosis, with specificity reported of up to 90%.

- Commonly used pulse sequences in the imaging of acute osteomyelitis include T1- and T2-weighted images supplemented with short STIR and gadolinium-enhanced T1-weighted acquisitions.
- Osteomyelitis appears as a focus of low signal on T1-weighted images and high signal on T2-weighted images, STIR, or fat-saturated sequences.
- Other findings supporting the diagnosis of osteomyelitis include cellulitis, sinus tracts, cortical disruption, sequestra, and soft-tissue and bone abscesses. MRI has a considerable advantage over CT in the evaluation of soft-tissue involvement and is helpful in differentiating primary cellulitis from osteomyelitis.
- Gadolinium contrast distributes preferentially to areas of inflammation, causing increased signal on T1-weighted images. As a result, gadolinium administration facilitates the detection of abscesses (enhancement of the granulation tissue in the abscess wall but not of the fluid within it), sinus tracts (lined by granulation tissue), and sequestra (nonenhancing necrotic bone surrounded by granulation tissue).

Treatment

Acute osteomyelitis is primarily treated with parenteral antibiotics. Early initiation of treatment, before significant bone destruction occurs, offers the best results and reduces the need for surgical débridement. Parenteral antibiotics must be administered for at least 4 weeks, and ideally 6, to ensure a good result. Primary empiric treatment generally consists of a penicillinase-resistant synthetic penicillin and a third-generation cephalosporin to cover the suspected organisms. Following identification of the organism and its sensitivity, the antibiotic regimen is revised.

Prognosis

The prognosis is variable, depending on prompt diagnosis and aggressive therapeutic intervention. During the course of treatment, the patient should be monitored closely for signs of worsening infection. Early antibiotic therapy produces the best results and reduces the risk of complications, such as chronic osteomyelitis, secondary septic arthritis, and pathologic fracture.

PEARL

- The classic radiographic appearance of an "aggressive" lesion should always raise infection as a possible differential, especially in the young, elderly, and immunocompromised.

PITFALL

- Approximately 30 to 50% of the involved bone must be destroyed to be detected on plain films, and radiographic changes are therefore frequently not manifested until 2 weeks after the onset of infection.

Suggested Readings

Cardinal E, Bureau NJ, Aubin B, Chhem RK. Role of ultrasound in musculoskeletal infections. Radiol Clin North Am 2001;39:191–201

Oudjhane K, Azouz EM. Imaging of osteomyelitis in children. Radiol Clin North Am 2001;39:251–266

Tehranzadeh J, Wong E, Wang F, Sadighpour M. Imaging of osteomyelitis in the mature skeleton. Radiol Clin North Am 2001;39:223–250

CASE 68

Sam Y. Chun, Ali Islam, Alison Spouge, Anthony G. Ryan, and Peter L. Munk

Clinical Presentation

A 15-year-old boy presented with a 6-month history of arm pain.

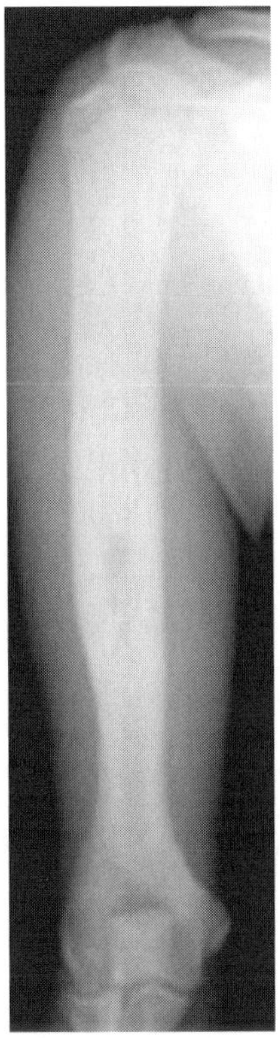

Figure 68A

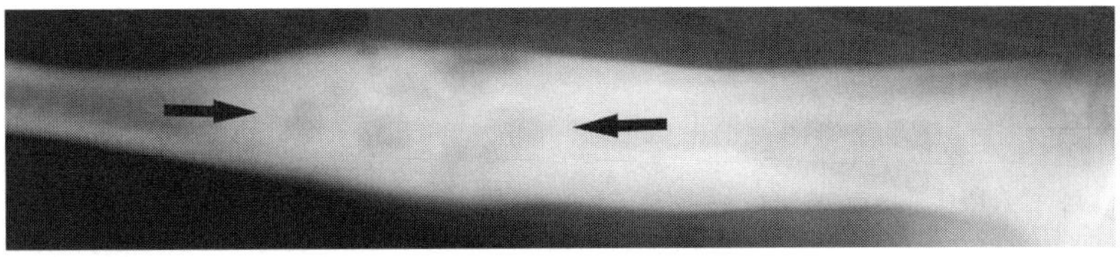

Figure 68B

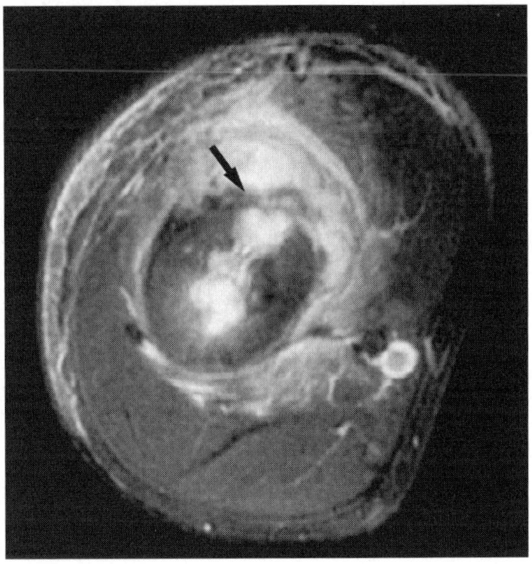

Figure 68C

Radiologic Findings

The anteroposterior (AP) radiograph of the humerus (**Fig. 68A**) shows extensive solid periosteal new bone in the diaphyseal region, with expansion and remodeling of the bone. An AP tomogram (**Fig. 68B**) shows irregular, well-defined lucencies in the medullary cavity and lateral cortex of the bone (arrows). An axial fast inversion recovery sequence (**Fig. 68C**) reveals discrete high signal intensity in the medullary cavity with cortical breakthrough anteriorly (arrow), consistent with a draining sinus track, in addition to cortical thickening and periosseous soft-tissue edema.

Diagnosis

Chronic osteomyelitis.

Differential Diagnosis

- Lymphoma
- Ewing's sarcoma
- Stress reaction/fracture
- Osteoid osteoma, if < 1.5 cm

Discussion

Background

Chronic osteomyelitis is prolonged infection of the bone (generally defined as lasting more than 6 weeks), typically affecting adults. It is most often a sequela of an open fracture and may also be associated with vascular insufficiency, inadequate treatment, or immune deficiency. Chronic osteomyelitis may be classified as active or inactive, but differentiating the two is often difficult. Active infection implies that the pathogens are viable, which may be detected radiographically by the presence of sequestra, abscesses, and subperiosteal fluid collections.

Brodie's abscesses may be seen in both subacute and chronic infections; however, this entity is discussed separately in case 69.

Etiology

Chronic osteomyelitis is usually the sequela of an acute infection; therefore, the same organisms are involved, particularly *Staphylococcus aureus.*

Clinical Findings

Patients with chronic osteomyelitis may present with localized bone pain, erythema, and draining sinus tracts. In chronic active osteomyelitis, the viable pathogens may remain isolated within the sequestrum and give rise to recurrent episodes of acute osteomyelitis. The patient may be asymptomatic between exacerbations.

Complications

Complications can be severe and sometimes fatal. Serious complications include septic arthritis, epiphyseal plate damage with secondary growth disturbances in children, and epidermoid carcinoma of the fistula. Epidermoid carcinoma, usually squamous cell carcinoma, occurs in 0.5 to 1.6% of patients with chronic osteomyelitis, with a 20- to 40-year latent period. Radiographic signs of malignant transformation include a lytic lesion superimposed on changes of chronic osteomyelitis, soft-tissue mass, and pathologic fracture.

Pathogenesis

Several factors may contribute to the progression of acute osteomyelitis into chronic osteomyelitis.

First, the pathogens are contained within the sequestrum surrounded by the bony involucrum, which acts as a barrier against both host immune defenses and antibiotics.

Second, the abscess cavity within bone cannot collapse like those in soft tissues, and the dead infected bone cannot be absorbed. In addition, host factors such as immunocompromised states, vascular disease, treatment compliance, and general tissue health can influence the course of the acute infection.

The pathologic findings depend on the phase of chronic infection. Sequestration is the characteristic finding in the active phase. A sequestrum is a segment of necrotic bone commonly located in the medullary cavity of tubular bones surrounded by granulation tissue and osteolysis of the adjacent bone. The healing phase is characterized by prominent periosteal sclerosis surrounding the involved cortex, with the marrow cavity gradually being replaced by granulation tissue, fibrous tissue, and cellular and fatty marrow.

Garré's sclerosing osteomyelitis is a rare form of chronic infection characterized by intense cortical thickening or periosteal reaction with no necrosis or purulent exudate and little granulation tissue. This entity most commonly involves the mandible and less often the diaphysis of long bones.

Chronic recurrent multifocal osteomyelitis (CRMO) is another rare form of osteomyelitis of unknown etiology that most often affects children and young adults, with a female-to-male ratio of 2:1. The clinical course is one of exacerbations and remissions over several years. CRMO is characterized by multifocal lytic lesions usually involving the metaphysis of long bones in a symmetric distribution. The lesions may be sclerotic if in the healing phase. The most common locations are the tibia, femur, clavicle, and fibula. Bone biopsies demonstrate nonspecific subacute/chronic osteomyelitis. There appears to be an association between this entity and certain dermatological conditions such as palmoplantaris pustulosis and psoriasis. As a result, the acronym SAPHO (synovitis, acne, pustulosis, hyperostosis, and osteitis) has been coined.

Imaging Findings

RADIOGRAPHY

Both phases of chronic osteomyelitis may demonstrate bone destruction and sclerosis. The most specific radiographic sign of the active phase is the detection of sequestra that commonly harbor virulent pathogens. However, sequestra are infrequently seen, in as low as 9% of cases in one series. The sequestra appear as radiodense bony spicules, which are often sharply defined from the surrounding osteolytic bone and granulation tissue. Other signs of active chronic infection are soft-tissue swelling, aggressive periosteal reaction, and progressive or poorly defined osteolysis.

Radiographic findings of the healing or inactive phase include cortical thickening, resolving osteolysis, and bone expansion/remodeling.

ULTRASOUND

Ultrasound can be useful in chronic osteomyelitis for the detection of soft-tissue abnormalities such as abscesses or fluid collections, which can be aspirated or drained under ultrasound guidance. Occasionally, a soft-tissue fluid collection can be seen extending to within the marrow cavity, which is highly suggestive of reactivated chronic osteomyelitis.

Ultrasound is particularly useful in assessing infectious complications following orthopedic surgery. Ultrasound allows evaluation of the soft tissues adjacent to the hardware without the metallic artifact that may be seen on both CT and MRI. Identification of a fluid collection next to hardware outside the immediate postoperative period is suspicious for infection and should be aspirated for diagnosis.

COMPUTED TOMOGRAPHY

Bony changes may be detected earlier on CT than on plain films; additionally, CI demonstrates sequestra, cloacae, and cortical destruction to advantage.

NUCLEAR MEDICINE

Technetium 99m diphosphate triple-phase bone scanning is often used in combination with gallium 67–labeled leukocytes or (more commonly) indium 111–labeled leukocytes for the detection of osteomyelitis. The combination of technetium 99m–methylene diphosphonate and gallium 67 has a reported sensitivity and specificity of 69 to 70% and 83 to 93%, respectively. Indium 111 is highly sensitive in the detection of acute infection but rather insensitive (~50%) for chronic infections, particularly those located in the axial skeleton.

MAGNETIC RESONANCE IMAGING

The classic MR findings in acute osteomyelitis (e.g., high signal intensity in the bone marrow on T2-weighted sequences) may not be seen in the chronic form. In acute osteomyelitis, the demarcation between normal and diseased marrow is usually poorly defined due to significant edema. In chronic osteomyelitis, a peripheral rim of fibrous tissue or sclerosis is often seen around the affected marrow, which is demonstrated as a well-defined rim of low signal intensity on all pulse sequences. This "rim" sign is seen in 93% of patients with chronic osteomyelitis.

Differentiation between the active and inactive forms of chronic infection can be difficult. MRI features of the active phase include the presence of sequestra, cloacae, abscesses, and subperiosteal fluid collections. Sequestra typically appear as low signal on all sequences that do not enhance with gadolinium. The sinus tracts or cloacae appear as curvilinear areas of high T2 signal involving both bone and soft tissue, which may demonstrate enhancement following administration of gadolinium because the walls are lined with granulation tissue. Inactive or healed osteomyelitis is characterized by fatty replacement of the marrow, which may be seen as increased signal intensity on T1-weighted sequences.

Follow-up evaluation of treated chronic osteomyelitis can also be difficult. Both postoperative changes and active infection may show increased signal intensity on T2-weighted sequences, but infection is suggested by increased signal intensity on T2-weighted sequences that becomes more prominent on serial imaging or persists more than 9 months following surgical débridement. In these postoperative cases, leukocyte-labeled scintigraphy may be useful.

Treatment

Initial treatment for acute osteomyelitis consists of parenteral antibiotics for 4 to 6 weeks. If the osteomyelitis is refractory to treatment and progresses to the chronic stage, surgical débridement in combination with a repeated 4- to 6-week course of parenteral antibiotics is generally required. Chronic osteomyelitis usually does not respond to antibiotic therapy alone.

Prognosis

Patients with chronic osteomyelitis usually require surgical débridement for a favorable long-term outcome.

PEARLS

- The "rim" sign (a well-defined rim of low signal intensity on all pulse sequences relating to the fibrous tissue or sclerosis around the affected marrow) is seen in 93% of patients with chronic osteomyelitis.

- Ultrasound permits evaluation of the soft tissues adjacent to orthopedic prostheses when infection is suspected without the metallic artifact that may be seen on both CT and MRI.

PITFALL

- Rarely (0.5 to 1.6%), chronic osteomyelitis is complicated by the development of squamous cell carcinoma, usually after a 20- to 40-year latent period. The development of a new lytic focus, soft-tissue mass, or pathologic fracture should raise this suspicion, rather than simply be ascribed to the underlying infection.

Suggested Readings

Boutin RD, Brossmann J, Sartoris DJ, Reilly D, Resnick D. Update on imaging of orthopaedic infections. Orthop Clin North Am 1998;29:41–66

Oudjhane K, Azouz EM. Imaging of osteomyelitis in children. Radiol Clin North Am 2001;39:251–266

Tehranzadeh J, Wong E, Wang F, Sadighpour M. Imaging of osteomyelitis in the mature skeleton. Radiol Clin North Am 2001;39:223–250

CASE 69

Sam Y. Chun, Ali Islam, Alison Spouge, Anthony G. Ryan, and Peter L. Munk

Clinical Presentation

A 15-year-old boy with knee pain diagnosed with osteochondritis dissecans (OCD) of the knee was sent for MRI evaluation of the OCD.

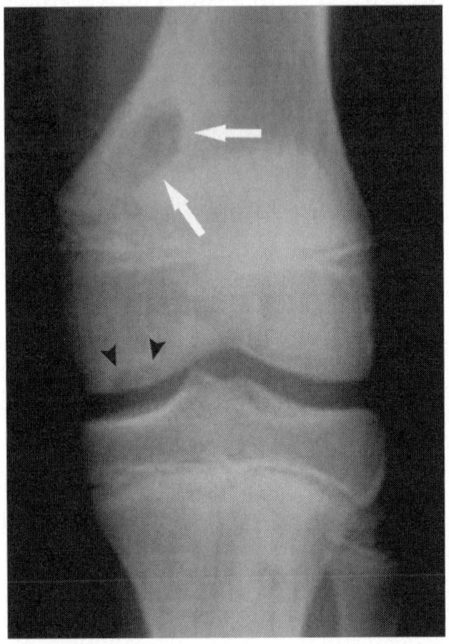

Figure 69A

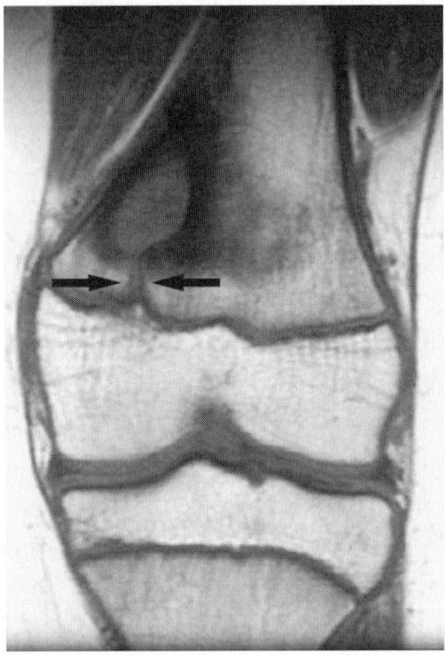

Figure 69B

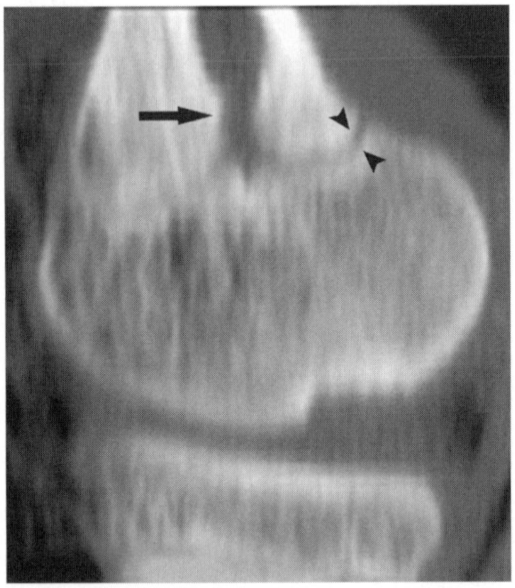

Figure 69C

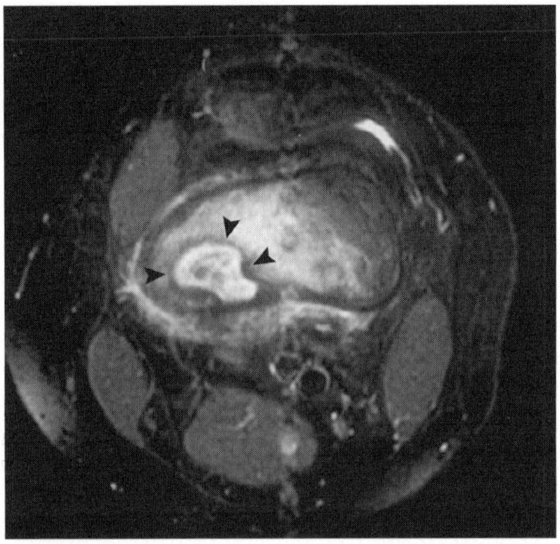

Figure 69D

Radiologic Findings

An anteroposterior radiograph of the knee (**Fig. 69A**) shows an area of OCD in the midmedial femoral condyle (arrowheads). A large geographic lytic area in the posteromedial distal femoral metaphysis is also evident (arrows), with marginal sclerosis fading peripherally. A coronal T1 spin-echo image (**Fig. 69B**) shows a corresponding area of extensive low signal intensity with a small track (arrows) extending caudally to the physeal plate.

A sagittal computed tomography reformat (**Fig. 69C**) shows the lower end of the low density lesion (arrow) to be in continuity with the physis, which is open posteriorly (arrowheads). Axial inversion recovery (**Fig. 69D**) shows the lesion to have a heterogeneous appearance (arrowheads) with areas of central intermediate and high signal intensity, surrounded by a low signal intensity rim with surrounding bone marrow and soft-tissue edema.

Diagnosis

Brodie's abscess.

Differential Diagnosis

- Nonossifying fibroma
- Osteoblastoma/osteoid osteoma (if < 1.5 cm)
- Fibrous dysplasia
- Eosinophilic granuloma

Discussion

Background

Brodie's abscess is named after the surgeon who first described the entity in prehistoric paleopathologic remains in 1832. These well-defined abscesses occur most commonly in children (particularly boys) and are typically associated with subacute osteomyelitis but may also be seen in chronic osteomyelitis.

Etiology

The most common organism is *Staphylococcus aureus*, although in up to 25% of the abscesses, no organisms are isolated.

Clinical Findings

Most patients present with localized pain, swelling, and erythema that may persist for weeks or months. Systemic signs and symptoms of infection may be absent.

Pathology

Brodie's abscess is typically an elongated avascular cavity 1 to 4 cm in diameter lined by granulation tissue and sometimes containing purulent or mucoid fluid. The cavity is usually surrounded by spongy bone eburnation. Abscess fluid cultures may not reveal the causative organism.

Pathogenesis

As with acute hematogenous osteomyelitis, the vascular metaphysis of long bones in children is the most commonly affected site, especially the tibia. The abscesses may also be seen in other tubular, flat, or irregular bones, including the vertebrae, the carpal and tarsal bones, and the diaphysis of long bones. The infection rarely crosses the avascular physis in children. In infants, where the physis is traversed by vessels, abscesses may occur at the epiphysis. It is uncertain why bone abscesses occur, but possible contributing factors include diminished pathogen virulence and increased host immune response to infection. If an acute infection is contained locally by host defenses, it can become surrounded by scar tissue and rim sclerosis, resulting in an abscess.

Imaging Findings

RADIOGRAPHY

- Brodie's abscess classically appears as a well-defined radiolucent metaphyseal lesion surrounded by a dense sclerotic rim that fades peripherally (**Fig. 69A**). Occasionally, a tortuous lucent tract may be seen extending from the lesion to the physis that is pathognomonic for Brodie's abscess and indicates the presence of an active infection (**Fig. 69B**).
- Other findings include periosteal bone formation and adjacent soft-tissue swelling. With appropriate antibiotic treatment, the metaphyseal lesion should diminish in size with diaphyseal migration of the radiolucent focus as the patient matures and new bone is laid down at the epiphysis.
- In the diaphysis, the abscess may be central, subcortical, or cortical in location. A cortical abscess may have a similar appearance to an osteoid osteoma, an eosinophilic granuloma, or a stress fracture. In the epiphysis, the lytic lesion may border on the chondro-osseous junction or the physis, where it may continue into the metaphysis.

COMPUTED TOMOGRAPHY

- The superior spatial resolution of CT permits the more exact evaluation of the size and location of the abscess, the presence of a radiolucent tract (**Fig. 69C**), and soft-tissue extension.
- These findings may help in planning for biopsy or surgical intervention.

MAGNETIC RESONANCE IMAGING

- Brodie's abscesses are well demonstrated with MRI.
- T1-weighted images demonstrate a well-defined lesion of low-intermediate signal intensity (**Fig. 69B**) with a peripheral rim of granulation tissue that enhances with gadolinium administration.
- T2-weighted images demonstrate a high signal intensity lesion surrounded by low signal sclerosis.
- Sinus tracts are usually more conspicuous on MRI, as they may show curvilinear high T2-signal intensity and gadolinium enhancement due to granulation tissue lining the tract walls (**Fig. 69D**). MRI is also useful for determining the extent of soft-tissue involvement.

Treatment

- Most cases are treated with surgical débridement in combination with parenteral antibiotics. The dead space created by débridement is commonly packed with antibiotic-impregnated beads.
- Larger abscesses may require bone grafting.
- Selected culture-positive cases may be managed with a 4- to 6-week course of parenteral antibiotics. Sterile abscesses usually do not require medical treatment and may be followed radiographically.

Prognosis

Prognosis is generally excellent with adequate treatment. One study that followed patients who were affected as children did not demonstrate significant growth disturbance at bone maturity.

PEARL

- Infection must be excluded in the presence of a lucent focus in the metaphysis of a young patient.

PITFALL

- Image-guided biopsy may be performed under fluoroscopic or CT guidance; however, cultures are frequently negative, which does not exclude the diagnosis.

Suggested Readings

Boutin RD, Brossmann J, Sartoris DJ, Reilly D, Resnick D. Update on imaging of orthopedic infections. Orthop Clin North Am 1998;29:41–66

Oudjhane K, Azouz EM. Imaging of osteomyelitis in children. Radiol Clin North Am 2001;39:251–266

Tehranzadeh J, Wong E, Wang F, Sadighpour M. Imaging of osteomyelitis in the mature skeleton. Radiol Clin North Am 2001;39:223–250

CASE 70

Sam Y. Chun, Ali Islam, Alison Spouge, Anthony G. Ryan, and Peter L. Munk

Clinical Presentation

A 24-year-old man presented with a 10-day history of right hip pain.

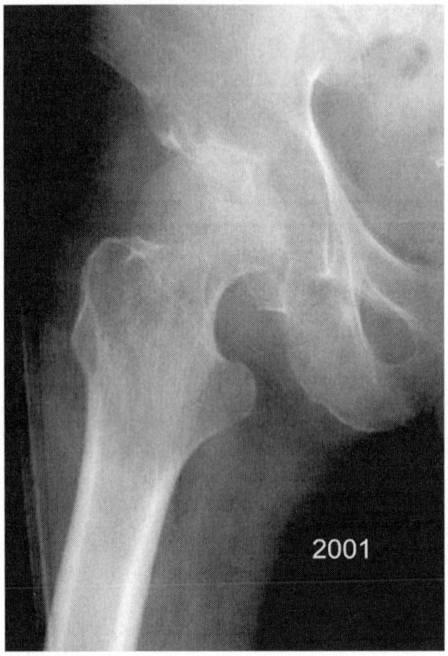

Figure 70A

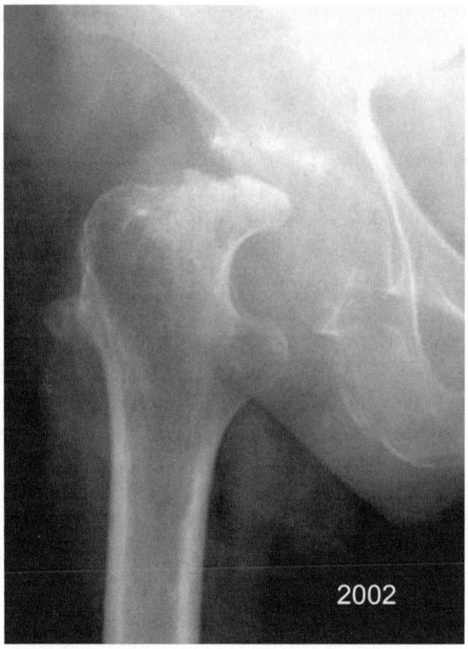

Figure 70B

Radiologic Findings

An anteroposterior radiograph of the right hip (**Fig. 70A**) at the time of presentation shows marked narrowing of the joint space with relative preservation of bone density. A radiograph 1 year later (**Fig. 70B**) shows extensive destruction of the right hip joint with near-complete loss of the femoral head and the articular portion of the acetabulum.

Diagnosis

Pyogenic (septic) arthritis.

Differential Diagnosis

- Nonpyogenic arthritis (tuberculosis, fungus)
- Viral arthritis
- Human immunodeficiency virus (HIV) infection

- Lyme disease
- Gout/pseudogout
- Rheumatoid arthritis

Discussion

Background

Pyogenic or septic arthritis is a rapidly progressive joint disease with destructive and debilitating consequences. In the general population, the incidence of septic arthritis is ~2 to 10 per 100,000. The outcome of the disease depends on the speed of diagnosis, the organism and joint involved, and the patient's preexisting health. Risk factors include advanced age, immunosuppression, sexually transmitted disease, diabetes, rheumatoid arthritis, joint trauma/injection, prosthetic joints, and intravenous drug abuse. Although the disease is usually monarticular, polyarticular disease occurs in up to 20% of cases.

Etiology

Staphylococcus aureus is the most common pathogen in adults, accounting for ~40% of cases. In some series, streptococci account for up to 30% and gram-negative rods up to 20%. *Neisseria gonorrhoeae* is the most common pathogen in young, sexually active patients, but it accounts for only 3.0 to 7.5% of overall cases. Children younger than 6 months of age are usually infected by vaginal flora that include gram-negative rods and gram-positive cocci. Between 6 months and 3 years, *Haemophilus influenzae* is common.

Following orthopedic procedures, both *S. aureus* and *S. epidermidis* are common causative agents.

Clinical Findings

Nongonococcal arthritis presents with a hot swollen joint that is painful throughout passive and active range of motion. Fever and signs of sepsis may also be present. Pain is present on both passive and active range of motion. The knee is the affected joint in over half of all cases in adults, followed by the hip, shoulder, wrist, ankle, elbow, and hand in order of decreasing frequency. Hip joint infections are more common in children. Infection of small joints is more common with intravenous drug abuse.

A primary source of infection can be found in almost half of all cases. The primary source is usually the skin or genitourinary or respiratory tract. Between 10 and 20% of infections are polyarticular, usually occurring in patients with collagen-vascular diseases such as rheumatoid arthritis.

A suspected septic joint is an orthopedic emergency, and joint aspiration should be expedited. Analysis of synovial fluid with Gram's stain, culture, microscopy, and cell count is of foremost importance. Negative blood culture and Gram's stain cannot exclude septic arthritis, especially if antibiotics have been initiated before testing. Serum white blood cell count and erythrocyte sedimentation rate can be elevated but are not sufficient to confirm or exclude septic arthritis.

Gonococcal arthritis presents with fever, migratory arthralgias, skin rash, and tenosynovitis of the hands and feet. Routine cultures of the pharynx, genitourinary tract, rectum, and blood should be performed.

Septic arthritis involving the foot is very common in diabetic patients. Differentiation from neuropathic arthropathy can be challenging, although the time course may be helpful if serial radiographs are available, as septic arthritis will progress more rapidly than neuroarthropathy.

Complications

- Osteomyelitis
- Abscess formation
- Joint ankylosis

Pathogenesis

Bacteria can infect the synovium and joint by multiple routes. Hematogenous spread can occur if there is a remote primary site of infection, intravenous drug use, or endocarditis. The absence of a basement membrane in the synovium allows bacteria to enter the joint. Direct inoculation can also occur through joint injection, arthroscopic procedures, or penetrating trauma. The joint can secondarily be infected by direct spread from adjacent bone or bursae, such as in osteomyelitis, septic bursitis, or cellulitis. This commonly occurs in the diabetic foot. Perioperative wound contamination can cause early-onset septic arthritis in prosthetic joints. Delayed-onset infection is from hematogenous spread of bacteria.

Bacterial toxins and mediators released by polymorphonuclear cells that infiltrate the synovium begin to cause changes in cartilage and synovium within hours. Proteolytic enzymes and cytokines cause necrosis of synovium, which leads to the breakdown of collagen and proteoglycans in cartilage. The type of organism influences the type of cellular and biochemical host defense, which in turn influences the degree of joint damage (e.g., typically the degree of joint destruction is less with *N. gonorrhoeae* compared with *S. aureus*).

Pathology

Septic arthritis causes rapid changes within a joint. Debris and inflammatory cells may be found in joint effusions. Synovial hypertrophy, destruction of cartilage within the joint capsule, and erosion of bone within the joint capsule in areas unprotected by overlying cartilage (marginal erosions) are features of septic arthritis. As cartilage loss progresses, central erosions in the subchondral bone are seen.

Imaging Findings

RADIOGRAPHY

- Fat plane distortion and soft-tissue swelling due to joint effusion or synovial hypertrophy are an early finding.
- In small joints or joints with a tight capsule, such as the pediatric hip, widening of the joint space can occasionally be seen.
- Intra-articular gas due to the vacuum phenomenon excludes the presence of a joint effusion.
- Marginal erosion of bone uncovered by overlying cartilage within the joint is the next finding with maintenance of bone mineralization. Loss of the definition of the white cortical rim over a lengthy continuous segment of bone is the main feature.
- Joint space narrowing due to cartilage destruction is the next finding, in contrast to tuberculous arthritis, in which the joint space is preserved. Central erosions begin to appear at this stage.

BONE SCAN

- Increased tracer uptake in all three phases of technetium scanning is seen. There is elevated joint line uptake on both sides of the joint. Technetium scanning is sensitive but nonspecific.
- Technetium uptake in the epiphysis of pediatric patients is a normal finding. Thus, in children, scanning with gallium may be helpful.

ULTRASOUND

- Ultrasound has a high sensitivity for detecting joint effusion and can be used to aid joint aspiration, especially in the pediatric group, obviating the utilization of ionizing radiation.

COMPUTED TOMOGRAPHY

- Ideal for detecting cortical bone loss and bony erosions

MAGNETIC RESONANCE IMAGING

- MRI is highly sensitive, even early on in the disease, but is nonspecific. Joint effusions show increased signal intensity on T2-weighted sequences and are easily identified. The effusions may contain fluid-fluid levels because of precipitation of intra-articular debris.
- Bone erosions show low signal intensity on T1-weighted images. Articular cartilage can demonstrate focal or diffuse irregular contour and signal heterogeneity.
- Subarticular marrow edema manifested by low signal intensity on T1- and high intensity on T2-weighted sequences may be seen.
- Synovial thickening may be present showing prominent enhancement with gadolinium.

Treatment

- Antibiotic therapy is initiated as soon as the diagnosis is strongly suspected. The treatment is modified when the synovial or blood culture results are obtained. Antibiotic choice is influenced by the clinical setting, especially if cultures are negative.
- There is controversy regarding the role of joint decompression in the management of septic arthritis. Some authors advocate open surgical drainage of infected joint contents, whereas others advocate repeated joint aspiration in selected settings. The hip joint as well as joints that are difficult to aspirate should be managed surgically. Arthroscopy or arthrotomy allows removal of gross debris, inflamed synovium, intra-articular loculations, and adhesions. Surgical therapy is indicated in those patients with generalized sepsis, who are refractory to more conservative therapy, or who are immunocompromised.
- Early-onset prosthetic joint infections can sometimes be eradicated by local débridement and 6 weeks of parenteral antibiotics without resorting to hardware removal, which is performed with delayed-onset infections followed by replacement arthroplasty.

Prognosis

Despite improvements in antibiotics and imaging, the outcome of septic arthritis has not changed significantly in the last few decades. The overall mortality in septic arthritis remains near 10 to 15%, with permanent joint damage occurring in 25 to 50% of all patients.

PEARLS

- Intra-articular gas due to vacuum phenomenon excludes the presence of a joint effusion.
- A suspected septic joint is an orthopedic emergency, and joint aspiration should be expedited.

PITFALL

- Technetium uptake in the epiphysis of pediatric patients is a normal finding; thus, in this setting, a gallium- or indium-labeled white cell scan is recommended.

Suggested Readings

Goldenberg DL. Septic arthritis. Lancet 1998;351:197–202

Learch TJ, Farooki S. Magnetic resonance imaging of septic arthritis. Clin Imaging 2000;24:236–242

Turpin S, Lambert R. Role of scintigraphy in musculoskeletal and spinal infections. Radiol Clin North Am 2001;39:169–189

CASE 71

Anthony G. Ryan, Peter L. Munk, and Alison Spouge

Clinical Presentation

A 4-year-old boy presented with slowly progressive swelling and worsening pain on the ulnar aspect of his hand. Clinical examination revealed obvious swelling on the ulnar aspect and of the hypothenar eminence in general. The skin was erythematous but was not hot.

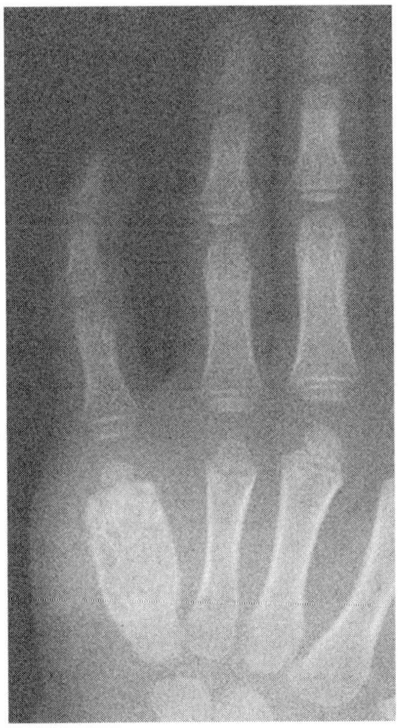

Figure 71A

Radiologic Findings

An anteroposterior radiograph of the left hand (**Fig. 71A**) shows obvious soft-tissue swelling centered on the fifth metatarsal which is expanded and sclerotic, with marked loss of corticomedullary differentiation. The remaining bones are normal.

Diagnosis

Tuberculous dactylitis (tuberculous osteomyelitis).

Differential Diagnosis

- Pyogenic osteomyelitis
- Sarcoidosis

Discussion

Background

In industrialized nations, a recent upswing in the numbers of patients infected with tuberculosis has occurred. Tuberculosis is still the most common opportunistic infection in patients with human immunodeficiency virus (HIV), and the elderly remain vulnerable, with patients in the United States over 65 accounting for 26% of cases despite being only 6% of the population. Globally, tuberculosis poses a significant challenge, affecting nearly one third (1.9 billion people) of the world's population.

Musculoskeletal manifestations of tuberculosis are relatively rare, occurring in only 1.5 to 3.0% of infected patients. Only 50% of patients with osteoarticular tuberculosis have a history of pulmonary infection, with a higher association seen in children. Osteoarticular tuberculosis affects both genders equally and is seen in all age groups. In endemic areas, however, children are more commonly affected.

Tuberculous infection can affect any bone, but the most common site is the spine (50% of cases), followed by articular involvement of the hip and pelvis (12 to 15%), knee, wrist, and elbow. Historically, extra-axial osteoarticular tuberculosis was more frequently reported in the larger joints of the lower extremities, but there has been a recent trend toward a more peripheral distribution, especially in the elderly and the young.

Etiology

Although *Mycobacterium tuberculosis* is the most common cause of mycobacterial infection, atypical acid-fast bacilli, for example, *Mycobacterium avium-intracellulare* and *Mycobacterium fortuitum,* can also affect the bone and joints.

Pathogenesis

Musculoskeletal tuberculosis generally occurs by hematogenous spread from a primary nonosseous site. Reactivation tuberculosis may be seen infrequently in the hip.

Tuberculous osteomyelitis is a disease of childhood, essentially unheard of in the adult population. In long bones, the epiphysis is the most commonly affected site, secondary to either transphyseal spread from metaphyseal involvement or adjacent tuberculous arthritis. This is in contradistinction to pyogenic osteomyelitis, where metaphyseal infection is more common and transphyseal spread is rare. The diaphysis is rarely involved in tuberculosis.

Tuberculous arthritis usually arises from adjacent osteomyelitis. The slowly progressive nature of the joint destruction is in part due to the lack of proteases in the exudate compared with pyogenic septic arthritis.

In the adult, the first site of extraspinal osseous involvement is typically a large weight-bearing joint leading to tuberculous arthritis.

Clinical Findings

Tuberculous osteomyelitis in childhood usually presents as a painless swelling of the hand or foot.

In the adult, the diagnosis of osteoarticular tuberculosis is often difficult and is delayed on average 16 to 19 months from presentation, at which time the symptoms may have been present for months or years.

Clinical findings are generally insidious, nonspecific, and slowly progressive. Patients, who are typically middle-aged or elderly, may present with chronic localized pain, boggy swelling, and weakness. They may have weight loss and fever. Muscle wasting may be obvious on examination, and there may also be associated lymphadenopathy, a draining sinus, or a cold abscess.

Ancillary tests such as the tuberculin skin test and chest x-rays may be of benefit. However, a positive tuberculin test is commonly seen in endemic areas or in those who have received the bacille Calmette-Guérin vaccine. A negative test provides more diagnostic information, but negative tests are being reported more frequently in immunosuppressed and elderly patients. A negative chest x-ray in an adult does not exclude tuberculosis, as only 50% of patients with skeletal tuberculosis have pulmonary involvement. It is thought that a negative chest x-ray in a child effectively excludes the diagnosis of concomitant musculoskeletal tuberculosis.

Definitive diagnosis requires specimen culture from aspiration or preferably biopsy of bone or synovium. In endemic areas, subacute or chronic osteomyelitis is treated as tuberculosis until proven otherwise.

Complications

- Weight loss
- Bursitis
- Tenosynovitis
- Cold abscess
- Draining sinus
- Joint ankylosis

Pathology

GROSS

In hematogenous seeding, the tubercle is formed in the marrow, which results in resorption of surrounding trabeculae. The tuberculous exudation and necrosis may then spread through the medullary and cortical bone, with penetration through the periosteum. Whitish gray necrotic material is typical of the appearance of a bone biopsy in such cases. Alternatively, the infection may advance toward the epiphysis and penetrate the articular cartilage into the joint space.

When tuberculosis affects the joint first, tuberculous granulation tissue may be seen involving the synovium and penetrating through the articular cartilage. The thickened synovium tends to be covered by a fibrinous exudate. Once the subchondral bone is exposed, destruction of the underlying bone ensues.

Sinus tracts may form in soft tissues, resulting in abscesses, or extend to the skin surface as a draining fistula.

MICROSCOPIC

Definitive diagnosis requires biopsy- or aspiration-obtained tissue specimens demonstrating acid-fast bacilli in culture. The classic finding in tuberculosis is the presence of tubercles: epithelioid granulomas with central caseous necrosis and Langhans' multinucleate giant cells. Musculoskeletal tuberculosis ultimately results in destruction and necrosis of bone, cartilage, and soft tissues. Among other factors, the lack of proteases as expressed by pyogenic organisms accounts for the indolent nature of the infection.

Imaging Findings

RADIOGRAPHY

Tuberculous osteomyelitis

The initial appearance is similar to that seen with pyogenic osteomyelitis.

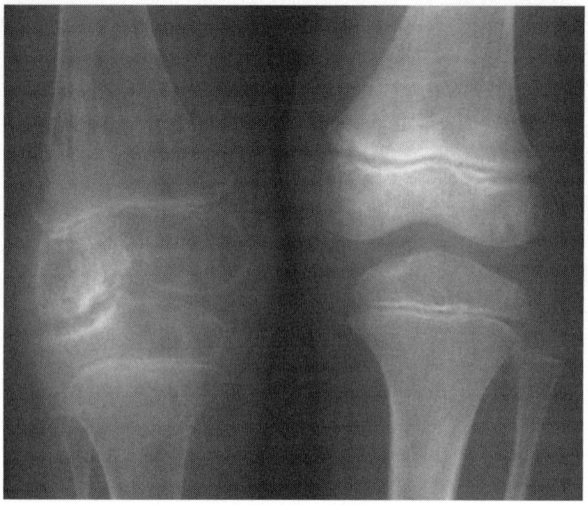

Figure 71B Bilateral knee radiograph in a young girl with tuberculous osteomyelitis complicated by tuberculous arthritis. Overgrowth of the femoral and tibial epiphyses with consequent limb length discrepancy is shown as is diffuse osteoporosis. In addition, large lateral compartment "kissing" erosions of the femoral and tibial surfaces are demonstrated; joint space (although reduced) remains relatively well preserved, considering the advanced nature of the other changes.

The findings include the following:

- Osteolytic foci, which are usually round and poorly defined initially, are seen with no reactive sclerosis.
- Variable amounts of periostitis and soft-tissue swelling/effusion may be present.
- In children, hyperemia associated with osteomyelitis may result in epiphyseal overgrowth similar to that seen in juvenile rheumatoid arthritis or hemophilia (**Fig. 71B**) or, alternatively, limb shortening secondary to early physeal closure.
- Sequestra are less commonly seen than in pyogenic infections.

Two types of tuberculous osteomyelitis require special mention:

Cystic tuberculosis is characterized by multifocal well-marginated lytic lesions that may involve one or multiple bones. This entity is more commonly seen in children, in whom the lesions usually affect the metaphysis of peripheral tubular bones, may be symmetrically distributed, and usually lack sclerosis. In the adult, the skull, shoulder, pelvis, and spine are most frequently affected, and sclerosis is more frequently seen.

Tuberculous dactylitis affects the short tubular bones of the hands and feet, and may affect multiple bones simultaneously in 25 to 35% of cases. More commonly seen in children, this entity is characterized by fusiform expansion of the bone secondary to endosteal cortical erosion and resultant periostitis, leading to a solid exuberant periosteal new bone formation (**Fig. 71A**). Variable soft-tissue swelling and sinus tracts may be evident. Although sequestra are uncommon, if present they may be extruded via the sinus tracts. The historical term *spina ventosa* means "spinelike, puffed full of air."

Tuberculous arthritis

- Typically monoarticular
- Early in the process, prominent juxta-articular osteoporosis is typical, with no erosion or soft-tissue abnormality evident.
- As the disease progresses, opposing cystlike erosions appear on the non-weight-bearing aspect of the joint.
- There may be little or no joint space narrowing until late in the disease (after months).
- Subchondral bone erosion occurs earlier in joints with large opposing articulating surfaces (e.g., hips and shoulders) (**Fig. 71C**). Prior to frank erosion, the cortex may appear "smudged."
- Infection of subchondral bone forming "kissing sequestra" (**Fig. 71D**)
- When the knee is involved, widening of the intercondylar notch secondary to erosion has been frequently described (**Fig. 71E**).

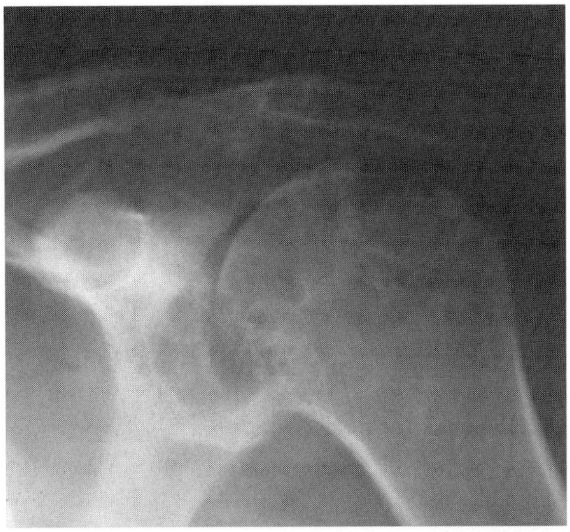

C

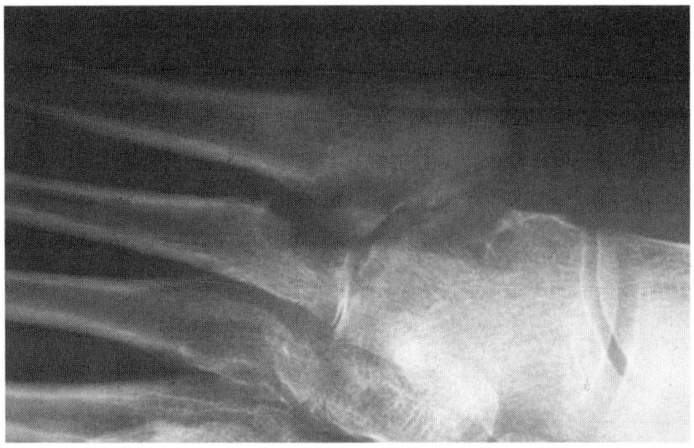

D

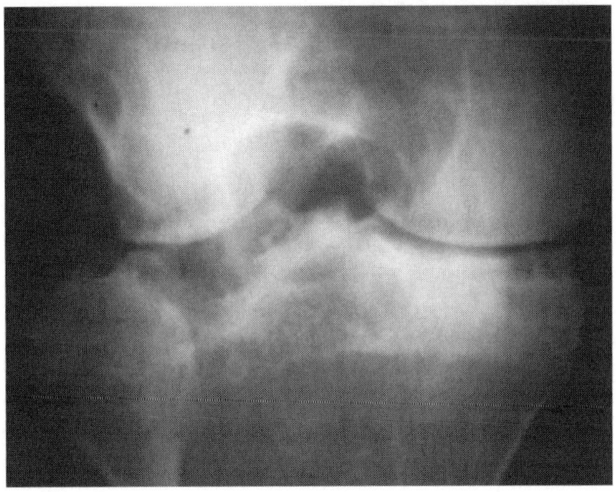

E

Figures 71C An anteroposterior shoulder radiograph shows multiple subchondral erosions affecting the articular and nonarticular surfaces of the joint, with a particularly large marginal erosion evident superiorly just below the acromion process. **71D** Tuberculous arthritis of the cuboid fifth-fourth metatarsal articulation. Oblique radiograph shows a marked, well-marginated erosion of the lateral aspect of the base of the fourth metatarsal and subchondral destruction of the cuboid-fifth articulation with a contained "kissing" sequestrum composed primarily of a portion of cuboid subchondral bone. **71E** Tuberculous arthritis of the knee. Tunnel view shows the lateral compartment and intercondylar notch erosions, the latter giving rise to the classic "widening." This erosion is seen to extend superiorly to the insertion of the posterior cruciate ligament. A small sequestrum is revealed in the subchondral bone of the lateral tibial plateau.

- Fibrous joint ankylosis may occur as an end-stage phenomenon.
- When the sacroiliac joints are involved, sclerosis tends to be a relatively early feature.
- When treatment has commenced, healing may be evident as sclerosis in the bone and extensive soft-tissue calcifications.

The classic description of a tuberculous joint also includes the following, known as Phemister's triad:

- Juxta-articular osteoporosis
- Marginal erosions
- Gradual narrowing of the joint space (**Fig. 71B**)

COMPUTED TOMOGRAPHY

- Utilized in the detection and characterization of paraspinal and sacroiliac collections, which tend to be much larger than a corresponding pyogenic infection
- Invaluable in the detection and characterization of early erosions and sclerosis in relation to tuberculosis sacroiliitis and sternoclavicular involvement
- The ability of CT to clearly identify calcifications in relation to abscesses is superior to that of MRI.
- Sequestra are clearly seen.

MAGNETIC RESONANCE IMAGING

- MRI findings in osteoarticular tuberculosis are nonspecific and similar to that seen with pyogenic musculoskeletal infections.
- MRI readily shows joint effusions and contained rice bodies, nodular synovitis, and cold abscesses.
- MRI also allows earlier detection of marrow edema and infiltration, which may expedite diagnosis and treatment.
- Gadolinium administration may better demonstrate soft-tissue fistulae, sinus tracts, and abscesses.

BONE SCAN

- Bone scanning with technetium is nonspecific and is likely to show a pattern of multifocal uptake similar to metastatic disease or cold spots, even in the presence of active disease. These cold foci are thought to represent avascular areas related to abscesses.

Treatment

- Treatment of osteoarticular tuberculosis is primarily medical, usually requiring long-term administration (between 12 and 18 months) of a combination of three drugs. The typical combination consists of isoniazid, rifampin, and pyrazinamide.
- If there is ongoing active disease after 4 to 6 months of continuous treatment, multidrug resistance should be suspected.
- Surgery for abscess drainage may be required.
- In cases where there is extensive joint destruction at the time of diagnosis, surgery in the form of synovial resection, arthrodesis, and/or arthroplasty may be required.
- Arthroplasty is generally reserved for those with secondary degenerative changes subsequent to tuberculous arthritis. Pre- and postoperative antibiotic therapy is required to avoid the potential disaster of placing a prosthesis in an infected space.

Prognosis

If there is no joint space loss at the time of diagnosis, medical therapy alone should suffice. The key to a favorable outcome is early diagnosis. When treated early and adequately, bone and joint infections tend to resolve with almost complete restoration of function. However, due to the indolent and nonspecific nature of its clinical presentation, the diagnosis of osteoarticular tuberculosis can be difficult and is often delayed, leading to significant morbidity. Residual pain and limitation of motion are common sequelae.

PEARLS

- When presented with a case of osteomyelitis with concurrence of both epiphysis and metaphysis in a child, it is most likely to be tuberculous, as transphyseal spread rarely occurs in pyogenic infections.
- The gradual destruction of cartilage and subchondral bone in tuberculous arthritis is in contradistinction to the rapid destruction seen in pyogenic arthritis.
- The maximum weight-bearing surfaces of the joint are typically affected only late in the process compared with pyogenic arthritis.

PITFALLS

- Early radiographs may be normal and do not exclude the disease; thus, in the appropriate clinical setting, one should have a high index of suspicion.
- Early juxta-articular osteoporosis is characteristic of tuberculous arthritis compared with pyogenic arthritis, in which osteoporosis tends to occur later.
- A negative chest x-ray in an adult does not exclude tuberculosis, as only 50% of patients with skeletal tuberculosis have pulmonary involvement. It is thought, however, that a negative chest x-ray in a child effectively excludes the diagnosis of concomitant musculoskeletal tuberculosis.

Suggested Readings

Moore SL, Rafii M. Imaging of musculoskeletal and spinal tuberculosis. Radiol Clin North Am 2001;39:329–342

Rathakrishnan V, Mohd TH. Osteo-articular tuberculosis: a radiological study in a Malaysian hospital. Skeletal Radiol 1989;18:267–272

Resnick D. Osteomyelitis, septic arthritis, and soft tissue infection: organisms. In: Resnick D, ed. Diagnosis of Bone and Joint Disorders, 4th ed. Philadelphia: WB Saunders; 1996;684–716

Watts HG, Lifeso RM. tuberculosis of bones and joints. J Bone Joint Surg Am 1996;78:288–298

CASE 72

Sam Y. Chun, Ali Islam, Alison Spouge, Anthony G. Ryan, and
Peter L. Munk

Clinical History

A 45-year-old man presented with a 1-month history of chest pain.

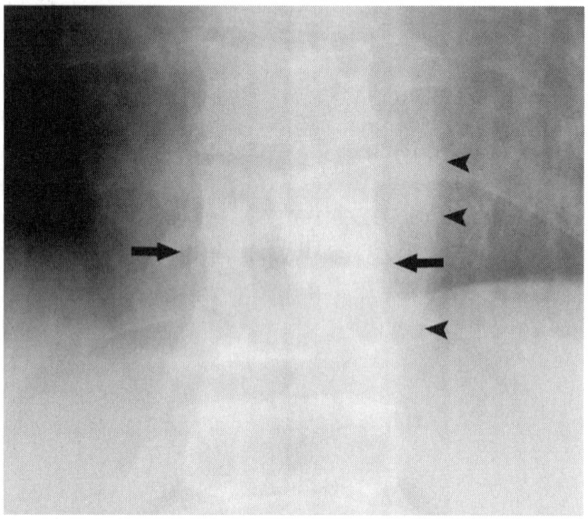

Figure 72A

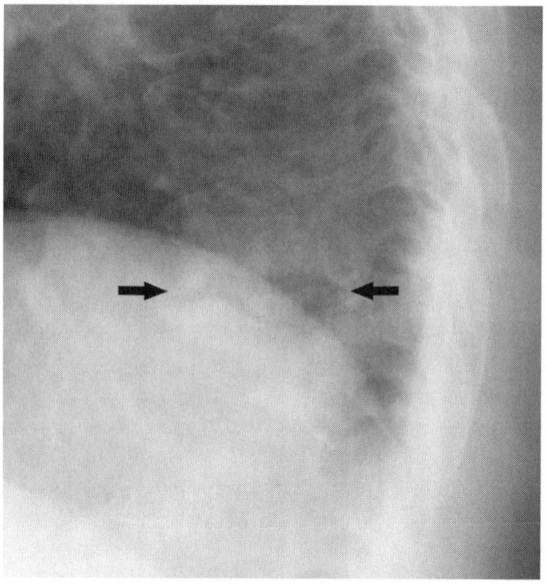

Figure 72B

Radiologic Findings

Anteroposterior (AP) (**Fig. 72A**) and lateral (**Fig. 72B**) views of the lumbar spine show destruction of the end plates at the T11/T12 disk space (arrows), with narrowing of the intervertebral disk space and mild irregular sclerosis. The AP view shows a left-sided paraspinal soft-tissue mass (arrowheads).

Diagnosis

Pyogenic diskitis.

Differential Diagnosis

- Pott's disease
- Chronic degenerative disk disease
- Metastatic disease

Discussion

Background

Diskitis refers to infection of the intervertebral disk space that occurs more often in children than in adults. It commonly involves the end plates of adjacent vertebral bodies and is thus also termed spondylodiskitis. Predisposing factors for spontaneous diskitis include concomitant infection at a primary site and immunocompromised states, such as advanced age, renal failure, and diabetes mellitus. Diskitis can also occur in the postoperative setting in up to 3% of spinal surgery cases.

Etiology

Pyogenic diskitis can be due to a variety of different organisms but is most frequently secondary to *Staphylococcus aureus.*

In the setting of endocarditis, *Streptococcus* is the most frequent causative agent, whereas *Pseudomonas aeruginosa* predominates among intravenous drug abusers.

Clinical Findings

The most common presenting features are back pain, localized tenderness, stiffness, and fever. These symptoms may occur following infections of the genitourinary, gastrointestinal, or respiratory tract. The lumbar spine is more often affected than the thoracic spine. Neurologic symptoms such as sciatica and paraparesis may also be present. Symptoms can be insidious, and diagnosis is often delayed for weeks or months.

Positive Gram's stain, blood culture, and erythrocyte sedimentation rate are supportive tests. Disk biopsy is confirmatory but may require multiple attempts and does not always yield a positive culture.

Pathogenesis

In childhood, vascularity of the disk allows for direct hematogenous infection. The intervertebral disks become avascular in adulthood, however, and in spontaneous diskitis, the initial site of infection occurs in the subchondral bone of the anterior aspect of the vertebral body from hematogenous spread of a primary infection, which then spreads to the adjacent disk. Spread of infection from the vertebral body to the adjacent disk is aided by local hyperemia of the inflamed end plate. The periphery of the disk is usually affected first. Once seeded, the avascular nature of the disk shelters it from immune defenses, facilitating spread of infection and destruction of the disk.

Complications

Infection of the intervertebral disk can lead to disruption of the anulus fibrosus and loss of disk height. Disk fragments that enter the spinal canal may cause spinal cord or nerve root compression. End plate destruction and osteolysis may also occur. Reparative bone formation in the vertebral body occurs after several weeks. Chronic infection can cause scoliosis or kyphosis.

Paravertebral or epidural abscess is an uncommon complication of diskitis.

Imaging Findings

RADIOGRAPHY

Radiographs in the initial stage of the infection may be normal. Irregularity of the adjacent end plates and loss of intervertebral disk height are the earliest findings, but these may take 2 to 3 weeks to become apparent. If the diskitis leads to vertebral osteomyelitis, almost half of the mineralized bone must be destroyed before osteopenia becomes evident. Chronic diskitis can lead to vertebral fusion that results in kyphoscoliosis.

BONE SCAN

Both technetium and gallium scanning are sensitive but nonspecific. Unlike technetium scans, gallium scans quickly become negative following treatment.

COMPUTED TOMOGRAPHY

CT accurately delineates end plate and vertebral body destruction and may detect paravertebral abscesses. End plate destruction is characterized by erosions and fragmentation. The intervertebral disk may show a central low attenuation area during early diskitis.

MAGNETIC RESONANCE IMAGING

MRI is the modality of choice in the assessment of diskitis and associated paravertebral disease. Both the infected disk and the adjacent end plates typically show hypointense signal on T1-weighted images and hyperintense signal on T2-weighted sequences. The abnormal vertebral marrow signal reflects the spread of edema and inflammatory infiltrates. End plate irregularity can also be identified. Early diskitis may have atypical signal characteristics and may not initially involve both adjacent end plates.

In children, low signal intensity on T1-weighted sequences may be more challenging to detect because the vertebral bodies contain a relatively larger amount of red marrow in children than in adults, resulting in a background of low to intermediate signal intensity on T1-weighted images.

The enhancement pattern of the disk following gadolinium administration is variable in diskitis and can be complete and homogeneous, heterogeneous, or peripheral. In the vertebral body, focal areas of osteolysis and abscesses show peripheral enhancement.

Treatment

The usual treatment for diskitis involves antibiotics and anti-inflammatory drugs along with external immobilization for 6 to 12 weeks. When empiric, antibiotic coverage should include gram-positive organisms such as *Staphylococcus aureus*. If diskitis is complicated by paravertebral abscess formation, percutaneous drainage may also be necessary. Surgical débridement may be necessary infrequently when there are signs of progressive neurologic impairment due to spinal cord or nerve root compression, or unremitting symptoms. Internal immobilization or spinal fusion is rarely necessary.

Prognosis

The prognosis of treated diskitis is usually favorable. In a study of 35 children followed for an average of 17 years, fewer than 50% had residual back pain, and more than 90% had normal flexion. Although residual pain and limited mobility can occur, recurrences are uncommon, and mortality is rare. The incidence of residual back pain is higher in elderly patients.

Even if untreated, many patients recover spontaneously. However, spinal fusion and kyphoscoliosis may occur in this setting.

PEARL

- Unlike technetium scans, gallium scans quickly become negative following treatment.

PITFALL

- Although Modic type I end plate changes produce T2-weighted high signal intensity changes within the end plates adjacent to a disk space, the disk itself will be dessicated; that is, it will show low signal intensity and will not demonstrate the rim enhancement seen with diskitis.

Suggested Readings

Friedman JA, Maher CO, Quast LM, et al. Spontaneous disc space infections in adults. Surg Neurol 2002;57:81–86

Maiuri F, Iaconetta G, Gallicchio B, Manto A, Briganti F. Spondylodiskitis: clinical and magnetic resonance diagnosis. Spine 1997;22:1741–1746

Ozuna RM, Delamarter RB. Pyogenic vertebral osteomyelitis and postsurgical disc space infections. Orthop Clin North Am 1996;27:87–94

CASE 73

Ali Islam, Alison Spouge, Anthony G. Ryan, and Peter L. Munk

Clinical Presentation

A 38-year-old woman presented with left lower quadrant abdominal pain and a background of chronic back pain. Clinical examination revealed a palpable mass within the left lower quadrant and a vague swelling in her back just cephalad to her iliac crest.

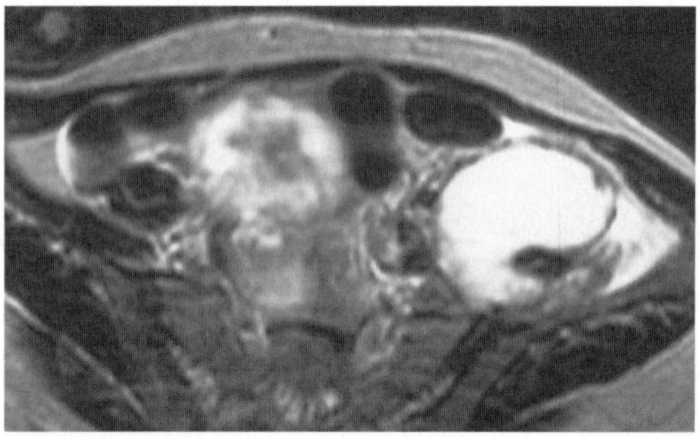

Figure 73A

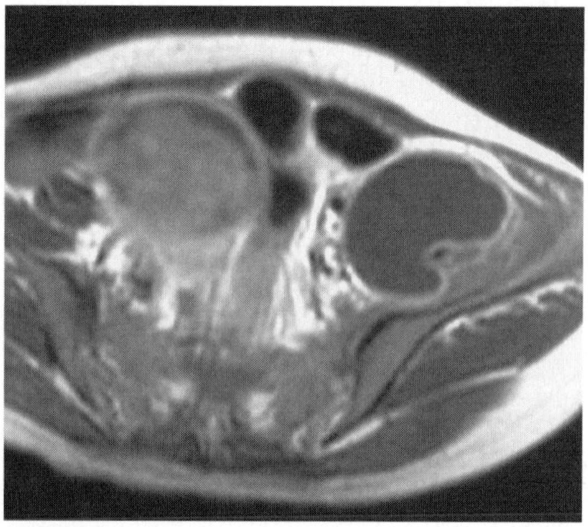

Figure 73B

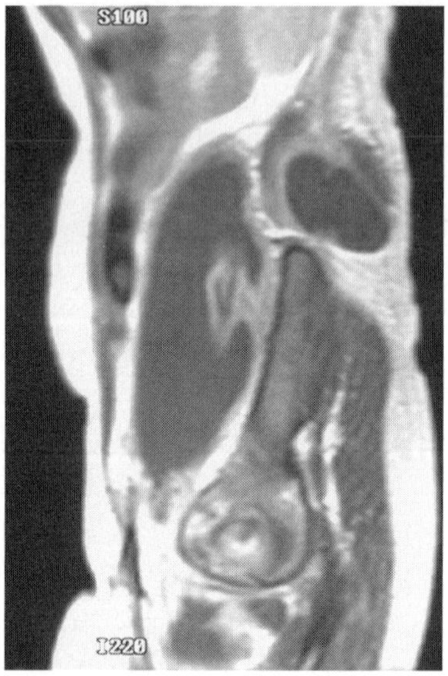

Figure 73C

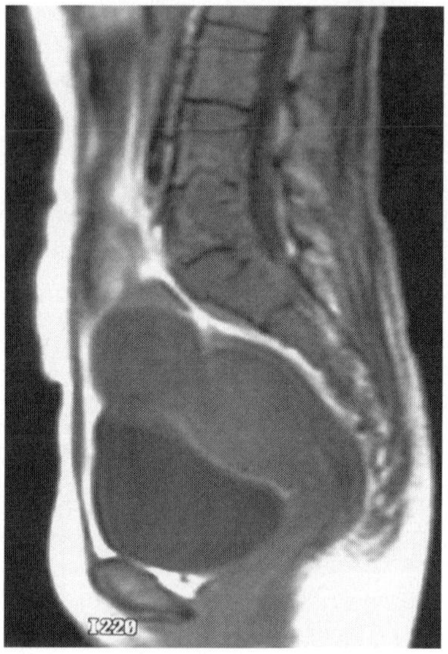

Figure 73D

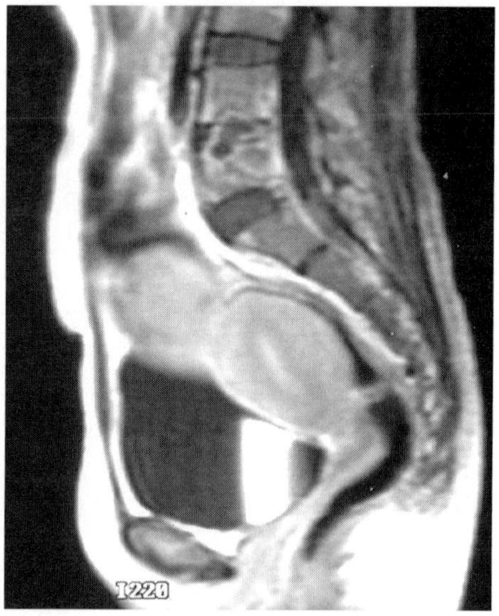

Figure 73E

Radiologic Findings

A transaxial T2-weighted image (**Fig. 73A**) through the pelvis shows a high signal collection, which on T1-weighted image postgadolinium (**Fig. 73B**) reveals a hypointense center and an enhancing rim.

A parasagittal T1-weighted image postgadolinium (**Fig. 73C**) shows the same collection in longitudinal section. Extension of the collection posterior to the spine above the iliac crest can be seen.

A sagittal T1-weighted image (**Fig. 73D**) reveals an ill-defined lobular lesion within the vertebral body of L5, which crosses the disk space superiorly into L4 and inferiorly into the back of the S1 vertebral body. Although the center of the lesion is hypointense, it demonstrates some internal heterogeneity. Most of the L4/L5 disk space is obliterated.

A sagittal T1-weighted image postgadolinium (**Fig. 73E**) shows rim enhancement of the lesion with heterogeneous enhancement of the surrounding vertebral bodies.

Diagnosis

Pott's disease (tuberculosis [TB] of the spine).

Differential Diagnosis

- Pyogenic spondylodiskitis
- Metastatic disease
- Fungal infection
- Sarcoidosis

Discussion

Background

Tuberculosis infects nearly 2 billion people worldwide, of which musculoskeletal infection accounts for nearly 2%. Tuberculosis of the spine (accounting for up to 60% of all musculoskeletal tuberculosis), or Pott's disease, as described by Percival Pott in 1779, is one of the most dangerous forms of tuberculous infection, as it may cause paraplegia and vertebral body destruction and collapse. It accounts for roughly half of the cases of musculoskeletal infection.

Tuberculosis is endemic in the population of many developing nations, and Pott's disease is common in children living in these areas. There is no gender predilection. In the developed world, risk factors for Pott's disease include human immunodeficiency virus (HIV), immunosuppression, alcoholism, homelessness, drug abuse, and residence in long-term care facilities and prisons.

Etiology

Pott's disease is characterized by infection with the acid-fast bacillus *Mycobacterium tuberculosis*. The spinal infection is usually secondary to a preexisting primary extraspinal source, commonly pulmonary tuberculosis.

Clinical Findings

The most common presenting symptoms of Pott's disease are back pain, weight loss, fever, and neurologic manifestations including paraplegia. The thoracolumbar spine is most commonly involved, followed by the lumbosacral and cervical spine. The constellation of symptoms depends on the level of disease and whether other organ systems are involved. Patients may present with abscesses or sinus tracts. Symptoms can be insidious and diagnosis is often delayed for weeks or months.

A negative tuberculin skin test does not exclude the diagnosis of Pott's disease. Diagnosis can be made by blood culture, percutaneous aspiration, or bone biopsy.

Pathogenesis

Pott's disease usually results from reactivation of quiescent primary tuberculosis at a distant site via hematogenous spread to epiphyseal vessels. The vessels typically responsible are the veins of Batson's paravertebral plexus rather than spinal arteries, as infection generally begins at the corners, particularly the anterior corner, of vertebrae. Because disks are avascular, their involvement is secondary. Local spread is via blood vessels and subligamentous channels.

Pathology

GROSS

The classic description of Pott's disease is that of end plate destruction of two adjacent vertebral bodies, along with involvement of the intervening disk and a paraspinal mass, as in the reference case above. However, an atypical form of the disease characterized by spondylitis without disk involvement is becoming more commonly recognized.

Vertebral body involvement can be paradiscal, anterior, or central. In the most common form (paradiscal), infection in the vertebral metaphysis erodes the end plate and the disk. In the anterior form, infection deep to the anterior longitudinal ligament can elevate periosteum, devascularize bone, and spread to multiple levels. In the central form, the entire body is involved, and severe vertebra plana deformity can occur.

Collapse of the anterior elements may result in kyphosis. Neurologic involvement may be due to dural invasion or mass effect on spinal nerves by abscess, granulation tissue, bone, or disk sequestra.

Abscesses are common and may track along tissue planes, into the epidural compartment, or rupture through the skin.

MICROSCOPIC

Seen on microscopic examination are tuberculous caseating granulomata consisting of giant and epithelioid cells with variable calcification, surrounded by a rim (mantle) of lymphocytes, progressing to abscess formation.

Imaging Findings

RADIOGRAPHY

- Erosions, irregular end plates at two (or more) contiguous levels, loss of vertebral body height, disk space narrowing, sequestra, and paravertebral soft-tissue swelling may be identified on conventional radiographs.
- Reactive sclerosis is an uncommon feature of Pott's disease.
- A sharp kyphosis, or gibbus deformity, may present acutely.
- The entire vertebral body is not usually involved.
- Narrowing of the intervertebral disk spaces occurs early in the disease due to herniation into weakened end plates.

BONE SCAN

- Technetium scanning is sensitive but nonspecific in the diagnosis of Pott's disease.
- Radionuclide scanning is useful in screening for additional sites of osseous involvement.

COMPUTED TOMOGRAPHY

- CT is the modality of choice for detecting bony sequestra within the paraspinal tissues and is used to guide percutaneous biopsy.
- CT also shows end plate and vertebral body destruction and may detect paravertebral abscesses.
- The pattern of destruction is usually fragmentary but may be diffusely osteolytic and less commonly sclerotic.

MAGNETIC RESONANCE IMAGING

- MRI is the modality of choice for visualizing the entire spine and central canal, as it can accurately assess for cord or nerve compression, meningeal disease, and paraspinal abscess formation.
- Diseased vertebrae and disks typically demonstrate hypointense signal on T1-weighted sequences and show heterogeneously hyperintense signal on T2-weighted images.
- Chronic tuberculosis may have hypo- or hyperintense signal on T1-weighted images. Abscesses, which in Pott's disease are typically large, will show central necrosis and peripheral enhancement following gadolinium administration (**Fig. 73E**) and can thus be distinguished from granulation tissue on T1 sequences.

Treatment

- The primary treatment of choice is 6 months of antibiotic therapy. Current recommendations are treatment with four drugs for 2 months, followed by 4 months of treatment with two drugs. Revised recommendations may extend medical therapy to 12 months.
- Surgery is performed if there is involvement of the posterior elements, instability, recurrent neurologic deficit, or persistent active infection.
- Immediate surgery is indicated when there is acute paraplegia, acute kyphosis, or severe neurologic impairment.
- The approach and type of surgery performed vary between centers. Anterior débridement with spinal fusion is advocated most often to prevent kyphosis.

Prognosis

- Although tuberculosis kills nearly 3 million people each year, Pott's disease can be treated and cured. The best indicator of healing Pott's disease is spontaneous fusion between vertebral bodies following antibiotic treatment.
- More than 90% of patients who receive adequate therapy will recover, with additional surgical intervention required in ~25% of cases.
- The recovery rate from paraplegia is highly variable and is unlikely to improve if paralysis is persistent for more than 6 months.

PEARLS

- Abscesses, which in Pott's disease are typically large, will show central necrosis and peripheral enhancement following gadolinium administration and can thus be distinguished from granulation tissue on T1 sequences. Paravertebral abscesses may be calcified.

- Reactive sclerosis is an uncommon feature of Pott's disease.
- The best indicator of healing Pott's disease is spontaneous fusion between vertebral bodies following antibiotic treatment.

PITFALLS

- The indolent nature of the disease can be deceptive, and in the presence of ongoing clinical symptoms, further investigations should be pursued in the presence of normal initial radiographs (a normal chest radiograph in a child suggests that musculoskeletal tuberculosis is very unlikely).
- Although it makes the diagnosis less likely, a negative skin test does not exclude the diagnosis.
- In the presence of a spondylodiskitis with prominent sclerotic reaction, tuberculosis is unlikely and an alternative diagnosis should be sought, such as more common pyogenic organisms or other atypical organisms (e.g., brucellosis).

Suggested Readings

Boachie-Adjei O, Squillante RG. Tuberculosis of the spine. Orthop Clin North Am 1996;27:95–103

Moon MS. Tuberculosis of the spine: controversies and a new challenge. Spine 1997;22:1791–1797

Weaver P, Lifeso RM. The radiological diagnosis of the adult spine. Skeletal Radiol 1984;12:178–186

CASE 74

Sam Y. Chun, Ali Islam, Alison Spouge, Anthony G. Ryan, and
Peter L. Munk

Clinical Presentation

A 45-year-old woman with a 1-week history of increasing anterior knee pain and swelling presented to us. Physical exam showed focal soft-tissue swelling and erythema over the front of the knee.

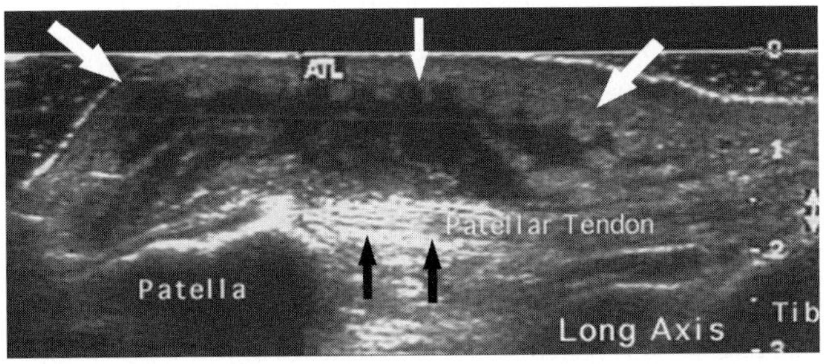

Figure 74A

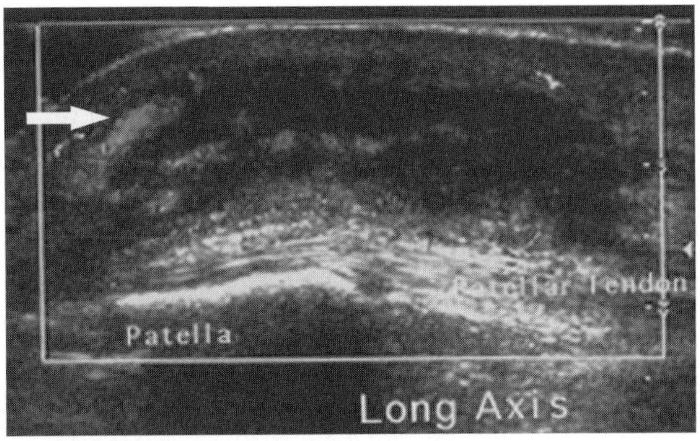

Figure 74B (See also **Figure 74B** in color insert.)

Radiologic Findings

A long axis sonogram at the anterior aspect of the knee (**Fig. 74A**) shows a large, irregular fluid- and debris-containing collection (white arrows) with thick, irregular walls. The deep surface of the collection contacts the anterior aspect of the patella and patellar tendon (black arrows).

A long axis sonogram (**Fig. 74B**) in the same location as **Fig. 74A** with color Doppler shows prominent hyperemia (white arrow).

Diagnosis

Septic prepatellar bursitis.

Differential Diagnosis

- Infected versus noninfected bursitis
- Cellulitis
- Hematoma/seroma
- Abscess

Discussion

Background

Bursae are sacs lined by endothelial cells that serve to reduce friction at sites where tendons, muscle, and bone glide over each other. Constant bursae are formed during normal development, and adventitious bursae are formed when there is abnormal friction and stress, causing myxomatous degeneration of fibrous tissue at pressure points. Deep bursae frequently communicate with the adjacent joint.

Risk factors for bursitis include occupations requiring repetitive motion, increased age, gout, rheumatoid arthritis, and concurrent bacterial infection. In athletes, the incidence of bursitis has been reported to be as high as 10%, and in the general population, it accounts for < 0.5% of visits to primary-care facilities.

Common sites for bursitis include the shoulder (subacromial/subdeltoid bursa, subscapular bursa), olecranon bursa, iliopsoas bursa, ischiogluteal bursa, greater trochanter bursa, prepatellar bursa, deep and superficial infrapatellar bursae, Baker's cyst, and retrocalcaneal and pre-Achilles' bursae. Adventitious bursae are found in sites where there are pseudoarthroses, exostoses, or malalignment of a joint, such as hallux valgus.

Etiology

There are many causes for bursitis. Some of the most common causes are trauma, infection, and crystal deposition. Traumatic bursitis may be related to hemorrhage or inflammation from repetitive injury. Infectious bursitis is usually due to staphylococcal or streptococcal species. Tuberculous bursitis is rare. Crystal deposition within bursae may be due to gout, pseudogout (calcium pyrophosphate deposition), autoimmune disease such as rheumatoid arthritis, or metabolic conditions such as hyperparathyroidism.

Clinical Findings

The onset of symptoms is variable, ranging from acute pain to chronic low-grade irritation. The range of motion in the adjacent joint is often limited due to pain. Chronic bursitis can lead to muscle atrophy. Bursitis can be a difficult clinical diagnosis because symptoms are often vague and nonspecific and because they can be related to multiple adjacent structures. Specific physical findings depend on the location of the bursa.

A history of trauma, infection, or arthropathy related to crystal deposition can be helpful. In the setting of infectious bursitis, fever, cellulitis, local warmth, and bacteremia can suggest the diagnosis.

Serum leukocyte count and erythrocyte sedimentation rate may be elevated but are nonspecific markers. Bursal fluid can be analyzed by microscopy, cell count, Gram's stain, and culture to establish the exact etiology, given the clinical overlap in presentation of noninfectious and infectious bursitis. Septic bursitis is less common in children.

Pathogenesis

Synovial cells present in constant bursae secrete fluid containing proteoglycans and collagen. The synovial fluid produced is of sufficient volume to reduce friction. Overproduction of fluid due to various reasons can cause effusion and inflammatory changes in bursae.

Inflammatory bursitis from repetitive microtrauma is due to local hyperemia and altered vascular permeability that allows extravasation of fluid and proteins into the bursa. The presence of extravasated proteins or crystal deposited within the bursa initiates a cytokine- and leukocyte-induced inflammatory response that may cause synovial lining hypertrophy and villous hyperplasia. Chronic bursitis can lead to formation of fibrous tissue.

Distended fluid-filled bursae increase friction and impede the motion of tendons, skin, bone, and muscle. Viscous fluid due to infection or hemorrhage also has fewer lubricant qualities.

Bursitis can occur in various locations: subcutaneous, subfascial, subtendinous, submucosal, or interligamentous.

Superficial bursae are more prone to infection and are also prone to hemorrhage from direct trauma. Deep bursae often communicate with the adjacent joint, such as the knee.

Imaging Findings

ULTRASOUND

- Sonography is the primary modality for the diagnosis of bursitis, as it is readily available, inexpensive, and highly sensitive in detecting and localizing fluid in superficial and most deep bursae.
- It provides additional information regarding the severity of inflammation using color Doppler.
- It may be used to guide needle aspiration.

MAGNETIC RESONANCE IMAGING

- MRI is very accurate in establishing the diagnosis of bursitis and is most useful as a problem-solving tool when ultrasound fails to yield a diagnosis or if visualization is suboptimal for deeper sites of involvement.
- Fluid within bursae is usually uniformly low signal on T1- and bright on T2-weighted images, unless hemorrhage or purulent debris is present.

COMPUTED TOMOGRAPHY

- CT can be particularly helpful if infection is suspected in the underlying bone.

NUCLEAR MEDICINE

- An active bursitis will be markedly hyperintense and focal.
- More widespread activity suggests an accompanying cellulitis of the overlying subcutaneous soft tissues.
- No increased radiopharmaceutical uptake on the delayed images helps to exclude underlying osteomyelitis.

Treatment

ASEPTIC BURSITIS

- Conservative management with rest, elevation of the involved extremity, hot or cold compresses, and nonsteroidal anti-inflammatory drugs
- Occasionally, aspiration of bursa and intrabursal injection of steroids is performed.
- For chronic bursitis, intrabursal injections of sclerosing agents can be considered.
- Surgical correction of tendon or bony abnormality contributing to the bursitis can also be considered.

SEPTIC BURSITIS

- Antibiotics are initiated immediately even before culture results from the bursal aspirate become available.
- Initial coverage should include staphylococcal and streptococcal species. Most patients are treated on an outpatient basis for 10 to 14 days.
- Surgical débridement is performed if there is a failure to respond to adequate treatment.

Prognosis

- Patients treated for septic bursitis take an average of 40 days to recover normal function, although the bursal fluid is often sterilized within 4 days of starting antibiotics.
- In contrast, patients treated for aseptic bursitis may take weeks or months to recover.
- Chronic bursitis and muscle atrophy can be avoided by improving flexibility and performing range of motion exercises. Steroid injections should not be given more than three times a year and should be spaced apart by at least 1 month to avoid complications such as tendon rupture, fat atrophy, and infection. Close to 50% of patients have improvement in symptoms with steroid injection within 2 weeks.

PEARL

- Radionuclide imaging is the best single investigation to exclude underlying osteomyelitis and may help identify deep cellulitis not initially suspected clinically.

PITFALL

- Care should be taken to ensure there is no history of penetrating injury, as a subcutaneous abscess secondary to retained foreign body may be indistinguishable from a septic bursitis.

Suggested Readings

Biundo JJ Jr, Irwin RW, Umpierre E. Sports and other soft tissue injuries, tendinitis, bursitis, and occupation-related syndromes. Curr Opin Rheumatol 2001;13:146–149

Stell IM. Management of acute bursitis: outcome study of a structured approach. J R Soc Med 1999;92:516–521

Zimmermann B III, Mikolich DJ, Ho G Jr. Septic bursitis. Semin Arthritis Rheum 1995;24:391–410

CASE 75

Sam Y. Chun, Ali Islam, Alison Spouge, Anthony G. Ryan, and Peter L. Munk

Clinical Presentation

A 40-year-old diabetic patient presented with sudden onset of arm pain, swelling, and erythema. The patient was afebrile with a normal leukocyte count.

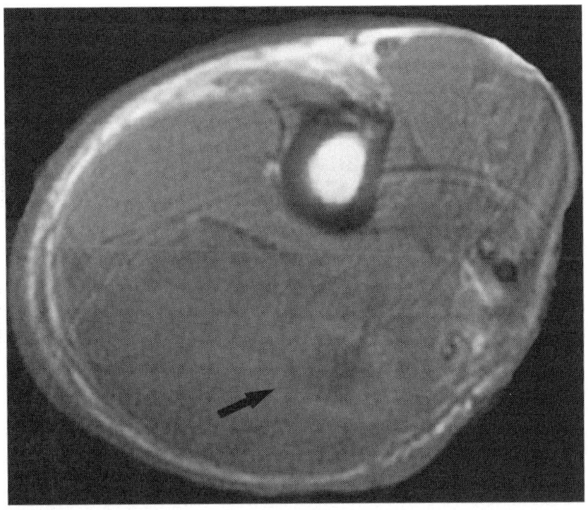

Figure 75A

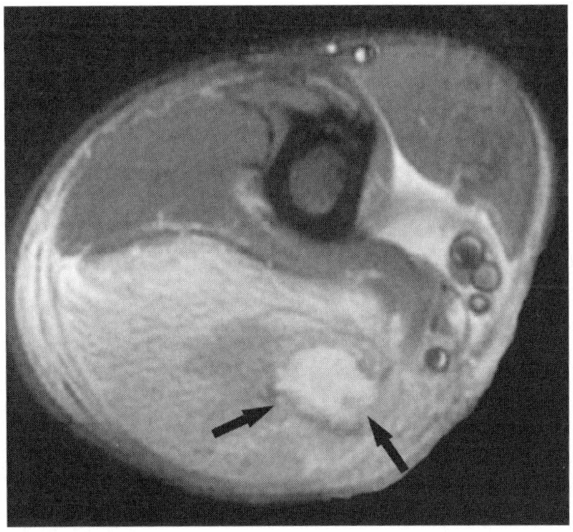

Figure 75B

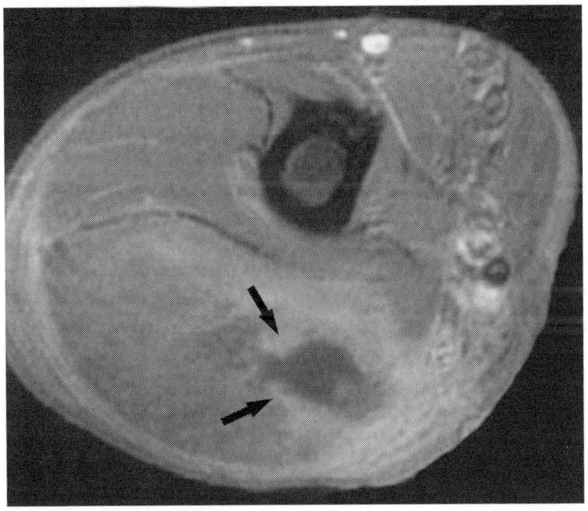

Figure 75C

Radiologic Findings

An axial spin-echo T1-weighted image (**Fig. 75A**) shows diffuse low signal intensity within the triceps muscle, with a more focal region of hypointensity (arrow). Extensive high signal intensity is present on the inversion recovery sequence (**Fig. 75B**), with a focus of particularly high intensity (arrows) corresponding to the hypointense region on the T1 image. Fat-saturated T1-weighted image postgadolinium (**Fig. 75C**) shows rim enhancement of the area consistent with abscess formation (arrows).

Diagnosis

Pyomyositis.

Differential Diagnosis

- Necrotizing fasciitis
- Cellulitis
- Idiopathic inflammatory myositis

Discussion

Background

Diagnosis of soft-tissue infections has markedly improved with the advances in cross-sectional imaging modalities, particularly MRI. Soft-tissue infections can be generally classified as

1. Primary infections, including cellulitis, pyomyositis, abscesses, and necrotizing fasciitis
2. Secondary infections associated with septic arthritis or bursitis
3. Soft-tissue infections related to underlying osteomyelitis
4. The diabetic foot
5. Parasitic infections
6. Miscellaneous

Here we will focus on primary soft-tissue infections, that is, cellulitis, necrotizing fasciitis, and pyogenic myositis (pyomyositis).

Etiology

CELLULITIS

Group A *Streptococcus* is the most common causative organism, followed by *Staphylococcus aureus*. Other inciting organisms include *Haemophilus influenzae*, *Streptococcus pneumoniae*, *Neisseria meningitidis*, and *Cryptococcus*.

NECROTIZING FASCIITIS

Although the majority of cases are polymicrobial, group A *Streptococcus* and/or *S. aureus* are commonly the initial infecting bacteria. Other aerobic and anaerobic organisms may be present, including *Bacteroides*, *Clostridium*, *Peptostreptococcus*, Enterobacteriaceae, coliforms, *Proteus*, *Pseudomonas*, and *Klebsiella*.

PYOMYOSITIS

Infectious myositis can be caused by a variety of pathogens, including bacteria, viruses (e.g., influenza, coxsackie), protozoa, and parasites. Pyogenic myositis is most frequently caused by *Staphylococcus aureus*; less common causative bacteria include *Mycobacterium tuberculosis*, *Nocardia*, *Streptococcus pyogenes* and *viridans*, and *Cryptococcus*.

Clinical Findings

CELLULITIS

Cellulitis generally refers to an acute spreading infection of the dermis and subcutaneous tissues that presents with signs and symptoms of inflammation (pain, swelling, erythema, and heat). Other clinical findings may include regional lymphadenopathy and fever. If the cellulitis becomes more extensive or spreads to other structures, complications such as necrotizing fasciitis, osteomyelitis, and septic arthritis may arise. Aspiration of the wound is rarely useful, as the cultures are positive only one third of the time.

NECROTIZING FASCIITIS

Necrotizing fasciitis is a relatively rare but rapidly progressive condition, with an associated mortality rate of 30 to 70%. It is characterized by extensive necrosis of the subcutaneous tissues, fascia, and surrounding soft tissue. Predisposing risk factors include immunocompromised conditions such as diabetes, cancer, and vascular disease. There is often a history of recent trauma or surgery to the involved area. Necrotizing fasciitis in its early stages may be difficult to diagnose, as patients may have a nonspecific presentation of pain, swelling, and fever. The clinician should be suspicious of this condition in patients whose pain is out of proportion with physical signs. The infection can spread rapidly over the course of hours or days as a growing area of indurated, erythematous skin that eventually becomes a dusky or purplish color. The pain may progress to anesthesia due to necrosis of nerve fibers. The most important physical findings include tissue necrosis, putrid discharge, bullae and blisters, severe pain, crepitus, rapid undermining of the fascial planes, and relative lack of the classical inflammatory signs. The degree of deep-tissue necrosis is usually more severe than clinical findings suggest. The patient may rapidly progress to septic shock and multiorgan failure.

PYOMYOSITIS

Pyomositis is a serious infection of the muscles that most commonly affects children and young adults living in the tropics. The condition is becoming more prevalent in temperate climates, especially among the immunocompromised and intravenous (IV) drug users. The patient presents with muscle pain and tenderness with hard induration of the overlying skin. Other clinical findings include fever, malaise, and muscle spasm and contracture. The muscles of the lower extremities, particularly in the thigh and buttocks, are the most commonly affected. Blood work demonstrates leukocytosis and an elevated erythrocyte sedimentation rate, but serum creatine kinase (marker of muscle damage) and blood cultures are usually negative. Early detection is important to prevent myonecrosis and sepsis, but pyomyositis can be difficult to diagnose. Because the infections are deep-seated, the clinical presentation is often vague and nonspecific and may resemble other more common conditions, such as deep venous thrombosis, septic arthritis, and malignancy.

Pathogenesis

Primary infections of the soft tissues generally result from direct contamination following penetrating trauma or any other process that disrupts skin integrity. Hematogenous route of infection is less common. In some cases, no discernible skin injury can be found. Predisposing risk factors include IV drug abuse and systemic debilitating disease, such as diabetes and peripheral vascular disease.

CELLULITIS

Most bacterial soft-tissue infections begin as cellulitis. The infection can remain localized or spread to other structures, giving rise to fasciitis, myositis, and osteomyelitis. Cellulitis due to *Staphylococcus aureus* tends to spread centripetally from a localized infection such as an abscess or folliculitis, whereas *Streptococcus pyogenes* cellulitis usually spreads more rapidly and diffusely, with associated fever and lymphangitis.

NECROTIZING FASCIITIS

Necrotizing fasciitis is characterized by rapid spread of infection along fascial planes and through the vascular and lymphatic systems. This results in extensive necrosis of subcutaneous tissues, fascia, and surrounding soft-tissue structures such as muscle.

PYOMYOSITIS

Most patients with pyomyositis do not have a history of penetrating trauma. However, the disease is most prevalent in the tropics, where the lack of footwear may predispose to minor trauma and insect bites, resulting in local infection. The majority of tropical cases are associated with foot pyoderma. Because skeletal muscle is relatively resistant to infections, particularly via the hematogenous route, the pathogenesis of pyomyositis is unclear. It is thought that an initial muscle insult may be required for local seeding of infection and subsequent development of abscesses.

Pathology

- *Cellulitis* is seen as acute inflammation of the skin, subcutaneous tissue, and underlying fascia.
- *Necrotizing fasciitis* is characterized by extensive inflammation and necrosis of the subcutaneous tissues, fascia, and sometimes muscle. The deeper fascial planes between muscle bundles tend to be affected in necrotizing fasciitis but not commonly in cellulitis.
- *Pyomyositis* is characterized by inflammation and widespread necrosis of muscle fibers, perimysium, and blood vessels, resulting in single or multiple intramuscular abscesses. Usually, only one muscle group is affected, but infection of multiple muscles is occasionally seen.

Imaging Findings for Cellulitis

ULTRASOUND

- Ultrasound is a readily accessible imaging modality that can quickly evaluate soft-tissue infections. Under ultrasound, the characteristic subcutaneous edema of cellulitis appears as hypoechoic strands between hyperechoic fat lobules, often in a cobblestone pattern. This is a nonspecific finding, as subcutaneous edema of any cause can have the same appearance.
- Ultrasound may also identify larger fluid collections or abscesses, which can be aspirated under sonographic guidance for diagnostic purposes.

NUCLEAR MEDICINE

- Three-phase bone scan can help to differentiate between cellulitis and osteomyelitis. In cellulitis, increased activity is seen on the blood flow and immediate images, with only mildly increased or normal uptake on the delayed scan. Osteomyelitis demonstrates increased uptake on all three phases.

COMPUTED TOMOGRAPHY

Because cellulitis is generally a clinical diagnosis, imaging is usually not required. Plain film findings are subtle and nonspecific, consisting mainly of soft-tissue swelling or haziness of the subcutaneous fat. If gas is present, small lucent foci may be identified. If necrotizing fasciitis is a concern, CT and MRI may be utilized for early detection.

CT findings of cellulitis include

- Thickening of the skin
- Septation of the subcutaneous fat
- Thickening of the underlying fascia
- All of the above may demonstrate enhancement with contrast administration.

MAGNETIC RESONANCE IMAGING

- MRI findings are similar to those seen with CT except that the abnormal structures demonstrate high T2 signal intensity and enhancement with gadolinium administration.
- Surrounding soft-tissue edema is better appreciated with MRI.

Imaging Findings for Necrotizing Fasciitis

RADIOGRAPHY

- Plain film findings are similar to those of cellulitis (soft-tissue swelling), but serial films will demonstrate rapid changes over a relatively short period of time. In some cases, gas is identified in the soft tissues, which is highly suggestive of necrotizing fasciitis.

ULTRASOUND

- Ultrasound findings are similar to those of cellulitis (subcutaneous edema), with the addition of gas bubbles and involvement of the deep fascial plane between muscle bundles.

COMPUTED TOMOGRAPHY

- CT has been advocated for the early detection of necrotizing fasciitis, as it can readily demonstrate asymmetric fascial thickening, gas, and abscesses.

MAGNETIC RESONANCE IMAGING

- On MRI, T2-weighted images demonstrate increased signal intensity in the subcutaneous tissues (similar pattern to cellulitis) as well as high signal intensity tracking and thickening in the deeper fascial planes.
- Occasionally, low signal intensity foci representing gas are seen within the abnormal high signal background. Ill-defined edema may be present in the neighboring muscle.
- On T1-weighted images, gadolinium administration demonstrates enhancement of diseased tissue similar to that seen on T2-weighted images. However, necrotic tissue enhances minimally or only at the periphery of the infected area.
- Although MRI is a reliable means of detecting and evaluating necrotizing fasciitis, it can be a time-consuming procedure, which may endanger the critically ill patient who requires immediate treatment.

Imaging Findings for Pyomyositis

RADIOGRAPHY

- Plain film findings in pyomyositis are often absent but may show soft-tissue swelling and obliteration of deep fat planes.

ULTRASOUND

- Ultrasound may be used for the imaging of pyomyositis. In the early stages of infection, the muscle is edematous and hypoechoic in appearance. This stage of infection can usually be treated with intravenous antibiotics alone. If left untreated, intramuscular abscesses develop that manifest as hypoechoic fluid collections, often containing mobile hyperechoic debris.
- Color Doppler characteristically demonstrates increased vascularity around the abscess without any flow within it. After the abscess has been identified, ultrasound-guided aspiration may be performed for diagnostic and/or therapeutic purposes.

COMPUTED TOMOGRAPHY

- CT readily demonstrates muscle edema and focal fluid collections representing abscesses that show rim enhancement after contrast administration. In addition, fluid aspiration may be attempted under CT guidance. CT, however, often underestimates the degree of muscle involvement.

MAGNETIC RESONANCE IMAGING

- MRI can more accurately demonstrate the full extent of infection and even identify foci of disease not detected on CT.

- On T1-weighted images, the affected area typically demonstrates slightly higher signal intensity than normal muscle and is often surrounded by a rim of increased signal intensity.
- On T2-weighted images, the involved muscles demonstrate heterogeneously increased signal intensity, which may be associated with foci of high signal intensity fluid. These fluid collections are usually surrounded by a low T2 signal intensity rim that enhances with gadolinium administration.
- Other MRI findings include reticulation of the subcutaneous fat and thickening of the fascial planes and overlying skin. These findings can also be seen with diabetic myonecrosis, which classically presents with a sudden onset of extreme muscle pain.

Treatment

CELLULITIS

- Mild cases can usually be treated by oral antibiotics, typically consisting of a penicillinase-resistant synthetic penicillin or a first-generation cephalosporin. Patients who do not improve may require parenteral antibiotics.

NECROTIZING FASCIITIS

- Early detection is vital for any chance of successful treatment, which consists of urgent aggressive surgical débridement of all necrotic tissue in addition to antibiotic therapy. Repeated débridement may be necessary to ensure that all the necrotic tissue is excised.
- Antibiotic regimens must have coverage for aerobic and anaerobic bacteria. Differentiation from uncomplicated cellulitis can be difficult but is imperative because cellulitis is treated nonsurgically.

PYOMOSITIS

- Early diagnosis and treatment help prevent myonecrosis and sepsis.
- Antibiotics are the mainstay of treatment, usually starting with parenteral agents until clinical improvement is noted, which is followed by oral agents for a total course of 3 weeks.
- Abscess drainage under ultrasound or CT guidance may be required, especially for larger abscesses.

Prognosis

CELLULITIS

- Prognosis is excellent, as the antibiotic regimens are > 90% effective.

NECROTIZING FASCIITIS

- Prognosis is generally poor, with an overall morbidity and mortality of 70 to 80%. Life-threatening complications are septic shock with cardiovascular collapse and renal failure. Survivors are often left with disfiguring scarring and/or amputations.

PYOMYOSITIS

- Prognosis is usually good with prompt treatment. Potential life-threatening complications include sepsis and toxic shock syndrome (strep infection).

PEARL

- Three-phase bone scan helps to differentiate between cellulitis and underlying osteomyelitis. In cellulitis, increased activity is seen on the blood flow and immediate images, with only mildly increased or normal uptake on the delayed scan. Osteomyelitis demonstrates increased uptake on all three phases.

PITFALL

- In the ultrasound assessment of pyomyositis, a significant amount of muscle damage and infiltration may occur before frank abscess formation is evident. In the appropriate setting, hypoechoic, edematous-appearing muscle should raise the suspicion of infection. At this stage of infection, intravenous antibiotics are the treatment of choice and aspiration is not indicated. Visible abscesses should, of course, be aspirated for culture and sensitivity.

Suggested Readings

Boutin RD, Brossmann J, Sartoris DJ, Reilly D, Resnick D. Update on imaging of orthopedic infections. Orthop Clin North Am 1998;29:41–66

Cardinal E, Bureau NJ, Aubin B, Chhem RK. Role of ultrasound in musculoskeletal infections. Radiol Clin North Am 2001;39:191–201

Struk DW, Munk PL, Lee MJ, Ho SG, Worsley DF. Imaging of soft tissue infections. Radiol Clin North Am 2001;39:277–303

CASE 76

Anthony G. Ryan and Peter L. Munk

Clinical Presentation

A 45-year-old man presented with chronic left hip pain exacerbated by exercise, status post subcapital fracture, which had been acutely pinned and appeared radiographically healed. The patient's range of motion was limited by pain.

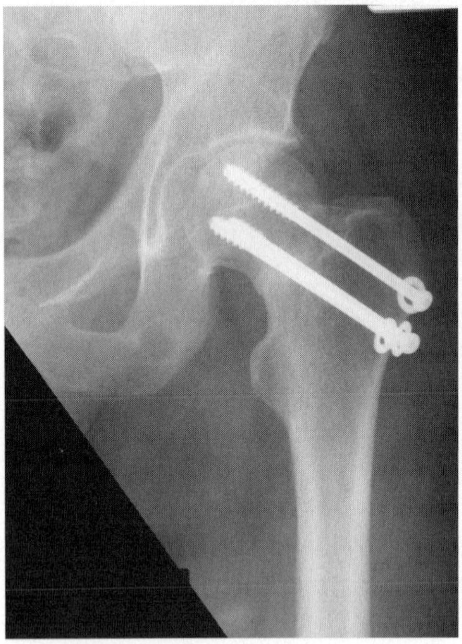

Figure 76A

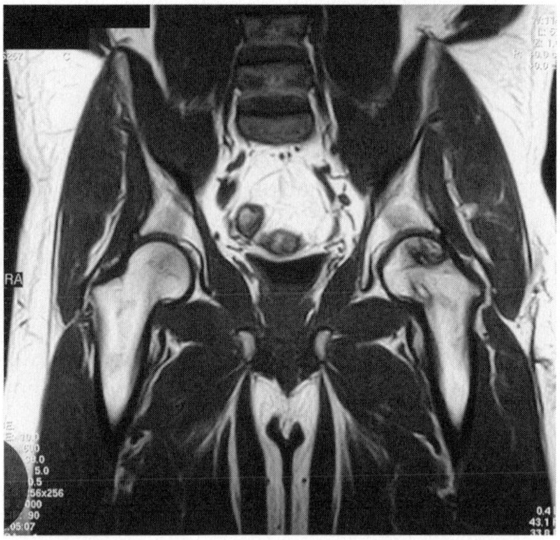

Figure 76B

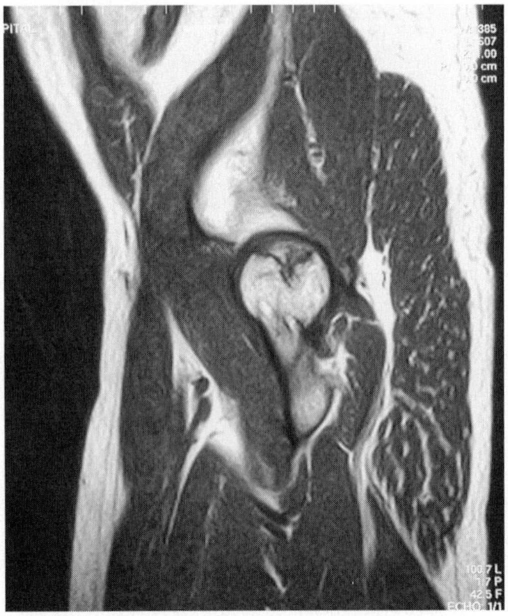

Figure 76C

Radiologic Findings

An anteroposterior radiograph of the left hip with fixation screws in situ shows some joint space narrowing and acetabular articular sclerosis, but no other significant abnormality (**Fig. 76A**). A coronal T1-weighted image taken 3 months later (**Fig. 76B**) shows a crescentic low signal intensity line undermining the superolateral femoral head with heterogeneity of the cephalad fragment, which itself contains multiple low signal intensity lines. Loss of continuity of the cortical margin is evident laterally. Irregularity of the articular surface of the femoral head and adjacent acetabular articular surfaces is evident.

Similar findings are demonstrated on the accompanying sagittal T1-weighted image (**Fig. 76C**), which shows the loss of joint space and articular surface irregularity with greater conspicuity. The prominent, well-demarcated low signal intensity line assumes a triangular margin in this plane.

Diagnosis

Avascular necrosis (AVN) of the femoral head.

Differential Diagnosis

None.

Discussion

Etiology

Interruption of the blood supply to bone may occur secondary to trauma to, or obstruction of, the vessels supplying the bone by intravascular elements, vasculitis, or extravascular compromise.

In the adult, traumatic arterial interruption is typically caused by fracture of the femoral neck or, less commonly, by hip joint dislocation. Intravascular causes of arterial obstruction include hemoglobinopathies and caisson disease ("the bends").

Vasculitic causes include connective tissue disorders and radiation exposure. Increased intraosseous pressure may arise secondary to accumulation of abnormal cells, such as histiocytes in Gaucher's disease on fat cells secondary to steroid usage.

The mechanism by which alcohol abuse causes AVN has not been clearly identified. It is thought that pancreatitis causes AVN by a combination of the above, for example, vasculitis associated with abnormal intravascular cells.

A cause for avascular necrosis is not identified in as many as 25% of cases.

The femoral head is at particular risk for necrosis by virtue of the tenuous blood supply to the femoral epiphysis via the medial circumflex and lateral epiphyseal arteries.

Pathophysiology

The hallmark of AVN is, as its name suggests, an ischemic insult producing interruption (of varying duration, depending on the etiology) of the blood supply to the affected bone or portion of bone. The radiologic features of fragmentation, collapse, sclerosis, and eventual reossification of the involved bone correlate well with the pathologic progress and repair of the resultant osteonecrosis. Disruption of the blood supply, sufficient to cause anoxia, causes death of hematopoietic cells in 6 to 12 hours, bone cell death within 12 to 48 hours, and marrow fat cell death after 48 to 60 hours.

The central zone of cell death is surrounded by a region of less complete ischemic injury, at the margin of which is a zone of hyperemia secondary to thrombosed vessel recanalization and concurrent neovascularity.

Clinical Findings

The typical patient is between 20 and 50 years of age, presenting with a combination of hip, groin, thigh, or knee pain, usually ongoing for months, with a limited range of motion on examination.

Stages of Disease

Based on clinical and imaging findings:

Stage 0 Suspected clinically, normal radiographs
Stage 1 Clinical findings, abnormal nuclear medicine studies
Stage 2 Osteopenia, cysts, bone sclerosis
Stage 3 Crescent sign secondary to subchondral fracture but without collapse
Stage 4 Flattening of the femoral head with a retained joint space
Stage 5 Joint narrowing and changes on the acetabular aspect of the joint

Complications

Accelerated degenerative joint disease, including

- Cartilage destruction
- Intra-articular loose bodies
- Subchondral cyst formation
- Rarely, malignant transformation

Pathology

GROSS

- Subchondral fractures
- Fragmentation and collapse of the femoral head
- Cartilaginous fragmentation
- Femoral head remodeling

MICROSCOPIC

The cascade of cell death leads eventually to the most resilient (ischemia-resistant) cells dying, that is, the fat cells as evinced by the death of fat cell nuclei and the formation of fat cysts, both of which are taken as features of established osteonecrosis. Subsequently, there is infiltration by mesenchymal cells, which, when differentiated into osteoblasts, produce new bone on the remnants of the necrotic trabeculae. Concurrent capillary infiltration results in neovascularization.

Imaging Findings

The radiologic findings parallel the evolution of the disease process. Thus, at the time of cell death, conventional radiographs will be normal, as will radionuclide studies.

RADIOGRAPHY

With subsequent ischemia and reactive hyperemia, osteopenia will be evident; however, it takes between 2 and 5 months for this to be demonstrable radiographically.

Other intermediate signs include

- Fragmentation of the femoral epiphysis
- Variable femoral head sclerosis as reossification occurs
- Calcification within the devascularized cartilage
- Demineralization cysts, seen in the lateral metaphysis in one third of cases

At 9 to 10 months, the "crescent" sign becomes visible, often with associated subchondral collapse, the crescent representing the presence of a subchondral fracture, most frequently occurring on the anterosuperior aspect of the femoral head.

Femoral head remodeling (e.g., resulting in flattening) becomes evident at 18 months. Early degenerative changes as evinced by reduced joint space may subsequently become evident.

RADIONUCLIDE STUDIES

- Reduced uptake may be evident in the blood pool phase in the initial stages, reflecting the reduced blood supply.
- In the later stages, there is increased uptake, reflecting osteoblastic remodeling activity. A persistent cold spot may be evident centrally (within the zone of increased uptake), giving rise to the so-called doughnut sign.
- Later still, increased uptake in both the femoral head and the acetabulum may be demonstrated if complicated by secondary degenerative disease.

ULTRASOUND

- Synovial swelling and increased joint space may be demonstrable acutely.

MAGNETIC RESONANCE IMAGING

- Greater sensitivity for the earlier changes of the disease, when death of marrow fat cells may be detected, permitting earlier diagnosis
- Permits direct assessment of articular cartilage
- Useful in the evaluation of femoral head coverage

T1

- Irregular, subchondral low signal: low signal foci or linear signal within the epiphysis that extends to the subchondral bone (**Figs. 76B–76D**)

T2/T2 STIR/fat-saturated

- The "double line" sign: an inner hyperintense line corresponding to acute granulation tissue and an outer hypointense line corresponding to developing fibrosis and sclerosis (**Fig. 76E**)
- Increased physeal signal (**Fig. 76E**)

T2 gradient

- Initially, increased cartilage thickness, which decreases in later stages
- The coronal and sagittal planes are most useful to assess the congruity of the joint and femoral head coverage.
- The use of subtraction gadolinium-enhanced magnetic resonance angiography to evaluate femoral head vascularity has been proposed as a potentially useful early predictor of outcome.

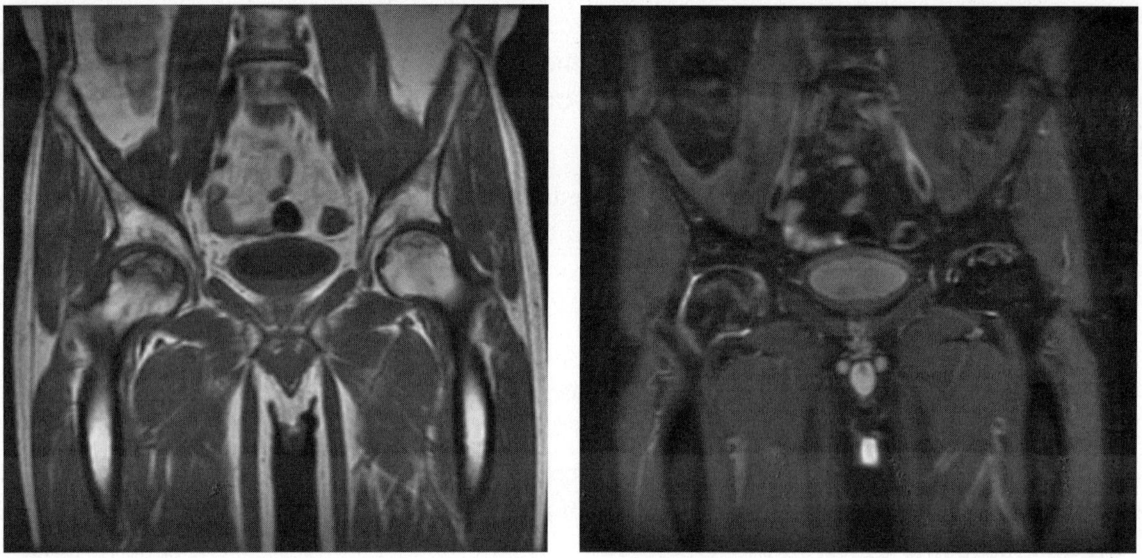

D E

Figures 76D A coronal T1-weighted image shows bilateral femoral head avascular necrosis (AVN) (in the presence of AVN of one hip, the risk to the contralateral hip increases to 70%), as evinced by bilateral low-signal crescentic lines with further low signal lines extending to the subchondral bone, indicating fragmentation (more severe on the right). **76E** A coronal STIR image of the same patient as in **76C** shows the "double line" sign, that is, an inner high signal intensity line and an adjacent outer low signal intensity line (best seen on the left). A small joint effusion is evident in addition. Physeal hyperintensity is shown on the right.

Treatment

- "Unloading" the hip with non-weight-bearing crutches
- Core decompression
- Varus derotation osteotomy

In the adult, joint replacement is frequently required in an effort to reduce the probability of developing accelerated degenerative joint disease.

Prognosis

- Dependent on the amount of femoral head involved; if $>$ 20% of the head is extruded laterally the prognosis is poor.
- AVN of one hip increases the risk of involvement of the other side to 70%.

PEARLS

- The crescent sign, that is, a curvilinear subcortical lucency corresponding to the presence of a subchondral fissure fracture, is best seen on the frog-leg view.
- The presence of apparent femoral head osteoarthritis in the absence of joint space loss should alert the radiologist to the possibility of AVN.
- When performing nuclear medicine studies, imaging with radiocolloid as opposed to diphosphonates is more sensitive.

PITFALLS

- No cause is identified in as many as 25% of cases.
- Although nuclear medicine studies are more sensitive than plain films, they are less sensitive than MRI; thus, the latter should be performed if the results of plain films and radionuclide studies are normal or equivocal in the presence of a high clinical index of suspicion.
- An isolated epiphyseal fracture may mimic AVN; however, a fracture is usually evident as a focal defect or depression on the cortical surface in association with a linear hypointense fracture line. A close temporal relationship between the onset of symptoms and recent trauma is also more likely to be present.

Suggested Readings

Radke S, Kirschner S, Seipel V, Rader C, Eulert J. Magnetic resonance imaging criteria of successful core decompression in avascular necrosis of the hip. Skeletal Radiol 2004;33:519–523

Stevens K, Tao C, Lee SU, et al. Subchondral fractures in osteonecrosis of the femoral head: comparison of radiography, CT, and MR imaging. Am J Roentgenol 2003;180:363–368

Uberoi R, Tai G, Hughes PM. Gadolinium-DTPA-enhanced MRI in the evaluation of osteonecrosis. Clin Radiol 1994;49:645–648

CASE 77

Anthony G. Ryan and Peter L. Munk

Clinical Presentation

A 35-year-old woman with chronic medial knee joint pain was referred for magnetic resonance arthrography (MRA).

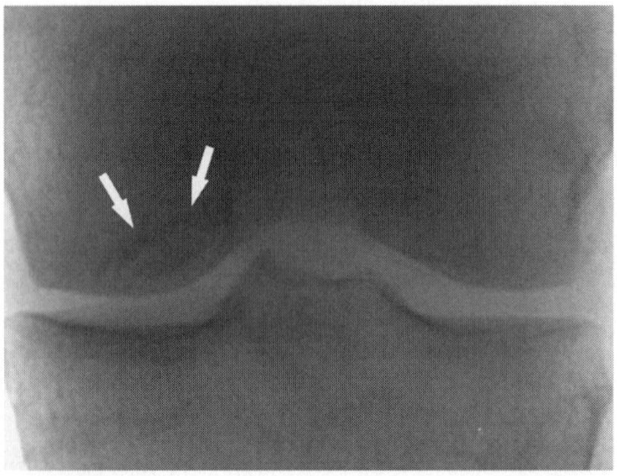

Figure 77A

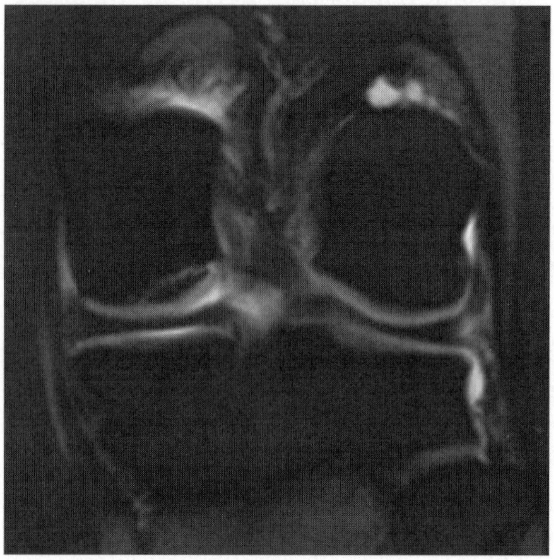

Figure 77B

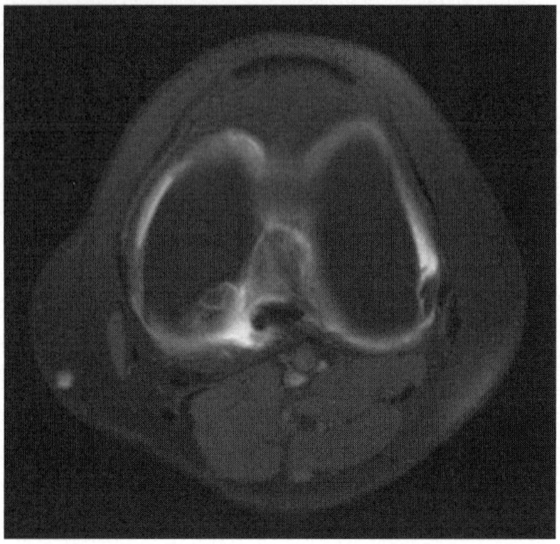

Figure 77C

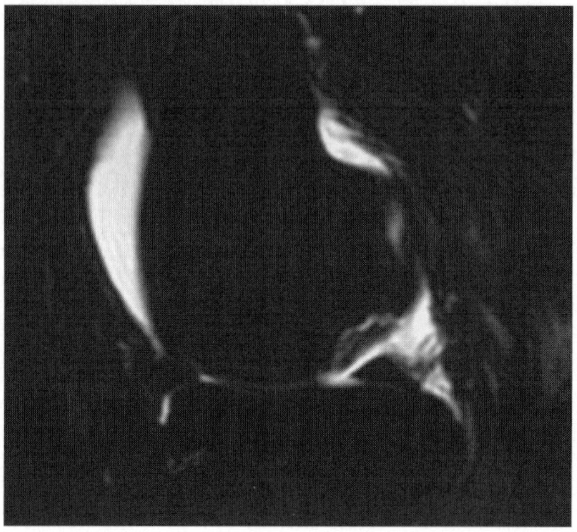

Figure 77D

Radiologic Findings

A "grabbed" fluoroscopic image (**Fig. 77A**) shows a convex sclerotic rim cephalad to an ovoid radiodensity, which is surrounded by a radiolucent line projected through the lateral aspect of the medial femoral condyle. T1 fat-saturated images after intra-articular injection of dilute gadolinium (**Figs. 77B**, coronal; **77C**, transaxial; and **77D**, sagittal) show a discrete fragmented lesion of bone and cartilage in the posterolateral aspect of the medial condyle. Gadolinium is seen to undermine the fragment over ~75% of its surface area, especially posteriorly. A subtle linear low-signal alteration is evident within the cartilage at the medial margin of the lesion, whereas the cartilage is discontinuous laterally (**Fig. 77B**). The sagittal image reveals osseous discontinuity anteriorly and posteriorly.

Diagnosis

Osteochondritis dissecans (OCD).

Differential Diagnosis

Spontaneous osteonecrosis.

Discussion

Background

Osteochondritis dissecans is the title given to a posttraumatic osteochondral fracture comprising variable osseous and chondral components, thought to be complicated by ischemia, the subsequent devascularization producing a focal transchondral or subarticular osteonecrosis.

The lesion occurs most frequently (75%) in the non–weight-bearing surface (lateral aspect) of the medial femoral condyle, from which comes the acronym LAME: lateral aspect medial epicondyle.

Less commonly, the medial aspect of the medial femoral condyle, the lateral aspect of the lateral condyle (5%), and rarely the anterior femoral condyle are affected.

When osteochondritis dissecans occurs elsewhere in the skeleton, it affects the bone on the convexity of the affected joint (e.g., talar dome, capitellum, head of first metatarsal) almost exclusively, with rare exceptions, such as the tibial plafond and the glenoid.

The condition is bilateral in 20 to 30% of patients.

Etiology

Proposed etiologies include

- Chronic repetitive trauma
- Ischemia, similar to avascular necrosis
- Idiopathic

Some authorities describe osteochondritis dissecans as a subtype of avascular necrosis of bone, with which it may form a continuum, that is, a more focal manifestation of an ischemic insult rather than necrosis of a complete epiphysis. A history of trauma is found in ~50% of cases, however, and pathologic examination of the osteochondral lesions favors a traumatic etiology over avascular necrosis.

Osteochondritis dissecans of the femoral head occurs as a rare complication in the late onset of Legg-Calvé-Perthes disease, possibly secondary to a persistent loose fragment or the weakening induced during the revascularization phase.

Pathophysiology

Repetitive trauma produces a subchondral fatigue fracture, secondary to shearing or tangential forces, which is subsequently complicated by devascularization, resulting in focal osteonecrosis, whereby a segment of articular cartilage and subchondral bone dies and becomes partially or totally separated from the underlying bone. The fragments may thus consist of cartilage alone or cartilage and underlying bone, may remain firmly attached and eventually heal, or may partially or completely detach.

Cysts may form deep to the lesion (**Figs. 77E,77F**) secondary to the influx of synovial fluid into the fracture site and the increased joint pressure as a result of the articular surface irregularity. The presence of cysts is associated with a higher incidence of instability, as is evidence of fluid imbibing within the fragment (native effusion or positive contrast introduced at arthrography) and the remainder of the underlying bone. New bone forms over the defect, which may unite with the underlying bone; however, if subjected to repetitive forces (e.g., if the condition is not recognized or immobilization is inadequate), unstable fragments develop, which do not unite. Fragments may, of course, be unstable de novo.

When the lesion occurs at the capitellum (in younger patients with a short duration of symptoms, prior to physeal closure), localized subchondral bone flattening without fragmentation is occasionally seen. Subsequent new bone formation and fragment reunification are seen with adequate immobilization in this group.

In the talar dome, a history of forced inversion and dorsiflexion is noted to produce a lateral lesion (40% of cases), whereby the lateral margin of the talar dome is forced against the fibular styloid. These lesions are typically found in the mid to anterior portion of the talar dome.

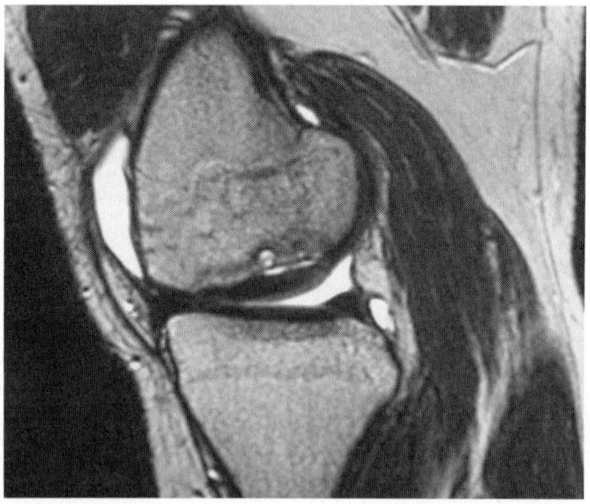

E

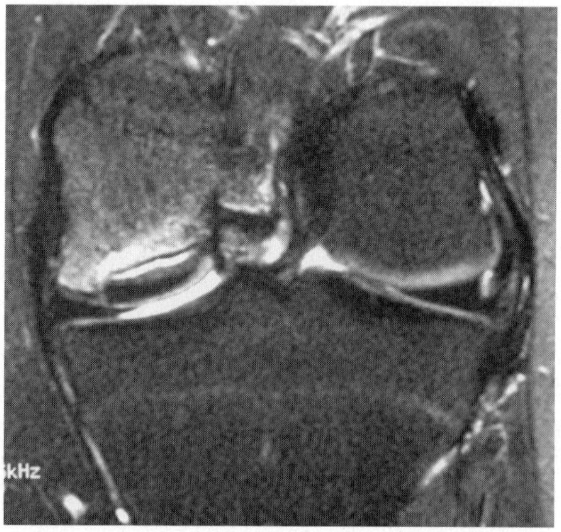

F

Figures 77E Sagittal T1-weighted image after intra-articular gadolinium shows thickening and sclerosis of the femoral condylar subchondral cortex, gadolinium signal intensity deep to the cortex, and a clearly defined cyst within the underlying medullary bone. Ill-defined low signal intensity is demonstrated within the medullary bone surrounding the cyst, suggesting edema. **77F** A coronal STIR image after intra-articular gadolinium shows the same osteochondral fragment as in **77E**. The cortex is again seen to be thickened and sclerotic, the overlying cartilage is thinned, the condylar cortex is irregular, and fluid is seen imbibed deep to the osteochondral fragment. High signal intensity within the condyle is consistent with surrounding edema.

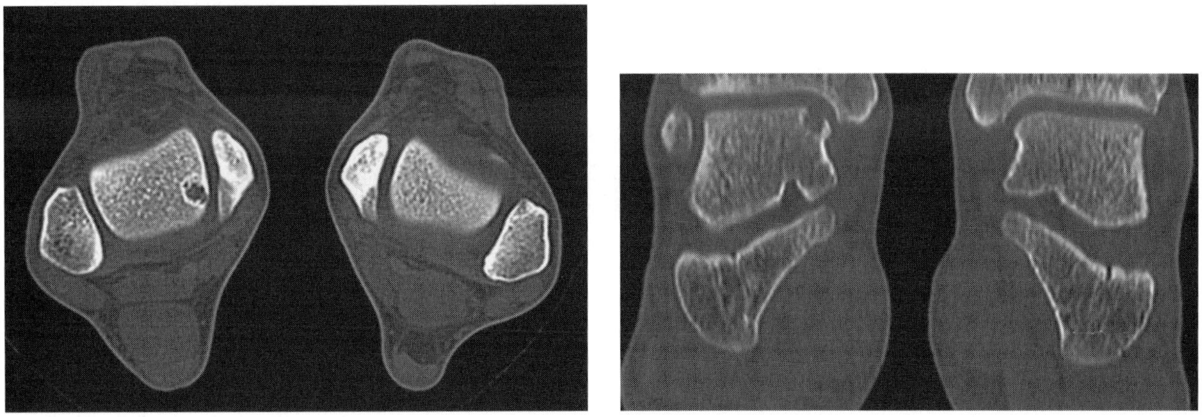

G H

Figures 77G and **77H** CT images (**77G**, transaxial acquisition; **77H**, coronal reformat) show the typical appearance of a posteromedial talar osteochondral lesion, with a cup-shaped defect and a well-defined prominent sclerotic margin. Although this was an established lesion, no new bone formation is evident in the roof of the defect.

Forced inversion and plantar flexion with external rotation of the tibia cause medial lesions (60% of cases) secondary to impact between the posteromedial portion of the tibia and the medial talar margin. Medial lesions, usually cup-shaped and deeper (**Figs. 77G,77H**) than lateral lesions, are less frequently associated with a history of trauma, as are lateral lesions, which tend to be wafer-shaped and thin.

Clinical Findings

This is a painful, usually unilateral disease, typically occurring in adolescence (second and third decades, mean age 15), with males affected to a greater degree than females (2 to 3 times more frequently).

There is a history of trauma in up to 50% of cases, although the inciting event may not be recalled by the patient, and the condition may be labeled idiopathic.

Although usually painful, the condition may be asymptomatic or have vague, nonspecific complaints. There may be clicking, locking, and limiting of motion of the affected joint, and as the condition progresses, there may be progressive swelling with pain aggravated by movement.

Stages of Disease

The lesions are described in four stages, based on the size of the osteochondral lesion and the thickness of the surrounding sclerotic rim.

Stage 1 The lesion measures ~1 to 3 cm in diameter, and the articular cartilage overlying the defect is intact.

Stage 2 The articular cartilage demonstrates a cleft or fissure that extends to the cortex, but there is no evidence of loosening of the fragment.

Stage 3 Partial detachment of the osteochondral defect with a large cleft extending into the subchondral bone

Stage 4 The fragment is loose within the crater.

Stage 5 The fragment is completely free within the joint as a loose body, and the empty crater is evident.

The staging of talar lesions based on conventional radiographs include the following:

Stage 1 Subchondral compression fracture with no ligamentous sprain; normal radiographs; may be painless

Stage 2 Partially detached osteochondral fragment with a hinge or flap of articular cartilage. T2-weighted MRI may be necessary to identify the osteochondral fragment.

Stage 3 A complete nondisplaced fracture remains within the bone crater.

Stage 4 A detached fragment with a loose osteochondral portion

Stages 2 to 4 are usually associated with sprain or rupture of the collateral ankle ligament.

Complications

- Nonunion of the fracture
- Loose body; osteochondral lesions are the most common cause of loose body in the adolescent age group
- Locking of the joint, particularly with a larger bone fragment
- Degenerative (posttraumatic) arthritis: if treatment is delayed or does not occur secondary to lack of diagnosis, arthritis develops in ~50% of patients.

Pathology

GROSS

- There is a bony defect or fragmentation of subchondral bone. The defect may be a surface hole, or the defect may be filled with fibrous tissue or fibrocartilage.
- The fragments comprise cartilage alone or bone and cartilage in variable proportions. The fragments may be partially attached or firmly attached with fibrous tissue to the underlying bone.

MICROSCOPIC

- 50% of specimens consist of articular cartilage only with no attached subchondral bone.
- Degenerative secondary calcification of articular cartilage
- New bone formation secondary to revascularization
- Calcification in new surface layers of cartilage and bone in the loose body

Imaging Findings

RADIOGRAPHY

If the lesion consists purely of cartilage, radiographs are frequently normal, although a joint effusion may well be demonstrable even in the absence of an osseous fracture.

One of the earliest features of osteochondritis dissecans in the capitellum is subchondral bone flattening, over which new bone subsequently forms, producing sclerosis of the subchondral cortex.

If there is an osseous component, the bony defect or fragmentation of the subchondral bone may be demonstrable, the fracture line tending to parallel the joint surface. In the chronic state, the donor site may be visible on the articular surface as a pit with a variable sclerosed margin (**Fig. 77I**). If the fragment remains attached, a radiolucent line separating the osteochondral body from the underlying bone (sclerotic margin) may be evident (**Figs. 77A** and **77J**; see also **Fig. 77K** for comparison).

If the fragment (attached or detached) is radiodense, it may be due to

- An attached osseous component (subchondral bone) (**Fig. 77L**)
- Secondary degenerative calcification of the articular cartilage

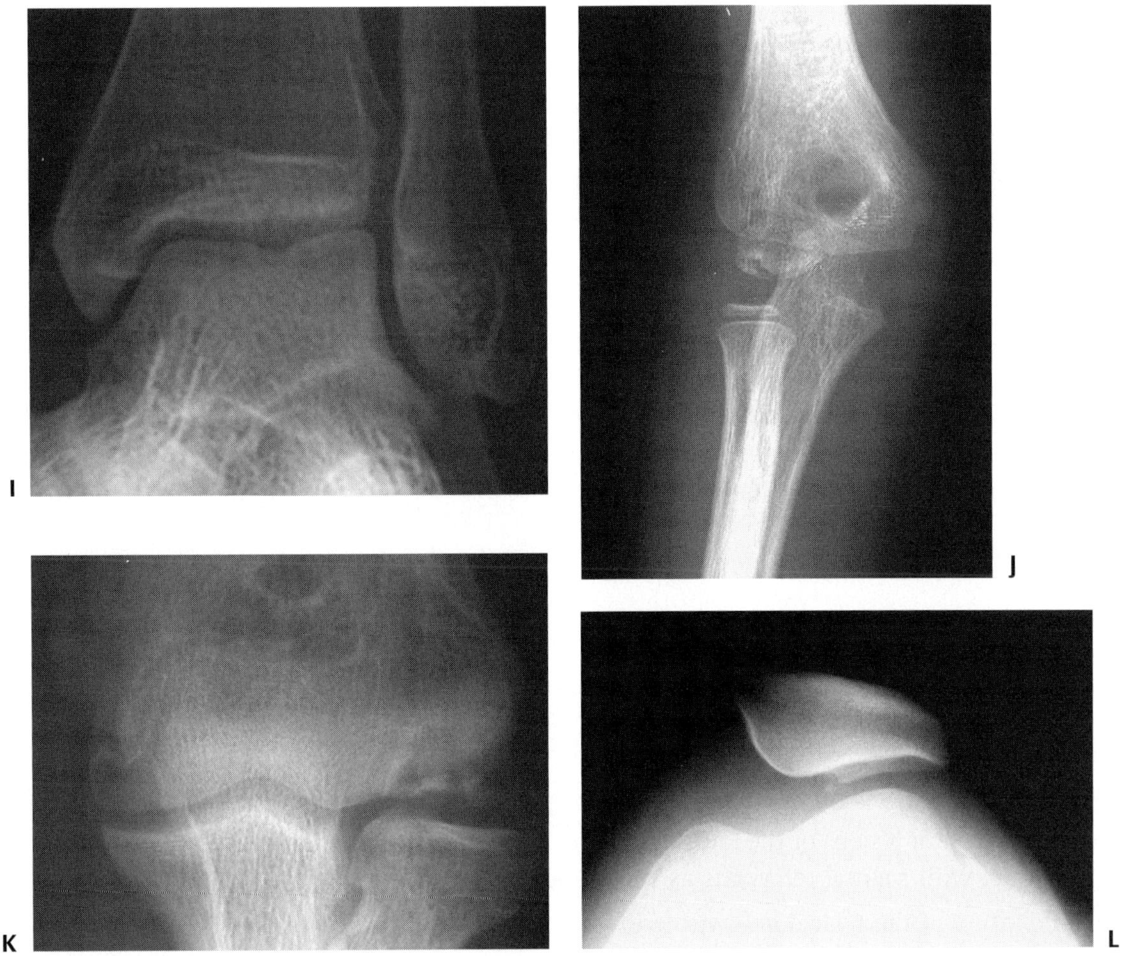

Figures 77I Oblique ankle radiograph shows an osteochondral lesion of the midtalar dome with a minimal sclerotic reaction. **77J** An anteroposterior (AP) radiograph of the elbow shows an osteochondral fragment separated from the underlying bone by a radiolucent line. A sclerotic margin is evident on the donor aspect of the lesion. Comparison should be made with **77K**. **77K** An AP radiograph of the elbow in a patient with osteonecrosis of the capitellum (typically posttraumatic, but if idiopathic, is known by the eponym "Panner's disease"). The capitellum is collapsed and fragmented. **77L** "Skyline" view of the patella in a teenage girl after recurrent dislocation shows a radiodense fragment at the dorsal apex consisting of both osseous and cartilaginous components.

- New bone formation secondary to revascularization
- Calcification in new surface layers of cartilage and bone in the loose body

Radiodense loose bodies are found in typical locations within the affected joint:

- Knee joint: the posterior joint space
- Elbow: the olecranon fossa
- Glenohumeral joint: the axillary/subscapular recess

The lesion size and the thickness of the sclerotic margin are good predictors of instability of the fragment.

ULTRASOUND

- In the evaluation of the capitellum, sonography performed with a 7.5-MHz probe has been demonstrated to have a greater sensitivity than radiography in the assessment of the presence and stability of capitellar lesions.

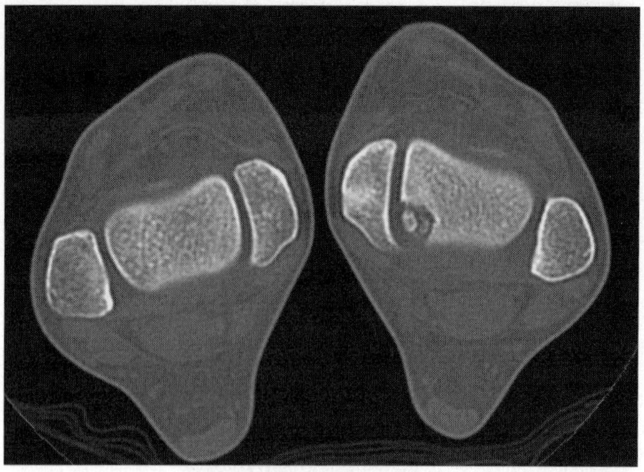
M

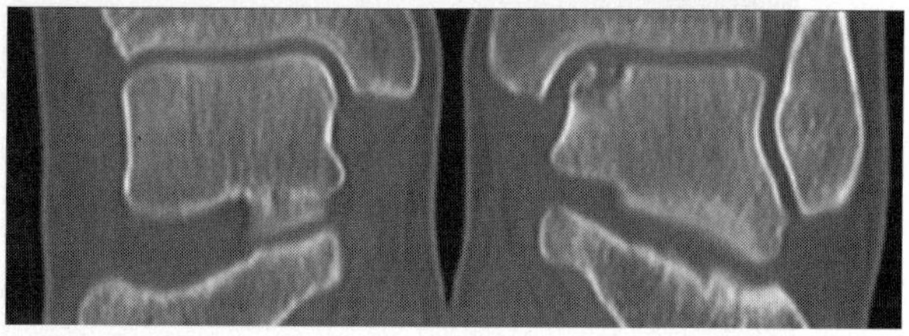
N

Figures 77M and **77N** Transaxial (**77M**) and coronal reformat (**77N**) CT images show a posteromedial tibial osteochondral lesion with fragmentation not displaced from the donor site.

COMPUTED TOMOGRAPHY

A classification exists for lesions of the talus based on CT performed in the direct transverse or coronal planes at 1.5 mm, with sagittal reformats as shown below.

Stage 1 Cystic lesion of the talar dome with an intact roof.
Stage 2A Cystic lesion with communication to the talar dome surface (**Figs. 77G,77H**)
Stage 2B Open articular surface lesion with an overlying nondisplaced fragment (**Figs. 77K–77N**)
Stage 3 Nondisplaced lesion with low attenuation
Stage 4 Displaced fragment

The addition of direct coronal CT arthrography adds further information regarding the degree of attachment of the osteochondritic fragment. However, MRI remains the investigation of choice to examine the cartilage.

MAGNETIC RESONANCE IMAGING

MRI is the most accurate technique for the demonstration of the osteochondral complex, particularly in the detection of radiographically occult lesions, for staging detected lesions, and in defining the stability of any fragments present. MRI classification is as follows:

Stage 1 Subchondral compression (flattening)
Stage 2A Subchondral cyst
Stage 2B Incomplete separation of the fragment (roof of cyst)
Stage 3 Fluid around an unattached nondisplaced fragment
Stage 4 Displaced fragment

On T1-weighted images, the bone defect will demonstrate low (synovial fluid) to intermediate (fibrous tissue) signal intensity (**Figs. 77O–77Q**). When the lesion is established, the defect has a well-demarcated sclerotic rim that extends to the articular surface, shown as peripheral areas of low signal intensity on both T1- and T2-weighted images. Ongoing necrosis within the bone is typically evinced by hypointensity within the focus, reflecting increased bone density and surrounding demineralization secondary to hyperemia.

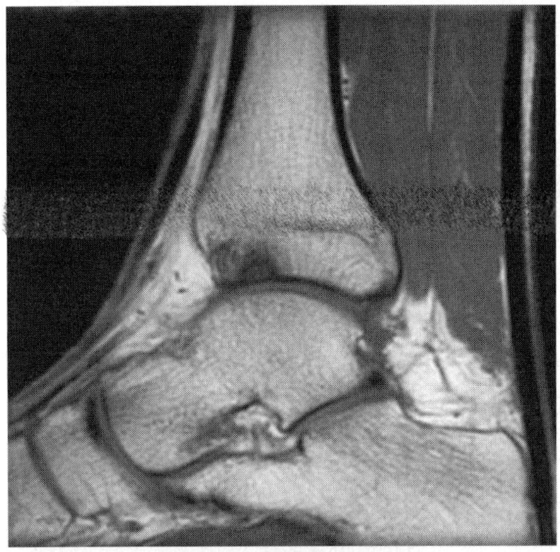
O

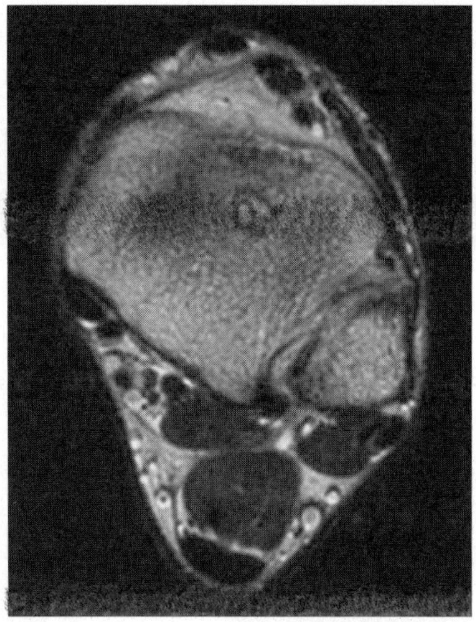
P

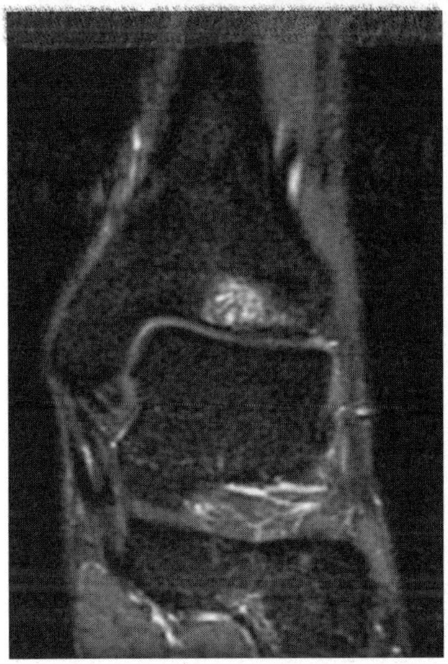
Q

Figures 77O–77Q Sagittal T1-weighted (**77O**), axial T2-weighted (**77P**), and coronal STIR (**77Q**) images show a thin, low-signal rim on both T1- and T2-weighted views, representing a sclerotic margin. The osseous defect is a mixture of low and intermediate signal intensity, seen on both T2-weighted and STIR images to be predominantly high signal, consistent with synovial fluid imbibed into the cystic defect. The subchondral cortical bone is thinned and irregular, as is the overlying cartilage. A faint low-signal "halo" is present around the lesion on the T1-weighted sagittal image, seen on the STIR to be high signal, representing a small amount of marrow edema.

Adjacent subchondral marrow edema or hyperemia (usually more extensive than the osteochondral defect) will be hyperintense on STIR/fat-suppressed T2-weighted images, correlating with the low signal intensity observed on T1-weighted images (**Figs. 77E,77F**).

Normal hyaline articular cartilage shows intermediate signal intensity on T1- and T2-weighted images, low to intermediate on fat-suppressed T2-weighted images, and high signal intensity on gradient sequences. In cases of doubt, gradient (T2-weighted) images are particularly sensitive to small foci of cartilaginous disruption. The cartilage overlying the bony defect may be deformed or focally bowed away from the surface of the bone without disruption.

- T2-weighted images may detect high signal intensity fluid surrounding the osteochondral fragment, with a potential pitfall being that of granulation tissue simulating free fluid (**Figs. 77R–77T**).
- Partially attached fragments have an irregular high-signal zone on T2-weighted images at the fragment/bone interface (**Figs. 77E,77F**).

Fat-suppressed T2-weighted and STIR images are more specific and sensitive than T2-weighted images alone in the detection of fluid transgressing articular cartilage (**Figs. 77R–77T**).

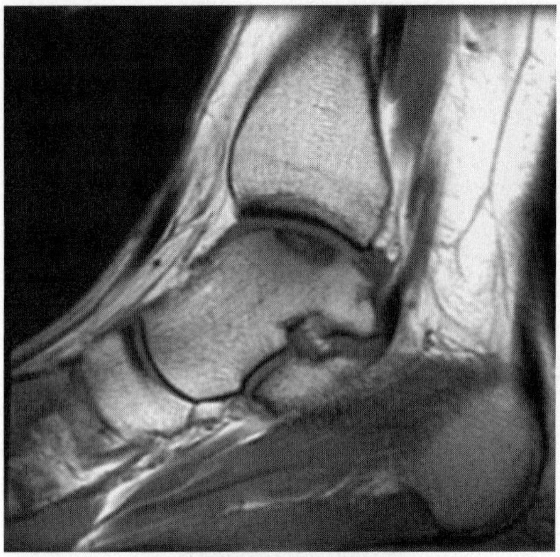

R

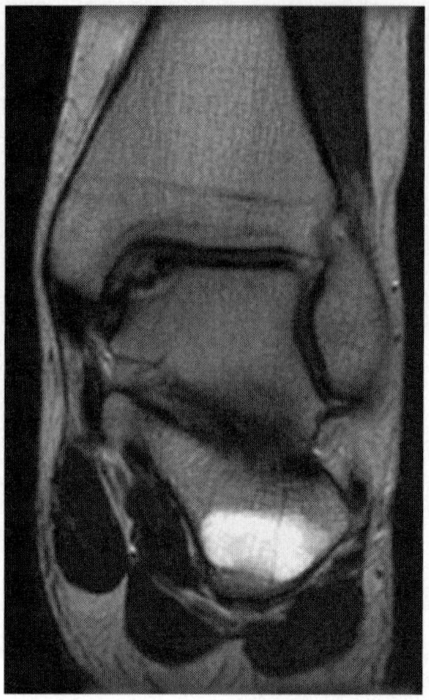

S

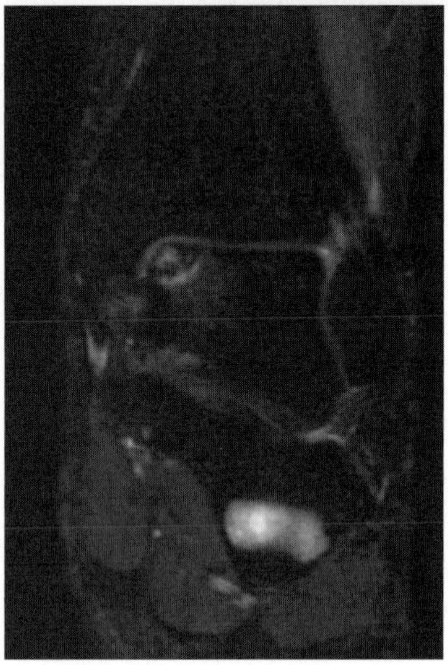

T

Figures 77R–77T Sagittal T1-weighted (**77R**), coronal T2-weighted (**77S**), and coronal STIR (**77T**) images of the same lesion as in **77R** and **77S** show a faint low-signal intensity margin consistent with sclerosis on T1- and T2-weighted views. A rim of high signal intensity is also demonstrated on the T2-weighted image, raising the possibility of fluid beneath the fragment; however, the appearances also raise the differential of granulation tissue. The STIR resolves the issue, clearly demonstrating the high signal to be fluid intensity, which, taken with all the other findings, is indicative of a partially attached fragment. The STIR also shows edema in the surrounding marrow, which the T2-weighted image did not demonstrate clearly. Clinically and on the basis of sequential imaging, this lesion had been stable over a period of a year. Incidental note is made of a unicameral cyst in the calcaneus.

- A complete ring of fluid signal intensity surrounds the lesions in unattached fragments. At direct MRA, fat suppression is used to directly evaluate the flow of contrast material over the articular surface (**Figs. 77B–77D**).
- A detached cortical fragment will remain low in signal intensity on all sequences.

Four MRI signs of fragment instability (based on studies of the talar dome and femoral condyles) are as follows:

1. High signal intensity line (seen beneath 72% of lesions)
2. Cystic area beneath the lesion
3. High signal intensity line through the articular cartilage
4. Focal articular defect

Signs 2 to 4 are found in 22 to 31% of unstable lesions.

The presence of any one sign indicates instability, the most frequent sign being an underlying high signal intensity line.

NUCLEAR MEDICINE

- Compared with conventional radiographs, bone scintigraphy is more sensitive and specific in determining the mechanical stability of OCD lesions.

Treatment

Lesions that are large, have fluid extending into the interface with the adjacent bone, or have overlying disrupted articular cartilage and underlying cystic changes are more prone to eventual detachment and are treated more aggressively, that is, with drilling.

Thus, in combination with the duration of symptoms and the imaging findings, arthroscopy is performed to probe and assess the chondral fragment.

Arthroscopic Classification

This classification was based on the appearance of overlying cartilage on arthroscopy.

Grade 1 Intact, firm, shiny articular cartilage
Grade 2 Intact but soft cartilage
Grade 3 Frayed cartilage

- Loose fragments are either fixated with absorbable pins, K-wires, or screws or excised with subsequent drilling of the base. Drilling or abrasion promotes fibrocartilaginous ingrowth and healing of the defect.
- Primary chondral lesions without attached bone are excised with débridement and drilling or abrasion.
- If the osteochondral fragment remains attached, it may respond to drilling (to decompress and relieve the pressure on an already tenuous blood supply), which may promote reattachment of the separated portion.
- Cystic areas are treated with bone grafting if the overlying cartilage is intact; if not, the cyst is corrected with drilling or abrasion of the base.

Prognosis

In the femoral condyle, a good clinical outcome is likely when the growth plate is open, when the lesion is small (< 160 mm^2 in area), and when the lesion is stable by MRI.

When a cartilage fracture or articular defect is found on MRI, the patient is likely to have a poor outcome, with degenerative arthritis a likely result.

PEARLS

- It is important to recognize the expected irregularity of the normal ossification center of the posterior condyle of the femur (which can mimic OCD) and true OCD.
- Radiographically, the tunnel view, which visualizes the posterior aspect of the intracondylar notch, detects a posterior lesion to best advantage.
- In contrast to avascular necrosis of the talus, marrow hyperemia associated with the osteochondral lesion is usually less extensive and directly radiates from the lesion. The articular surface may appear thinned, bowed, nodular, or disrupted. The accumulation of high signal intensity joint fluid at or undermining the cartilage surface indicates small fissures or breaks.

PITFALLS

- The area of OCD may not be readily apparent on routine radiographs; therefore, a high index of suspicion is necessary for diagnosis.
- Although CT scanning may be performed in the follow-up of a known osteochondral lesion, if the lesion has not been previously diagnosed, MRI is the better investigation for the patient with ankle pain of unknown origin.
- MRI is the most accurate technique for establishing the stability of a lesion. T2-weighted images may detect high signal intensity fluid surrounding the osteochondral fragment, with a potential pitfall being that of granulation tissue simulating free fluid.

Suggested Readings

De Smet AA, Fisher DR, Graf BK, Lange RH. Osteochondritis dissecans of the knee: value of MR imaging in determining lesion stability and the presence of articular cartilage defects. Am J Roentgenol 1990;155:549–553

Mesgarzadeh M, Sapega AA, Bonakdarpour A, et al. Osteochondritis dissecans: analysis of mechanical stability with radiography, scintigraphy, and MR imaging. Radiology 1987;165:775–780

Milgram JW. Radiological and pathologic manifestations of osteochondritis dissecans of the distal femur: a study of 50 cases. Radiology 1978;126:305–311

Peiss J, Adam G, Casser R, Urhahn R, Gunther RW. Gadopentetate-dimeglumine–enhanced MR imaging of osteonecrosis and osteochondritis dissecans of the elbow: initial experience. Skeletal Radiol 1995;24:17–20

CASE 78

Hema N. Choudur, Anthony G. Ryan, and Peter L. Munk

Clinical Presentation

A patient with systemic lupus erythematosus (SLE) presented complaining of right knee pain. An MRI was performed to exclude an internal derangement of the knee.

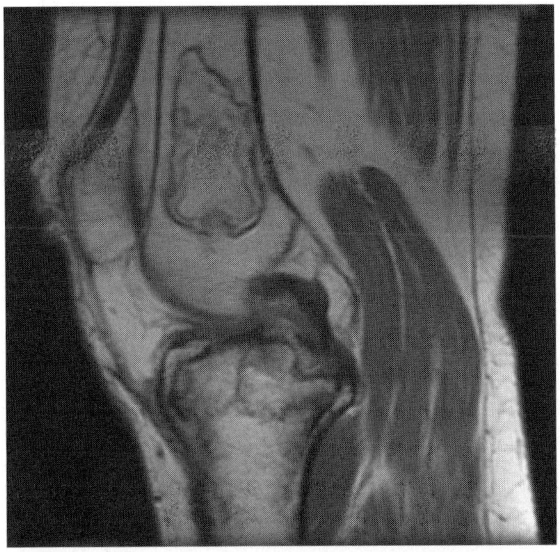

Figure 78A

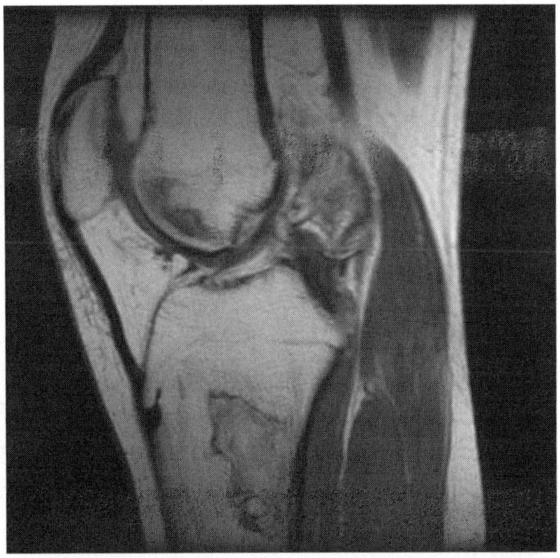

Figure 78B

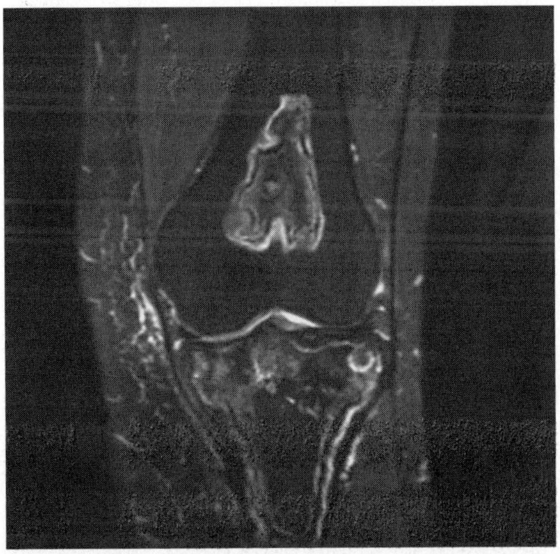

Figure 78C

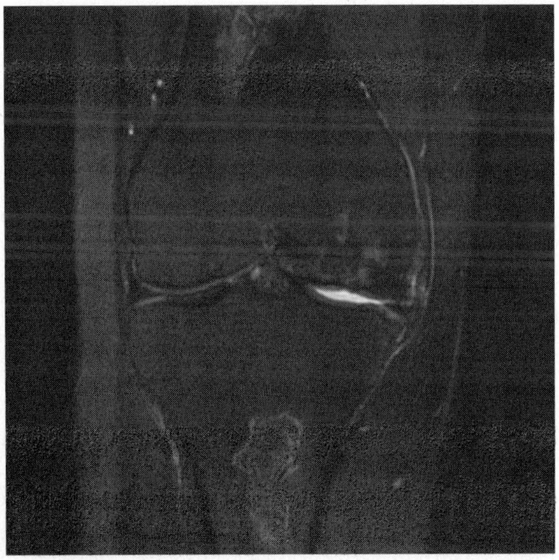

Figure 78D

Radiologic Findings

A well-defined oval area of altered signal intensity is shown in the distal femoral diametaphysis that is isointense to bone on T1-weighted images with a hypointense serpiginous rim (**Figs. 78A,78B**, T1 sagittal); hypointense on T2-weighted, fat-saturated images with a bright, hyperintense rim; and heterogeneously hyperintense on STIR sequences (**Figs. 78C,78D,** coronal STIR).

Diagnosis

Medullary bone infarct.

Differential Diagnosis

- Infectious, metabolic, or neoplastic processes
- An encysted medullary infarct must be differentiated from a brown tumor, unicameral bone cyst, eosinophilic granuloma, and, uncommonly, an intraosseous ganglion.

Discussion

There are two types of bone infarcts. The first involves only the diametaphyseal medulla with loss of the trabecular pattern and is usually clinically silent. The second involves the epiphyseal cortex and medulla, is usually subchondral and painful, and is often referred to as osteonecrosis or avascular necrosis, characteristically involving the femoral and humeral heads.

Background

Due to loss of blood supply, there is ischemic death of the marrow cellular elements. The extent and location of the lesion varies. It usually occurs in the long bones, frequently in the humeral and femoral shafts. Before the advent of MRI, bone marrow infarction was diagnosed with the use of conventional radiography and bone marrow scanning. Conventional radiographs show no acute changes, and areas of marrow ischemia are present only on follow-up examinations. Scintigraphic studies may not allow differentiation of acute from chronic marrow infarction. On MRI, acute marrow infarcts are often seen as focal marrow abnormalities.

Etiology

Focal marrow ischemia may arise secondary to intrinsic or extrinsic compression of the blood vessels or a combination of both. In the red marrow, cell death occurs in ~12 hours following anoxia, in the fatty marrow, it occurs within 5 days.

The causative anoxia may be idiopathic, but trauma, dysbaric osteonecrosis, SLE, rheumatoid arthritis, scleroderma and collagen vascular diseases, sickle cell and other hemoglobinopathies, hemophilia, Gaucher's disease, infection, pancreatitis, steroid intake, and diabetes are among the other causes.

Of patients undergoing radiation therapy for breast cancer, 1 to 3% develop bone infarcts in the shoulder girdle. Hyperlipidemias are found to be associated with osteonecrosis in 80% of patients. The lesions may be unilateral, as in trauma or infection, or bilateral, as in caisson disease.

In SLE, as in our case, the most commonly affected sites are the humeral head, femoral condyles, tibial plateaus, and talus. An unusual feature is the involvement of small bones of the wrist, hands, and feet.

Pathophysiology

The dead bone cannot be resorbed and remains radiographically opaque, but the surrounding bone undergoes secondary hyperemic changes with osteoclastic activity and therefore appears lucent on radiographs and hyperintense on T2-weighted MRIs.

Repair occurs in two phases. While macrophages engulf the dead marrow cells, the surrounding capillaries grow between areas of the dead bone. Mesenchymal cells then differentiate into either fibroblasts or osteoblasts, depending on how favorable the environment is (e.g., the local oxygen tension). New bone is laid over dead trabeculae, accounting for the increasing patchy sclerosis on radiographs.

Clinical Findings

Although most of the medullary infarcts are incidentally detected on radiographic studies, some present with localized bony pain. The degree of pain is less than in juxtachondral osteonecrosis.

Stages of the Disease

The earliest plain radiographic evidence of anoxic cell death is irregular medullary sclerosis. This is followed by scavenging of dead cells by macrophages, with capillary ingrowth seen as areas of radiographic lucency. New bone laid over dead trabaculae is less commonly appreciated as serpiginous calcific sclerosis within the lesion.

MRI and radionuclide bone scans pick up medullary anoxia in its early stages.

Complications

Rarely, sarcomatous malignant degeneration has been reported in medullary bone infarcts. It occurs in the 40- to 70-year-old age group and is more common in males. Typically, the distal part of the femur or proximal tibia is involved, although other sites may be affected as well. The radiographic appearance is that of a soft-tissue mass associated with bone destruction at a previous site of bone infarction.

Cystic degeneration within the infarct is differentiated from cystic bone lesions by the fact that there is no cortical involvement.

Pathology

GROSS

- The dead medulla appears yellow with occasional flecks of calcium surrounded by a grayish collagenous capsule or granulation tissue.

MICROSCOPIC

- Macrophages with engulfed dead fatty marrow cells are seen interspersed with ingrowing capillaries. Surrounding fibroblasts or, in more favorable conditions, osteoblasts are noted with new bone laid over the scaffold of dead trabaculae.

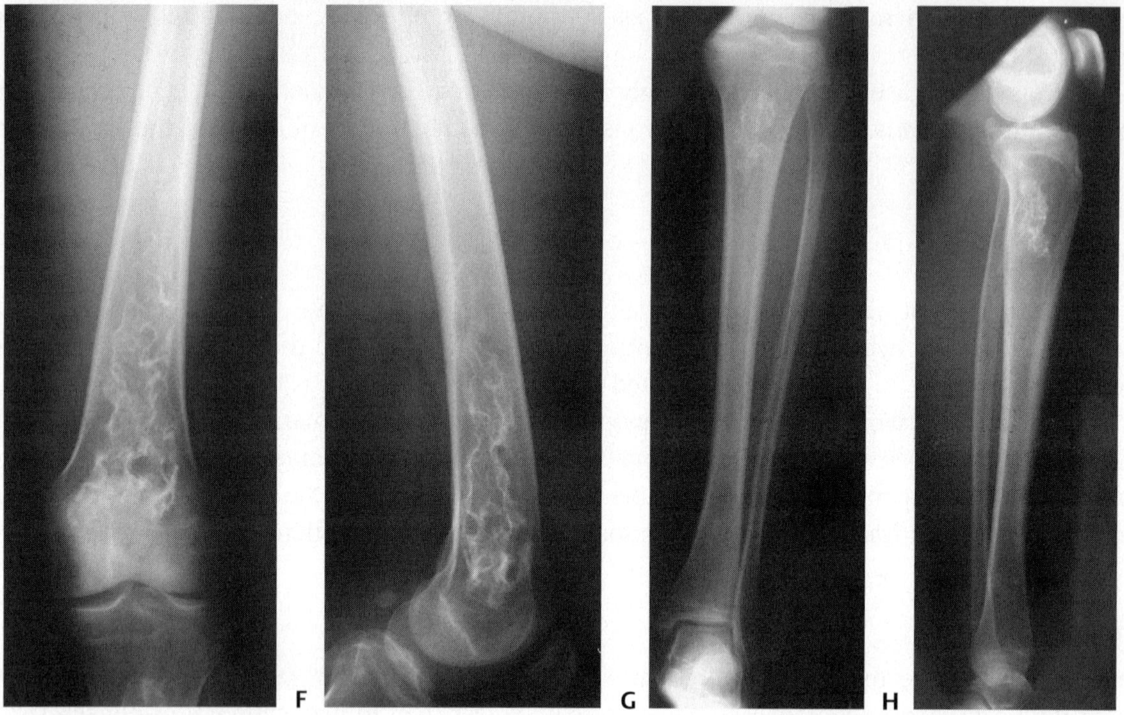

E F G H

Figures 78E–78H Plain radiographs of the distal femur anteroposterior (AP; **78E**) and lateral (**78F**) views and tibia/fibula AP (**78G**) and lateral (**78H**) views reveal well-defined metadiaphyseal intramedullary serpiginous calcific densities.

Imaging Findings

RADIOGRAPHY

Radiographs are insensitive to medullary infarcts, with several months elapsing before focal irregular sclerosis is noted within the metaphysis or diaphysis of long bones, frequently the femur or humerus.

Later, serpiginous sclerosis is evident, with the dead trabaculae being thickened by overlying new bone formation. Rarely, the lesion appears lucent with a sclerotic rim. A shell of calcification is infrequently visualized and is typical of a bone infarction. No involvement of the cortex is demonstrated at any stage (**Figs. 78E–78H**).

ULTRASOUND

Some centers use ultrasound to differentiate soft-tissue involvement in osteomyelitis from medullary bone infarction in patients with sickle cell anemia undergoing a crisis. The findings are then correlated with bone scans.

COMPUTED TOMOGRAPHY

CT is not very specific for the diagnosis of medullary bone infarcts but is sometimes used to differentiate osteomyelitis and bone neoplasms. Decreased attenuation may be seen earlier than in the plain radiographs.

MAGNETIC RESONANCE IMAGING

Ischemia may be demonstrated at an early stage using MRI. Red marrow ischemia is seen much earlier (6–12 hours). Fatty marrow takes longer, about 5 days, to become visible. Acute lesions appear as intermediate or low on T1- and high on T2-weighted and inversion recovery sequences. Chronic lesions show more defined borders and a fibrous interface.

MRI characteristics of bone infarction are variable focal abnormalities and are commonly demonstrated as patchy areas of low signal intensity on T1-weighted spin-echo images. The most characteristic appearance of avascular necrosis, the "double line" sign, consists of a hyperintense inner ring and a hypointense outer ring; on T2-weighted sequences, it is not seen in medullary infarcts. This finding reflects the reactive interface between ischemic and nonischemic bone.

On T1-weighted sequences, this interface appears as a low-signal intensity line, reflecting the combination of granulation tissue and sclerotic bone, findings which are in fact demonstrable in medullary infarcts. MRI in immature infarcts reveals a central area with high or intermediate signal with a serpentine, thin, low-signal border on T2 images.

NUCLEAR MEDICINE

Uptake of technetium 99m diphosphonate may be delayed by ~72 hours following avascular necrosis. Focal osteopenia is initially documented. Increased uptake occurs once there is revascularization and new bone formation. However, studies have revealed that medullary fat cells are resistant to ischemia, dying 5 days after the initial insult. In such cases, though MRI findings may be negative, findings from isotopic scans may become positive during this period.

Gallium 67 citrate scintigraphy has proven to be more useful in differentiating photopenic infarcts from early osteomyelitis.

Imaging characteristics of a bone infarct per se are nonspecific, and increased activity can be caused by a variety of conditions, such as fractures, infections, inflammations, and metabolic and neoplastic processes. Photon-deficient bone lesions may occur with early osteomyelitis, plasmacytoma, histiocytosis X, bone metastases, and sickle cell crises.

Treatment

Once devitalized, the nonprogressive infarct remains quiescent for a lifetime, with some initial reparative attempts made by the body's defense mechanisms. No treatment is indicated for medullary infarcts, though a sarcomatous transformation is appropriately treated.

Prognosis

A bone infarct may occasionally dedifferentiate to osteogenic sarcoma, fibrosarcoma, or malignant fibrous histiocytoma. The described association of angiosarcoma with a bone infarct is extremely rare.

PEARLS

- Medullary bone infarcts occur most commonly at the proximal humerus, femur, tibia, and talus.
- These lesions may be differentiated from infection and metabolic and neoplastic processes by their characteristic radiological appearance of a well-defined medullary lucency with serpiginous sclerosis.
- A soft-tissue swelling at the site of a previous infarct should raise the suspicion of malignant change.

PITFALLS

- Clinically, bone infarcts may mimic bone abscess (especially in sickle cell disease). MRI is especially invaluable in this setting.

- Incidentally detected silent medullary infarcts are rarely a cause for concern; however, patients presenting with recent onset of pain in previously quiet lesions must be investigated for evidence of malignant degeneration.

Suggested Readings

Armas RR, Goldsmith SJ. Gallium scintigraphy in bone infarction: correlation with bone imaging. Clin Nucl Med 1984;9:1–3

Furey JG, Ferrer-Torrer-Torells M, Reagan JW. Fibrosarcoma arising at the site of bone infarcts. J Bone Joint Surg Am 1960;42-A:802–810

Mankad VN, Yang YM, Williams JP, Brogdon BG. Magnetic resonance imaging of bone marrow in sickle cell patients. Am J Pediatr Hematol Oncol 1988;10:344–347

Munk PL, Helms CA, Holt RG. Immature bone infarcts: findings on plain radiographs and MR scans. Am J Roentgenol 1989;152:547–549

CASE 79

Hema N. Choudur, Anthony G. Ryan, Peter L. Munk, and Laurel O. Marchinkow

Clinical Presentation

A young boy presented with severe wrist pain after having fallen on his outstretched hand while playing soccer.

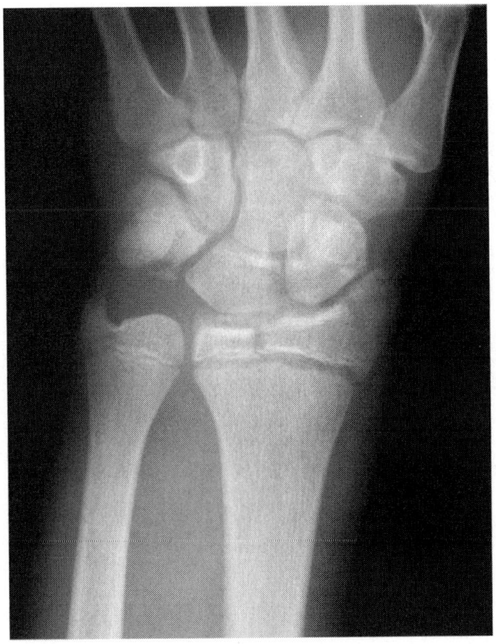

Figure 79A

Radiologic Findings

An anteroposterior radiograph of the wrist (**Fig. 79A**) shows a fracture of the distal radial epiphysis with widening of the radial aspect of the distal radial growth plate. A fracture of the triquetrum is also evident.

Diagnosis

Salter-Harris fracture (type 3).

Differential Diagnosis

None.

Discussion

Salter-Harris fractures are fractures of the growth plate and are therefore seen only in the pediatric population, prior to growth plate closure. They are classified as fractures of the physis with variable involvement of the epiphysis and metaphysis.

Etiology

These fractures usually occur secondary to horseplay or sports injuries.

Pathophysiology

Nutrition is supplied to the growth plate from the distal to the proximal epiphyseal end by the epiphyseal vessels. The growth plate itself is avascular. The cartilage cells transform as they progress from the germinal layer toward the metaphysis to form the zone of provisional calcification. Neovascularization occurs from the metaphyseal end of the growth plate.

Fractures that result in apposition and consequently compression of the vascular beds on both sides of the growth plate halt further growth. Those that occur through the growth plate with no fracture displacement do not impede growth. Disruption of the vascularity at either end of the growth plate may hamper growth.

Clinical Findings

The child usually complains of pain or points to the affected bone following the injury. There is swelling and variable bruising at the site of the injury.

Complications

- Premature fusion of the growth plate in type 5
- Shortening of the affected bone
- Arthropathy from intra-articular extension
- Limb deformity

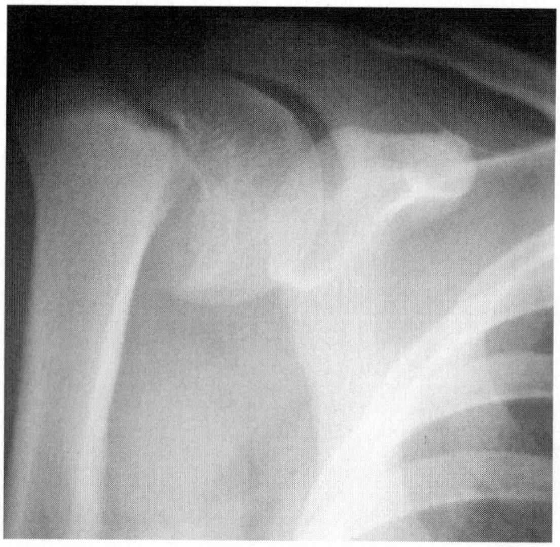
B

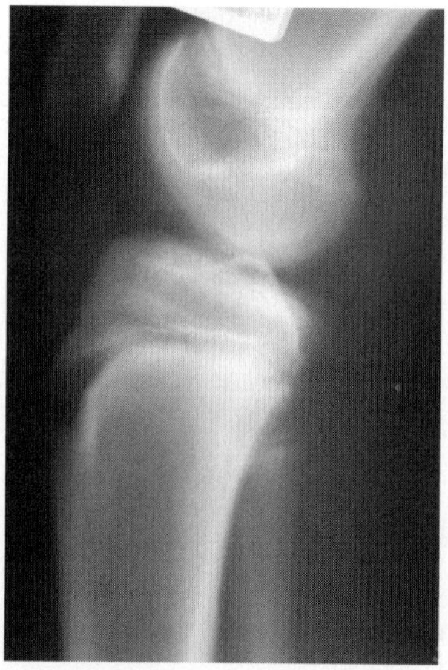
C

Figures 79B Salter-Harris type 1 fracture involving the proximal humeral growth plate with considerable displacement. **79C** Salter-Harris type 1 fracture of the proximal tibia.

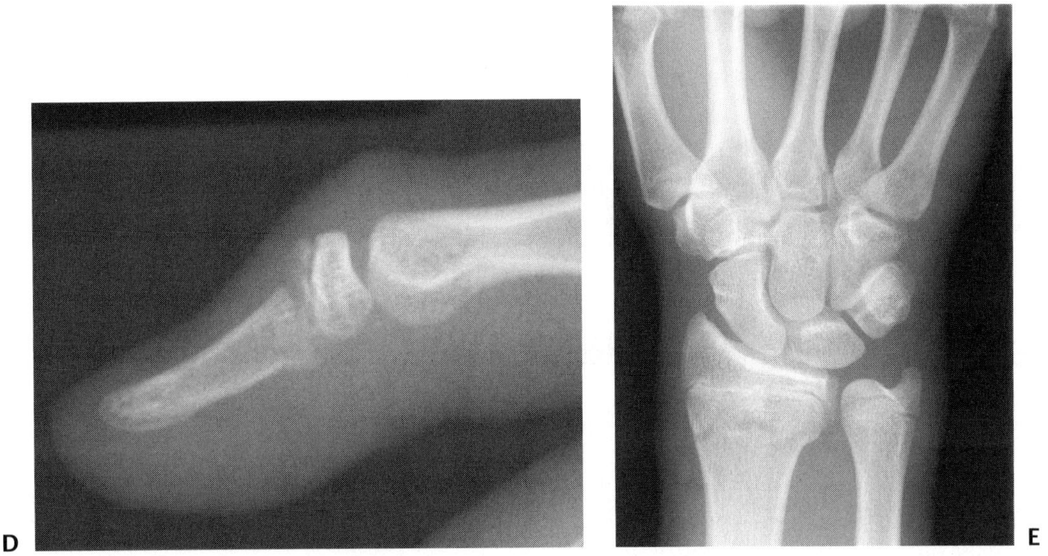

Figures 79D Salter-Harris type 2 fracture of the distal phalanx of the thumb. **79E** Salter-Harris type 2 fracture of the distal radius.

Imaging Findings

RADIOGRAPHY

The plain radiographic findings can be classified in the following way.

Type 1 Widening of the growth plate due to a transverse fracture (**Figs. 79B,79C**). The growing zones, however, are not affected.

Type 2 This is the most common subtype, a fracture through the physis and metaphysis (**Figs. 79D,79E**), resulting in a variable metaphyseal fragment, the latter referred to as the Thurston-Holland fragment. The epiphysis is not involved. These fractures may be complicated by mild residual shortening following fusion but no gross functional impairment typically.

Type 3 A fracture through the physis and epiphysis extending to the articular surface, exemplified by the Tillaux fracture of the ankle (anterolateral tibial epiphysis avulsion fracture). The metaphysis is not involved. These fractures may produce chronic disability due to arthropathy (as the fracture extends to the articular surface) and deformity.

Type 4 The fracture involves the epiphysis, physis, and metaphysis. There is premature fusion of the growth plate. There is resultant shortening, deformity, and arthropathy.

Type 5 This is a crush/compression injury of the growth plate secondary to excessive axial loading. No involvement of the epiphysis or metaphysis is seen. The prognosis is poor, as the diagnosis is usually delayed, made only after premature fusion of the growth plate. Initial radiographs may only reveal soft-tissue swelling at the growth plate.

Figures 79F to **79K** are line drawings of a normal growth plate and Salter-Harris fracture types.

COMPUTED TOMOGRAPHY

- Usually unnecessary; however, in complex cases with comminution and rotational displacement, multiplanar reformats can aid in planning reconstructive surgery

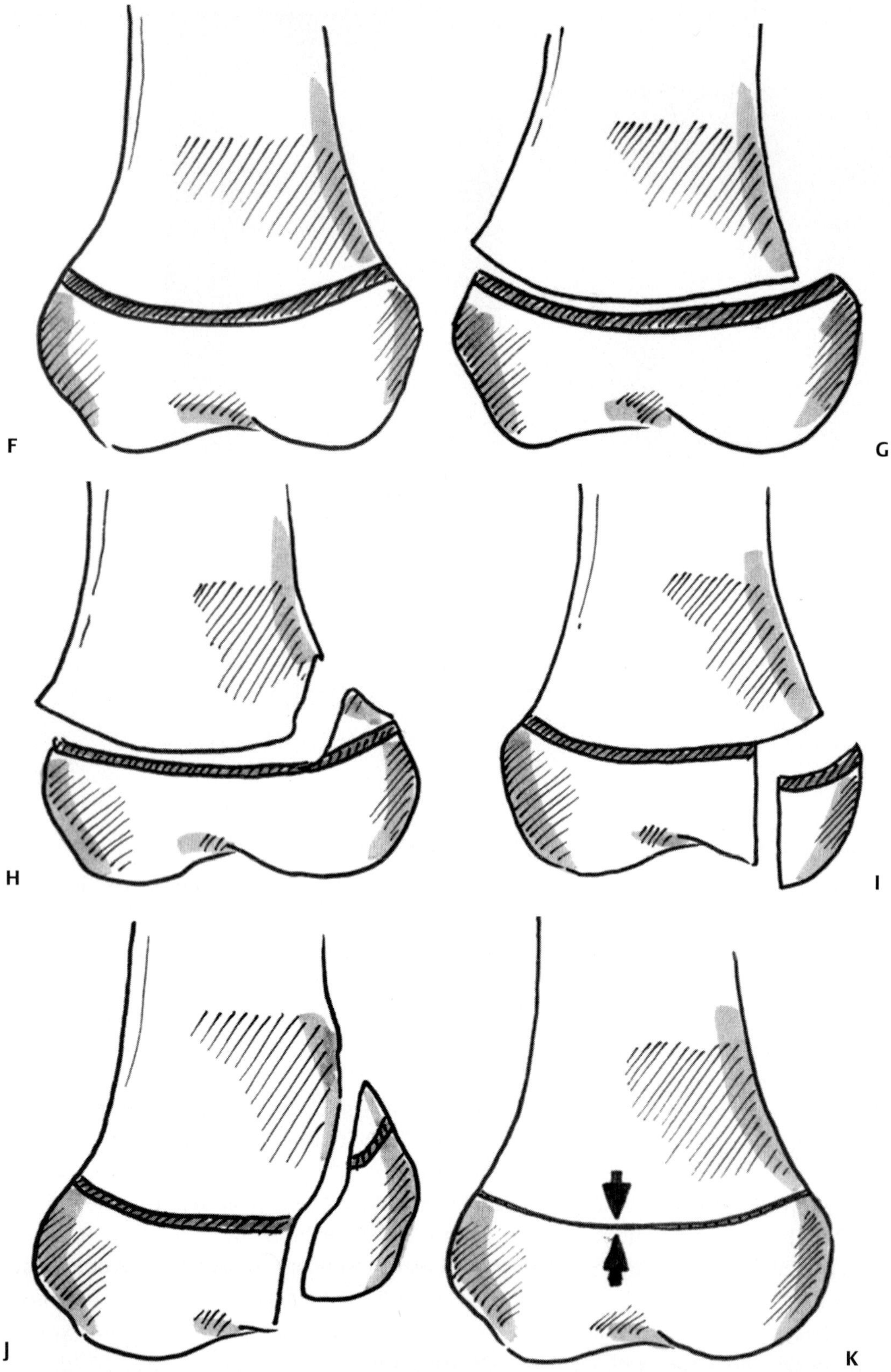

Figures 79F–79K Line diagrams of a normal growth plate, or epiphysis (**79F**), Salter-Harris I fracture through the plate (**79G**), Salter-Harris II fracture through the plate extending into metaphysis (**79H**), Salter-Harris III fracture through the plate extending into the epiphysis (**79I**), Salter-Harris IV fracture vertically through the plate (**79J**), Salter-Harris V impaction of the epiphysis (**79K**),

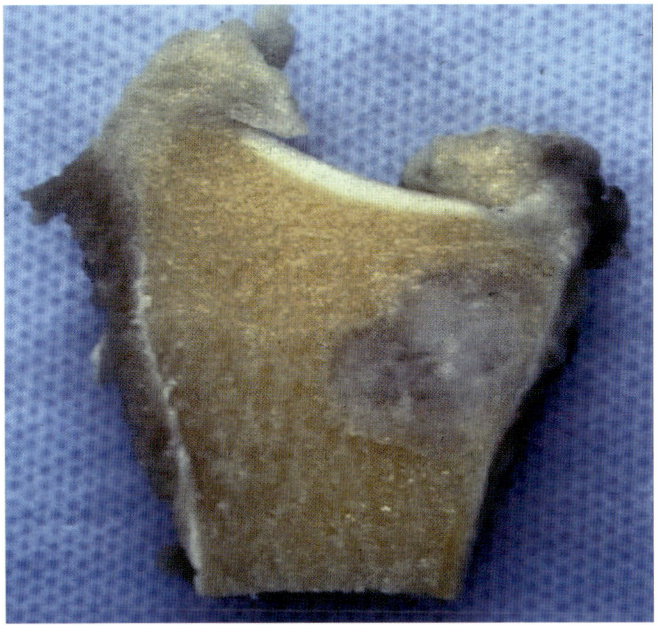

Figure 51D (See **Figure 51D**, page 273.)

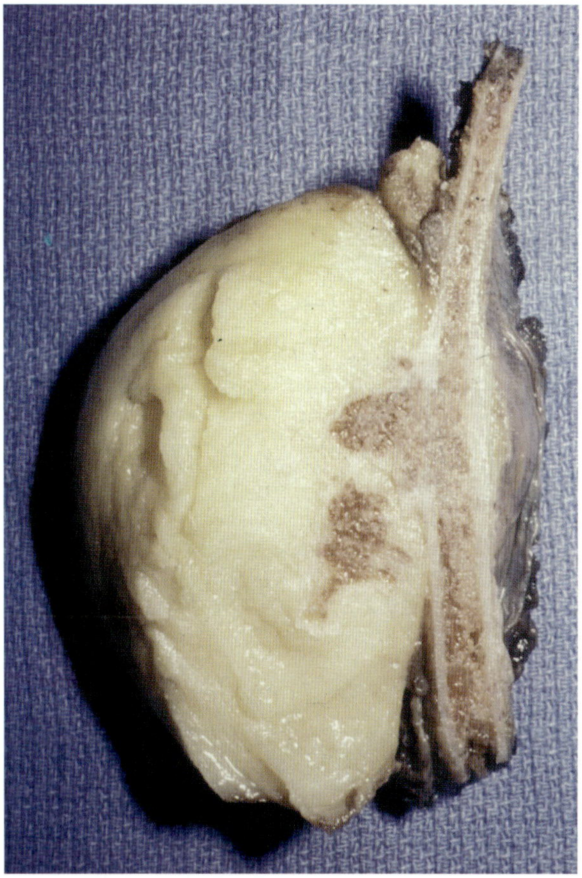

Figure 53F Gross specimen demonstrating an osseous excrescence arising from the lateral aspect of a rib with no corticomedullary continuity surrounded by a fatty mass. (See **Figure 53F**, page 288.)

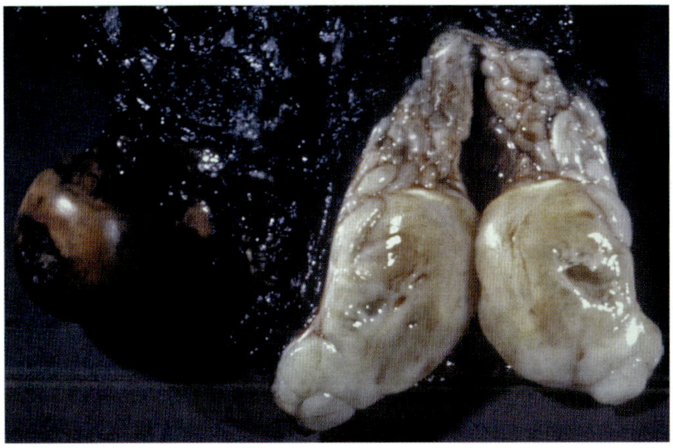

Figure 59O A cut surgical specimen is depicted. (See **Figure 59O**, page 318.)

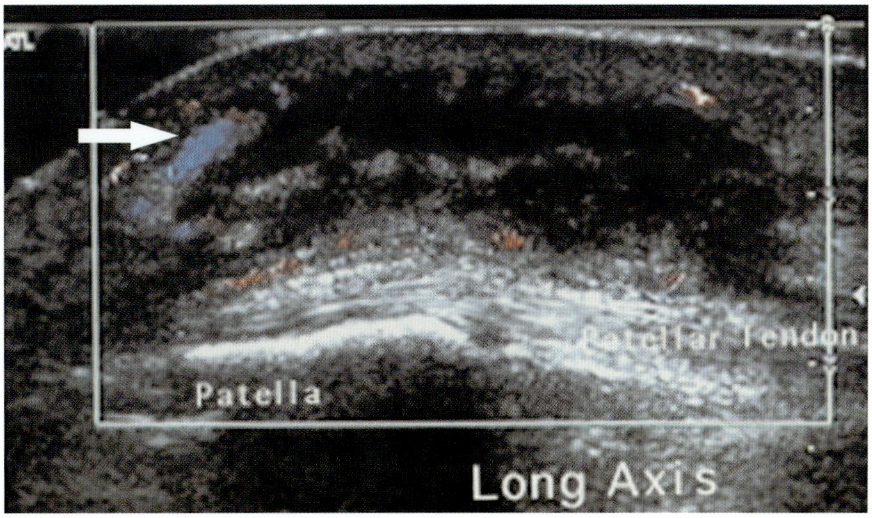

Figure 74B (See **Figure 74B**, page 393.)

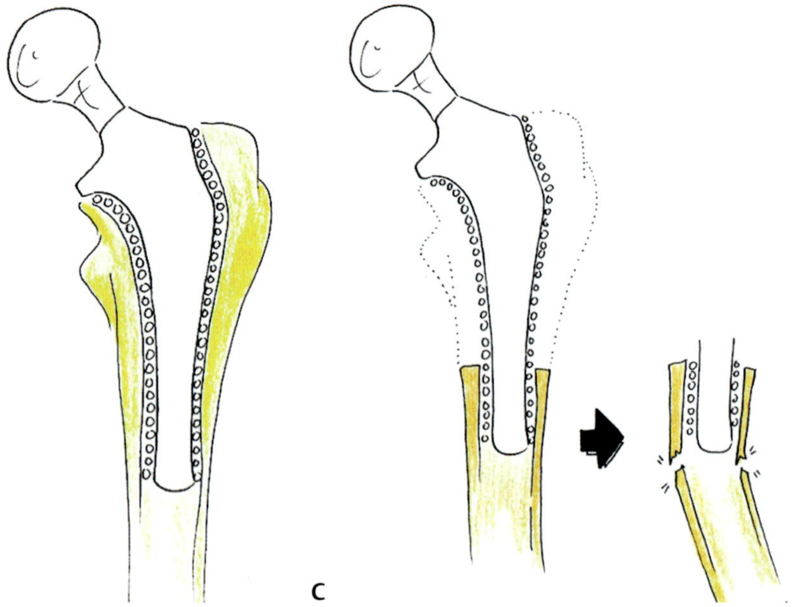

Figures 130B Stress shielding diagram shows the femoral component in place. **130C** Stress diagram shows relative thinning of the femoral cortex, yielding a periprosthetic fracture at the level of the tip. (See **Figures 130B, 130C**, page 731.)

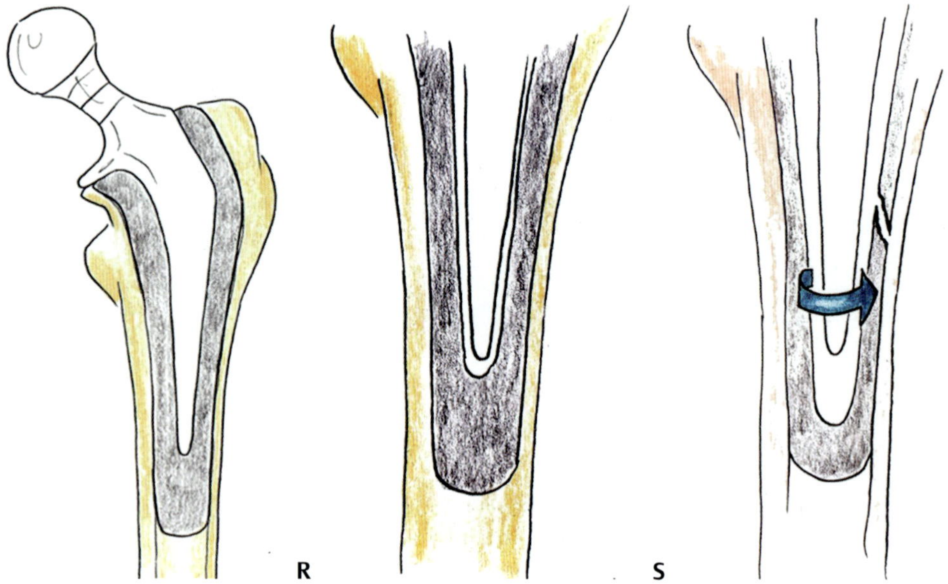

Figures 130Q A line diagram shows the expected immediate postoperative appearances of a cemented prosthesis, that is, close apposition of bone–cement and cement–prosthesis. **130R** Line diagram showing the interval development of lucency between the prosthesis and the cement. **130S** Line diagram showing how the increased periprosthetic space permits a degree of prosthetic movement, building considerable torque forces that can give rise to cement fractures, as shown. (See **Figures 130Q, 130R, 130S**, page 735.)

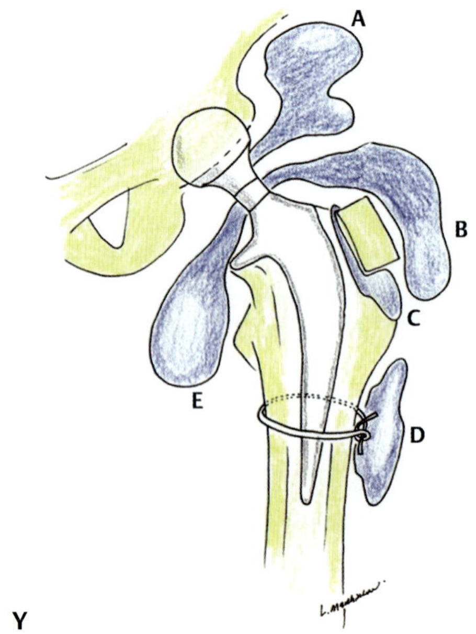

Figures 130Y Line diagram showing the bursae and pseudobursae that may be seen on arthrography of a total hip arthroplasty. A, supra-acetabular; B, trochanteric; C, subtrochanteric; D, sutural; E, iliopsoas bursa. (See **Figure 130Y**, page 737.)

MAGNETIC RESONANCE IMAGING

- MRI has an important role in the evaluation of acute pediatric growth plate injuries, particularly when diagnostic uncertainty persists following conventional radiographs. MRI allows detection of occult fractures, may alter Salter-Harris staging, and consequently may alter patient management.
- Salter-Harris fractures are of low signal intensity on T1- and of high signal intensity on T2-weighted images with adjacent marrow edema. The three-dimensional MPGR is valuable in the evaluation of physeal injuries, given its elegant depiction of cartilage.

Prognosis

- Usually good with no functional impairment despite mild deformity in types 2 and 3, arthropathy in types 3 and 4
- Type 5 fractures have a poor prognosis, secondary to delayed diagnosis and consequent premature closure of the growth plate.

PEARLS

- Type 2 injuries are by far the most common.
- In equivocal cases, especially where type 5 injuries are suspected, the greater sensitivity of MRI may disclose evidence of injury not demonstrated radiographically.

PITFALLS

- A high degree of clinical and radiological suspicion should be present to detect these injuries, especially type 5.
- Whenever the growth plate appears widened or narrowed compared with the opposite side, particularly in association with adjacent soft-tissue swelling, the diagnosis should be presumed, the limb immobilized, and follow-up radiographs arranged, looking for the presence of sclerosis and/or a more conspicuous accompanying fracture line.

Suggested Readings

Carey J, Spence L, Blickman H, Eustace S. MRI of pediatric growth plate injury: correlation with plain film radiographs and clinical outcome. Skeletal Radiol 1998;27:250–255

Close BJ, Strouse PJ. MR of physeal fractures of the adolescent knee. Pediatr Radiol 2000;30:756–762

Petit P, Panuel M, Faure F. Acute fracture of the distal tibial physis: role of gradient-echo MR imaging versus plain film examination. Am J Roentgenol 1996;166:1203–1206

CASE 80

Peter L. Munk and Anthony G. Ryan

Clinical Presentation

A 30-year-old man presented with chronic wrist pain after a fall on his hand 24 months previously.

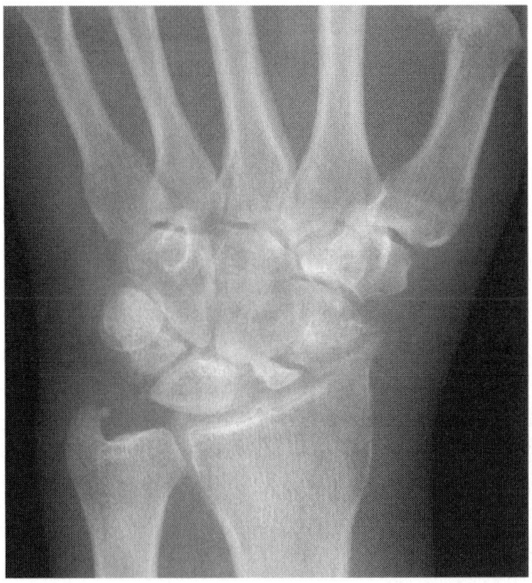

Figure 80A

Radiologic Findings

An anteroposterior (AP) wrist radiograph (**Fig. 80A**) shows reduced joint space and osteophyte formation at the radioscaphoid articulation and an increased scapholunate interval. A dense triangular bony fragment is evident on the radial aspect of the lunate.

Diagnosis

Avascular necrosis of the proximal pole of the scaphoid with collapse.

Differential Diagnosis

None.

Discussion

Background

Scaphoid fractures represent approximately three quarters of all carpal bone fractures. This bone is critical to proper functioning of the wrist, and the morbidity of a poorly healed or unhealed fracture is significant. Although uncommon, fractures of the scaphoid in children tend to be avulsions of the distal pole, the latter accounting for 75%, with 20% of the waist and 5% of the proximal pole.

Etiology

The typical mechanism for a fracture is a fall on the outstretched hand.

Pathophysiology

In adults, the most common site for a fracture is through the waist (**Figs. 80B,80C**), where ~70 to 75% occur. Twenty percent of fractures occur in the proximal third of the bone, with the remainder occurring in the distal portion (**Fig. 80D**), including the tuberosity (**Figs. 80E,80F**). These fractures are often quite subtle, particularly as the fracture plane is transverse or slightly oblique.

The blood supply of the scaphoid enters via the distal pole via dorsal and volar branches from the radial artery. Fractures through the waist or proximal portion therefore isolate the proximal pole

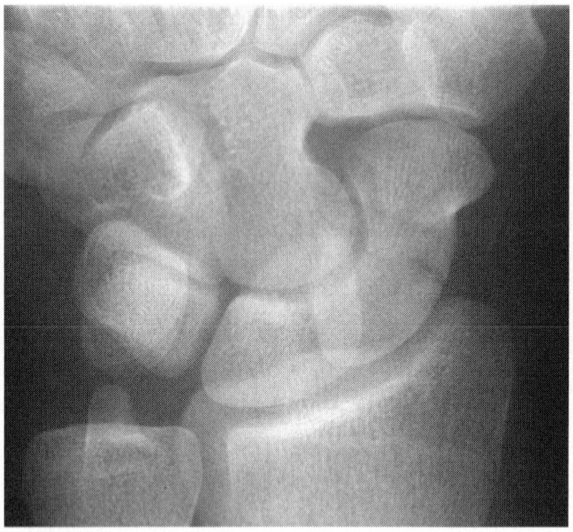
B

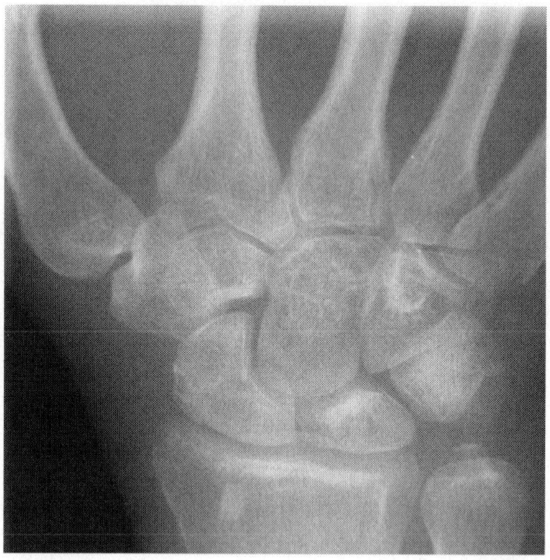
C

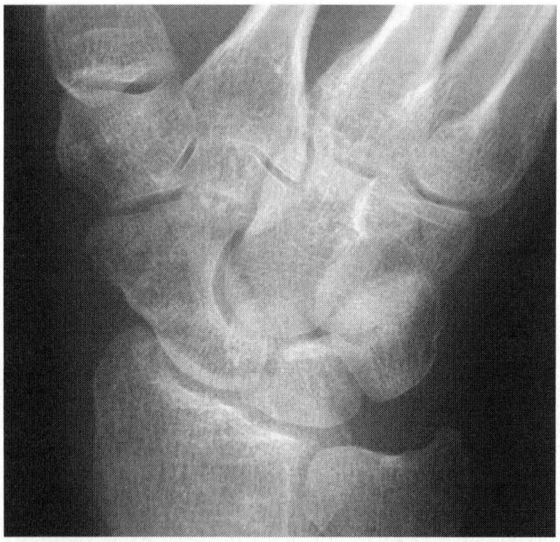
D

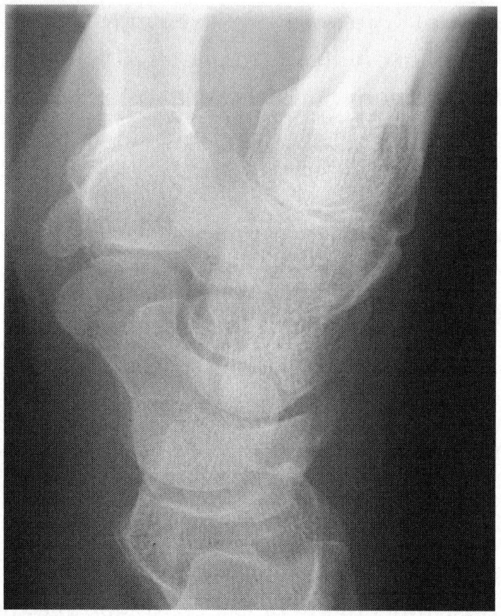
E

Figures 80B–80E An undisplaced fracture through the waist of the scaphoid. **80C** A minimally displaced fracture of the waist of the scaphoid; a cortical step is evident on the radial aspect of the scaphoid. **80D** A minimally displaced fracture of the proximal pole of the scaphoid; a cortical step is evident proximally at the scapho-trapezium articulation. **80E** A minimally displaced fracture of the distal pole of the scaphoid through the base of the scaphoid tubercle, frequently seen best on a lateral view, as in this case.

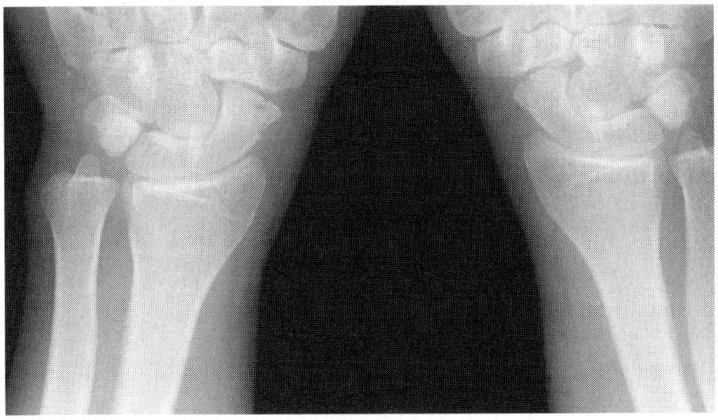

Figure 80F An AP radiograph of both wrists demonstrating bilateral scaphoid tubercle fractures.

from most of its blood supply, and it may become avascular. The more proximal a fracture, the more likely avascular necrosis is to occur.

This is usually manifest as increased density of the proximal pole relative to the surrounding bones, which retain normal perfusion (**Fig. 80A**). Avascular necrosis may at times go on to heal if collapse does not occur.

With time, the isolated fragment may collapse, producing a malalignment in the proximal carpal row. Numerous fragments may function as loose bodies, interfering further with wrist motility and promoting chondrolysis.

Clinical Findings

Scaphoid fractures are most frequently found in young active individuals between 5 and 40 years of age, secondary to a fall on the outstretched hand. In the younger age group, they are far more common in male adolescents than female. In the older age group, that is, above 50 years, a fall on an outstretched hand typically results in a fractured distal radius.

Complications

- Malunion, nonunion
- Avascular necrosis of the proximal pole
- Collapse of the proximal pole
- Chondrolysis secondary to malalignment or loose bodies
- Secondary degenerative change

Imaging Findings

RADIOGRAPHY

- Often these fractures are virtually undisplaced, and multiple projections are required to delineate the fracture with conventional radiographic imaging. They are usually best seen on an AP view with ulnar deviation or a semipronated oblique view.
- Not infrequently, a satisfactory demonstration requires ancillary imaging methods, such as tomography (**Fig. 80G**), CT, MRI, or nuclear medicine bone scanning.
- Should these imaging modalities not be immediately available, an acceptable alternative would be immobilization of the suspected fracture, with repeat radiography at 7 to 10 days. At this time, some resorption of mineral around the fracture line will have occurred, and the fracture will be

evident on radiographs. It should be remembered that up to 25% of fractures can be occult at the time of radiography.
- The presence of a scaphoid fat stripe has been advocated as a useful ancillary sign in ruling out the presence of a scaphoid fracture, although in cases with strong clinical suspicion, this should not be relied on to definitively exclude the presence of a fracture, and additional imaging should be secured.
- Avascular necrosis is usually manifest as increased density of the proximal pole relative to the surrounding bones, which retain normal perfusion (**Fig. 80A**). Avascular necrosis may at times go on to heal if collapse does not occur.

COMPUTED TOMOGRAPHY

- CT is ideally performed in the coronal (**Fig. 80H**) or sagittal planes, as this tends to be more perpendicular to the fracture line. Sections as thin as possible, for example, 1.0 to 1.25 mm, should be obtained.

MAGNETIC RESONANCE IMAGING

- MRI is particularly helpful in the demonstration of undisplaced fractures, as the fracture line itself is usually of low signal intensity, but with extensive surrounding edema in the bone marrow (**Fig. 80I**). Diffuse edema without a low signal linearity may be the only evidence of a fracture.

NUCLEAR MEDICINE

- Standard technetium bone scans are also very useful, as these demonstrate increased radiopharmaceutical uptake around the fracture line.

Treatment

IMMOBILIZATION

- For tubercle fractures: 3 to 4 weeks
- Fractures of the waist: 10 to 12 weeks with the wrist in a cast after closed reduction of the proximal fragment (if displaced) with radial deviation of the wrist

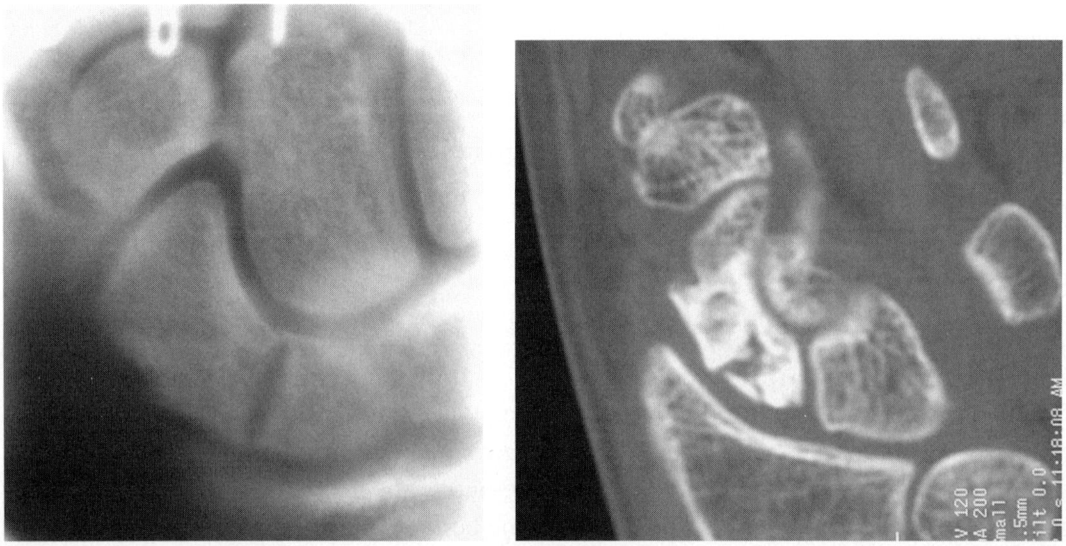

G H

Figures 80G,80H A tomogram on day 10 after injury of an undisplaced waist of scaphoid fracture, which was inconspicuous on initial radiographs. **80H** A coronal CT clearly shows the sclerosis of the proximal scaphoid with fragmentation of collapse of the proximal pole secondary to avascular necrosis.

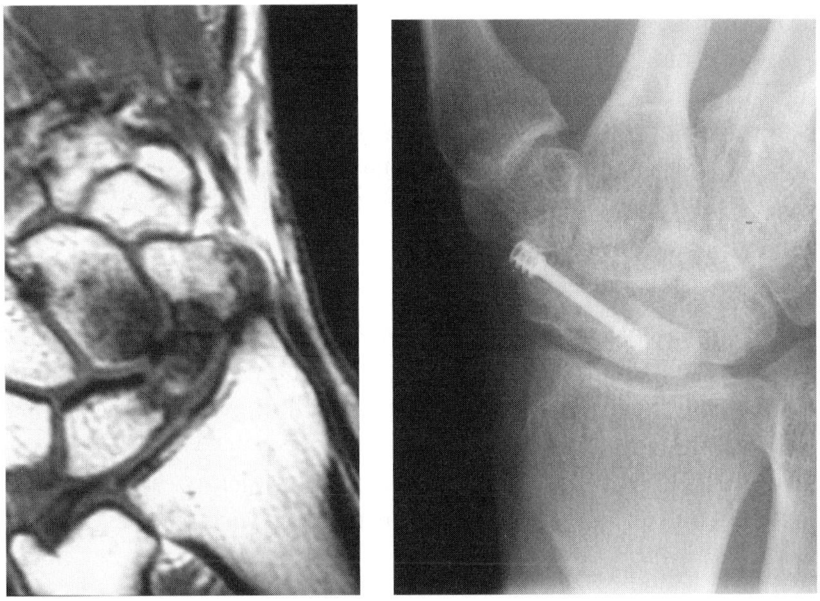

I J

Figures 80I,80J A coronal T1-weighted image shows a chronic fracture of the waist of the scaphoid as a low signal intensity line and sclerotic change within the adjacent scaphoid and the capitate. Reduced joint space is evident at the scaphocapitate articulation and the radioscaphoid articulation, with further sclerosis evident at the tip of the radial tuberosity. **80J** A Herbert screw fixation of a proximal pole fracture thought to be undergoing avascular necrosis; note the relative sclerosis of the proximal pole. The proximal pole ultimately survived after this intervention.

- Healing should be evidenced as disappearance of the fracture line and restoration of trabecular continuity.

OPEN REDUCTION AND FIXATION

- Bone grafting of nonhealing fractures has been successful, but if this fails, arthrodesis may be necessary.

Prognosis

- 95% of scaphoid fractures heal satisfactorily with standard cast immobilization.
- Fixation of scaphoid fractures that are significantly displaced or those that appear to be undergoing avascular necrosis is reported to improve long-term prognosis (**Fig. 80J**).
- If no healing is evident after 6 months of immobilization, further immobilization will not be effective.
- Poor prognostic factors include
  - Displacement during treatment
  - Increasing visibility of the fracture line
  - Early cystic changes

PEARLS

- CT is ideally performed in the coronal or sagittal planes, as this tends to be more perpendicular to the fracture line.

- At 10 to 14 days after the initial trauma, resorption of mineral around the fracture line will have occurred, rendering the fracture line more conspicuous on radiographs.
- Falls on the outstretched hand have different outcomes, depending on the age of the victim: in children, a distal radial buckle fracture tends to be the outcome, whereas in young adults, the scaphoid tends to fracture; in older adults, a Colles' fracture of the distal radius tends to occur.

PITFALLS

- It should be remembered that up to 25% of fractures can be occult at the time of radiography.
- It can be relatively easy to overlook the subtle differences in density between the scaphoid and the remaining carpal bones in the early stages of avascular necrosis, and these differences should be looked for critically in every case.
- It is vital to avoid "satisfaction of search" having identified a scaphoid fracture, as other carpal injuries, such as trans-scaphoid perilunate dislocation, may be present. Such injuries are more easily diagnosed on the lateral wrist view.

Suggested Readings

Brydie A, Raby N. Early MRI in the management of clinical scaphoid fracture. Br J Radiol 2003;76:296–300

Kozin SH. Incidence, mechanism, and natural history of scaphoid fractures. Hand Clin 2001;17:515–524

Munk PL, Lee MJ, Logan PM, et al. Scaphoid bone waist fractures, acute and chronic: imaging with different techniques. Am J Roentgenol 1997;168:779–786

CASE 81

Hema N. Choudur, Anthony G. Ryan, and Peter L. Munk

Clinical Presentation

A middle-aged woman slipped on snow, landing on her outstretched hand. In the ensuing hours, she had severe pain, swelling, and tenderness in the shoulder with decreased mobility of the right arm.

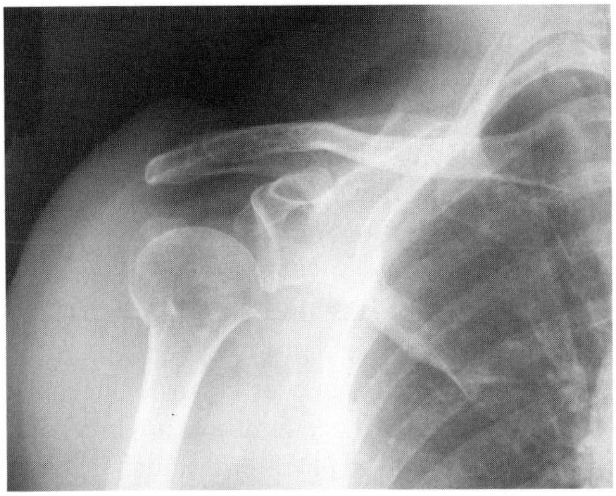

Figure 81A

Radiologic Findings

An anteroposterior (AP) upright view radiograph of the right shoulder (**Fig. 81A**) shows a two-part fracture comprising an undisplaced fracture of the surgical neck of the humerus and a minimally displaced fracture of the greater tuberosity. An associated fat-fluid level is shown within the shoulder joint. The glenohumeral and acromioclavicular articulations are normal.

Diagnosis

Undisplaced proximal humeral fracture involving the surgical neck of the right humerus and greater tuberosity with associated lipohemarthrosis.

Differential Diagnosis

Dislocation must be differentiated from pseudosubluxation, and true fractures from pathologic, insufficiency, and stress fractures.

Discussion

Background

Proximal humeral fractures are not uncommon and account for 5 to 10% of fractures. Although nondisplaced and minimally displaced fractures are the most common and are fairly easy to treat, grossly displaced fractures pose a challenge.

Etiology

The most common etiology is a fall on the outstretched hand. The humerus is severely abducted, resulting in a fracture. Direct blows on the arm can sometimes result in similar fractures. These fractures are more common in women than men and are usually secondary to osteopenia in the elderly. Younger individuals can present with similar injuries secondary to sports-related trauma.

Pathophysiology

The type and extent of the fracture depend on the age of the patient and the mineralization of the bones. Physeal injuries occur in childhood. Dislocations are more common in younger individuals and proximal humeral fractures in the middle-aged and elderly.

Most of these fractures are undisplaced or minimally displaced due to the protection offered by the rotator cuff and surrounding muscles, capsule, and periosteum. Following a proximal humeral fracture, the upper fragment is usually abducted and externally rotated by the external rotators, while the lower fragment is adducted and internally rotated by the internal rotators.

Comminuted and significantly displaced fractures of the neck can cause injury to the blood supply of the humeral head. The main blood supply to the humeral head arises from the anterolateral branch of the anterior humeral circumflex artery. This vessel passes lateral to the long head of the biceps and forms the arcuate artery. The arcuate artery arises from the ascending branch of the anterior humeral circumflex artery as it penetrates bone. It enters into the humeral head in the area of the intertubercular groove and gives branches to the lesser and greater tuberosities. It perfuses the entire epiphysis of the humeral head.

The posterior circumflex artery supplies only a small area in the posteroinferior aspect of the humeral head.

Clinical Findings

As the shoulder is surrounded by a bulk of muscles, radiographic assessment is essential to rule out a clinically suspected fracture. Pain, tenderness, focal swelling, and inability to move the arm are the common presenting complaints following either a fall or a sports-related injury.

The clinical examination also helps to rule out a vascular/nerve injury. If the arm is swollen and red, axillary artery compromise is suspected, and an angiogram is indicated. Other vessels that can be injured are the anterior and posterior circumflex arteries and the ascending humeral circumflex artery. The brachial plexus and axillary nerve may also be injured.

Complications

LIPOHEMARTHROSIS

The fat that escapes into the joint, from the bone marrow, following the fracture is seen as a lucent layer over the radiodense blood-fluid layer because of its lighter weight (**Fig. 81B**).

Inferior subluxation is often seen after an intra- or extra-articular fracture of the proximal humeral head, due to the pressure exerted by the joint effusion on the underlying head, causing it to subluxate or displace inferiorly (**Fig. 81C**). However, with gradual resorption of the fluid, the head returns to its normal articulation.

DELAYED UNION AND NONUNION

Delayed union and nonunion are associated with considerable morbidity. Patients complain of pain, stiffness, and disability in association with shoulder dysfunction. In some studies, patients who

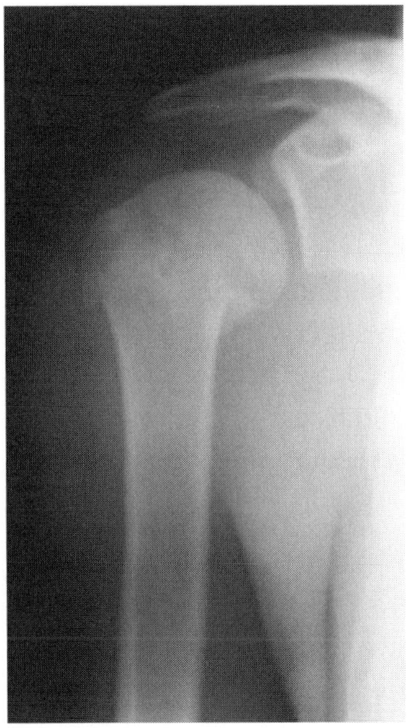

B

Figures 81B,81C Impacted fracture of right humeral surgical neck with lipohemarthrosis. **81C** Inferior pseudosubluxation of the left humerus following an impacted fracture of the humeral surgical neck.

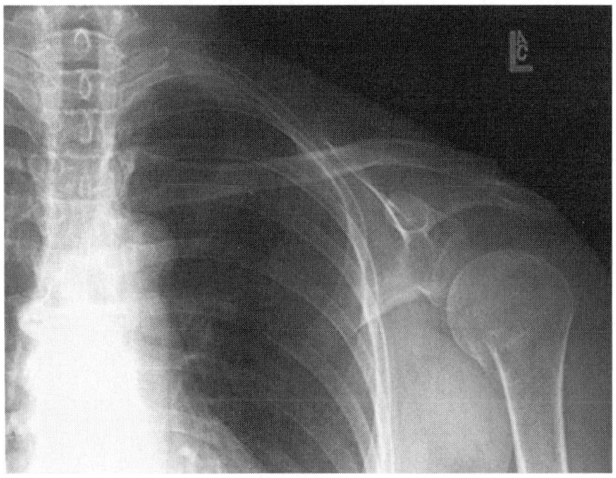

C

decline surgical treatment can have nonreamed intramedullary nails but have limited shoulder motion and pain without union. Patients treated with proximal humeral hemiarthroplasty have relief of pain but limited motion despite rotator cuff reconstruction. The best results of treatment occur after ORIF and bone grafting. A tension band reconstruction that fixes the rotator cuff and proximal humerus to a plate/shaft composite is also used successfully in some patients.

OSTEONECROSIS

Osteonecrosis is most often seen in fractures involving the articular surface or in four-part fractures. There is loss of blood supply to the head from the muscle insertions, and the arcuate branch of the medial humeral circumflex artery. Osteonecrosis is found in 7 to 50% of cases. It is seen as patchy sclerosis and lucency within the head, close to the articular surface.

OSTEOARTHRITIS

Osteoarthritis following fractures involving the articular surface is another complication, in addition to heterotopic ossification surrounding the capsule and rotator cuff tears. Brachial plexus and axillary artery injuries can result from anterior fracture dislocations due either to traction or to impaction by the fractured fragment.

Imaging Findings

RADIOGRAPHY

Anteroposterior and axillary views are mandatory, in addition to the transcapular Y view. If the arm cannot be positioned for the axillary view, a Velpeau axillary view is performed. Axillary is the most important view for proximal humeral fractures, because it shows the most angulation and displacement.

The fractures per Neer's classification may involve any of the four components—the articular head (fracture through the anatomical neck), the greater tuberosity, the lesser tuberosity, and the surgical neck. A displaced fracture is one with $>$ 1 cm of displacement and $>$ 45 degrees of angulation. Associated anterior or posterior dislocation may be present.

One-part fractures

Nondisplaced and minimally displaced fractures are considered one-part fractures and account for 80% of proximal humeral fractures. Almost no angulation is noted in one-part fractures.

Two-part fractures

These fractures can involve any two of the mentioned four components, with one part displaced significantly from the other three. They account for ~15% of all proximal humeral fractures. The most common is a fracture of the surgical neck with impaction or anterior angulation. Anterior and medial displacement may be seen due to the tug of the pectoralis major on the shaft. The most difficult to diagnose are the undisplaced fractures involving the articular head.

Two-part fractures involving the greater tuberosity cause a longitudinal tear of the rotator cuff, best visualized on MRI. Lesser tuberosity fractures result in a medial displacement of the lesser tuberosity secondary to the pull of the subscapularis.

Three-part fractures

These involve displacement of two of the four components. These fractures usually involve the surgical neck with displacement of either the greater or lesser tuberosity. They account for 3 to 4% of all proximal humeral fractures. When the greater tuberosity is fractured, the subscapularis causes a posterior rotation of the head. When the lesser tuberosity is fractured, the supra- and infraspinatus rotate the head anteriorly.

Four-part fractures

Four-part fractures occur when all four components are displaced. They involve displacement of the surgical neck and both tuberosities and account for 3 to 4% of total proximal humeral fractures. Typically, a fracture of the anatomical neck is combined with lesser and greater tuberosity fractures and results in ischemia of the head.

The term *fracture-dislocation* is used when the articular segment is displaced beyond the joint space.

COMPUTED TOMOGRAPHY

- CT is sometimes indicated to evaluate the degree of articulation of the head and the degree of displacement of the tuberosities and to evaluate the degree and pattern of comminution prior to surgery.

MAGNETIC RESONANCE IMAGING

- Surrounding soft-tissue involvement, especially of rotator cuff tears, is best assessed at MRI. Brachial plexus injuries can also be evaluated by MRI.

Treatment and Prognosis

ONE-PART FRACTURES

Early immobilization in a sling with gradual exercises after a week in nondisplaced and minimally displaced fractures results in near preinjury mobility.

TWO-PART FRACTURES

Two-part fractures of the greater tuberosity are assessed best on lateral axillary views and CT. The avulsion of the rotator cuff is best evaluated on MRI. Such fractures are usually treated with heavy, nonabsorbable interfragmentary sutures with repair of the cuff.

In two-part fractures of the surgical neck, the shaft is displaced anteriorly and medially with an anterior angulation in valgus or varus, depending on the position of the arm. Closed reduction with percutaneous pinning is indicated in patients with good bone quality and minimally comminuted or noncomminuted fractures. Open reduction and internal fixation (ORIF) is indicated in patients with severely comminuted fractures or poor bone quality. Intramedullary Enders rods plus interfragmentary sutures are used in patients with advanced osteoporosis.

Two-part fractures of the lesser tuberosity are very rare. These fractures are not well demonstrated on plain radiographs but are clearly seen on CT. A two-part fracture can be rendered one part by treating the glenohumeral articulation.

THREE-PART FRACTURES

Three-part fractures are treated with ORIF, using interfragmentary sutures, intramedullary rod or plate, and screws. With poor bone stock or severely comminuted fractures stock, hemiarthroplasty is indicated.

FOUR-PART FRACTURES

Four-part fractures are usually treated with hemiarthroplasty; otherwise, the chance of an avascular necrosis is 90%. ORIF is attempted in younger individuals.

In valgus-impacted four-part fractures, closed reduction with pinning is done. Such fractures are best evaluated in the AP view.

PEARL

- An articular surface undisplaced fracture may be missed on plain radiographs, and a CT scan is often needed when there is suspicion of the same. Also, in such cases, follow-up radiographs for avascular necrosis are recommended.

PITFALLS

- The pseudosubluxation from joint fluid must not be mistaken for a true dislocation. Follow-up radiographs reveal the head returning to its normal position as the joint effusion is resorbed.
- It is imperative to check for adjacent rib fractures, with or without pneumothorax (**Fig. 81D**).

D
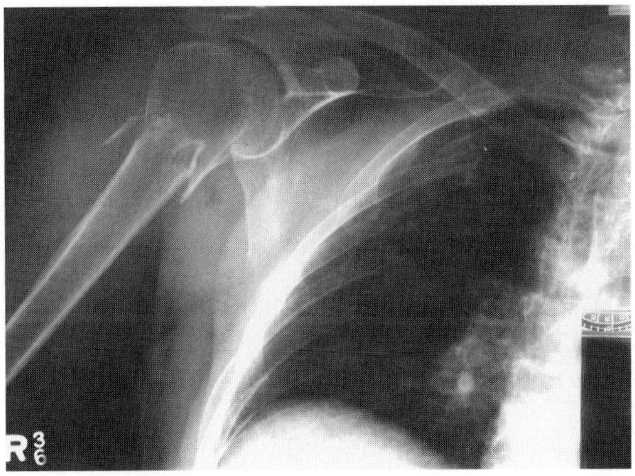

Figure 81D Rib fractures without obvious pneumothorax in an impacted fracture of the humeral surgical neck.

Suggested Readings

Bernstein J, Adler LM, Blank JE, et al. Evaluation of the Neer system of classification of proximal humeral fractures with computerized tomographic scans and plain radiographs. J Bone Joint Surg Am 1996;78:1371–1375

Neer CS II. Displaced proximal humeral fractures. I. Classification and evaluation. J Bone Joint Surg. 1970;52:1077–1089

Resnick D. Bone and Joint Imaging. 2nd ed. Philadelphia, PA: WB Saunders; 1996:758–760

Rogers LF. The shoulder and humeral shaft. In: Radiology of Skeletal Trauma, 3rd ed. Winston-Salem, NC: Churchill Livingstone, Wake Forrest Univ., 2002:593–582

CASE 82

Anthony G. Ryan and Peter L. Munk

Clinical Presentation

An unconscious 24-year-old woman presented after a high-velocity motor vehicle impact. The driver of the vehicle was found dead at the scene. The patient had been an unrestrained front-seat passenger, had been expelled from the vehicle, and was found by the ambulance personnel with the lower half of her body trapped beneath the vehicle.

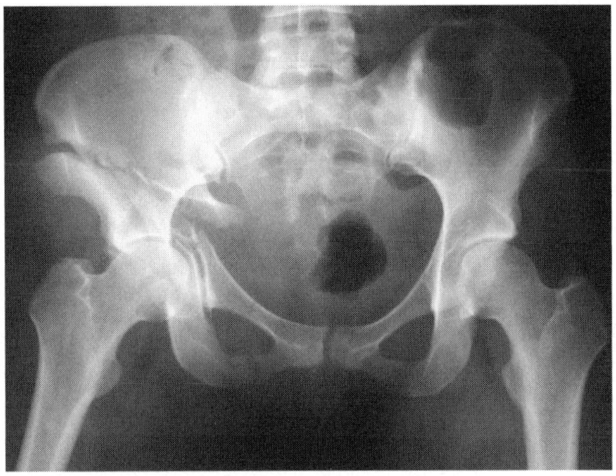

Figure 82A

Radiologic Findings

A plain film of the pelvis (**Fig. 82A**) performed as part of the initial examination shows multiple fractures of the right pelvic rings, including the superior and inferior pubic rami and diastasis of the right sacroiliac joint (the right iliac wing is seen completely en face). There is a complete transverse fracture of the iliac wing exiting between the anterior superior and inferior iliac spines. A butterfly fragment in relation to this fracture is present, displaced centrally. Both the iliopectineal and ilioischial lines are disrupted.

Diagnosis

Combined modality pelvic fracture (AP compression predominant) with severe complex acetabular fracture.

The plain film shows a severely comminuted fracture involving the anterior and posterior columns, evinced by disruption of both iliopectineal and ilioischial lines. The acetabular articular surface is split at its apex.

Concomitant transaxial CT at the level of the acetabulum (**Fig. 82B**) confirms the fractures of the anterior and posterior columns, with a further infratectal transverse component (running in the AP direction and caudad to the larger transverse fracture seen on the plain film). In addition to the posterior column fracture, the posterior wall of the acetabulum is fractured. A breach of the quadrilateral plate is seen as well, with an associated pelvic side wall hematoma.

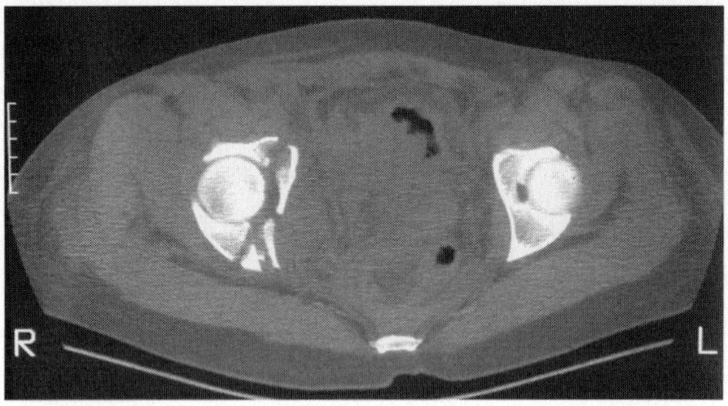

Figure 82B

Differential Diagnosis

None.

Discussion

Background

Acetabular fractures are relatively common, comprising 25% of all pelvic fractures, with fractures of the acetabular wall most common.

Given its weight-bearing function, the most clinically important part of the acetabulum is the roof, formed and supported by the anterior and posterior columns, which meet to form an inverted Y with a 60-degree angle between the divergent limbs. Fractures involving the roof, one or both columns, or any combination of the above will be discussed below.

Etiology

These fractures occur as a result of high-energy trauma, for example, secondary to high-speed motor vehicle accident or a fall/jump from a great height, as in an attempted suicide or an unopened parachute accident. The mechanism of injury frequently results in complex fractures with comminution and components in multiple planes.

Pathophysiology

Fractures disrupting the acetabular articular surface result in two fundamental injuries: to the articular cartilage and to the supporting skeleton of the joint.

Cartilage injury may result in alteration of the proteoglycan matrix and in some cases can cause chondrocyte death, leading to further degeneration of the articular surface in addition to the focal direct cartilaginous trauma experienced.

Unreduced or malaligned fractures result in articular surface irregularity secondary to the osseous disruption and concomitant cartilaginous destruction, which in turn causes significant increases in peak contact pressures, the latter promoting the development of degenerative arthritic changes.

Clinical Findings

These fractures are found predominantly in young male patients involved in incidents as described above. They are frequently in hemorrhagic shock on arrival at the emergency room. If there is a concomitant hip dislocation, the affected leg will be in internal rotation. Accompanying sciatic nerve injury is indicated by paresis of the hamstrings and forelimb muscles and by paresthesias of the foot.

Stages of Disease

Acetabular fractures are often complex, with multiple fragments and secondary fracture lines. Four injury patterns make up 75% of all acetabular fractures: posterior wall, transverse, combined transverse, and posterior wall and fractures of both columns. The use of the classification system devised by Judet in 1964 and modified by Letournel in 1980 led to improved management of such injuries.

Fractures are divided into two main types: elementary, which consist of injuries to a single structural component, and associated, which are combinations of the elementary types.

The five elementary fracture types are

- Posterior acetabular wall (27%)
- Transverse acetabular (9%)
- Anterior column (disrupting the iliopubic line) (5%)
- Posterior column (disrupting the ilioischial line) (4%)
- Anterior acetabular wall (2%),

The five associated fracture types, which involve a combination of the elementary entities, are

- Transverse and posterior wall (20%)
- Fractures of both columns (19%)
- T-shaped (6%)
- Anterior wall and posterior hemitransverse (5%)
- Posterior column and posterior acetabular wall (3%)

The individual fractures and their combinations are considered in more detail below.

ELEMENTARY FRACTURES

Posterior acetabular wall fracture

A posterior acetabular wall fracture is typically caused by the impact on the knee of a flexed, abducted hip against the dashboard in a motor vehicle accident. The size of the resultant fracture is directly proportional to the degree of abduction of the hip. The greater the degree to which the hip is flexed, the more inferior the fracture will be located on the acetabular rim.

If displaced, the fragment is usually driven posteriorly; however, posterior marginal impaction can occur, which is more difficult to diagnose. If unrecognized preoperatively, this will limit the success of reduction and fixation.

Transverse acetabular fracture

Transverse fracture of the acetabulum, as the name implies, bisects the joint in the transaxial plane, dividing the hemipelvis into two halves: inferior (which is also usually anterior) and superior. The fracture is rarely truly transverse, with a tendency to angulation in the craniocaudal direction, higher medially than laterally. On transaxial CT slices, the fracture line may thus be seen to follow a lateral course from above inferiorly, which may be confused for a vertically oriented fracture. Multiple plane radiographs or multiplanar reformats of CT data may be required to establish the orientation.

Transverse fractures may be further subclassified by virtue of their exact relationship with the acetabular roof: juxtatectal, transtectal, or infratectal. Infratectal fractures cross below the level of the acetabular roof.

The transtectal transverse fracture line crosses the roof of the articular surface, whereas the juxtatectal fracture line crosses the acetabulum at the junction of the roof of the acetabulum and the cotyloid fossa, which, while not disrupting the articular surface directly, may give rise to secondary surface irregularity.

Anterior column fracture

The iliopubic column rarely fractures in isolation and is usually associated with posterior column or transverse fractures. These fractures usually begin on the anterior ilium at or between the level of the anterior spines and exit through the ischiopubic ramus.

Anterior column fractures occur secondary to an impact on the greater trochanter, with the hip in internal rotation. Because they are vertically oriented, they are generally easily seen on standard transaxial images.

Posterior column fracture

This occurs like a posterior wall fracture but with sufficient force and abduction to separate the posterior column from the remainder of the hemipelvis as a result of an additional fracture through the ischiopubic ramus. The presence of the latter is necessary for the fracture to be defined as a true posterior column fracture.

Anterior acetabular wall fracture

The least common elementary fracture, this occurs secondary to impact on the greater trochanter, driving the head of the femur against the anterior margin and giving rise to separation of the anterior articular margin with detachment of the adjacent iliopubic column. The fracture line originates on the anterior rim and exits through the superior pubic ramus (**Figs. 82C–82E**), thus differentiating it from an anterior column fracture.

ASSOCIATED FRACTURES

Transverse and posterior wall fracture

A combination of transverse and posterior wall fractures is the most common associated fracture complex.

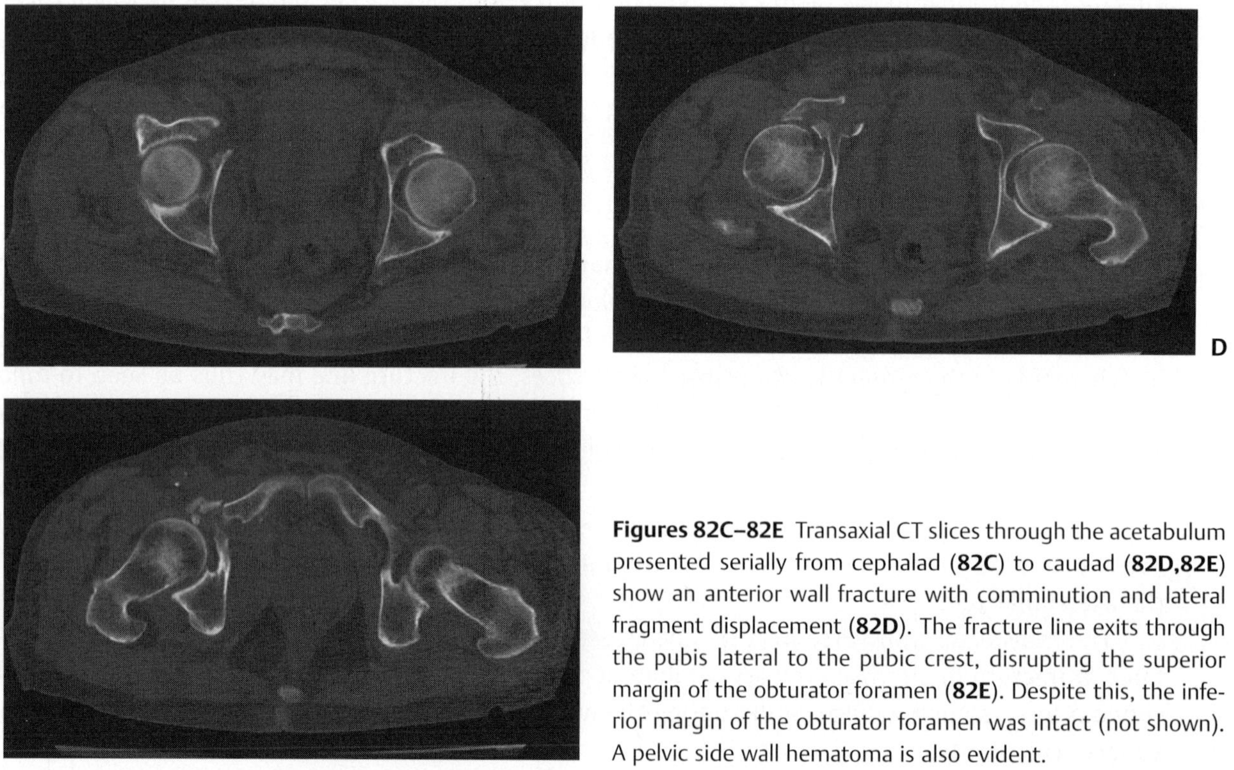

Figures 82C–82E Transaxial CT slices through the acetabulum presented serially from cephalad (**82C**) to caudad (**82D,82E**) show an anterior wall fracture with comminution and lateral fragment displacement (**82D**). The fracture line exits through the pubis lateral to the pubic crest, disrupting the superior margin of the obturator foramen (**82E**). Despite this, the inferior margin of the obturator foramen was intact (not shown). A pelvic side wall hematoma is also evident.

Fracture of both columns

A fracture of both columns is the most complex of the acetabular fractures, resulting in extensive comminution, rotation, and displacement. The posterior column component is similar to an isolated fracture. The fracture extends from the greater sciatic notch through the acetabular fossa and the ischiopubic ramus. The anterior component typically begins on the anterior ilium, descends vertically, and meets the posterior fracture line, usually in the region of the acetabulum.

Because both of these fragments are essentially free, they do not retain their usual relationship and may thus displace considerably. This is in contradistinction to the elementary transverse fracture, in which the portions retain their relationship.

The important clinical implication of this combination is that no part of the weight-bearing acetabulum is stable.

T-shaped fracture

The T-shaped fracture is a transverse fracture combined with a vertical component extending inferiorly through the acetabulum, exiting at the obturator foramen and through the ischiopubic ramus.

Anterior wall and posterior hemitransverse fracture

This is a combination of anterior wall and transverse fractures. The significance of this injury is that, operatively, the fracture must be approached anteriorly, whereas a posterior approach is required for a T-shaped fracture.

Posterior column and posterior wall fracture

The uncommon posterior wall fracture complicates matters by virtue of contributing multiple fragments that can become impacted into the innominate bone, which would require arthrotomy for complete reduction.

Complications

- Posttraumatic arthritis
- Sciatic nerve injury
- Superior gluteal artery disruption
- Although femoral head avascular necrosis and osteochondral injuries of the femoral head occur secondary to acetabular fractures, they most commonly occur secondary to hip dislocation.
- Femoral nerve palsy associated with an associated posterior wall transverse acetabular fracture has been reported, presumably secondary to the inciting anterior impact.
- Acetabular fractures during pregnancy are associated with high maternal (9%) and fetal (35%) mortality rates.
- Associated injuries are seen with the iliopsoas muscle, iliopsoas tendon, and inguinal canal.
- Although other pelvic fractures, such as pubic symphysis diastasis, sacroiliac diastasis, and sacral, iliac, and pubic rami fractures, are associated with bladder rupture, isolated acetabular fractures do not correlate with rupture.
- Bowel perforation secondary to a severely comminuted acetabular fracture is a very rare complication.
- Late complications include nonunion, wound infection, and heterotopic bone formation.

Imaging Findings

RADIOGRAPHY

Anterior (more medial on an AP radiograph) and posterior rim lines mark the acetabular margins. The iliopectineal line and ilioischial lines represent the anterior and posterior columns, respectively.

Although relatively few fractures and dislocations are missed on plain radiographs (10%), a very large proportion (80%) of intra-articular fragments in the hip joint associated with acetabular fractures will be missed on plain films. For these reasons, in addition to the difficulties of achieving satisfactory Judet views (including pain and loss of time in an emergent state), CT is recommended in all cases of acetabular fracture.

COMPUTED TOMOGRAPHY

CT is now the investigation of choice to fully evaluate acetabular fractures, especially where multiple fracture planes coexist. It is also useful postoperatively in assessing fracture alignment and the presence of free intra-articular fragments (acetabular or femoral head) or transcortical extension of fixation screws. CT can assist in directing fixation of femoral fractures.

The initial assessment must address the following:

- Disruption of the acetabular columns
- Incongruity of the fracture lines
- Size, relationship, and displacement of resultant fragments

Column and transverse fractures have particular CT findings:

- Column fractures are oriented in a medial to lateral direction, and are thus best analyzed on the coronal reformats. These fractures involve the obturator foramen.
- Transverse fractures split the innominate and are oriented AP. They are best assessed in the sagittal plane.

The transverse fracture divides the hemipelvis into two halves: inferior (which is also usually anterior) and superior. Because transverse fractures may occur in the transaxial plane and are thus parallel to the plane of CT acquisition, they can give rise to some confusion when axial slices are viewed without recourse to multiplanar reformats.

The fractures are rarely truly transverse, however, and there is a tendency to angulation in the craniocaudal direction, typically higher medially than laterally. On transaxial CT slices, the fracture line may thus be seen to follow a lateral course from above inferiorly, which may be confused for a vertically oriented fracture.

Minimally displaced fractures do not require complex reconstructions. More complex fractures resulting in considerable displacement and rotational deformity undoubtedly benefit from multiplanar and occasionally three-dimensional reconstructions, the latter perceived to be very helpful by the operating surgeon.

Three-dimensional images have demonstrated utility in complex displaced fractures by fully depicting the fracture plane and its orientation (never in a single true orthogonal plane).

Orthopedic surgeons find the latter particularly helpful in viewing the spatial relationships of fragments and planning their operation to restore articular congruity. In addition, 3D CT is a useful teaching tool for demonstrating the different types of acetabular fractures.

However, despite the above advantages, plain radiographs and conventional transaxial CT images are more sensitive than the 3D images in detecting undisplaced fractures. In addition, intra-articular fragments (including intra-articular protrusion of fixation screws) are more likely to be appreciated on axial images rather than reconstructions (including orthogonal reformats) as a result of the reduced spatial resolution of the latter.

CT provides accurate assessment of the inevitably associated soft-tissue damage.

MAGNETIC RESONANCE IMAGING

The superior soft-tissue contrast of MRI permits more accurate assessment of associated soft-tissue injuries and also allows detection of bone contusion.

A study directly comparing MRI with CT and intraoperative assessment (Potter et al., 1994) showed the following:

- Whereas MRI showed the acetabular fractures adequately and revealed a femoral head fracture not seen on concomitant CT, intra-articular fragments that were readily apparent on CT were often missed.
- MRI showed subchondral contusion of the femoral head in 65% of cases, all of which had appeared normal on CT.
- Postgadolinium examination of the sciatic nerve showed intraneural or perineural enhancement in all patients with either changes in baseline sensory evoked potential or preoperative neurologic deficit.

Thus, subclinical injury of the sciatic nerve and occult injuries of the femoral head not readily apparent on CT are demonstrated on MRI.

Treatment

The primary goal of treatment is to stabilize the patient. Pelvic fractures are often associated with potentially fatal retroperitoneal hemorrhage and/or visceral injuries. If the patient is unstable, emergent external fixation and transfer to angiography is indicated to curtail destabilizing hemorrhage. Angiography permits direct embolization of injured arteries, such as the superior gluteal, inferior pudendal, or lateral sacral artery, the latter especially at risk in the presence of a diastased sacroiliac joint, as in the reference case. Placement of an inferior vena cava filter and central venous access may be performed during the same visit to the angiographic suite.

If the patient is stable, CT allows for the most expeditious investigation of both visceral and osseous lesions, with embolization indicated if active extravasation of contrast is seen.

The secondary goal of treatment is to preserve hip function (preventing early arthrosis) and return the patient to early mobility by restoring articular surface alignment and congruity.

The tertiary goals are to treat and prevent complications, for example, deep venous thrombosis.

These goals may be achieved by

- Conservative methods
- Percutaneous fixation in situ
- Open reduction
- Acute total hip arthroplasty

Intra-articular fragments are an indication for an operative approach.

Displaced acetabular fractures are an indication for an operative approach unless specific criteria for nonoperative management are present:

- A congruent hip joint on the AP and oblique (Judet) radiographs
- An intact weight-bearing surface (as defined by roof arc and subchondral arc measurements on CT scans)
- A clinically stable joint

A nonoperative approach may also be taken if the acetabulum is destroyed, especially in the elderly, as the risk of operation will far outweigh the chances of successfully reconstructing the joint. In these cases, a conservative approach is taken initially, followed by elective joint replacement.

Percutaneous screw fixation of acetabular fractures with CT guidance has been described.

Prognosis

Anatomic reconstruction of the innominate bone, and indirectly the articular surface, is associated with a higher incidence of return of normal or near-normal hip function. Interestingly, although anatomic reduction does not restore prefracture load patterns, significant increases in contact pressure and contact area were not observed.

Symptomatic posttraumatic arthritis developed in 35% of cases with nonanatomic reduction.

Late complications that may occur after nonoperative or operative treatment include

- Posttraumatic arthritis
- Nonunion
- Wound infection
- Heterotopic bone formation

Displaced both column fractures with secondary congruence have better results than other displaced fractures.

PEARLS

- Because both of the fragments in a combined anterior and posterior column fracture are essentially free, they do not retain their usual relationship superiorly and may thus displace considerably. This is in contradistinction to the elementary transverse fracture, in which the superior portions retain this relationship.
- Although other pelvic fractures (e.g., pubic symphysis diastasis, sacroiliac diastasis, and sacral, iliac, and pubic rami fractures) are associated with bladder rupture, isolated acetabular fractures do not correlate with rupture. Thus, CT cystography is not recommended as a routine imaging technique.
- Postgadolinium examination of the sciatic nerve showed intraneural or perineural enhancement in all patients with either changes in baseline sensory evoked potential or preoperative neurologic deficit. Thus, subclinical injury of the sciatic nerve and occult injuries of the femoral head not readily apparent on CT are demonstrated on MRI.

PITFALLS

- If angiography is anticipated, cystography must be avoided, so as to avoid contrast in the bladder or pelvis secondary to leakage obscuring extravasation at angiography.
- Because transverse fractures occur in the transaxial plane and are thus parallel to the plane of CT acquisition, they can give rise to some confusion when axial slices are viewed without recourse to multiplanar reformats.
- On transaxial CT slices, a transverse fracture that is not in the "true" transaxial plane is seen to follow a lateral course from above inferiorly, which may thus be confused for a vertically oriented fracture.
- Overemphasis on the 3D reconstructions must be avoided, as fragments are more likely to be appreciated on axial images rather than reconstructions as a result of the reduced spatial resolution of the latter. Plain radiographs and conventional CT scans were more sensitive than the 3D images in detecting undisplaced fractures.

Suggested Readings

Brandser E, Marsh JL. Acetabular fractures: easier classification with a systematic approach. Am J Roentgenol 1998;171:1217–1228

Burk DL Jr, Mears DC, Kennedy WH, Cooperstein LA, Herbert DL. Three-dimensional computed tomography of acetabular fractures. Radiology 1985;155:183–186

Judet J. Fractures of the acetabulum. Scalpel (Brux) 1963;116:791

Letournel E. Acetabulum fractures: classification and management. Clin Orthop Relat Res 1980;151:81–106

Potter HG, Montgomery KD, Heise CW, Helfet DL. MR imaging of acetabular fractures: value in detecting femoral head injury, intraarticular fragments, and sciatic nerve injury. Am J Roentgenol 1994;163:881–886

Saks BJ. Normal acetabular anatomy for acetabular fracture assessment: CT and plain film correlation. Radiology 1986;159:139–145

Shirkhoda A, Brashear HR, Staab EV. Computed tomography of acetabular fractures. Radiology 1980; 134:683–688

CASE 83

Hema N. Choudur, Anthony G. Ryan, and Peter L. Munk

Clinical Presentation

A young man who fell from a three-story building was brought to the radiology department on a stretcher, unable to move.

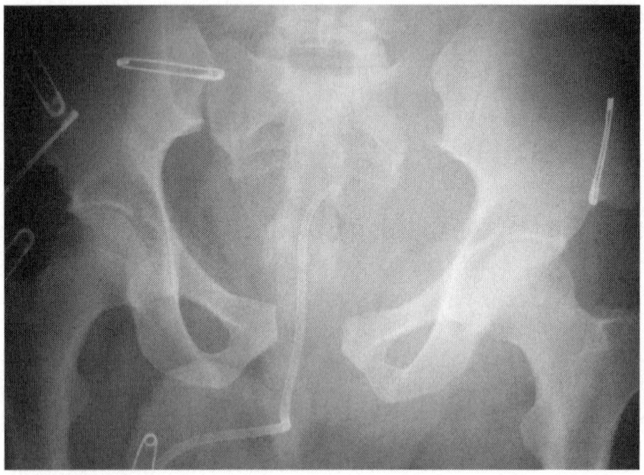

Figure 83A

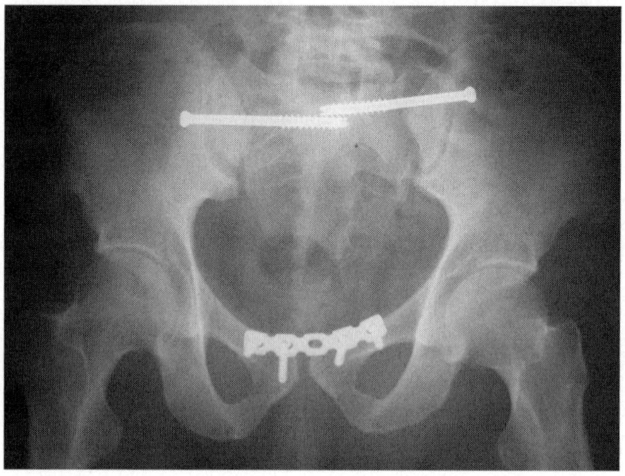

Figure 83B

Radiologic Findings

An anteroposterior (AP) radiograph of the pelvis (**Fig. 83A**) shows the pubic symphysis to be widely diastased, with an accompanying disruption and displacement of the right sacroiliac (SI) joint. There is an additional vertical fracture through the left sacral ala parallel to the SI joint.

The fractures were successfully treated with internal fixation (**Fig. 83B**).

Diagnosis

Pelvic shear fracture type 3.

Differential Diagnosis

None.

Discussion

Background

Fractures of the pelvis account for 3% of all fractures. The classification of these fractures is based on the direction of the vector and the degree of disruption resulting from applied force. These fractures are classified as lateral compression, AP compression, vertical shear, and combined mechanical injury.

Etiology

These injuries occur as a result of road traffic accidents or falls from a height. A high-impact vector directs the type of injury.

Pathophysiology

The major types of fractures are due to the following:

1. External rotation resulting in an open-book type of fracture: the pubic symphysis is diastased due to an externally rotating force acting on the femora and anterosuperior iliac spines. The anterior SI joint ligaments may be severed, but not the posterior. The force may also be applied to the posterosuperior iliac spines.
2. Vertical shear force acting perpendicular to the posterior pelvis may cause anterior and posterior pelvic fractures in addition to soft-tissue injury (bladder, urethra, etc).
3. A lateral compression force causes an internal rotation of the hemipelvis, resulting in fractures of the pubic rami and SI joint on the same side of the sacrum. Sometimes, an impaction can occur at the sites of the fracture and at the SI joints.
4. Complex injury may result from a combination of all of the above.

Clinical Findings

There is pain, swelling, and inability to move following the fracture. Extensive damage to bladder and pelvis vessels is not uncommon.

Complications

These injuries result in a high degree of mortality and morbidity. Complications such as pelvic hemorrhage are more frequent in vertical shear injuries due to pelvic vascular injury, but multiorgan failure and associated head injuries can result in high mortality rates. The urethra, urinary bladder, and peripheral nerves can be injured (**Figs. 83C** to **83F**).

Imaging Findings

RADIOGRAPHY

AP and oblique views are usually taken to delineate the fractures optimally, provided the necessary positioning causes no discomfort to the patient in the subacute phase. Radiographs of the pelvis with the patient standing on one limb are used to evaluate pubic symphyseal instability in the subocular phase.

Type 1 injury

No disruption of the pelvic ring is noted with fractures at only one site (e.g., avulsion fractures at musculotendinous origins). They account for 30% of the injuries of the bony pelvis. In the elderly, a single ramus fracture is often noted following a minor fall. Fractures of the iliac wing (Duverney's fracture) and transverse sacral fractures are the other examples.

Type 2 injury

A type 2 injury is a break of the pelvic ring at one site, either the ipsilateral pubic rami, the pubic symphysis, or near the SI joint. Subluxations of the pubic symphysis or the SI joint are also classified as type 2 fractures.

Type 2 fractures are typically seen in pregnant women and those riding horses.

Type 3 injury

Disruption of the pelvic ring at anterior and posterior sites (double breaks in the pelvic ring) indicate a type 3 injury.

Straddle fractures

Bilateral vertical pubic rami fractures or unilateral pubic rami fractures with pubic symphyseal diastasis are called straddle fractures. Urethral and visceral injuries are common (40%).

Malgaigne fractures

Malgaigne fractures are bilateral anterior fractures of the pubic rami or pubic symphyseal dislocation associated with posterior SI joint dislocation or fracture of the sacrum or ilium. These fractures account for 15% of pelvic injuries.

ULTRASOUND

Ultrasound functions as a complementary modality to rule out abdominal visceral injury.

COMPUTED TOMOGRAPHY

CT is often recommended to evaluate for additional fractures and to access visceral injury and hemorrhage.

MAGNETIC RESONANCE IMAGING

- MRI is rarely utilized due to the patient's hemodynamic instability and inability to lie in the magnet for the necessary length of time.

ISOTOPE SCANS

- Isotope scans are often helpful in detecting additional acute fractures not detected on plain radiographs.

Treatment

Suspected urinary complications are investigated with a retrograde urethrogram, cystogram, intravenous pyelogram, or combination thereof (**Figs. 83C** to **83F**). Catheterization of the bladder should not be attempted prior to urethral injury.

Hemorrhage is treated with blood transfusions, arteriography, and embolization of bleeding arteries. Fractures are treated using external or internal fixation.

Prognosis

Morbidity and mortality rates are higher in patients with a completely unstable pelvic ring injury. Emergency department stabilization and reconstruction of the pelvic ring with optimal operative techniques in these patients can reduce these rates. Anterior and posterior internal fixation results in satisfactory clinical outcomes.

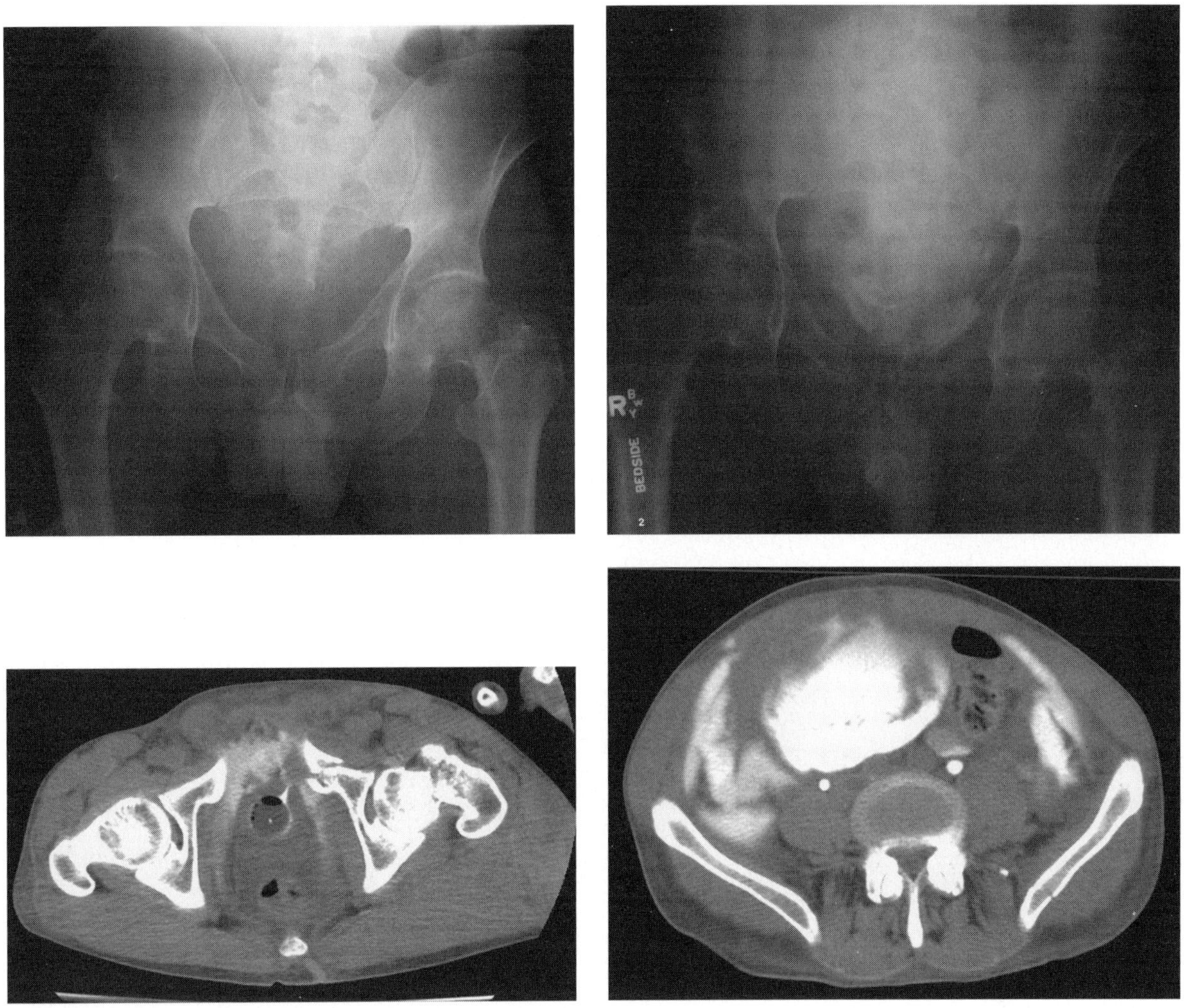

C D E F

Figures 83C–83F Radiographs show a left pubic ramis and anterior column fracture (**83C**) with bladder rupture (**83D**). Radiographs, cystogram, and CT scans (**83E,83F**) show the extraperitoneal bladder rupture with contrast extravasation. Also visible is the left femoral neck fracture (**83E**).

PEARLS

- Oblique views of the pelvis may reveal hidden fractures, especially of the acetabulum.
- When a single break in the pelvic ring of a severe magnitude is seen, always look for additional fractures along the line of the force.
- Never catheterize the bladder unless urethral injuries are ruled out.

PITFALL

- On conventional radiographs, overlying bowel loops may obscure fractures of the sacrum and ilium and diastasis of the SI joint. A CT scan may often be necessary to evaluate such clinically suspected fractures.

Suggested Readings

Falchi M, Rollandi GA. CT of pelvic fractures. Eur J Radiol 2004;50:96–105

Gansslen A, Giannoudis P, Pape HC. Hemorrhage in pelvic fracture: who needs angiography? Curr Opin Crit Care 2003;9:515–523

Kabak S, Halici M, Tuncel M, Avsarogullari L, Baktir A, Basturk M. Functional outcome of open reduction and internal fixation for completely unstable pelvic ring fractures (type C): a report of 40 cases. J Orthop Trauma 2003;17:555–562

Resnick D. Bone and Joint Imaging. 2nd ed. Philadelphia, PA: WB Saunders; 1996:2917–2924

CASE 84

Hema N. Choudur, Anthony G. Ryan, and Peter L. Munk

Clinical Presentation

A young boy sustained an injury while playing soccer, after which he was unable to extend his knee. Painful swelling along the anterior aspect of the knee followed in the ensuing hours, with extreme tenderness overlying the patella.

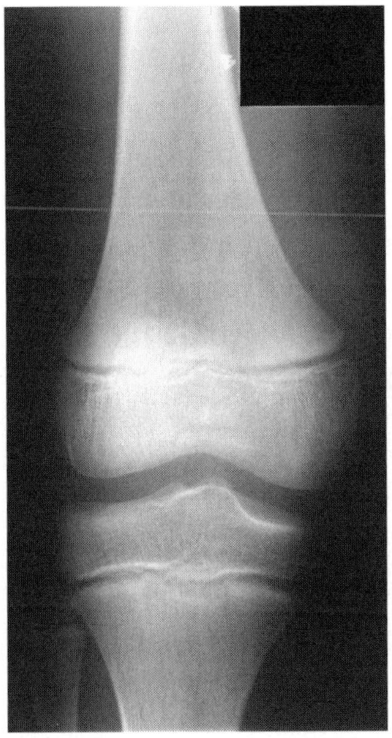

Figure 84A

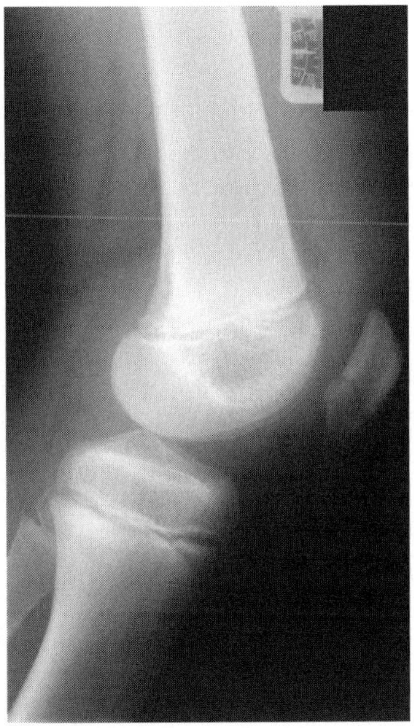

Figure 84B

Radiologic Findings

Anteroposterior (AP) and lateral radiographs of the knee (**Figs. 84A,84B**) reveal a transverse distal third patellar fracture with no significant displacement of the fractured fragments.

Diagnosis

Transverse patellar fracture.

Differential Diagnosis

Bipartite patella is usually seen at the superolateral edge of the patella and is unilateral in 57% and bilateral in the remainder, with a male:female predilection of 9:1. It is usually asymptomatic but may result in pain following a fracture or fibrous nonunion. On plain radiographs, the margins are smooth and corticated.

Dorsal defect of the patella is usually 1 cm in diameter, well defined, located in the superolateral aspect of the patella, and covered by articular cartilage.

Sinding-Larsen-Johansson disease, which is defined as osteochondrosis of the distal pole of the patella/tendinous junction, is related to chronic traction injury. This syndrome may mimic a stress fracture of the patella, an osteochondral sleeve fracture, or nonunited ossification center. It is well-differentiated on MRI, with high signal on inversion recovery sequences in the inferior aspect of the patellar tendon.

Old healed injuries of the patella are seen on MRI as thickened patellar tendon.

Insufficiency fractures of the patella are best differentiated on MRI with a low signal on all sequences.

Discussion

The patella is the largest sesamoid bone in the body and is present in the quadriceps tendon. The tendon includes contributions from the rectus femoris, vastus intermedius, medialis, and lateralis. It is anchored mainly to the tibial tuberosity. The medial retinacula attach the superomedial border of the patella to the medial tibial condyle, and the lateral retinacula, to the superolateral border and to the lateral condyle of the tibia. Overlying the patella is skin, subcutaneous fat, and the prepatellar bursa, making it a very superficial bone and consequently prone to direct injuries. It is lined posteriorly by articular cartilage. Usually, one ossification center is present, but this may vary up to three, seen between the ages of 2 to 6 years.

Background

Patellar fractures constitute 1% of all injuries. They may be transverse, vertical, marginal, or osteochondral (**Figs. 84C** to **84E**). The diagnosis of each specific type is important as the management varies.

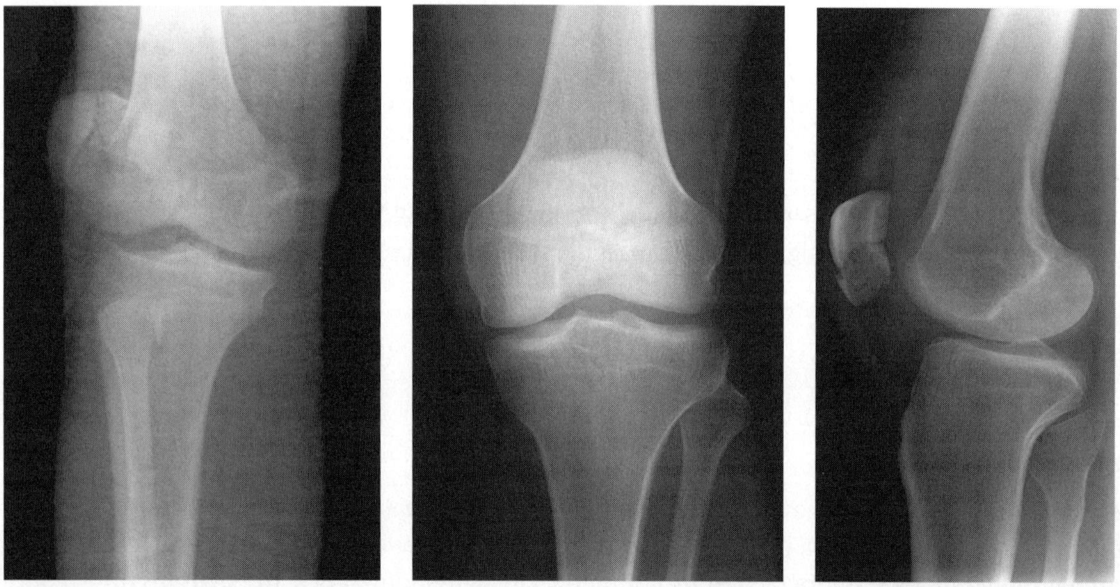

C–E

Figures 84C–84E AP and lateral views show a transverse patellar fracture requiring surgical treatment. Note that the fracture is barely discernible on the AP view, demonstrating the necessity of an accompanying lateral view.

Etiology and Pathophysiology

Patellar fractures can result from direct or indirect forces. When a force is directly thrust on the patella, it results in a comminuted fracture with little displacement of the fractured fragments, unlike an indirect injury such as occurs with momentary sudden flexion against a contracted patella. In the former, there is a greater degree of articular cartilage damage.

Clinical Findings

The most common presenting complaint is a sudden crack felt in the anterior knee after an acute flexion, as occurs while jumping, followed by pain and swelling over the patella with inability to move the knee. There may be a history of a direct blow to the knee followed by pain, swelling, and decreased range of motion.

Imaging Findings

The fracture through the patella is best seen in orthogonal views. The AP view often does not reveal the fracture line clearly due to bony overlap. A lateral view is therefore mandatory. The skyline view is helpful in some cases of vertical/marginal fractures to differentiate it from a bipartite patella.

Overlying soft-tissue swelling and joint effusion are accompanying findings.

The main types of fractures found on imaging are the following:

1. *Transverse fracture* Usually through the mid- or distal patella but may rarely occur in its proximal portion; usually due to an indirect injury
2. *Vertical fracture* Usually through the midpatella and is rarely seen
3. *Marginal fracture* Occurs at the edge of the patella, leaving the extensor mechanism of the knee intact (**Fig. 84F**)
4. *Osteochondral fracture* Involves the bony patella, adjacent articular cartilage, and retinaculum (**Fig. 84G**). This complex of associated injuries is seen in 5% of patellar dislocations and frequently occurs in children. It may be the result of a direct or indirect injury.

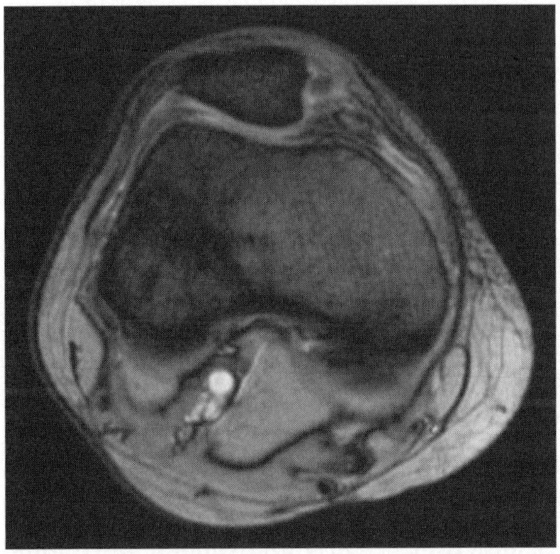

F

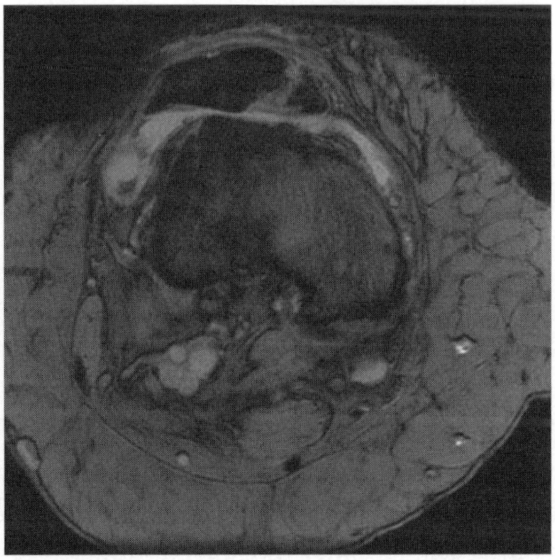

G

Figures 84F,84G **84F** MRI demonstrates a marginal patellar fracture following a dislocation. **84G** A tear of the medial retinaculum is seen with injury to the articular cartilage.

5. *Sleeve fracture with avulsed articular surface* Can involve either the medial, lateral, superior, or inferior aspects of the patella. With inferior sleeve fractures, in which the knee is flexed with the quadriceps contracted at the time of injury, a large superior fragment is separated from a smaller inferior fragment, with the fracture involving the articular cartilage and retinacula. It is best seen in the lateral view evinced by a high-riding patella and joint effusion.
6. *Avulsion fractures* May involve the superior pole, medial aspect, as in patellar dislocations, or the lateral aspect due to chronic stress at the insertion of the vastus lateralis
7. *Following an anterior cruciate ligament reconstruction,* in which the patellar tendon is used as an autogenous graft. This injury is commonly seen in the first 2 to 3 months of rehabilitation, as the patella is weakened by the removal of the inferior pole.

COMPUTED TOMOGRAPHY

CT is useful in cases where the plain radiographs are normal despite a high clinical suspicion. It also reveals any intra-articular fragments, especially in osteochondral fractures. Furthermore, the orientation and separation of the fragments are better visualized on CT with reconstruction in all planes.

MAGNETIC RESONANCE IMAGING

MRI is useful in depicting soft-tissue injury, bone marrow edema, and articular cartilage damage. Occult fractures are of low signal intensity on all sequences.

BONE SCAN

Nonvisible fractures on plain radiographs are picked up earliest by bone scans. A negative bone scan obtained 1 week after trauma excludes an occult patellar fracture.

Complications

Delayed union, malunion, and nonunion occur as with other fractures. A distance of more than 3 mm between the fractured fragments on x-rays is considered a risk for nonunion.

A badly comminuted fracture and an osteochondral fracture are at risk for nonunion. Degenerative patellofemoral changes may result from articular damage and bony surface irregularity. In the immediate postfixation period, infection and hardware failure are the other complications.

Treatment

- *Conservative* for all undisplaced fractures with a separation of < 3 mm and for fractures with a step of ~ 2 mm
- *Surgical* for fractures with separation of > 3 mm and a step of > 2 mm. Tension banding with or without threaded screws and Kirschner wires are used to transfix the fractured fragments (**Figs. 84H** to **84K**). Partial and, rarely, total excision are sometimes necessary.

Prognosis

Asymptomatic nonunion or delayed union can be treated conservatively with preservation of function. Operative treatment is necessary for those symptomatic postfracture knees for restoration of adequate function. The results of anterior tension band wire fixation are acceptable even in severely comminuted fractures. Partial excision provides satisfactory results, provided that at least three fifths of the patella can be preserved. Total excision is sometimes clearly unavoidable but should be preceded by careful deliberation when considered an alternative to internal fixation.

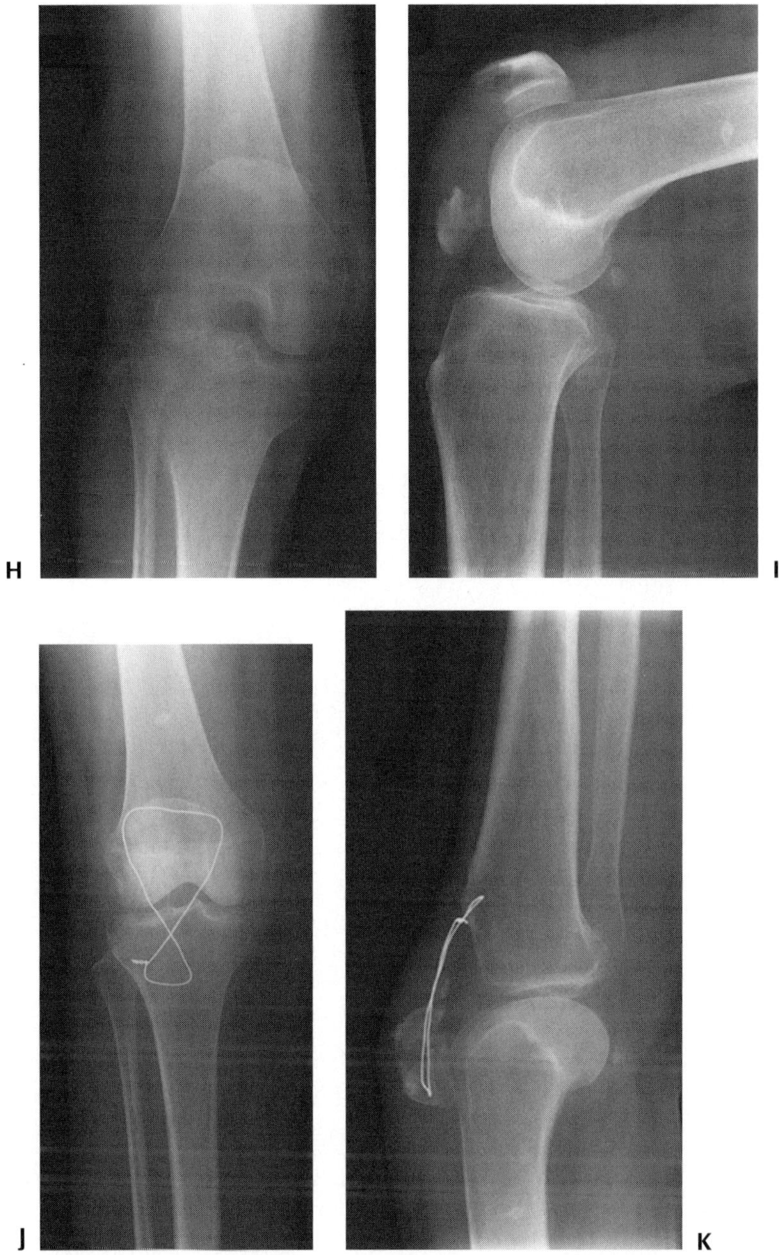

Figures 84H–84K AP (**84H**) and lateral (**84I**) views of a transverse patellar fracture that needs surgical fixation. AP (**84J**) and lateral (**84K**) views of a figure-of-eight fixation are shown.

PEARLS

- A true lateral view is the single best view to visualize a patellar fracture. A skyline view is mandatory to delineate osteochondral and marginal fractures.
- MRI is the investigation of choice to exclude associated retinacular injuries.

PITFALL

- MRI is the best modality to evaluate the articular cartilage defects in sleeve fractures, which are frequently missed on plain radiographs alone.

Suggested Readings

Christian SR, Andersen MB, Workman R, Conway WF, Pope TL. Imaging of anterior knee pain. Clin Sports Med 2006;25:781–802

Sonin AH, Fitzgerald SW, Bresler ME, Kirsch MD, Hoff FL, Friedman H. MR imaging appearance of the extensor mechanism of the knee: functional anatomy and injury patterns. Radiographics 1995;15:367–382

Resnick D. Bone and Joint Imaging. 2nd ed. Philadelphia, PA: WB Saunders; 1996:780,783

CASE 85

Hema N. Choudur, Anthony G. Ryan, and Peter L. Munk

Clinical Presentation

A young man was playing a game of rugby and sustained an acute injury to the knee. In the ensuing hours, he developed severe anterior knee pain and swelling with decreased mobility of the joint. Clinical examination revealed acute tenderness along the medial aspect of the patella with suprapatellar effusion.

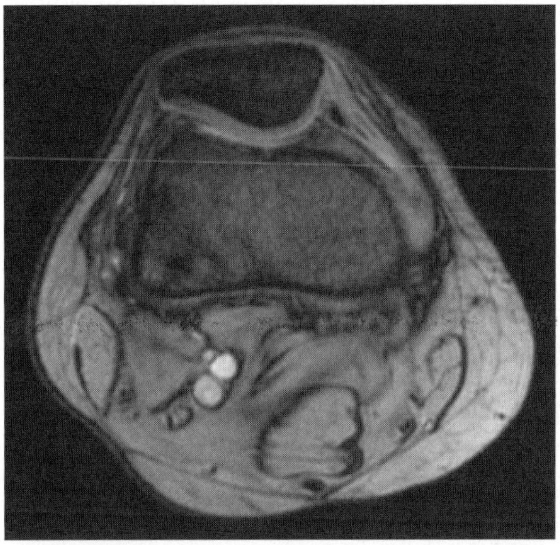

Figure 85A

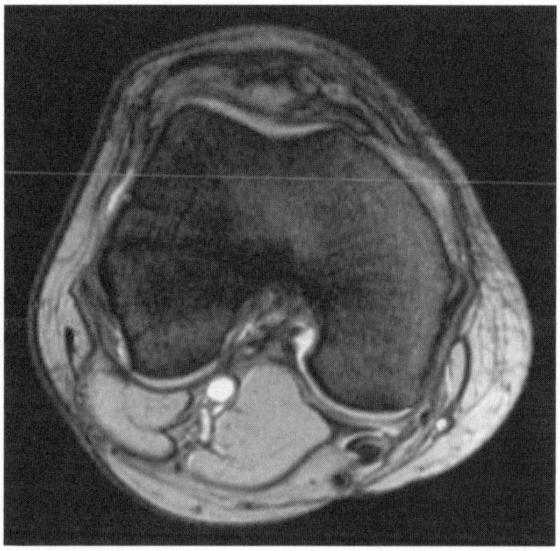

Figure 85B

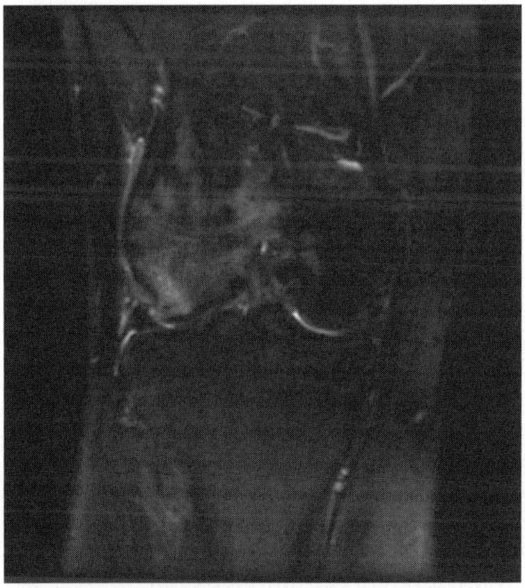

Figure 85C

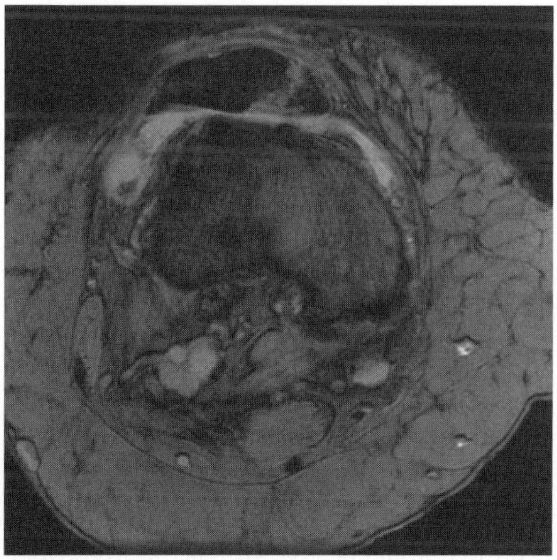

Figure 85D

Radiologic Findings

No plain radiographs were taken. The patient was sent directly for MRI to rule out internal derangement of the knee.

Axial MPGR (**Fig. 85A,85B**) and coronal STIR (**Fig. 85C**) images reveal medial retinacular tears and lateral femoral condylar fractures with associated bony contusion.

In the axial MPGR images, a tear of the medial retinaculum was clearly visualized, as were two lateral femoral condylar fractures seen as hypointense horizontal lines extending to the adjacent cortex. The patellofemoral cartilage was thinned out laterally and was almost absent medially. In addition, the fat-suppressed images revealed dramatic lateral femoral condylar edema suggestive of a contusion. Significant intra-articular effusion was seen on the T2 sagittal images.

In another case with a similar history (**Fig. 85D**), the axial MPGR images showed an osteochondral fracture of the medial patella with the medial retinaculum separated and retracted, indicative of a much greater force during injury. Almost-absent medial patellofemoral cartilage was clearly depicted.

Figure 85D shows an axial MPGR image that clearly depicts the osteochondral fracture of the medial patella with a tear of the patellofemoral cartilage and medial retinaculum.

Diagnosis

- Acute traumatic patellar dislocation with its characteristic sequelae of sprain/tear of the medial retinaculum. Most often, the medial patellofemoral ligament is torn off its femoral attachment but sometimes off the patellar attachment, as seen in this case.
- Contusion of the anterolateral femoral condyle/fracture of the anterolateral femoral condyle
- Medial patellar facet fracture/medial osteochondral junction fracture and/or associated articular cartilage loss.
- Concomitant joint effusion

Differential Diagnosis

- Medial synovial plica
- Patellar malalignment
- Multipartite patella
- Chondromalacia patella
- Quadriceps contracture
- Jumper's knee
- Patellar ligament rupture
- In children, Sinding-Larsen-Johansson disease

Discussion

Background

Patellar injury and lateral dislocation are common injuries in athletes and nonathletes. The ratio of men to women is higher in athletes; in the nonathletic group, women outnumber men.

Etiology

Acute injury by direct impact or even a sudden change of direction is the typical mechanism. The femur often medially rotates on a stabilized tibia, resulting in a sensation of "giving way" similar to that in anterior cruciate ligament injuries. This is a physiological protective mechanism as a result of quadriceps inhibition from pain. Rapid knee swelling and decreased mobility ensue.

Although high-energy mechanisms like motor vehicle accidents are often the cause, low-energy mechanisms such as sporting activities and minor falls also result in lateral patellar dislocations.

Pathophysiology and Biomechanics

The patella is the largest sesamoid bone in the body, residing within the complex of quadriceps and patellar tendons. It acts as both a lever and a pulley, magnifying the quadriceps force in extension and redirecting the quadriceps force medially in flexion.

Soft-tissue elements that stabilize the patella are the adjacent ligament and the capsular joint. The ligaments are continuous with the fibrous capsule encircling the patella. The synovial capsule of the knee joint attaches to the peripheral margins of the patella.

Often, after dislocation, the medial muscular (vastus medialis) attachments are strained or even torn. The medial retinacular complex is also damaged in a valgus injury, as was seen in this case.

Clinical Findings

Acute joint swelling and pain following the injury are the usual presentations. Flexion of the knee is very painful, with focal tenderness along the medial patella. This latter finding suggests that the medial retinacula are torn or bruised. Chondral injury after dislocation would result in superolateral patellar tenderness. Sometimes torn, thickened plicae may be palpable and tender.

Complications and Associated Injuries

- Osteochondral fracture of the lateral femoral condyle and/or patella
- Damage to the articular surface of the patella
- Pediatric patellar avulsion fractures
- Capsular avulsion of medial patellar origin
- Intra-articular fragments from patella and lateral femoral condyle

Imaging Findings

RADIOGRAPHY

Plain radiographs are not sensitive except for demonstrating bony fractures of the patella and, rarely, the lateral femoral condyle. Skyline views help to assess the extent of the dislocation/subluxation as well as fractures of the patella. Anteroposterior radiographs add information on femoral/tibial fractures.

MAGNETIC RESONANCE IMAGING

A thorough history and physical examination lead to the diagnosis, but a confirmation of the same, as well as the extent of soft-tissue and bony injury, is best performed with MRI.

In the axial gradient or proton density fat-suppressed sequences, the torn or strained medial retinacula are visualized with surrounding soft-tissue edema. Lateral patellar subluxation or dislocation and the presence of an anterolateral femoral condylar fracture are best evaluated on the axial sequences. Anterolateral femoral condylar edema, with or without a fracture at the site of patellar impaction, can be best seen on the coronal inversion recovery sequences.

Treatment

In the acute phase, nonsteroidal anti-inflammatory agents, physical therapy for quadriceps, iliotibial band strength exercises, and ice application are helpful. Reduction of pain and inflammation with rehabilitation exercises may result in complete recovery. Decreased loading by postural correction, activity modification, and shoe wear/orthotic management is very beneficial. However, in some patients, recurrent dislocations can occur, especially if the articular cartilage is damaged.

Surgical treatment is reserved for complicated dislocations with associated fractures. Medial patellar facet and lateral femoral condyle fractures are treated operatively. Arthroscopy can repair capsular avulsion of medial patellar origin and remove loose intra-articular fragments originating from the patella and lateral femoral condyle.

Prognosis

With conservative treatment, there is a 30 to 50% chance of continuing long-term symptoms of instability or pain. After 6 months of limited activity, including squatting, 60% of athletes may not be able to return to full preinjury-level activity.

PEARLS

- Patellar dislocation is almost always lateral.
- A careful history, clinical examination, and MRI findings of torn medial retinacula with anterolateral femoral condylar edema with or without a fracture are needed to determine lateral patellar dislocation.

PITFALLS

- In the absence of a clear history, symptoms may lead to the diagnosis of chondromalacia.
- Cartilage and osteochondral injury may complicate the dislocation and are best demonstrated with MRI, particularly the axial proton density fat-saturated sequence.
- The diagnosis may be missed if the typical pattern of bone contusion is not recognized in the anterolateral femoral condyle and medial patella.

Suggested Readings

Sanders TG, Morrison WB, Singleton BA, et al. Medial patellofemoral ligament injury following acute transient dislocation of the patella: MR findings with surgical correlation in 14 patients. J Comput Assist Tomogr 2001;25:957–962

Virolainen H, Visuri T, Kuusela T. Acute dislocation of the patella: MR findings. Radiology 1993;189:243–246

Warren LF, Marshall JL. The supporting structures and layers on the medial side of the knee: an anatomical analysis. J Bone Joint Surg Am 1979;61:56–62

CASE 86

Hema N. Choudur, Anthony G. Ryan, and Peter L. Munk

Clinical Presentation

A young athlete fell on an outstretched hand while skiing. She had acute pain and swelling along the distal aspect of the forearm. On examination, there was limitation of wrist movements. No sensory/motor deficit was elicited. The radial pulse was normal.

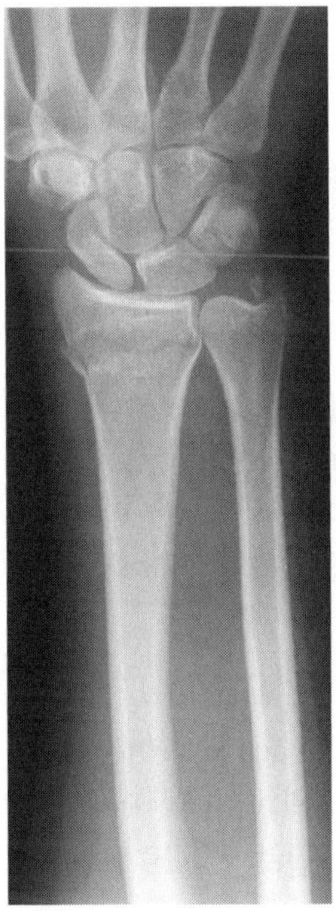

Figure 86A

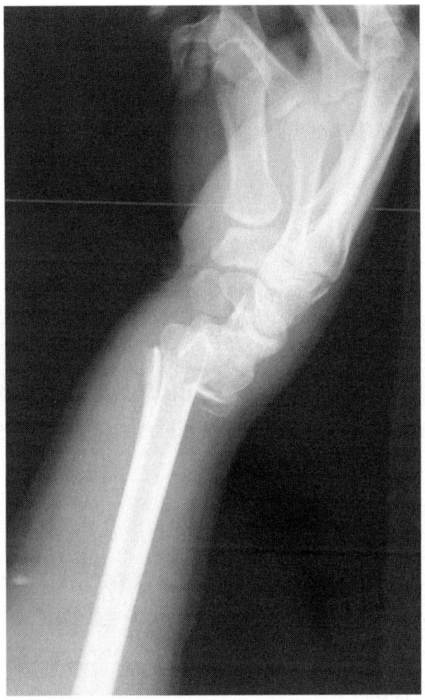

Figure 86B

Radiologic Findings

Anteroposterior (AP) and lateral views (**Figs. 86A,86B**) of the forearm show a transversely oriented fracture through the distal radial metaphysis with dorsal displacement of the distal fracture fragment. A concomitant ulnar styloid fracture is also present.

Diagnosis

Colles' fracture.

Differential Diagnosis

- Smith's fracture with volar displacement of the distal fractured fragment
- Barton's fracture, an intra-articular fracture of the dorsal aspect of the distal radius
- Chauffeur's fracture, base of the radial styloid fracture with intra-articular extension

Discussion

Background

Colles' fracture is the most common fracture in the region of the distal forearm and hand. It was first described by an Irish surgeon, Abraham Colles (1773–1843).

It is commonly seen in women with postmenopausal osteoporosis. Of note, elderly men with Colles' fracture are prone to future hip fractures and therefore should be investigated and, if necessary, treated for osteoporosis. Further, the morbidity/mortality following a hip fracture in men is higher than in women.

Etiology

Colles' fracture is mostly caused by a fall on an outstretched hand. It can also result from motor vehicle accidents. The injury is encountered in both sexes and in all age groups, but it is most common in postmenopausal women, osteoporosis being the predisposing factor. In the younger population, this injury is common to ice hockey, football, rugby, and handball players, as well as riders, wrestlers, and Alpine skiers.

Pathophysiology

A sudden force that dorsiflexes the hand or an axial force that forces the wrist against the distal radius can result in a fracture at the site of the distal flare of the radius. Due to muscle pull, the distal fragment is displaced dorsally. There may be an injury to the ligaments and cartilage at the wrist at the time of injury, or later due to wear and tear.

Clinical Findings

Clinical findings include a history of a fall on an outstretched hand, followed by acute pain, swelling, and inability to move the wrist joint and lift weights.

The primary types of Colles' fractures (based on a universal system of classification):

- *Type 1* is a nonarticular undisplaced fracture.
- *Type 2* is a nonarticular displaced fracture.
- *Type 3* is an intra-articular undisplaced fracture.
- *Type 4* is an intra-articular displaced fracture that is
  - Reducible, stable;
  - Reducible, unstable; or
  - Irreducible, unstable.

Follow-up postreduction films are taken to assess the accuracy of reduction and the adequacy of healing.

Complications

- Arthritis at the wrist joint due to unstable reduction or incongruity of joints or subluxation of the distal radioulnar joint

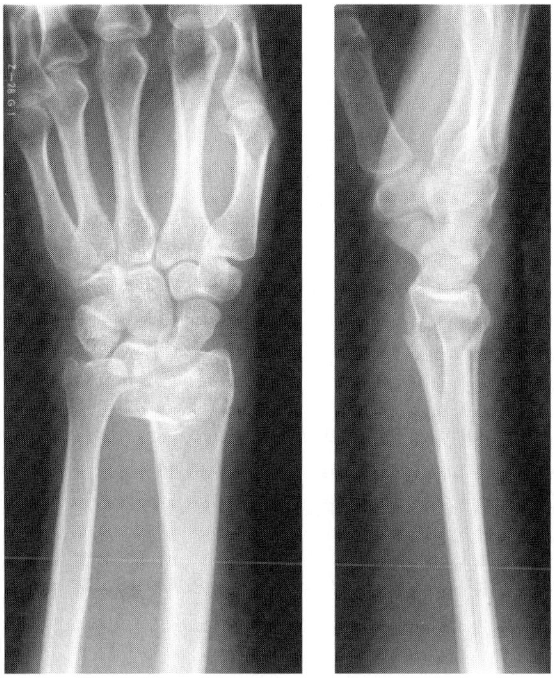

C D **Figures 86C,86D** AP (**86C**) and lateral (**86D**) views of a typical Colles' fracture as seen immediately following trauma.

- Tears of the triangular fibrocartilage from foreshortening of the radius, resulting in a positive ulnar variance
- Dorsal deformity from bony remodeling ("dinner fork" deformity)
- Compression of carpal and/or Guyon's tunnel structures, resulting in median and/or ulnar nerve neuropathy, respectively, or entrapment of the flexor tendons
- Rupture of the extensor pollicis longus tendon, reflex sympathetic dystrophy, carpal malalignment, and nonunion

Imaging Findings

RADIOGRAPHY

Routine AP and lateral views show fractures of the distal portion of the radius with dorsal displacement of the distal fractured fragment, varying degrees of radial displacement, angulation and shortening, presence or absence of intra-articular extension, ulnar styloid fracture in ~50 to 60% of cases, and associated injuries to the carpus, elbow, humerus, femur (in osteoporotic patients), and inferior radioulnar joint (**Figs. 84C** and **84D**). The initial transverse fracture line is usually well seen volarly, 2 to 3 cm proximal to the wrist joint.

Associated carpal bone injury and intercarpal ligament instability may also be present. If suspected, clenched wrist views are obtained, followed by an MR arthrogram to evaluate the triangular fibrocartilage and ligaments for tears in the subacute period.

COMPUTED TOMOGRAPHY

CT is usually performed to evaluate the position and alignment of comminuted fracture fragments prior to surgery. The physician evaluates for the presence of intra-articular loose fragments, intra-articular extension of the fracture, step deformities, inferior radioulnar displacement, and tendon injuries.

MAGNETIC RESONANCE IMAGING

MRI is used to evaluate triangular fibrocartilage and intercarpal ligament tears and to assess the structures of the carpal tunnel and tendons at the wrist.

Treatment

Treatment ranges from simple immobilization with a splint and sling to a lightweight fiberglass cast. If cast immobilization is insufficient to repair the fracture, surgical intervention with internal fixation with pins or a plate and screws may be necessary.

Prognosis

The undisplaced or mildly displaced two-component fractures heal well with immobilization, with normal return to activity in 6 to 12 months. Often, intra-articular fractures, comminuted fractures, and those that heal with foreshortening of the radius have chronic wrist pain with a decrease in functional status secondary to wrist arthropathy.

If the closed reduction is successful, there is mild comminution, dorsal angulation < 9 degrees, and radial shortening < 4 mm, and the fracture is considered stable. If the closed reduction is a failure, there is moderate comminution, dorsal angulation > 10 degrees, and radial shortening > 5 mm, and the fracture is considered to have secondary instability.

Unstable fractures show severe comminution, dorsal angulation > 20 degrees, and radial shortening > 10 mm.

PEARL

- Always carefully evaluate the follow-up radiographs after reduction for ensuing complications, such as foreshortening, malunion, nonunion, and wrist arthropathy, and advise an MRI if soft tissue injury is suspected to rule out cartilage and ligament tears.

PITFALLS

- Scaphoid fracture may accompany other fractures around the wrist and can easily be missed if not carefully searched for.
- Unless MR arteriogram is performed in cases of foreshortening of the radius, triangular fibrocartilage tears will be missed.

Suggested Readings

Haentjens P, Autier P, Collins J, Velkeniers B, Vanderschueren D, Boonen S. Colles' fracture, spine fracture, and subsequent risk of hip fracture in men and women: a meta-analysis. J Bone Joint Surg Am 2003;85:1936–1943

Kanterewicz E, Yanez A, Perez-Pons A, Codony I, Del Rio L, Diez-Perez A. Association between Colles' fracture and low bone mass: age-based differences in postmenopausal women. Osteoporos Int 2002;13:824–828

Rosenthal DI, Schwartz M, Phillips WC, Jupiter J. Fracture of the radius with instability of the wrist. Am J Roentgenol 1983;141:113–116

CASE 87

Hema N. Choudur, Anthony G. Ryan, and Peter L. Munk

Clinical Presentation

A woman with a known case of thyroid malignancy presented with acute right humeral pain with no history of trauma. She had tenderness and swelling along the proximal aspect of the arm with an inability to move her arm.

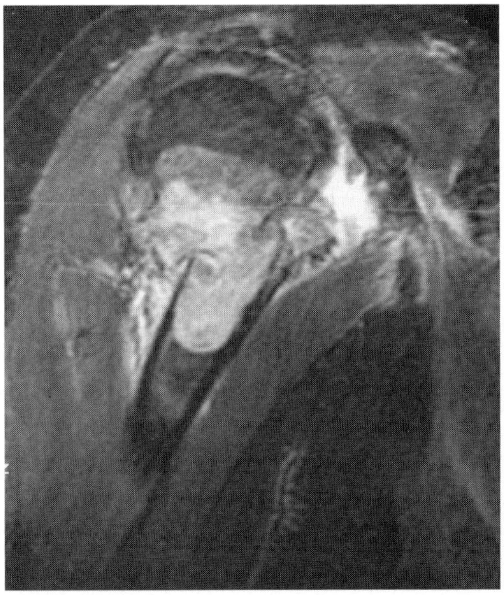

Figure 87A

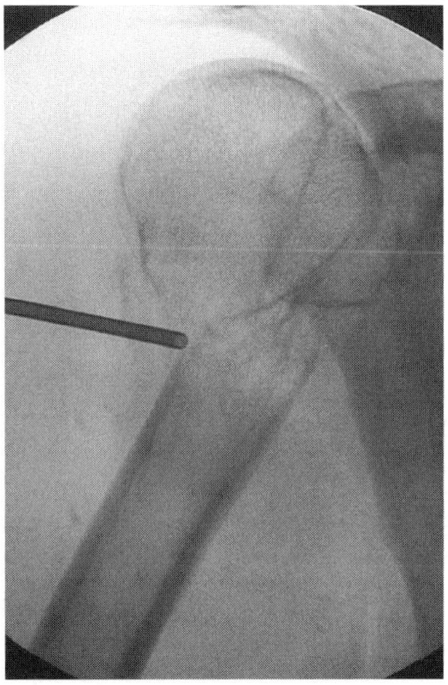

Figure 87B

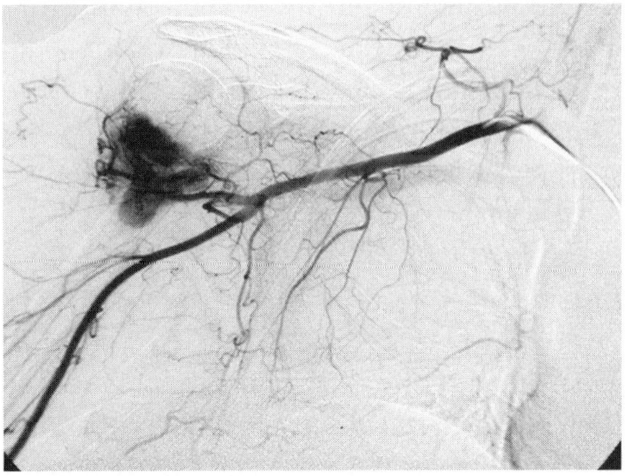

Figure 87C

Radiologic Findings

Inversion recovery MRI (**Fig. 87A**) shows gross cortical dusruption through an oval high signal intensity lesion involving the neck and proximal shaft of the right humerus with secondary joint effusion. There is moderate medial displacement of the distal tibial fragment. Fluoroscopy (**Fig. 87B**) at the time of biopsy demonstrated a fracture of the surgical neck with a lucent lesion in the adjoining bone. The angiogram (**Fig. 87C**) revealed a dense hypervascular "blush" at the site of the fracture.

Diagnosis

Pathologic fracture, secondary to metastasis.

Differential Diagnosis

- Traumatic fracture
- Stress fracture

Discussion

Etiology

Bone that is weakened by a preexisting condition, either primarily in the bone or secondary to a metastasis or primary tumor, can result in a fracture with trivial trauma. Usually the diagnosis is straightforward, given a history of malignancy or metabolic disease, but in other cases it may be the first indication of a malignancy. The histology and a directed search often lead to the primary malignancy.

Pathophysiology

There are numerous conditions that weaken the bone, making it susceptible to fracture. These conditions can be classified as generalized disorders causing osteopenia and focal bony lesions.

- Generalized disorders (e.g., osteogenesis imperfecta and rickets in children)
- Multiple myeloma, osteoporosis, carcinomatosis, and Paget's disease in the elderly
- Benign lesions that weaken bone (e.g., cysts and enchondromas)
- Osteomalacia, osteosclerosis, and hyperparathyroidism in adults

Clinical Findings

A pathologic fracture presents with acute pain, swelling, and inability to move the limb. In the absence of trauma and given the history of preexisting dull pain in an elderly patient, a pathologic fracture is suspected. The diagnosis is often suspected in patients with known metastases.

A biochemical evaluation of the blood and electrophoresis is helpful in evaluating for hematological malignancies, such as multiple myeloma and hyperparathyroidism.

Imaging Findings

RADIOGRAPHY

Conventional radiographs help to confirm the diagnosis. A fracture line through an area of rarified/mottled bone or through a well-defined bony lesion is suggestive of a pathologic fracture.

A large and aggressive lesion is more likely to produce a pathologic fracture than a small, nonaggressive one, unless there is gross cortical thinning. The fracture line in the long bones is usually transversely oriented (**Fig. 87D**).

COMPUTED TOMOGRAPHY

CT is often performed to evaluate the extent and nature of bony involvement and any soft tissue extension and to plan/perform guided biopsy.

MAGNETIC RESONANCE IMAGING

MRI reveals a hypointense fracture line, with the surrounding pathologic bone seen as a high signal intensity focus on the inversion recovery sequences.

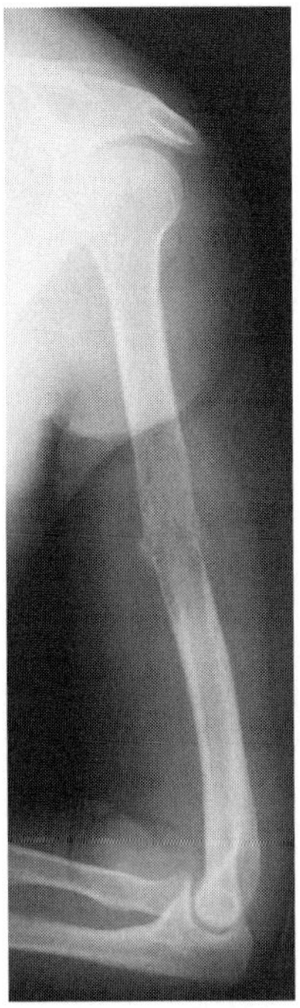

D

Figure 87D Radiograph of a woman with leiomyosarcoma of the uterus presenting with acute left arm pain reveals a mottled appearance and pathologic fracture of the mid humerus.

RADIONUCLIDE IMAGING

Bone scans delineate the multiplicity of bony lesions in metastases and systemic conditions.

Treatment

Treatment includes that of the fracture and, where appropriate, the underlying disease (**Fig. 87E** and **87F**). Internal fixation will help to establish the diagnosis, provide tissue for diagnosis where needed, and promote fracture healing.

The diagnosis is often confirmed by image-guided biopsy, fluoroscopy on CT, and occasionally ultrasound if there is a large soft-tissue component.

Prognosis

Most pathologic fractures secondary to a benign lesion are treated by surgical curettage and bone grafting, with excellent results. Most often, the fracture through a malignant lesion is treated with the intent of improving pain, quality of life, and mobility rather than cure.

In metastatic disease, surgical stabilization is frequently required to preempt a fracture. Prophylactic orthopedic surgery, consisting of excision of the bony lesion, depends on its size, location, age of the patient, level of activity, and individual disease process.

Although osteoplasty (the injection of polymethylmethacrylate bone cement) is primarily performed to alleviate pain, it may also confer a degree of strength to the weakened bone by stabilizing the innumerable microfractures associated with the main fracture line (**Figs. 87G** to **87I**).

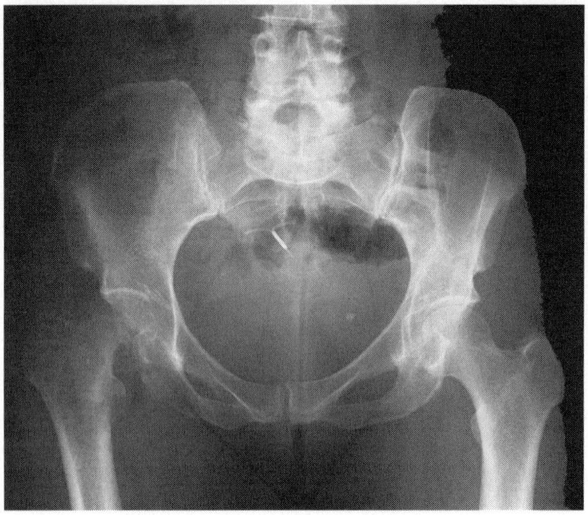
E

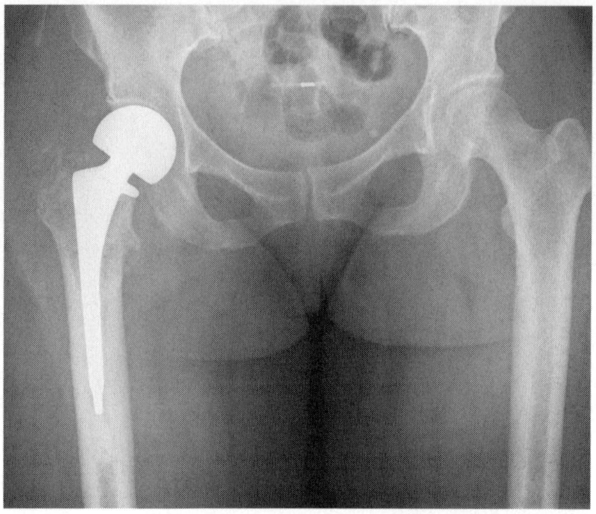
F

Figures 87E,87F Radiographs of a woman with breast cancer that had metastasized to the right femoral head and neck presenting with right hip pain (**87E**). The pathologic fracture was treated with a total hip replacement (**87F**).

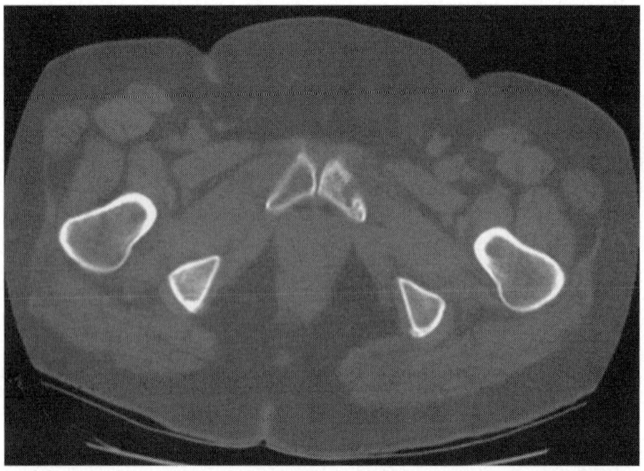
G

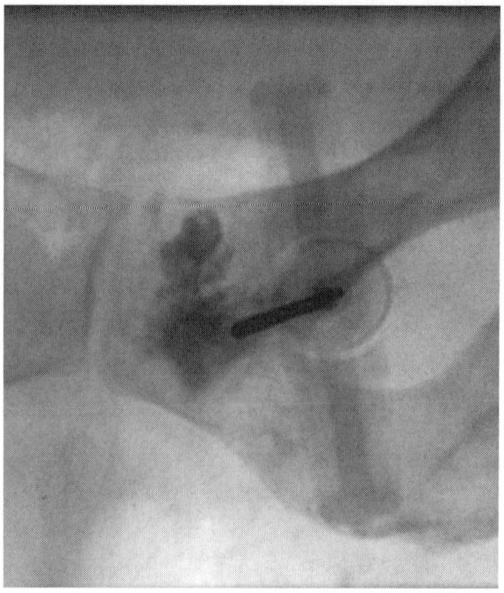
H

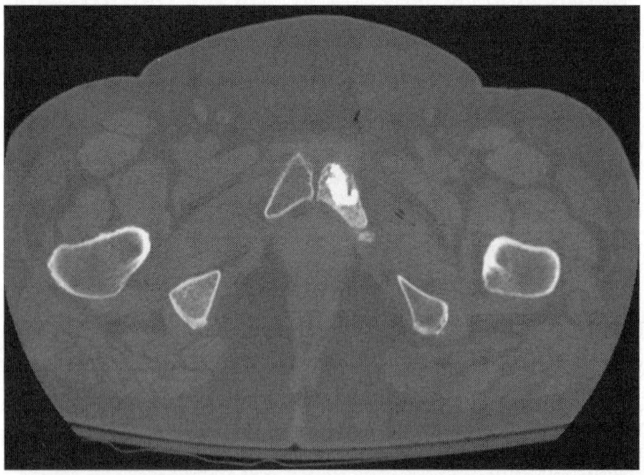
I

Figures 87G–87I Images before, during, and after osteoplasty performed to the pubis of a woman with metastatic breast cancer who had exceeded the maximum permitted radiation dose. In **87G,** a metastatic lesion resulting in a fracture of the left pubic ramus is noted. **87H** shows a vertebroplasty needle in the lesion immediately post-delivery of methylmethacrylate bone cement. The postprocedure CT (**87I**) shows filling of the fracture with cement.

PEARLS

- In the presence of decreased bone mineralization adjacent to the small fracture line, the diagnosis may be tricky. Absence of a history of trauma, painless swelling, and generalized bone pain may aid in making a diagnosis of a pathologic fracture.
- There is generalized demineralization of the bones in more diffuse conditions, such as hyperparathyroidism with a fracture through a brown tumor.
- The finding of intracortical tunneling, in addition to an apparent "permeative" pattern, favors the diagnosis of hyperparathyroidism and helps to differentiate the latter from malignant permeative conditions.

PITFALLS

- A fracture through a lession does not always indicate that metastatic disease is present. Biopsy is often helpful if any doubt exists.
- Pathologic fractures may be misdiagnosed as insufficiency fractures in the elderly with decreased bone mineralization.

Suggested Readings

Farad LM, Kamel IR, Kowamoto S, Bluemke DA, Frassica FJ, Fishman EK. Distinguishing stress fractures from pathologic fractures: a multimodality approach. Skeletal Radiol 2005;34:245–299

Hodge JC. Cementoplasty and the oncologic population. Singapore Med J 2000;41:407–409

Jensen ME, Kallmes DE. Percutaneous vertebroplasty in the treatment of malignant spine disease. Cancer J 2002;8:194–206

CASE 88

Hema N. Choudur, Anthony G. Ryan, and Peter L. Munk

Clinical Presentation

An elderly woman presented with pain in the right groin following a left hip arthroplasty and a greater trochanteric fracture fixation. Prior right hip arthroplasty had been performed several years previously. No abnormality was detected on clinical examination.

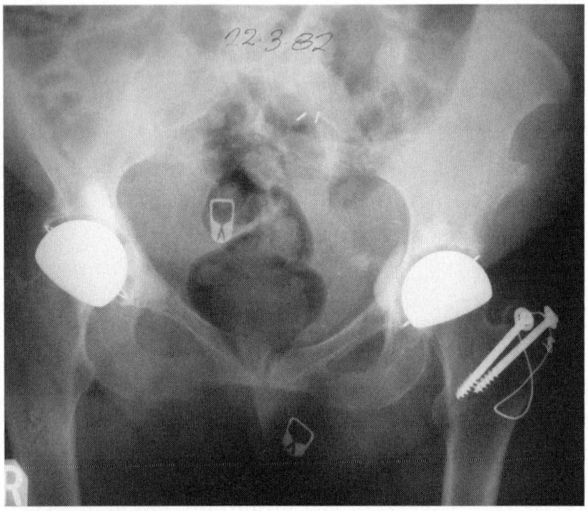

Figure 88A

Radiologic Findings

Plain radiograph of the pelvis (**Fig. 88A**) shows fractures through the right superior and inferior pubic rami following an arthroplasty. No other fractures are evident in the pelvic bones. Gross demineralization of the bones of the pelvis is evident.

Diagnosis

Insufficiency fractures of the right pubic rami.

Differential Diagnosis

- Pathologic fracture
- Stress fracture
- Traumatic fracture
- (Sometimes) malignant lesions

Discussion

Etiology

A fracture resulting from normal stress on abnormal bone is described as an insufficiency fracture. The abnormality is in terms of a generalized or focal demineralization of the bones, usually secondary to osteopenia. It must be differentiated from a pathologic fracture, which is through a primary or secondary bony lesion.

The most common sites of insufficiency fractures are the vertebral bodies. Other sites include the sacral ala, iliac bones, pubic rami, tibia, fibula, and calcaneus.

These fractures are more common in women than men, occur in 1 to 5% of any given population, and occur after 60 years of age.

Pathophysiology

When the bony trabaculae are lost, as in osteoporosis, the elasticity of the bone is reduced, resulting in a fracture, when the bone is no longer able to accommodate the stresses.

The most common cause of insufficiency fractures is postmenopausal or "senile" osteoporosis. Other causes include

- Pelvic irradiation
- Corticosteroid therapy
- Rheumatoid arthritis
- Vitamin D deficiency
- Fluoride therapy

Clinical Findings

Most patients present with groin, buttock, or low back pain. There is often no history of recognized trauma. There are often multiple sites of bony pain that can be severe enough to immobilize the patient.

A history of joint replacement may be noted, with the patient becoming more active following the surgery due to pain relief.

Imaging Findings

RADIOGRAPHY

Generalized gross demineralization of the bones is seen in the background of a fracture. The fracture line is rarely seen as a lucency with a cortical break, as in traumatic fractures, but instead is seen as a sclerotic line with exuberant callus and mild bony expansion and osteolysis.

COMPUTED TOMOGRAPHY

CT delineates these fractures very precisely, also showing the involvement of the sacral foramina. These sacral fractures are vertically oriented and lie parallel to the sacroiliac joints. They are frequently bilateral. Axially oriented fractures can, however, be missed on CT.

CT also helps to adequately evaluate compression fractures of the vertebral bodies and to rule out any retropulsion of the posterior bony margin into the spinal canal. This is mandatory prior to consideration for percutaneous vertebroplasty for stabilizing these osteoporotic compression fractures.

MAGNETIC RESONANCE IMAGING

In addition to showing the fracture at an early stage, MRI depicts the bone marrow/soft-tissue edema (**Figs. 88B** to **88F**). Subtle insufficiency fractures, for example, of the pubic rami, are sometimes incidentally picked up on MRI in the patient having pain referred to the hip.

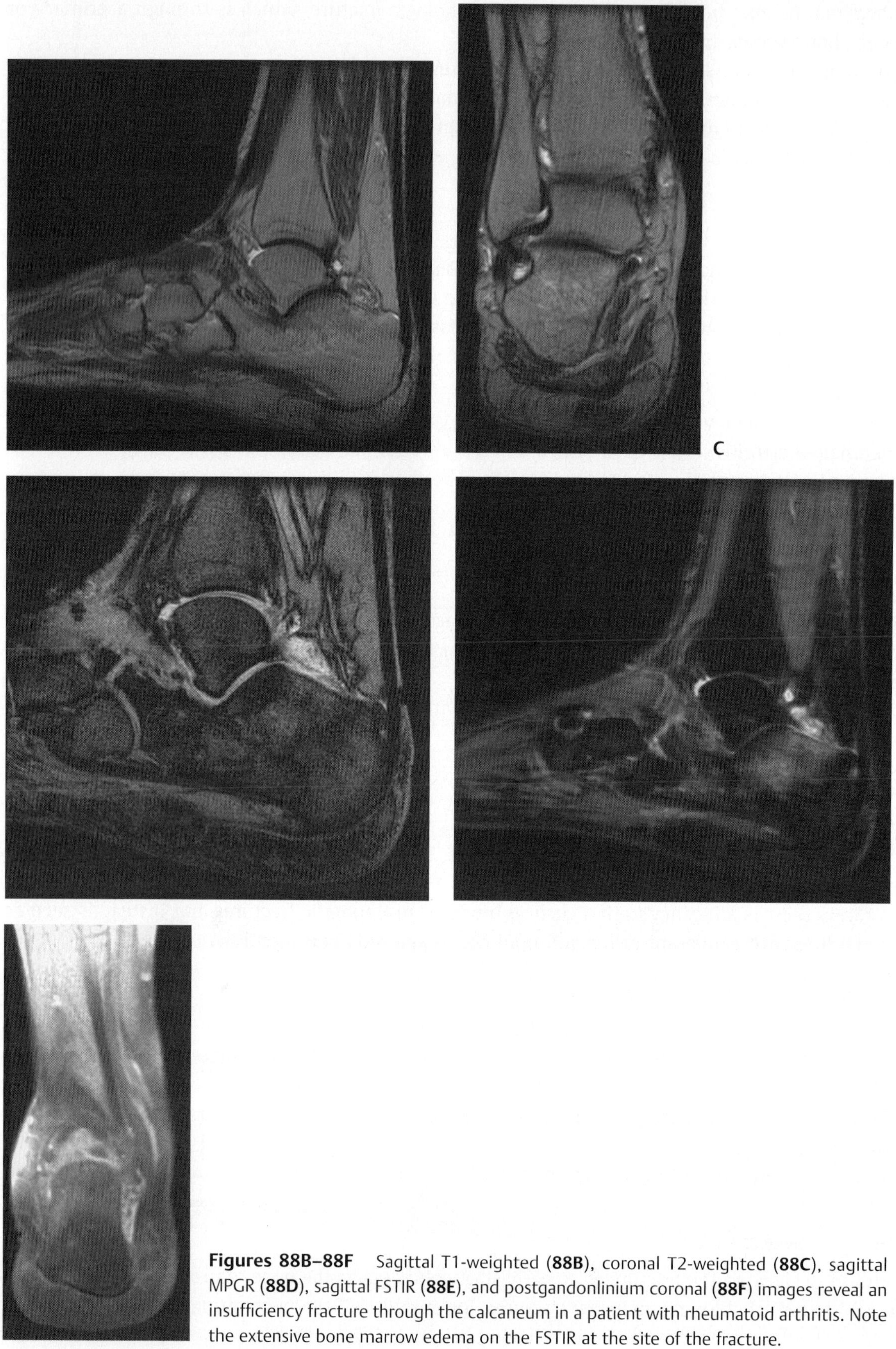

B C D E F

Figures 88B–88F Sagittal T1-weighted (**88B**), coronal T2-weighted (**88C**), sagittal MPGR (**88D**), sagittal FSTIR (**88E**), and postgandonlinium coronal (**88F**) images reveal an insufficiency fracture through the calcaneum in a patient with rheumatoid arthritis. Note the extensive bone marrow edema on the FSTIR at the site of the fracture.

BONE SCANS

Bone scans are usually the modality of choice in the absence of plain radiographic findings. The fractures are hot on the bone scans, assuming a typical pattern in the sacrum when bilateral. Scintigraphy also helps to evaluate the multiplicity of such fractures in the skeleton.

Treatment

Treatment is generally conservative with bed rest, analgesics, decreased weight bearing, and graded return to activity. Surgical stabilization is notoriously difficult, given the poor quality of the adjacent bone, making the secure placement of pins impossible in a significant proportion of cases. Intractable pain from sacral insufficiency fractures may thus be amenable to treatment by percutaneous osteoplasty. Polymethylmethacrylate injected at the fracture site under image guidance (sacroplasty) has shown promising results.

Prognosis

Prognosis is usually good, with return to normal activity in 4 to 6 weeks.

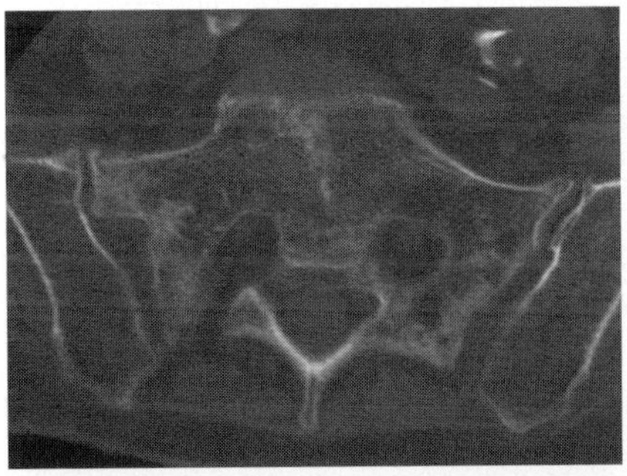

G

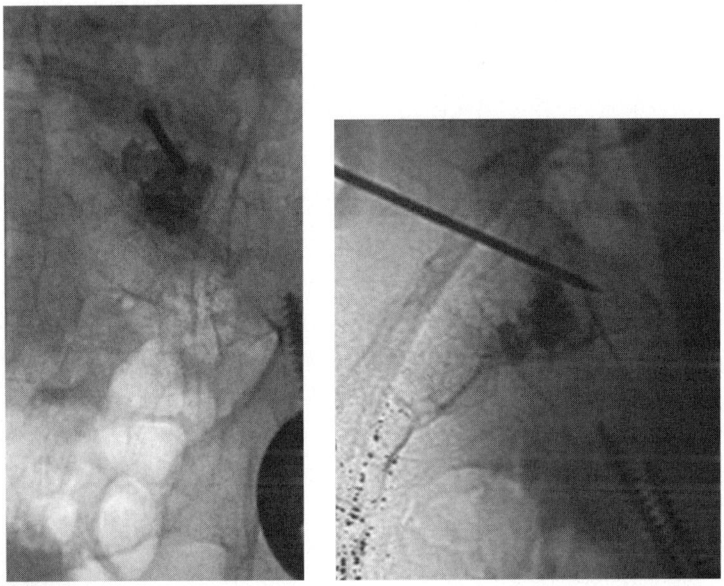

H,I

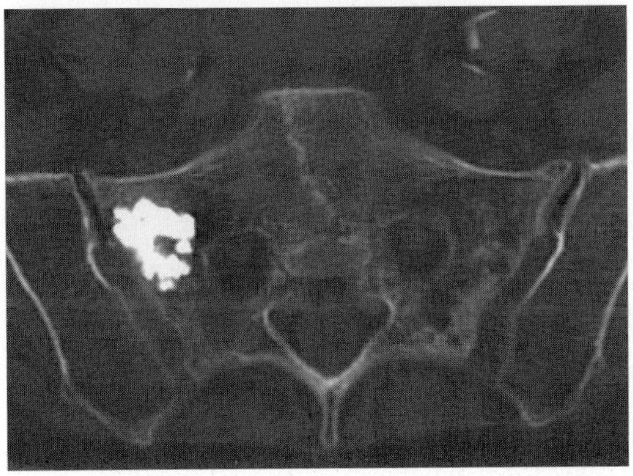

J

Figures 88G–88J Illustrate a sacral insufficiency fracture treated with osteoplasty. **88G** shows the sacral fracture on a preprocedure CT (AP view). **88H** and **88I** (lateral projection) show the injection of the cement under biplane fluoroscopic guidance. **88J** shows the postprocedural CT appearance.

PEARL

- With clinical suspicion of sacral, ilial, and supra-acetabular insufficiency fractures, not evident on plain radiographs, a bone scan, MRI, or CT is recommended to visualize the oft-missed fractures.

PITFALLS

- Insufficiency fractures require a high index of suspicion and can often be mistaken for other conditions, including infection.
- Sacral fractures are often difficult to diagnose on plain radiographs due to overlying bowel gas in a setting of decreased bone density.

Suggested Readings

Grangier C, Garcia J, Howarth NR. Role of MRI in the diagnosis of insufficiency fractures of the sacrum and acetabular roof. Skeletal Radiol 1997;26:517–524

Mammone JF, Schweitzer ME. MRI of occult sacral insufficiency fractures following radiotherapy. Skeletal Radiol 1995;24:101–104

Peh WC. Intrafracture fluid: a new diagnostic sign of insufficiency fractures of the sacrum and ilium. Br J Radiol 2000;73:895–898

CASE 89

Hema N. Choudur, Anthony G. Ryan, and Peter L. Munk

Clinical Presentation

A young marathon runner presented with severe pain in the right shin. There was no history of direct or indirect trauma.

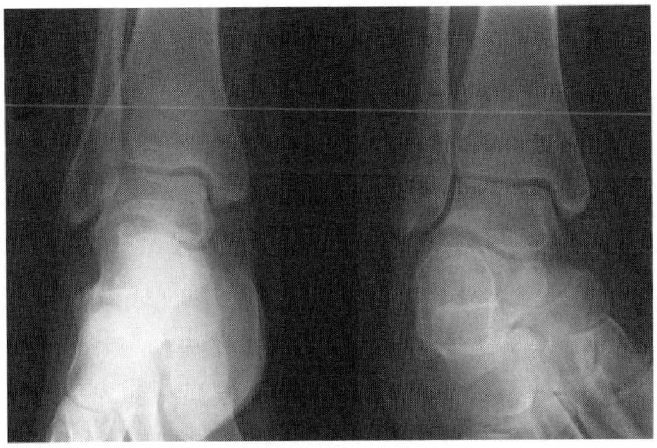

Figure 89A

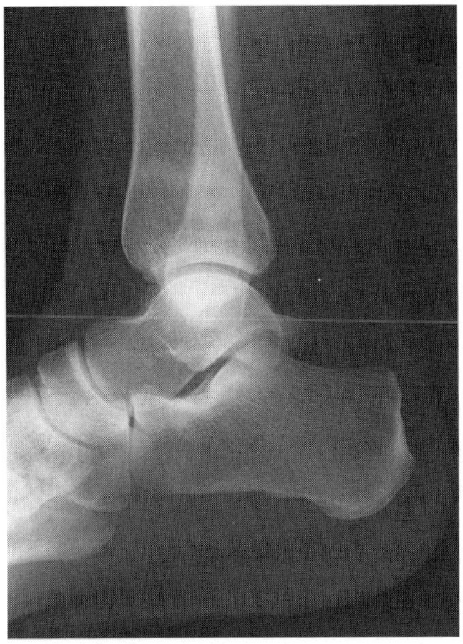

Figure 89B

Radiologic Findings

Anteroposterior and lateral views of the right tibia (**Figs. 89A,89B**) reveal a transverse sclerotic band in the distal tibia with no evidence of adjacent periosteal reaction or overlying soft-tissue swelling.

Diagnosis

Stress fracture.

Differential Diagnosis

- Traumatic fracture
- Insufficiency fracture

Discussion

Background

Stress or fatigue fractures result from excessive bone strain that causes microdamage to the bone, coupled with an inability to keep up with appropriate repair of the bone. They result from high-impact repetitive stress.

Etiology

The main cause of stress fractures is abnormal stress on a normal bone. This is often seen in athletes and military recruits who have suddenly started high-impact activity. Tennis, basketball, long-distance running, and gymnastics are activities in which the foot is constantly hit against a hard surface, resulting in stress fractures. Stress fractures are more common in females than males and are related to the triad of improper food habits with low calcium, amenorrhea, and osteoporosis. A sudden increase in the number of hours of activity, harder and flatter surfaces, and old and improper shoes are aggravating causes of stress fractures.

Stress fractures of the upper extremity, which are less common than lower extremity fractures, may occur in sports involving repetitive use of the arms, such as baseball and tennis. Stress fractures of the ribs occur in sports such as rowing.

Shin splints are vertically oriented stress fractures seen along the posteromedial tibial cortex, thought to be secondary to strain at the insertion of the soleus muscle on the underlying bone.

Tibial fractures are the most common lower extremity stress fractures and account for about one half of all such fractures in children and adults. In children, tibial stress fractures usually occur anteriorly in the proximal one third of the bone, whereas in adults, these fractures are more prevalent at the junction of the middle and distal one thirds. Anterior stress fractures of the tibia have a higher incidence of nonunion than anteromedial fractures.

Metatarsal fractures, accounting for approximately 25% of stress fractures, are most common in the distal second and third metatarsals and are least common in the fifth metatarsal. The former are called march fractures, as they are frequently seen in military recruits. Fifth metatarsal stress fractures must be distinguished from Jones fractures or avulsion fractures. Stress fractures of the calcaneum (**Fig. 89C**) and navicular are oriented in the sagittal plane.

Fibular fractures account for 10% of all stress fractures and are seen in the proximal fibula from jumping, and, in children in the distal fibula from running.

Femoral neck fractures (5%) are important to recognize because the rate of complications is high. They occur at the medial aspect of the femoral neck. Those that occur in the proximal neck are seen in older individuals as a lucent line and in the distal neck in younger athletic individuals as a focal area of callus formation; these are stable. Femoral neck fractures are less commonly seen in the infratrochanteric region, shaft, and supracondylar region of the femur.

Stress fractures of the ribs generally occur in the fifth to ninth ribs and are associated with periods of intensive training (e.g., rowing). Stress fractures can occur in the patella in both children and adults and should not be mistaken for a bipartite patella. They are seen in the coracoid in trapshooters, in the ulna in tennis players, baseball pitchers, and those in wheelchairs; in the phalangeal tufts in guitar players; and in the hook of the hamate and olecranon in baseball players.

Spondylolysis is a stress fracture of the pars interarticularis, most often seen at L5 in the lumbar spine and C6 in the cervical spine; they can be unilateral or bilateral. If unilateral, this fracture is often accompanied by sclerosis of the opposite pedicle and lamina secondary to weight-bearing stresses. It is depicted earliest on bone scans, which show a focal hot spot in that region. Axial CT slices show the pars defect very clearly.

Pathophysiology

When there is abnormal stress, the initial shock is absorbed by the muscles. When the muscles are no longer able to bear the brunt, the stress is transferred to the bones, which, after a particular threshold is reached, crack, resulting in stress fractures. Ischemia develops subcortically next to the cortical crack. The typical locations at which these fractures occur are the neck of the femur, the infe-

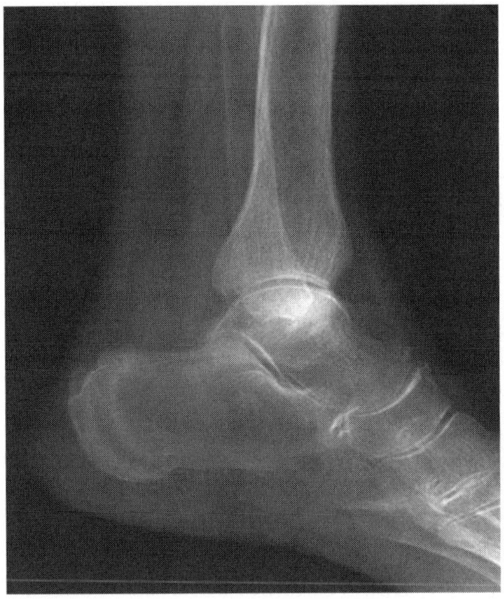

C

Figure 89C Radiograph of a stress fracture of the calcaneum. The fracture line is seen as a longitudinal lucency along the posterior aspects of the calcaneum.

rior tibia, and the lateral bones of the foot, especially the metatarsals. Fractures of the fibula and navicular are less common.

Male athletes have a relatively higher muscle mass and fare better than female athletes. Moreover, the width of the bones is larger. It has been shown that females who have a larger calf girth are less prone to stress fractures.

One theory holds that, during the initial increase in exercise, the osteoblastic activity lags behind osteoclastic activity by a few weeks, resulting in a period during which bone is more susceptible to injury. Another theory emphasizes strong and repetitive stress on bone at the insertion point of muscles, resulting in focal bending stresses beyond the ability of the bone to tolerate them.

Clinical Findings

Localized bone pain, especially with a history of increased physical activity, should raise the suspicion of a stress fracture. The pain is relieved by rest. Pain at the site of the fracture, for example, the groin, front of the knee, shin, or lateral aspect of the foot, is common. Tenderness to palpation typically is present at the injury site and is the hallmark of a stress fracture.

Imaging Findings

RADIOGRAPHY

Cortical radiolucency, focal periosteal reaction, endosteal thickening, increased callus formation, and sclerosis along the fracture lines are the plain radiographic findings of stress fractures. These findings are not seen before 2 weeks after the onset of symptoms.

Often three-phase bone scan, CT, or MRI are necessary to depict the fractures. Focal increase uptake of the radiotracer at the site of pain will help to make a diagnosis, though, less frequently, longitudinal fractures may be better delineated on MRI.

COMPUTED TOMOGRAPHY

CT demonstrates a radiolucent line seen easily with periosteal/endosteal thickening, medullary sclerosis, and adjacent soft-tissue swelling.

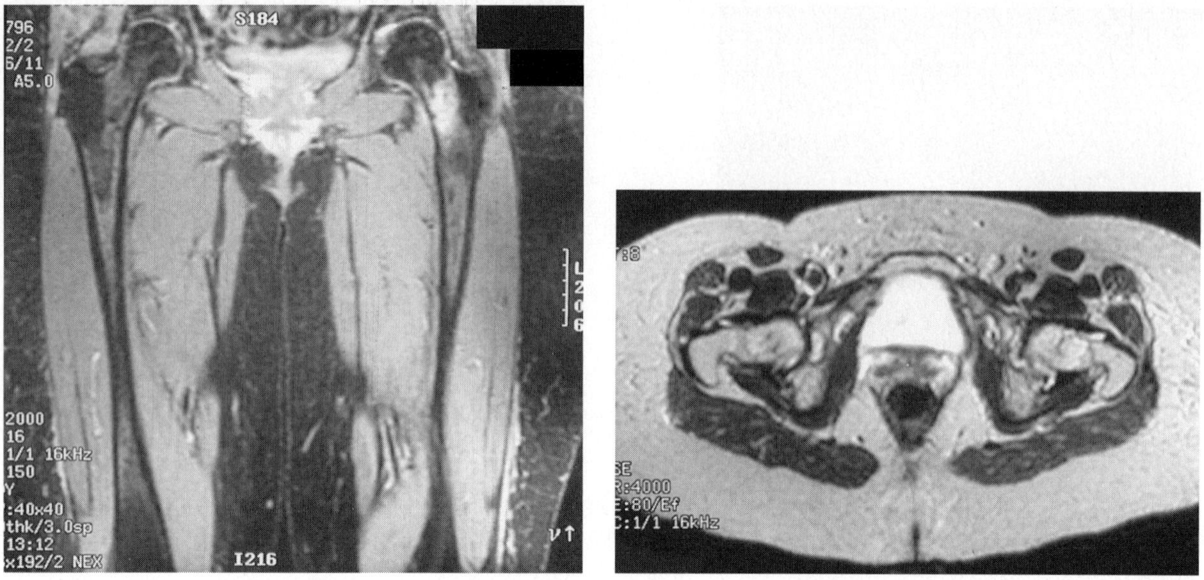

D E

Figures 89D,89E An inversion recovery sequence (**89D**) reveals the marrow edema at the site of the stress fracture in the left femoral neck. The T2-weighted axial image (**89E**) shows a high signal intensity at the site of the fracture.

MAGNETIC RESONANCE IMAGING

MRI typically reveals a low signal intensity line on T1-weighted images at the fracture site, with adjoining bone marrow edema seen well on T2-weighted images and inversion recovery sequences (**Figs. 89D,89E**).

RADIOISOTOPE SCANS

Radioisotope scans are useful for both diagnosis and follow-up of healing fractures, as the angiogram phase, blood pool phase, and delayed phase return to normal, in that order. Complete recovery takes 3 to 6 months or even 10 months.

Treatment

Rest with non–weight-bearing exercises for 4 to 6 weeks usually results in adequate healing of stress fractures. However, sometimes splinting/casting or even surgical treatment by an intramedullary rod or grafting may be necessary.

Prevention of stress fractures is most effectively accomplished by increasing the level of exercise slowly, adequately warming up and stretching before exercise, and using appropriate footwear.

Prognosis

When there is adequate compliance with medical advice, the vast majority of fractures will heal, and the patient will return to full activities. Approximately 60% of those with a stress fracture have had a previous stress fracture, suggesting the advice is not followed on return to training.

Complications

Progression to a complete fracture, nonunion, and avascular necrosis are more common in femoral neck fractures.

PEARLS

- Early stress fractures may be normal on plain radiographs, and, if clinically suspected, an isotope scan is mandatory to visualize the same.
- Focal bone marrow edema may be the only finding on MRI, and decreased level of activity is recommended until healing occurs.

PITFALL

- Radiographic findings may not be present for several weeks. Therefore, in many instances, a high index of suspicion is needed to make the diagnosis.

Suggested Readings

Boam WD, Miser WF, Yuill SC, Delaplain CB, Gayle EL, MacDonald DC. Comparison of ultrasound examination with bone scintiscan in the diagnosis of stress fractures. J Am Board Fam Pract 1996;9:414–417

Korpelainen R, Orava S, Karpakka J, Siira P, Hulkko A. Risk factors for recurrent stress fractures in athletes. Am J Sports Med 2001;29:304–310

Shearman CM, Brandser EA, Parman LM, et al. Longitudinal tibial stress fractures: a report of eight cases and review of the literature. J Comput Assist Tomogr 1998;22:265–269

CASE 90

Hema N. Choudur, Anthony G. Ryan, and Peter L. Munk

Clinical Presentation

While playing golf, a young man experienced sudden, agonizing pain along the ulnar aspect of his palm immediately after a forceful drive. Over the subsequent hours, swelling developed at that site with point tenderness, distal and radial to the pisiform bone. On examination, his grip strength was decreased, and there was weakness of the hypothenar muscles with paresthesia in the fourth and fifth fingers.

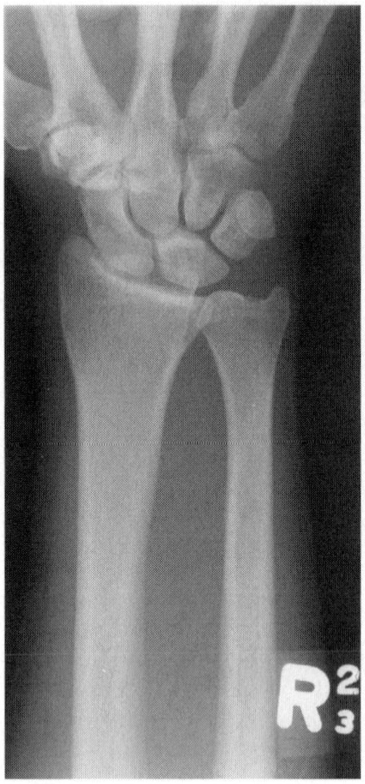

Figure 90A

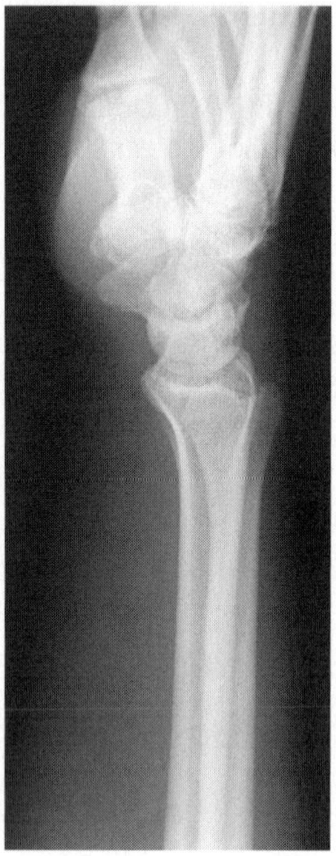

Figure 90B

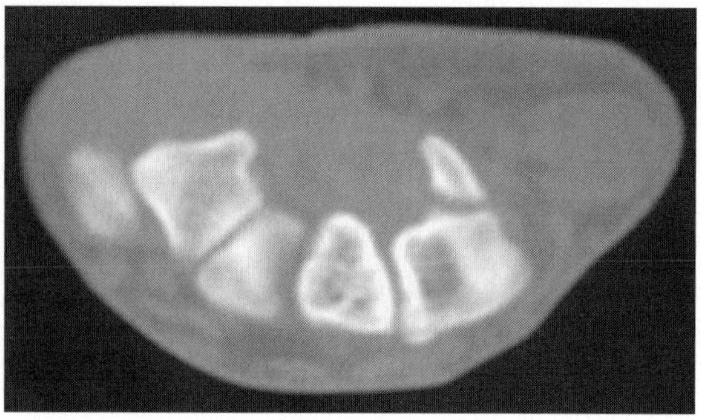

Figure 90C

Radiologic Findings

Except for soft-tissue swelling along the volar aspect of the wrist joint distally, no definite abnormality is noted on the plain radiographs (**Figs. 90A,90B**). Only on the subsequent CT (**Fig. 90C**) was the hook of hamate fracture convincingly demonstrated.

Diagnosis

Hook of hamate fracture.

Differential Diagnosis

Stress fractures of the hamate secondary to chronic repetitive trauma, as occurs in golf, hockey, and tennis.

Discussion

Hook of humate fractures result in high nonunion rates with conservative measures. Therefore, it is very important to detect and treat them. Using conventional x-ray projections, a sensitivity of 72%, a specificity of 88%, and an accuracy of 80% in detection of the fracture are typical. Using CT, the sensitivity is 100%, the specificity 94%, and the accuracy 97%; also, setup for CT scanning is less uncomfortable for the patient.

Fractures of the body of the hamate are much less common than fractures of the hook. They are often associated with fourth and fifth carpometacarpal fracture-dislocations. Fractures of the body may occur as a result of axial force transmitted through the metacarpals or from a direct blow to the ulnar aspect of the wrist.

Etiology

Hook of the hamate fractures are generally thought to result from two mechanisms: either from a fall on the wrist with the hand in dorsiflexion or by direct trauma. The latter mechanism is most commonly encountered with athletic injuries and is usually seen in sports that involve clubs or bats (golf, baseball). The fracture may result from repetitive stresses or from a direct blow when a club or racquet strikes the ground.

Fractures of the body of the hamate are associated with other injuries, such as a triquetral fracture or dorsal displacement of the fourth and fifth metacarpals.

Pathophysiology

The vessels supplying the hook enter it at its base radially and also at its tip, on the ulnar aspect. In addition, the radial and ulnar recurrent arteries supply the distal carpal row. There is no intraosseous anastomosis between the feeding arteries within the trapezoid and the hamate, so avascular necrosis can occur if the vessels are disrupted.

The hook of the hamate lies radial to the pisiform distally and forms the radial border of Guyon's canal. Therefore, the ulnar nerve and artery running in the canal are in close approximation to the hook.

Fractures can occur through the body or the hook or along the dorsal aspect distally. When the fourth and fifth metacarpals dislocate or sublux dorsally, a chip of the hamate dorsally is torn off in the coronal plane. Therefore, any chip of bone evident on plain radiographs should raise a suspicion of a hamate fracture, in addition to a triquetral fracture, especially if there is dorsal displacement of the metacarpals.

Clinical Findings

Following an acute injury, usually by means of a club or racquet, there is pain and soft-tissue swelling along the wrist the length of its ulnar aspect.

Complications

The patient usually returns to the preinjury level of activity following immediate removal of the fractured hook. Nonunion is a frequent complication due to delayed detection of this fracture. Ulnar neuropathy from compression of the adjacent ulnar nerve by the fractured hook results in pain and paresthesias in its distribution. Flexor tendon tears and ruptures secondary to abrasion from the sharp fracture margins tend to result in permanent disability despite surgical measures.

Imaging Findings

RADIOGRAPHY

Often fractures of the hook of the hamate are missed on routine orthogonal views of the wrist. A critical analysis of the posteroanterior view for absence of the hook, sclerosis of the hook, and discontinuity of the cortical outline may imply the presence of a fracture. A carpal tunnel view and a dedicated view with 15 degrees of tube tilt with the beam focused on the base of the fifth metacarpal will delineate the fracture.

COMPUTED TOMOGRAPHY

Thin-slice (1.5 mm), high-resolution CT with three-dimensional reformats will show the fracture very clearly, including the extent of displacement.

MAGNETIC RESONANCE IMAGING

- Excellent depiction of the fracture, especially in the axial orientation, with bone marrow edema, intervening fluid, and surrounding soft-tissue edema clearly evident
- Compression of the ulnar nerve in Guyon's canal and any tears of the flexor carpi ulnaris are clearly visualized.

Treatment

Fractures of the hook and body are usually nondisplaced, and they can be treated with cast immobilization. Intra-articular fractures with displacement > 1 mm are best treated with open reduction and internal fixation (ORIF). Displaced fractures that involve the distal aspect of the hook often result in nonunion if they are not treated with ORIF.

Immediate immobilization results in good healing, obviating the need for surgery. However, if treatment is delayed, nonunion is common and is treated with excision of the hook. Internal fixation for nonunion is associated with a poor outcome.

Distal carpal fractures associated with metacarpal dislocation are unstable injuries and usually require internal fixation. Anatomic reduction of hamate–fourth/fifth metacarpal joints is important, as they are the most mobile of the carpometacarpal joints.

Prognosis

The preinjury level of activity is often seen in immediately detected and adequately immobilized hook of hamate fractures. With delayed treatment and nonunion, surgical treatment may be successful, but long-term sequelae, such as pain and tendon tears, are frequent.

PEARL

- A systematic search for hamate fractures on orthogonal views and additional carpal tunnel view or CT in suspicious cases will prevent delay in treatment and associated complications.

PITFALLS

- Hook of hamate fractures can be slowly developing stress fractures. CT in these cases may show only sclerosis rather than a fracture line.

- The plain radiographic findings of hamate fracture may be very subtle, and the fracture may be missed unless a careful correlation with a clinical history is made. A CT scan is mandatory in suspicious cases.
- Fractures of the hook of the hamate are not detected on plain radiographs unless special views are taken following a high clinical suspicion.

Suggested Readings

Abbitt PL, Riddervold HO. The carpal tunnel view: helpful adjuvant for unrecognized fractures of the carpus. Skeletal Radiol 1987;16:45–47

Gillespy T 3rd, Stork JJ, Dell PC. Dorsal fracture of the hamate: distinctive radiographic appearance. Am J Roentgenol 1988;151:351–353

Norman A, Nelson J, Green S. Fractures of the hook of hamate: radiographic signs. Radiology 1985;154:49–53

CASE 91

Hema N. Choudur, Anthony G. Ryan, and Peter L. Munk

Clinical Presentation

Two patients presented with an inability to bear weight and pain, with swelling along the lateral aspect of the foot.

The child (case 1) had had a skiing injury a few weeks prior to his presentation, and the adult, a 52-year-old amateur tennis player (case 2), presented having sustained an inversion injury during a game.

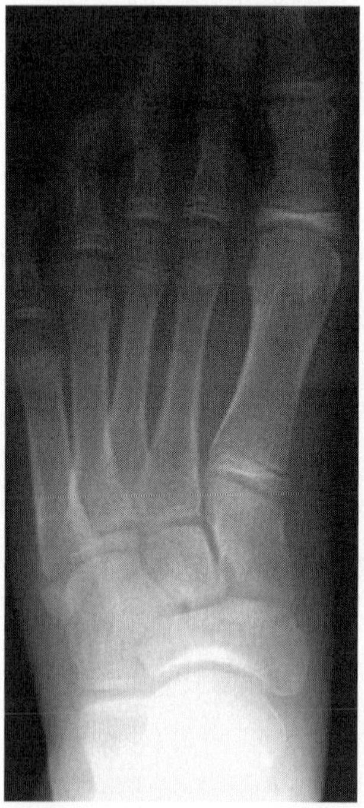

Figure 91A

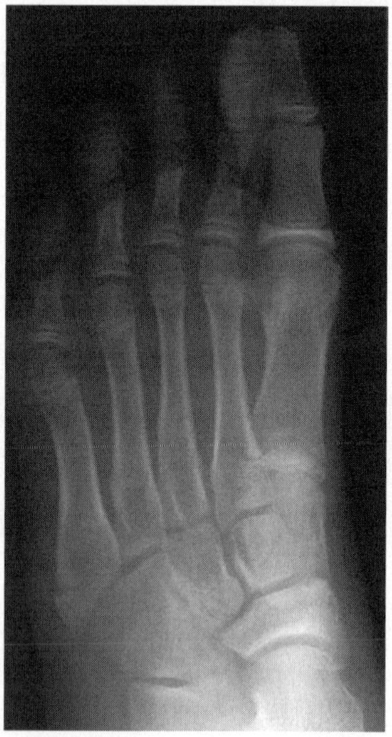

Figure 91B

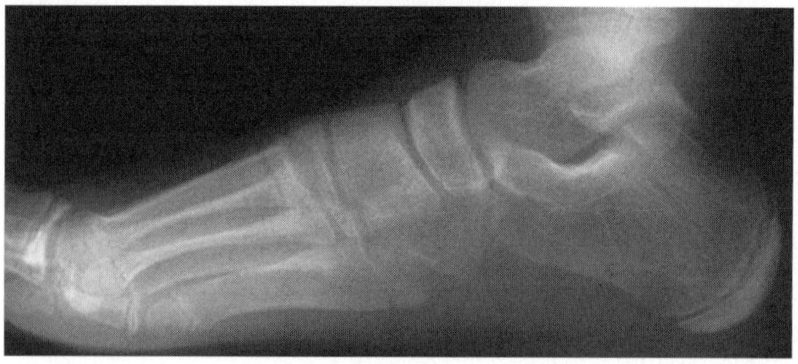

Figure 91C

Radiologic Findings

Case 1

Anteroposterior (AP), oblique, and lateral views of the foot (**Figs. 91A–91C**) show an undisplaced fracture through the base of the fifth metatarsal adjacent to the apophyseal growth plate.

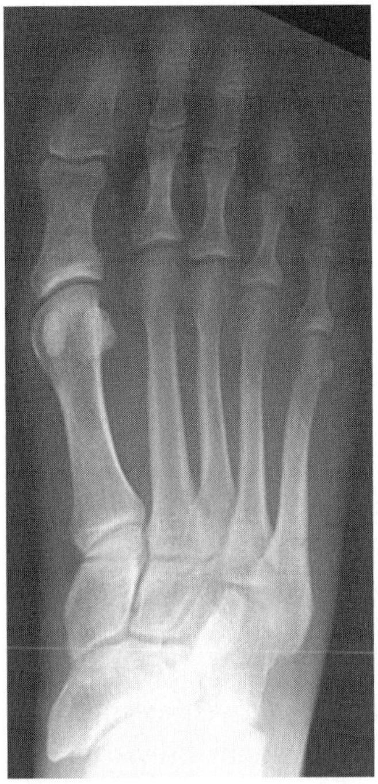

Figure 91D

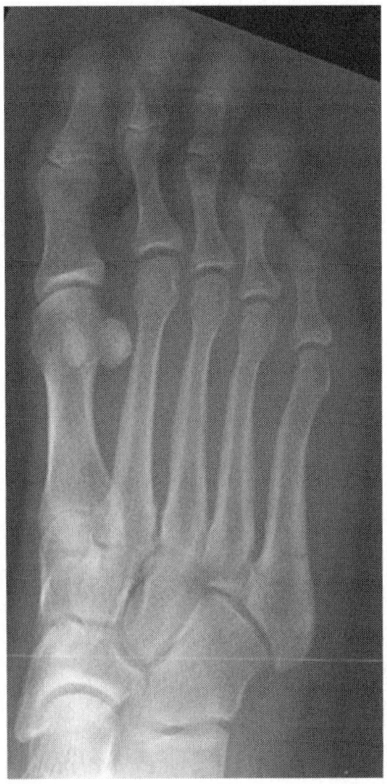

Figure 91E

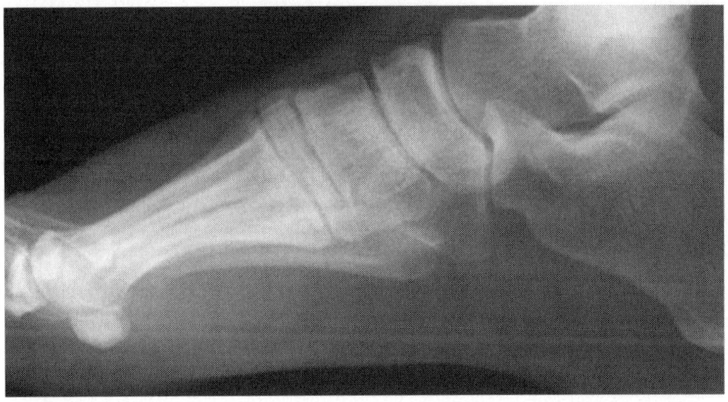

Figure 91F

Case 2

AP, oblique, and lateral views of the foot (**Figs. 91D–91F**) show a transverse fracture of the proximal shaft of the fifth metatarsal.

Diagnosis

Proximal fifth metatarsal fractures, as follows:

- *Case 1* Pseudo-Jones fracture
- *Case 2* Jones fracture

Differential Diagnosis

- Stress fracture

Normal variants include the following:

- An apophysis, an os in the peroneus brevis tendon, and an os vesalianum pedis may all mimic a fracture of the fifth metatarsal.

Discussion

Classical Jones fractures are common injuries causing pain during weight bearing. Unlike fractures caused by avulsion of the peroneus brevis tendon (pseudo-Jones, tennis, and dancer's fractures), true Jones fractures are due to a twisting inversion injury of the foot. However, all proximal fifth metatarsal fractures may look alike, and differentiating them is critical in initiating the correct management.

Etiology

Jones fractures are usually seen in athletes secondary to an inversion mechanism on the ankle or hindfoot. The more frequent avulsion injuries (dancer's fractures) occur without a twisting injury. In the past, these avulsions were thought to be associated with tearing at the peroneus brevis tendon insertion, but it is more likely that the injury occurs secondary to avulsion of the plantar aponeurosis.

Pathophysiology

Jones fractures occur when the ankle is plantar flexed and a strong adduction force is applied to the forefoot, as may occur in soccer, football, tennis, and other sports. Because of relatively poor vascularity and highly repetitive stresses at this site, Jones fractures are associated with a poor outcome.

The true Jones fracture, first described in 1902 by Sir Robert Jones, consists of a transverse fracture at the junction of the diaphysis and metaphysis between the points of insertion of the peroneus brevis and tertius tendons. To prevent confusion, only acute fractures in this precise location should be labeled Jones fractures.

A stress fracture, seen distal to the intermetatarsal ligaments due to excessive running loads, is never an acute injury.

Clinical Findings

Findings include pain, hematoma, and swelling along the lateral aspect of the foot with inability to bear weight.

Complications

Jones fractures may undergo fibrous union only. Other proximal fractures, such as stress and acute-on-chronic fractures, are also often associated with nonunion or delayed union.

Long-term immobilization and rest can lead to muscle atrophy and stiffness, hampering the patient's return to full athletic participation.

Imaging Findings

RADIOGRAPHY

- Fractures of the base of the fifth metatarsal should be interpreted based on the location and direction of the fracture line, as well as by the presence of intra-articular extension.

- The amount of sclerosis at the fracture site is helpful in discerning whether the fracture is acute or chronic.
- True acute Jones fractures are seen at least 1.5 cm distal to the tarsometatarsal joint line.
- The horizontal fracture line at the diametaphysis typically extends to the fourth to fifth metatarsal facet.
- Stress fractures are located distal to the proximal intermetatarsal ligaments and typically demonstrate a widened fracture line and varying degrees of medullary sclerosis.
- In avulsion injuries of the styloid process (as in case 1 above), the fracture line is transversely oriented proximal to the metatarsocuboid joint space on the lateral view. These fractures are almost always nondisplaced and involve the cortices and cancellous bone. These are differentiable from an apophysis, as the latter is smooth and separated by a vertical lucency at the base of the fifth metatarsal. The normal apophysis is seen between 9 and 14 years of age, and its line runs parallel to the metatarsal shaft along the inferior and lateral margin of the styloid process. No intra-articular extension is noted (unlike with the fracture), and it is always bilateral.
- Another differential is an ossicle, seen in 15% of the population within the peroneus tendon at the base of the fifth metatarsal. The rarer os vesalianum pedis is seen adjacent to the peroneus brevis insertion. Fractures typically have irregular or ragged margins, in contrast to the smooth, corticated border of an ossicle.
- If the injury is detected in a subacute setting, sclerosis of the fracture line with medullary sclerosis is seen, raising the possibility of a stress fracture. Stress fractures occur at the metadiaphyseal junction (the same site as a Jones fracture) but with marked intramedullary sclerosis, profound thickening of both the medial and lateral cortices, and a lucency in the lateral cortex. It should be noted that no radiologic evidence may be present in either an early Jones fracture or an early stress fracture.

COMPUTED TOMOGRAPHY

- When there is high clinical suspicion and the radiographs appear normal, subtle fractures can be delineated on CT, with multiplanar reformats occasionally helpful. Further, CT can help in differentiating a stress fracture from a Jones fracture by the exuberant callus and medullary sclerosis seen in the former.

MAGNETIC RESONANCE IMAGING AND BONE SCANS

- MRI and bone scans are often useful in detecting subtle fractures and stress fractures; however, marrow edema is noted in both Jones and stress fractures, making the two difficult to differentiate on these modalities.

Treatment

ACUTE JONES FRACTURE

- Nonoperative treatment is reserved for minimally displaced acute or subacute fractures. A non–weight-bearing cast for 6 to 8 weeks will result in adequate healing in 75% of cases.
- Operative treatment with cancellous screw fixation with or without a bone graft is considered in chronic, nonunited, and grossly displaced fractures.

AVULSION INJURIES

- Acute symptomatic treatment for dancer's fractures consists of limited weight bearing, modified activity, ice, and analgesics, followed by immobilization in a walking cast, with improvement expected in 3 to 4 weeks.
- If extensive intra-articular extension of the fracture line is seen with a large step deformity (> 2 to 3 mm) or a large intra-articular fragment is present, operative treatment is indicated. Nonunion is rare.

- Other proximal fractures, such as stress and acute-on-chronic fractures, are often associated with nonunion or delayed union. Such fractures are best treated by early operative intervention.
- Correct identification of stress and acute-on-chronic fractures of the fifth metatarsal is important because prompt surgical treatment shortens recovery and permits a quick return to sports activity, especially important in the professional athlete.

Prognosis

A prolonged healing course is seen with Jones fractures as compared with other metatarsal fractures with a high rate of nonunion.

The prognosis for avulsion fractures in this area is excellent, as they almost always heal within 4 to 6 weeks with conservative treatment.

PEARLS

- Fractures proximal to the metatarsal cuboid joint are avulsion injuries, and those located 1.5 cm distal to the joint line are either Jones fractures or stress fractures. Differentiation between the two is based on the history and radiographic features.
- In avulsion injuries of the styloid process (as in case 1 above), the fracture line is transversely oriented proximal to the metatarsocuboid joint space on the lateral view. These fractures are almost always nondisplaced and involve the cortices and cancellous bone. These are differentiable from an apophysis, as the latter is smooth and separated by a vertical lucency at the base of the fifth metatarsal. In addition, the line of the apophysis does not extend to the adjacent joint, unlike a fracture, and apophyses are always bilateral.
- Fractures typically have irregular or ragged margins, in contrast to the smooth, corticated border of an ossicle.
- CT can help in differentiating a stress fracture from a Jones fracture by the exuberant callus and medullary sclerosis seen in the former.

PITFALLS

- Oblique radiographs of the foot are essential to accurately assess these fractures, as they can easily be missed on standard AP projections, especially when undisplaced.
- It should be noted that no radiologic evidence may be present in an early Jones fracture or an early stress fracture.
- Although MRI and bone scans are often useful in detecting subtle acute fractures and stress fractures, marrow edema is noted in both, and thus it can be difficult to differentiate these entities on these modalities. The history should point to the correct diagnosis; however, if doubt remains, CT should resolve the issue.

Suggested Readings

Jones R. Fractures of the base of the fifth metatarsal bone by indirect violence. Ann Surg 1902;35:697–700

Karasick D. Fractures and dislocations of the foot. Semin Roentgenol 1994;29:152–175

Lawrence SJ, Botte MJ. Jones' fractures and related fractures of the proximal fifth metatarsal. Foot Ankle 1993;14:358–365

Nunley JA. Fractures of the base of the fifth metatarsal: the Jones fracture. Orthop Clin North Am 2001;32:171–180

Pao DG, Keats TE, Dussault RG. Avulsion fracture of the base of the fifth metatarsal not seen on conventional radiography of the foot: the need for an additional projection. Am J Roentgenol 2000;175:549–552

Preidler KW, Peicha G, Lajtai G. Conventional radiography, CT, and MR imaging in patients with hyperflexion injuries of the foot: diagnostic accuracy in the detection of bony and ligamentous changes. Am J Roentgenol 1999;173:1673–1677

Richli WR, Rosenthal DI. Avulsion fracture of the fifth metatarsal: experimental study of pathomechanics. Am J Roentgenol 1984;143:889–891

CASE 92

Anthony G. Ryan and Peter L. Munk

Clinical Presentation

A 20-year-old college football player presented with chronic anterior hip pain. Although he could recall no single acute event, there had been a period of intense preseason training 3 months previously.

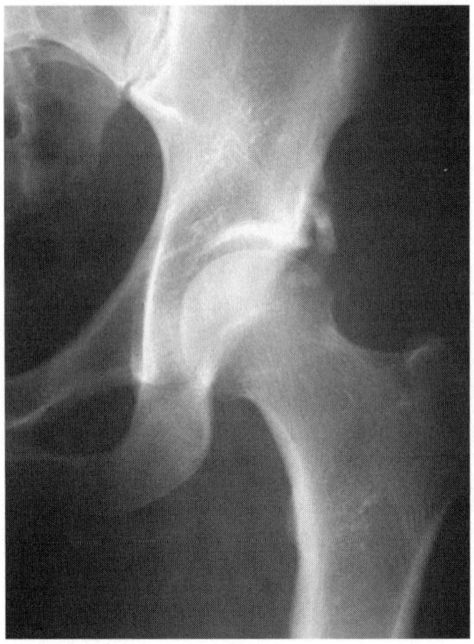

Figure 92A

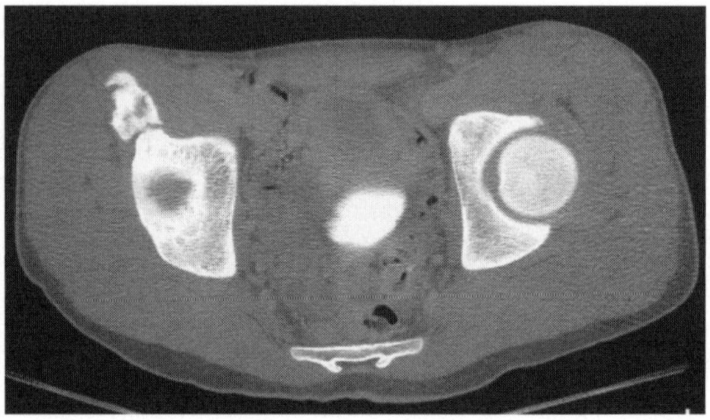

Figure 92B

Radiologic Findings

Radiograph of the left hip (**Fig. 92A**) reveals a thick, ossific, curvilinear density with smooth margins protruding from anterosuperior to the hip joint and projecting inferiorly.

A CT scan (**Fig. 92B**) shows an irregularly marginated, heterogeneously ossified density immediately anterior to the anterior inferior iliac spine, with some associated irregularity of the underlying bone but no soft-tissue mass.

Diagnosis

Chronic avulsion fracture of the anterior inferior iliac spine, origin of the straight head of the rectus femoris muscle

Differential Diagnosis

A differential diagnosis is inappropriate, as the history, location of the injury, and knowledge of the musculotendinous insertion anatomy yield the diagnosis.

Discussion

Background

When excessive stress is applied to the "muscle-tendon-bone" unit, the weakest link in the chain will give way. The point of greatest vulnerability varies with age; in the child or adolescent, the weak point is at the physis until it undergoes bony fusion (early to mid 20s). Thus, when excessive strain is applied through a muscle onto a bone underlying, which is an apophysis, the muscle-tendon-bone complex will break at the apophysis, giving rise to a characteristic avulsion fracture.

Although there is great variation in the spectrum of resultant avulsions, when typical, they pose no diagnostic dilemma. When their appearances are atypical, however, as they can be in the subacute or chronic states, they may mimic other, more aggressive lesions, such as neoplasms, or infection. Familiarity with the range of appearances of such lesions aids in the avoidance of inappropriate biopsy.

Around the pelvis, the most common sites for these avulsions are, in order of decreasing frequency:

- Ischial tuberosity (hamstring and adductor magnus) (**Fig. 92C**)
- Anterior inferior iliac spine (straight head of rectus femoris) (**Figs. 92A,92B**)
- Anterior superior iliac spine (sartorius, tensor fascia lata)
- Pubic symphysis, greater and lesser trochanters, inferior pubic ramus, and iliac crest (**Figs. 92D,92E**)

Etiology

The injuries may occur as a result of repetitive trauma or secondary to a single severe, usually eccentric, contraction during running, jumping, or kicking a ball, with subsequent healing of the acute fracture.

Pathophysiology

The sports most commonly producing the injuries are soccer, gymnastics, football, baseball, hurdling, cheerleading, and track athletics (sprinting, jumping).

C

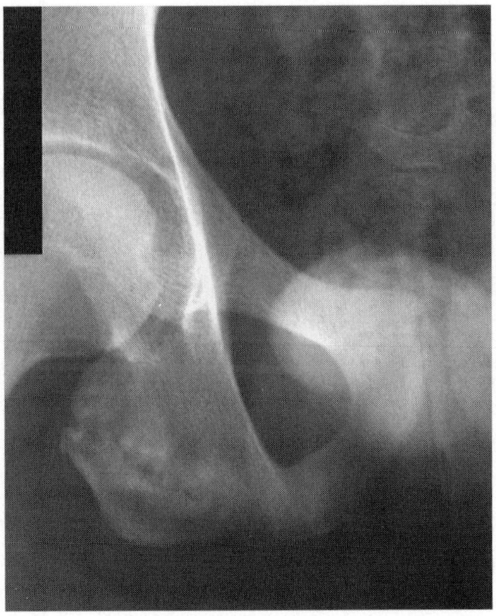

Figure 92C Chronic avulsion of the right ischial tuberosity in a 22-year-old soccer player. Plain film shows a large fragment partially fused with the underlying ischium, the irregular junction line characterized by an intermittent sclerotic pattern, partial fusion posterosuperiorly, and a persistent lucent line at the fracture interface.

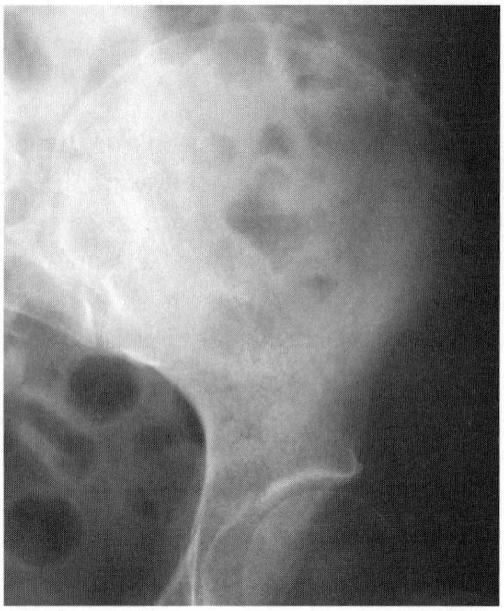
D

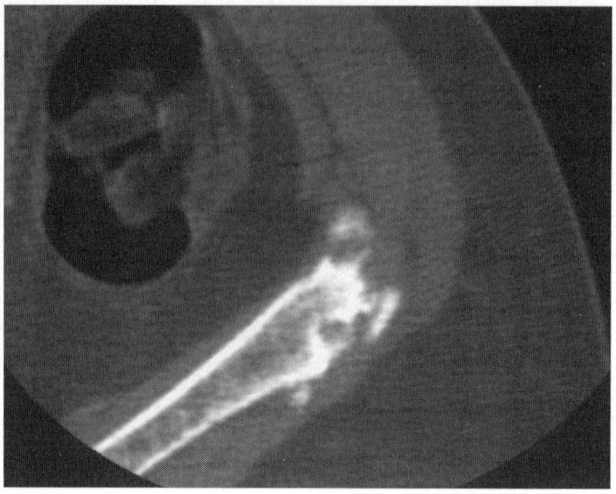
E

Figures 92D,92E Anteroposterior radiograph (**92D**) of the left ilium shows a faint radiodensity paralleling the iliac crest with apparent sclerosis of the underlying crest margin. A CT image (**92E**) confirms the presence of bony callus overlying the crest with associated sclerosis and irregularity of the underlying cortex, typical of an avulsive injury. No discernible mass or soft-tissue component is present.

The ischial tuberosity is most frequently injured by extreme active contraction of the hamstring muscles, such as may occur in sprinters, or extreme passive lengthening, as occurs in cheerleaders and dancers. The anterior superior iliac spine is typically injured by avulsion of the sartorius or tensor fascia lata in sprinters with forceful extension at the hip. The anterior inferior iliac spine is typically injured with forceful extension of the hip avulsing the apophysis underlying the attachment of the straight head of the rectus femoris.

Avulsions of the long or short adductors or gracilis produce lesions at the pubic symphysis, typically due to chronic overuse, rather than an acute injury, which can occur with forced contraction against resistance, for example, a forceful toe stub or a clash against another player. These injuries differ from the others in that bony fragments are rarely seen despite the often quite severe pain. A chronic avulsion at the pubis can cause prominent lysis that may have an apparent soft-tissue mass, which is, in fact, the associated retracted muscle fibers. These latter injuries are seen in almost all professional soccer players who come to imaging. It is thought these injuries occur in the earlier years of soccer apprenticeship while the skeleton is still maturing.

Iliac crest injuries are uncommon but occur as a result of abdominal muscular avulsion. When they do occur, there may be an underlying predisposition, for example, diabetics with dialysis-dependent renal failure, or there may be overuse, as in long-distance runners. Asymmetry of the crests will be evident, with an ossific rim over a variable distance of the crest (**Figs. 92D,92E**).

Lesser trochanteric avulsions are uncommon but occur in younger athletes with avulsion of the iliopsoas tendon. These are very painful lesions and can cause considerable disability.

The greater trochanter is injured with avulsion of the hip rotators (gluteus medius and minimus, internal obturator, gemellus, and piriformis), occurring as a result of a sudden directional change.

Clinical Findings

The patient is typically between the ages of 14 and 25. In cases of chronic avulsion, the inciting event may be forgotten by the time of presentation, or there may not have been a particular event, as in the case of overuse or chronic repetitive trauma. Patients with an acute ischial tuberosity avulsion can usually identify an inciting incident and report buttock pain and a limp. Injuries to the symphysis pubis and inferior pubic ramus are usually due to chronic overuse secondary to soccer, presenting with acute groin pain.

Complications

- Prominent callus formation or displaced fragments may cause local nerve irritation, such as sciatic pain in the setting of an ischial tuberosity injury, or interfere with adjacent bone growth, resulting in limb asymmetry in severe untreated cases.
- Nonunion with a symptomatic fibrous union is seen, particularly if there is a greater than 2 cm displacement of the fracture and it is not surgically reduced
- If union does not occur, these injuries can cause chronic disability as a result of the above mechanisms or resultant profound muscle atrophy.

Pathology

GROSS

Fracture with callus formation.

MICROSCOPIC

Inflammatory change combined with new bone formation, which, in the subacute phase particularly, can appear aggressive and give rise to a false-positive diagnosis of neoplasm.

Imaging Findings

RADIOGRAPHY

Acutely, the avulsed fragment may be clearly seen and the injury will be recognized as an acute fracture (**Fig. 92F**). However, especially in younger athletes, if the apophysis is undisplaced, the injury may be missed. Where the ischial tuberosity is concerned, the typical pattern is of round radiolucencies with associated callus formation at the lateral aspect of the ischial ramus (biceps insertion).

If the presentation is delayed, the appearances become less typical and may appear lytic and destructive, thus mimicking more aggressive pathology, particularly in the absence of a single traumatic event. In these cases, serial radiographs are likely to reveal the true nature of the lesion, whereas a cross-sectional study, particularly MRI, may in fact confuse matters. If a cross-sectional study is to be performed, CT is to be preferred as it is more likely to demonstrate the benign nature of the bony changes and help in excluding an associated mass.

COMPUTED TOMOGRAPHY

Chronic injuries tend to have prominent bone formation, with no clear history of trauma, an instance where CT is likely to be helpful (**Figs. 92B,92E**).

MAGNETIC RESONANCE IMAGING

- Edema (high signal intensity on T2-weighted images and low signal intensity on T1-weighted images) at the site of an injury or asymmetric findings will suggest the diagnosis if the apophysis is undisplaced on plain films, as mentioned above.

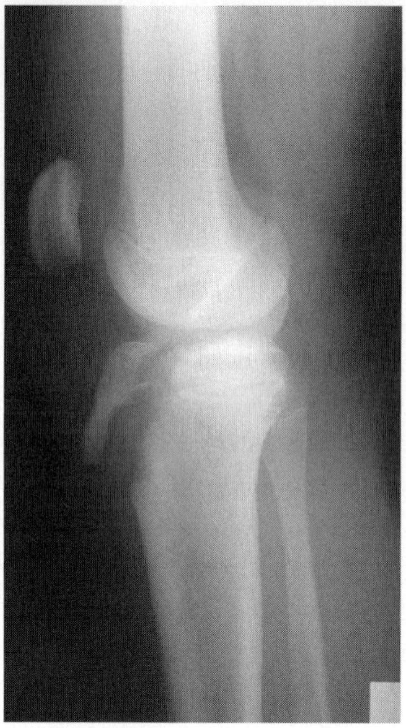

Figure 92F Lateral radiograph of the knee in a 16-year-old boy who had experienced severe anterior knee pain after missing the ball and kicking the ground with full force reveals avulsion of the tibial tuberosity (type 3 injury, according to the Watson-Jones classification, with displacement of the epiphyseal base and intra-articular extension of the fracture).

- If gadolinium is used, enhancement is expected, reflecting the local hyperemia.
- In the subacute and chronic stages, the MRI appearances of the involved bone may suggest an aggressive lesion and can thus be misleading.
- MRI is the investigation of choice, however, in the diagnosis of associated musculotendinous injuries.

Treatment

Undisplaced fractures are expected to heal with conservative management, for example, bed rest with hips and knees flexed, with subsequent progressive mobilization and eventual return to normal athletic activities.

Acute or early subacute injuries may be treated surgically if there is a > 2 cm displacement of the fracture. Leaving these untreated puts the region at risk of fibrous symptomatic union.

Prognosis

Prognosis depends to an extent on the site of injury:

- Ischial tuberosity: If union does not occur, these injuries can cause chronic disability, such as muscle atrophy, nerve (sciatic) irritation, and interference with adjacent bone growth.
- Iliac spines (superior and inferior): Return to full sporting activities is expected within 6 weeks.

PEARLS

- The weakest link in the muscle-tendon-bone chain is the physis until it undergoes bony fusion. Thus, when excessive strain is applied through a muscle onto a bone underlying, which is an apophysis, the muscle-tendon-bone complex will break at the apophysis, giving rise to a characteristic avulsion fracture.

- The patient's history is crucial in reaching the correct diagnosis. Also, knowledge of the musculotendinous anatomy of the pelvis is vital in recognizing the typical patterns. The location of musculotendinous insertions on the pelvic skeleton is given below:
  - Iliac crest: Abdominal musculature
  - Greater trochanter: Hip rotators
  - Lesser trochanter: Iliopsoas
  - Ischial tuberosity: Hamstring and adductor magnus
  - Anterior inferior iliac spine: Straight head of rectus femoris
  - Anterior superior iliac spine: Sartorius, tensor fascia lata
  - Pubic body and inferior pubic ramus: Adductors and gracilis
- If the presentation is delayed, the radiographic appearances become less typical and may appear lytic and destructive, thus mimicking more aggressive pathology, particularly in the absence of a single traumatic event. In these cases, serial radiographs are likely to reveal the true nature of the lesion, whereas a cross-sectional study, particularly MRI, may confuse matters further. If a cross-sectional study is to be performed, CT is to be preferred, as it is more likely to demonstrate the benign nature of the bony changes and help in excluding an associated mass.

PITFALLS

- The bony callus secondary to a healing avulsion fracture should not be misdiagnosed as an ossified or calcified neoplasm; the history, location of the injury, and knowledge of the musculotendinous insertion anatomy should yield the diagnosis. If any doubt exists, further radiographs after an interval with or without CT should resolve the dilemma.
- Ascribing a lesser trochanteric avulsion to simple trauma in a skeletally mature patient is dangerous without excluding the possibility of an underlying metastatic deposit.
- In the subacute and chronic stages, the MRI appearances of the involved bone can be quite aggressive and thus misleading. Reference should be made to the age, history, and location of the lesion to ensure that inappropriate biopsy is avoided.

Suggested Readings

Donnelly LF, Helms CA, Bisset GS 3rd. Chronic avulsive injury of the deltoid insertion in adolescents: imaging findings in three cases. Radiology 1999;211:233–236

Fernbach SK, Wilkinson RH. Avulsion injuries of the pelvis and proximal femur. Am J Roentgenol 1981;137:581–584

Heyse-Moore GH, Stoker DJ. Avulsion fractures of the scapula. Skeletal Radiol 1982;9:27–32

Khoury MB, Kirks DR, Martinez S, Apple J. Bilateral avulsion fractures of the anterior superior iliac spines in sprinters. Skeletal Radiol 1985;13:65–67

Rossi F, Dragoni S. Acute avulsion fractures of the pelvis in adolescent competitive athletes: prevalence, location and sports distribution of 203 cases collected. Skeletal Radiol 2001;30:127–131

Sundar M, Carty H. Avulsion fractures of the pelvis in children: a report of 32 fractures and their outcome. Skeletal Radiol 1994;23:85–90

CASE 93

Hema N. Choudur, Anthony G. Ryan, and Peter L. Munk

Clinical Presentation

An elderly woman sustained a fall when she inadvertently slipped on wet ground in her backyard. She was unable to pull herself up and was brought to the emergency department by her husband. On examination, she had pain and tenderness in her left groin and thigh and was unable to move her hip. The left lower limb was in external rotation. Her pulses and sensorimotor examination were normal.

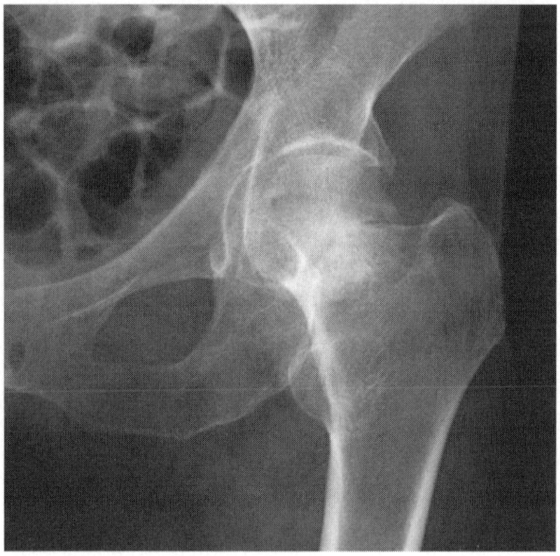

Figure 93A

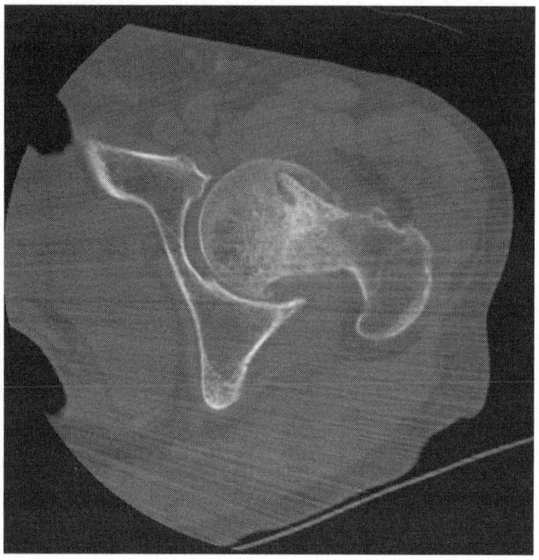

Figure 93B

Radiologic Findings

A plain radiograph (**Fig. 93A**) shows an impacted fracture of the left femoral neck. A CT scan (**Fig. 93B**) of the same patient delineates the undisplaced fracture line more clearly.

Diagnosis

Impacted fracture of the left midfemoral neck.

Differential Diagnosis

- Stress fractures in young athletes
- Pathologic fractures due to metastases or myeloma
- Insufficiency fractures due to osteomalacia or osteoporosis
- Paget's disease

Discussion

Background

Femoral neck fractures are very common and are associated with a high degree of morbidity and mortality; therefore, their diagnosis and treatment are of paramount importance. These fractures occur with a frequency of 1 in 1000 per year. One fourth of patients die within 6 months, and two thirds have persistent swelling and pain. Fewer than half return to preinjury level of function despite treatment.

Etiology

Whether a femoral neck fracture occurs or not depends on bone mineralization and the type of fall. Osteoporosis, osteomalacia, fatigue fractures, malignancy, and Paget's disease are the most frequently encountered etiologies of femoral neck fractures. The length of the femoral neck and the absence of osteoarthritis also have an influence.

For patients under the age of 55 years, femoral neck fractures are more common in men involved in road traffic accidents, but in patients over the age of 55, they are more common in women. After age 65, the increase is exponential in both sexes. These fractures are more common in Caucasian women than Black women.

Pathophysiology

The two proposed mechanisms in older individuals are a fall, producing a direct blow on the greater trochanter, and lateral rotation of the lower limb. A large direct force on the femoral shaft with or without a rotational component can cause similar injuries in young adults.

Even a minor trauma that goes unnoticed can cause a femoral neck fracture in an elderly osteoporotic woman. Osteopenia is by far the most common cause of femoral neck fractures, aside from Colles' and proximal humeral fractures.

Blood supply to the femoral head and neck involves two anastomotic rings: one extracapsular at the base of the neck, formed mainly by the medial and lateral circumflex femoral arteries posteroanteriorly, with contributions from the superior and inferior gluteal arteries, and the other a subsynovial intra-articular ring at the articular cartilage-neck junction formed by the retinacular arteries, which are branches of the ascending cervical arteries. The artery of the ligamentum teres in adults supplies only a small portion of the head, through its medial epiphyseal branches. The epiphysis is mainly supplied by the lateral and less so by the medial epiphyseal vessels and from the subsynovial ring. The metaphysis is supplied by the extracapsular ring, the ascending cervical arteries, and the subsynovial ring. Fracture may disrupt this blood supply. Because the head depends mainly on the retinacular vessels, avascular necrosis is an often-seen complication of femoral neck fractures. Inadequate reduction may also result in avascular necrosis from kinking or stretching of the supplying vessels. It is also important to note that the intracapsular neck does not heal by callus formation, as there is no cambium to its fibrous covering.

Clinical Findings

Inability to bear weight in the absence of any known trauma should prompt a clinician to evaluate the proximal femur in the elderly, as trivial trauma can result in unrecognized fractures.

The limb is held in external rotation, with pain, tenderness, and swelling in the region of the hip joint.

Imaging Findings

RADIOGRAPHY

Radiography delineates the fracture line or trabecular changes in most cases and fragment displacement/degree of comminution of the neck.

Common fracture types:

- *Subcapital fracture* The fracture line lies just below the femoral head.
- *Midcervical fracture* The fracture line lies in the mid neck (**Figs. 93C,93D**).
- *Basicervical fracture* The fracture line lies at the base of the femoral neck.
- *Subcapital and midcervical fractures* Intracapsular whereas the basicervical fractures are extracapsular. Intracapsular fractures are twice as common as extracapsular fractures.

Garden's is the most popular classification and is based on the degree of distortion of the medial trabecular lines. There are four types:

- *Type 1* Subcapital incomplete—stable injury with valgus configuration at the fracture site due to the externally twisted shaft
- *Type 2* Subcapital complete—no displacement, with the head in abduction. Stable fracture. Good prognosis
- *Type 3* Subcapital complete—partial displacement with the shaft externally displaced, and the head axially rotated and abducted. Head to neck in varus orientation
- *Type 4* Subcapital complete—complete displacement, with the head within the acetabulum, the shaft externally and proximally displaced in relationship to the head. Unstable with poor prognosis

Other types of proximal femoral fractures are the intertrochanteric and subtrochanteric, which occur along and below the intertrochanteric line, respectively. Although it may not always be easy to differentiate between these two fractures, the management plans for them do not differ markedly.

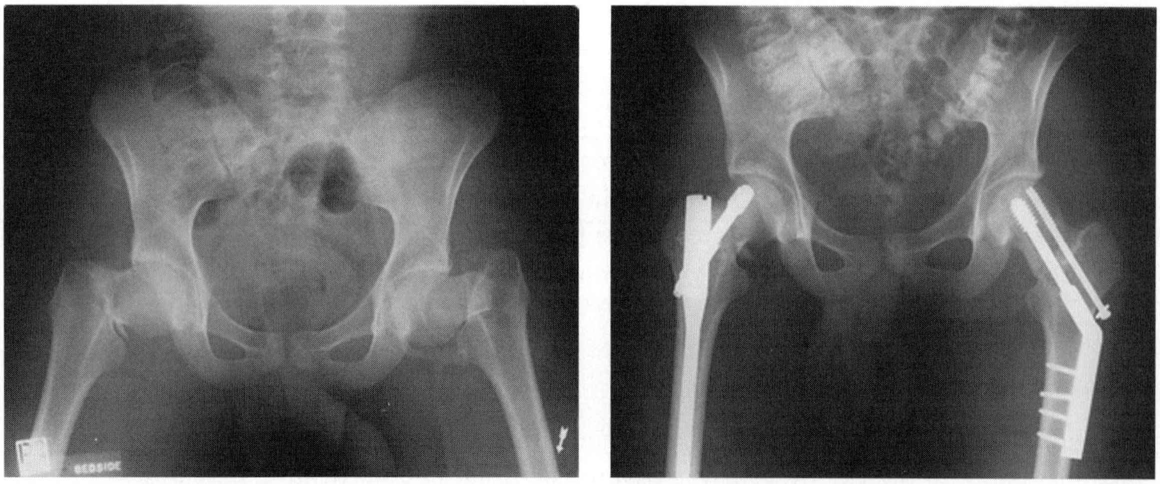

C D

Figures 93C,93D Bilateral cervical fractures of the femur before and after internal fixation.

Intertrochanteric fractures are seen frequently in older patients with osteopenia, usually after a direct or indirect trauma (**Figs. 93E–93G**). The fracture is considered stable if the medial cortices of the proximal and distal fragments are not comminuted, and there is no displacement of the lesser trochanter. Unstable fractures are those with comminution between the proximal and distal fragments, preventing their contact, and also posterior and medial displacement of the fractured fragments. Comminution of the greater trochanter and adjacent shaft and medial displacement of the distal fragment due to adductor pull render the fracture potentially unstable.

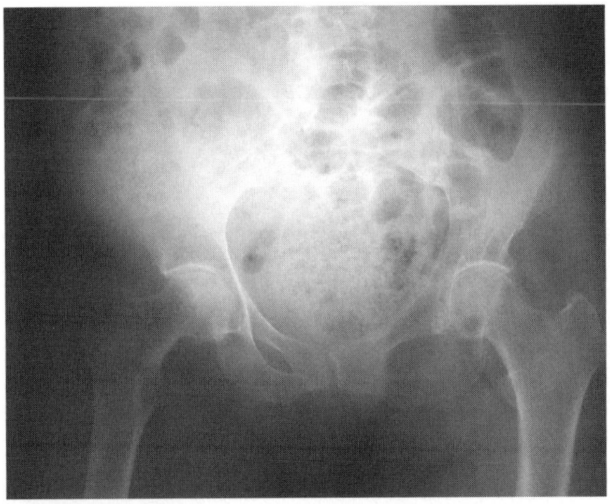

E

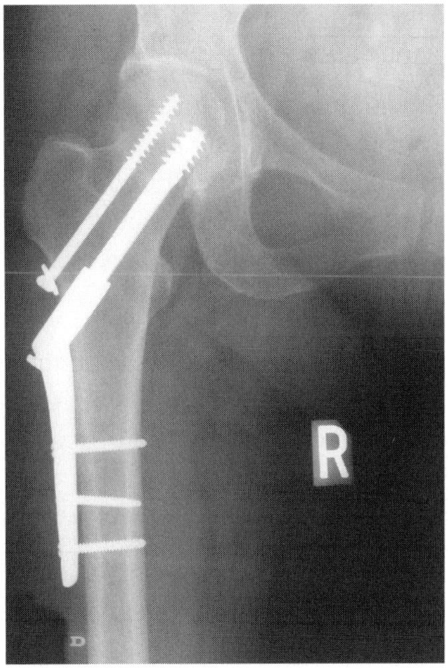

F

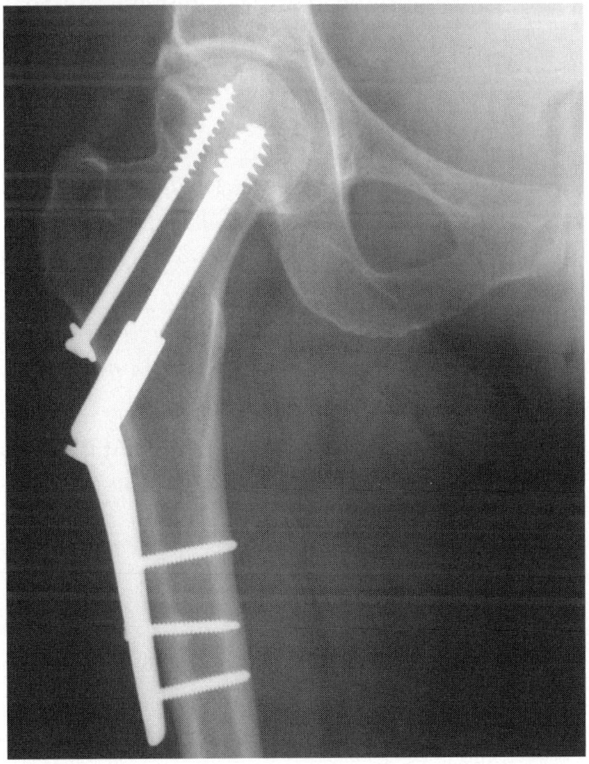

G

Figures 93E–93G An intertrochanteric fracture of the right femoral neck (**93E**) treated with a dynamic hip screw and additional pin (**93F**), complicated by avascular necrosis of the femoral head evinced by sclerosis, collapse, and partial fracture (**93G**).

Subtrochanteric fractures of the proximal femur occur in this region 5 to 30% of the time. They are seen in older individuals following minor trauma and younger persons following severe trauma. The degree of comminution is indicative of problems at fixation. The more distal the fracture, the greater is the tendency for nonunion and implant failure. **Figs. 93H** and **93I** show an unstable subtrochanteric fracture. The dynamic hip screw was replaced by a gamma nail, as there was no interval healing.

Isolated fractures of the greater trochanter can occur and are secondary to avulsion injuries in younger individuals or as a result of a direct force. In older persons, they often are the result of a fall. Lesser trochanter avulsion injuries occur in children. In the elderly, the latter should be suspected as representing a pathologic fracture.

COMPUTED TOMOGRAPHY

Although radiographs are the initial modality used in evaluating these fractures, stress fractures, subtle neck fractures (especially in osteoporotic bones), and some impacted fractures are best seen on CT. Also, the degree of comminution and the orientation of the fragments, as well as the relationship of the head and neck, are best evaluated by CT. CT is valuable in the follow-up of these patients in evaluating nonunion and avascular necrosis.

MAGNETIC RESONANCE IMAGING

- MRI is sometimes useful in early detection of occult fractures and stress fractures not visualized on plain radiographs. The fracture line is hypointense on T1-weighted images relative to marrow and hyperintense on T2-weighted images with edema around the site of fracture, better seen on inversion recovery sequences.
- MRI is also useful in detecting early avascular necrosis of the head following surgical treatment, in which case a prosthetic hip replacement is frequently required.

BONE SCANS

- Bone scans are positive 24 to 48 hours after the fracture and are as sensitive as MRI. They are best seen at 7 days, with 95% accuracy, and are also valuable in evaluating nonunion and avascular necrosis.

Treatment

Fixation of femoral neck fractures is performed with three screws aligned in the central portion of the head/neck, not reaching the subchondral surface, with a gap of at least 5 mm. This form of treatment is employed in younger, active patients and in older patients with a short life span or many medical problems.

Partial or total arthroplasty is indicated when there is a high risk of avascular necrosis or nonunion or following failure of screw fixation. It is also performed when the treatment is delayed, in chronically ill patients, and in those with severe disease in the native hip.

Basicervical, intertrochanteric, and subtrochanteric fractures are treated with plate and dynamic hip screw or and more displaced fractures with a gamma nail. These fractures carry a lower risk of avascular necrosis.

Complications

Complications include delayed union and nonunion (**Fig. 93K**). Normal union is evident in approximately 6 to 12 months. Nonunion occurs in 5 to 25% of the cases. There are many factors that lead to nonunion, including advanced age, demineralized bones, delayed fixation, improper reduction, and internal fixation, as well as posterior comminution of the fracture.

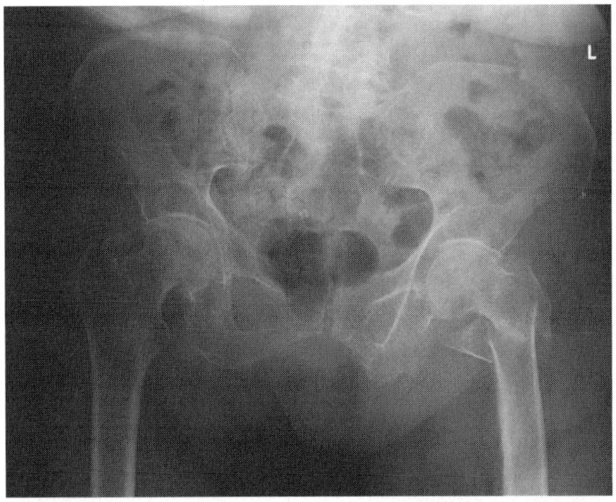

H

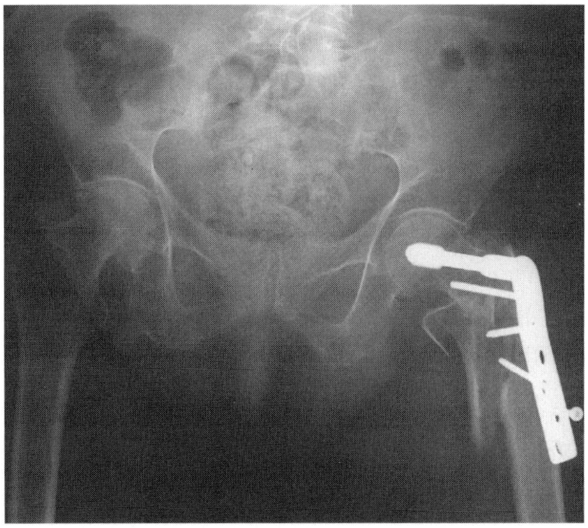

I

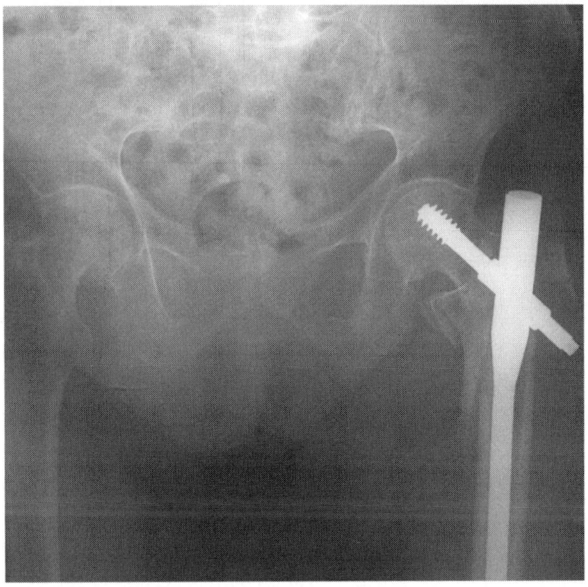

J

Figures 93H–93J Unstable, comminuted subtrochanteric fracture (**93H**), initially treated using a dynamic hip screw (**93I**) which was subsequently replaced by a gamma nail (**93J**), due to a lack of internal healing and persistent displacement.

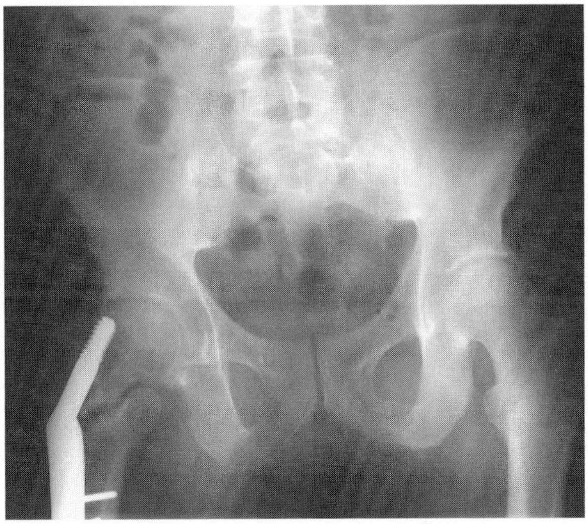

K

Figure 93K Image shows a basicervical/intertrochanteric fracture with loosening and displacement of the dynamic hip screw, resulting in nonunion.

Avascular necrosis is seen in 10 to 30% of cases, with increased risk following delayed treatment, damage to the blood vessels due to comminution, and displacement of the fracture. Persistent motion at the fracture site due to inadequate fixation is also cited as a cause of avascular necrosis.

Nonunion and avascular necrosis occur less often with intertrochanteric fractures.

Avascular necrosis is detected in follow-up radiographs as sclerosis of the head, a subchondral lucency, or irregularity of the articular surface (**Fig. 93G**). In later stages, the head may collapse. These changes may be seen from 3 months to 3 years following the fracture.

Posttraumatic thromboembolism, osteomyelitis following surgery, and septic arthritis are other complications.

Prognosis

One fourth of patients die within 6 months, and two thirds have persistent swelling and pain. Fewer than half of all patients return to preinjury level of function despite treatment.

PEARLS

- When an elderly woman is unable to bear weight, and plain radiographs are normal, a CT is mandatory, as a subtle fracture may be missed on plain radiographs.
- Bone scans become positive in 2 days to 1 week.

PITFALL

- Follow-up radiographs after fixation should be carefully evaluated for any avascular necrosis of the femoral head seen as increased density of the femoral head, subchondral lucency, or irregularity of the articular surface.

Suggested Readings

Caviglia HA, Osorio PQ, Comando D. Classification and diagnosis of intracapsular fractures of the proximal femur. Clin Orthop Relat Res 2002;399:17–27

Oakes DA, Jackson KR, Davies MR, et al. The impact of the Garden classification on proposed operative treatment. Clin Orthop Relat Res 2003;409:232–240

Pool FJ, Crabbe JP. Occult femoral neck fractures in the elderly: optimisation of investigation. N Z Med J 1996;109:235–237

CASE 94

Hema N. Choudur, Anthony G. Ryan, and Peter L. Munk

Clinical Presentation

A young person presented to the emergency department with severe pain and swelling in the medial aspect of the left clavicle, after being assaulted.

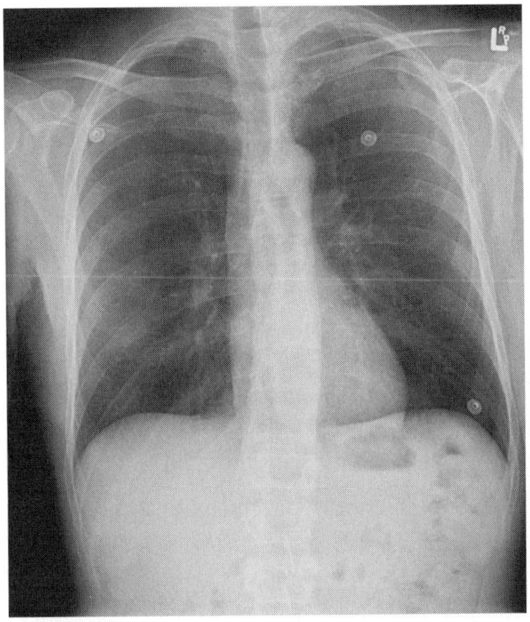

Figure 94A

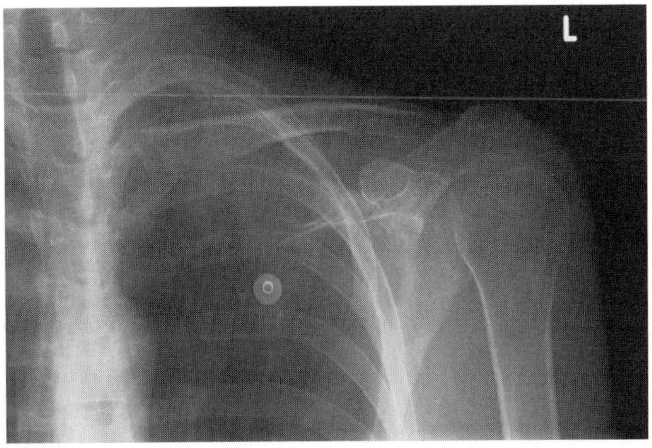

Figure 94B

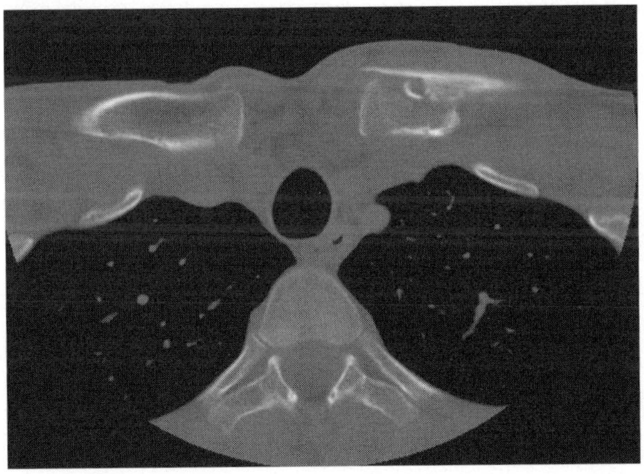

Figure 94C

Radiologic Findings

Plain radiographs of the chest (**Fig. 94A**) and left clavicle (**Fig. 94B**) show a subtle discontinuity of the interior cortex of the medial clavicle, suggestive of a fracture. The subsequent CT (**Fig. 94C**) confirms the minimally displaced fracture with no injury to the underlying structures. The sternoclavicular (SC) joint is seen to be congruent.

Diagnosis

Minimally displaced medial clavicular fracture.

Differential Diagnosis

Traumatic fractures must be differentiated from pathologic and stress fractures, the latter especially in gymnasts. Isolated SC dislocations can be differentiated with the help of CT.

Discussion

Medial clavicular fractures are fairly uncommon, accounting for only 5% of clavicular fractures. It is important to diagnose them accurately in view of the important mediastinal structures posteriorly.

Background

The clavicle is an S-shaped bony strut that connects the shoulder girdle to the axial skeleton. It is the first bone to ossify in utero by intramembranous ossification, with the medial and lateral endochondral ossifications occurring later. The medial epiphysis appears after age 12 years; it is the last ossification center to fuse in the entire skeleton and occurs around age 23 to 25. Many SC dislocations in young athletes are instead injuries of the medial physis of the clavicle. Of interest is the fact that the SC joint capsule is thought to be the strongest in the body.

The clavicle is attached securely to the medial aspect of the sternum and laterally to the scapula via the capsular and extra-articular ligaments, which maintain the width of the shoulders against gravity and muscle pull. The medial portion of the clavicle resists axial loading. It also protects the costoclavicular space, where the medial cord of the brachial plexus and the origin of the ulnar nerve are found. Fractures in this area put these structures at risk, as do clavicular nonunions and hypertrophic callus. The tubular shape of the medial clavicle and the flattened lateral clavicle place the medial clavicle at risk for fracture. In midclavicular fractures (**Figs. 94D,94E**), the sternocleidomastoid pulls the proximal fragment superiorly and posteriorly. The distal fragment is pulled inferiorly by the pectoralis major muscle and by gravity.

Etiology

The most common mechanism of injury is a direct blow secondary to contact sports or traffic accidents. Indirect mechanisms such as a fall on the outstretched arm or on the lateral border of the acromion can occur. In a fall on the acromion, the transmitted force passes across the acromioclavicular (AC) joint and clavicle medially to the SC joint. Failure can occur at any of these sites.

The muscles that originate or insert on the clavicle (deltoid, pectoralis major, trapezius, sternocleidomastoid, and subclavius) act as deforming forces after injury. Because the weakest point of the clavicle is the middle third, where it has the least support, fractures commonly occur at this site (80% of clavicular fractures). See **Fig. 94D**. Distal fractures account for about 15% and proximal fractures for only 5%.

Clinical Findings

Because the clavicle is a superficial bone, it can be examined easily, and emergency physicians can diagnose clavicular fractures with a high degree of certainty. In medial clavicular fractures, the diagnosis may be more difficult, with pain, soft-tissue swelling, and decreased mobility of the affected arm raising other differentials, such as SC dislocations and medial first rib fractures. Crepitus can usually be elicited at the site of fracture. Dyspnea from tracheal compression, pneumothorax, and dysphagia from esophageal compression can occur.

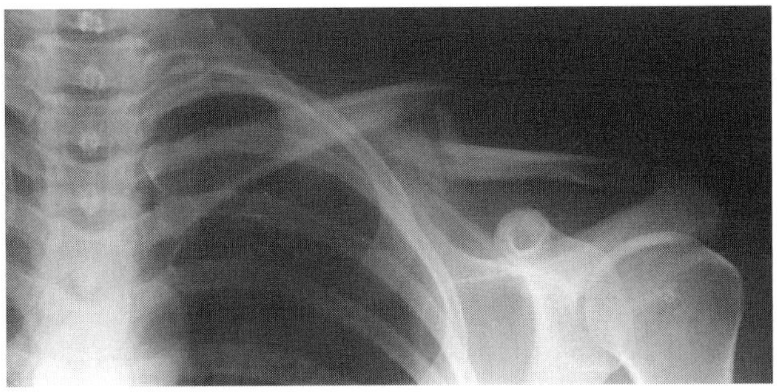
D

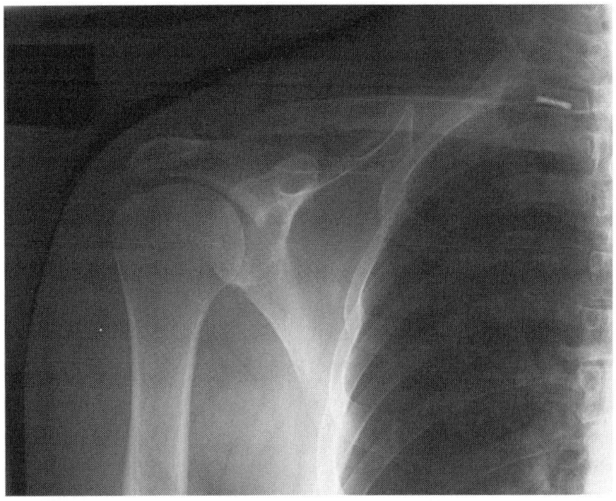
E

Figures 94D,94E Radiographs of a comminuted midclavicular fracture (**94D**) and a minimally displaced lateral clavicular fracture (**94E**).

Complications

Injury to the mediastinal vessels is the gravest complication of fractures of the medial third of the clavicle, especially with significant displacement. Fortunately, it is very rare. Associated SC joint dislocations, pneumothorax, and medial first rib injuries with compromise of the costoclavicular space can be ascertained with CT.

Imaging Findings

RADIOGRAPHY

Conventional anteroposterior radiographs may depict a displaced medial clavicular fracture; however, an undisplaced complete fracture of the medial clavicle may be missed unless an image is obtained with a 15-degree cephalic angulation.

In a skeletally immature person, a physeal injury may be mistaken for a SC dislocation. The position of the medial end of the clavicle may be higher than the normal side in anterior dislocations and lower in posterior dislocations at the SC joint. A CT scan will be helpful in differentiating the two.

In children, greenstick fractures, plastic bowing, and nondisplaced complete fractures can be visualized on radiographs supported by a good clinical history and examination.

ULTRASOUND

The usefulness of this modality lies in ruling out any damage to the superior mediastinal vessels by demonstrating normal color and duplex ultrasound. There are reports indicating ultrasound as a diagnostic tool for medial clavicular fractures in newborn infants following a birth injury. The fractured clavicle is visualized as a shorter echogenic line as compared with the normal side. Confirmation on plain radiographs or CT scan is, however, essential. Physeal injuries, which are similar to Salter-Harris fractures, are still a diagnostic dilemma.

COMPUTED TOMOGRAPHY

CT is essential in confirming equivocal undisplaced fractures of the medial clavicle. The degree of displacement is clearly depicted on the axial scans, as is the status of the superior mediastinal structures on contrast-enhanced images. Injury to the internal mammary, subclavian, and carotid vessels can be readily seen on CT. Also, the integrity of the trachea and esophagus can be well assessed.

Associated SC dislocations can be readily visualized, differentiating them from physeal injuries. Complicating pneumothorax can be easily diagnosed and dealt with by placement of a chest tube.

MAGNETIC RESONANCE IMAGING

There are reports in the literature on the use of MRI to rule out pathologic fractures of the clavicle, associated SC dislocations, and disruption of the neurovascular structures in the mediastinum. Fortunately, associated brachial plexus injuries, especially of the medial cord with ulnar nerve symptoms, are fairly uncommon.

Treatment

The uncomplicated, nondisplaced, or minimally displaced fractures of the medial clavicle are sufficiently dealt with by immobilization and support with a figure-8 bandage for about 4 to 6 weeks and appropriate pain management during the immediate period of injury. Comminuted fractures must be referred to the orthopedic surgeon for open reduction after evaluating the neurovascular status. Pneumothorax, vessel damage, and nerve palsy call for urgent consultation.

Prognosis

Return to normal activities is possible once the uncomplicated fracture has clinically and radiologically healed. However, contact sports are best avoided for 4 to 6 months. Prognosis is not as favorable in malunited/nonunited fractures with hypertrophic callus formation with pressure on the underlying structures. Débridement of the callus and open reduction are then indicated.

PEARLS

- A history of injury with focal pain over the medial clavicle should raise the suspicion of fracture.
- A CT helps to confirm the fracture in cases of doubt and to rule out an injury to the underlying vascular and neural structures when a fracture is present.

PITFALL

- Many undisplaced medial clavicular fractures are missed, as the plain radiographic findings are subtle and must be looked for carefully in the appropriate setting.

Suggested Readings

Sferopoulos NK. Fracture separation of the medial clavicular epiphysis: ultrasonography findings. Arch Orthop Trauma Surg 2003;123:367–369

Silloway KA, McLaughlin RE, Edlich RC, et al. Clavicular fractures and acromioclavicular joint dislocations in lacrosse: preventable injuries. J Emerg Med 1985;3:117–121

Stanley D, Trowbridge EA, Norris SH. The mechanism of clavicular fracture: a clinical and biomechanical analysis. J Bone Joint Surg Br 1988;70:461–464

CASE 95

Anthony G. Ryan and Peter L. Munk

Clinical Presentation

A 27-year-old man, traveling in the passenger seat of a car involved in a high-speed collision, presented with severe left-sided hip pain and an inability to move his left leg. An initial diagnosis of a posterior dislocation of the left hip was made, and closed reduction was performed emergently.

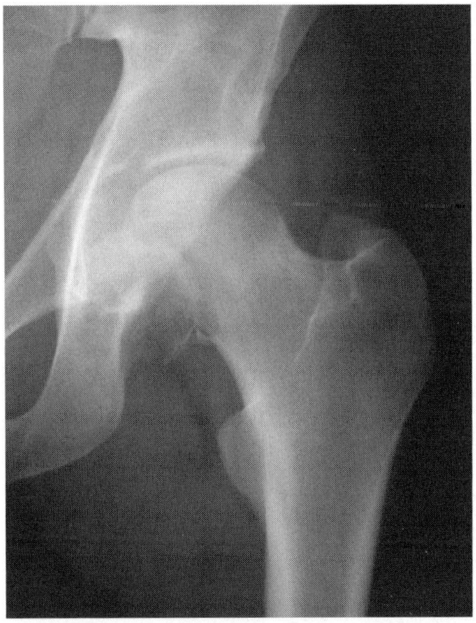

Figure 95A

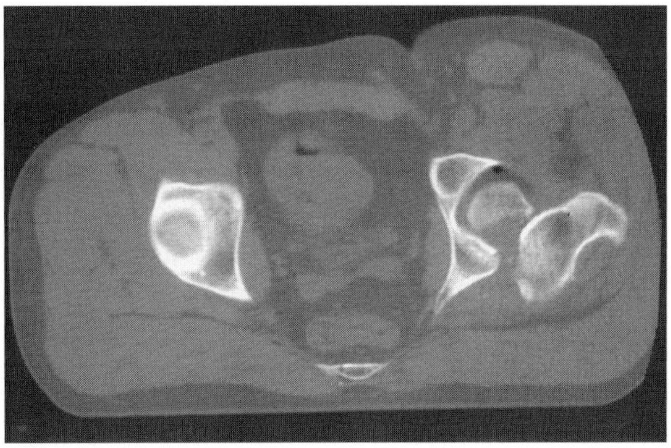

Figure 95B

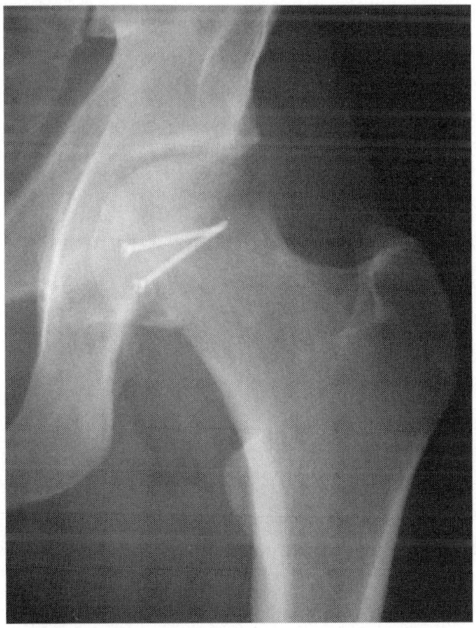

Figure 95C

Radiologic Findings

A coned anteroposterior (AP) radiograph of the left hip (**Fig. 95A**) shows a large crescentic radiodensity projected through the inferomedial half of the femoral head, which appears appropriately enlocated within the acetabulum.

The presence of the large free fragment prompted a decision to proceed to open reduction and internal fixation (ORIF), and radiology was consulted for a preoperative CT. A single slice from the CT (**Fig. 95B**) shows not only the large free fragment within the left hip joint but also that, despite the plain film appearances, the femoral head remains dislocated, necessitating formal relocation of the femoral head prior to reducing and fixating the large free fragment. A bubble of free nitrogen at the least dependent portion of the hip joint is evident, as is a subtle contained fluid-fluid level, the latter representing an intra-articular lipohemarthrosis. An AP radiograph of the subsequently relocated hip joint and fixated Pipkin fracture with 4.0-mm cancellous screws is shown in **Fig. 95C**.

Diagnosis

Hip dislocation complicated by Pipkin fracture and failed initial closed reduction, necessitating open reduction and fixation.

Differential Diagnosis

None.

Discussion

Background

Given the relative bony security of the joint, hip dislocation is uncommon, accounting for only 5% of all dislocations. Eighty to 85% of hip dislocations occur posteriorly (**Figs. 95A–95E**).

Posterior dislocations may be classified as two subtypes: those with and those without an accompanying fracture. The most common associated fracture is a single large fracture of the posterior acetabular rim, followed, in decreasing order of occurrence, by a comminuted fracture of the acetabular rim (**Fig. 99F**), a fracture of the acetabular rim and floor, and a fracture of the femoral head. Having passed through the sciatic notch, the femoral head usually occupies a position on the dorsum of the ilium.

Anterior dislocation occurs in about 5 to 10% of cases. The femoral head is displaced medially and toward the obturator foramen, pubis, or ilium. Anterior dislocations are further divided into superior and inferior subtypes: inferior dislocation occurring toward the obturator foramen and superior dislocation occurring toward the anterior superior iliac spine. There are two major types: the anterior obturator dislocation and the superoanterior pubic hip dislocation.

Central (internal) acetabular fracture dislocation refers to the head of the femur being driven medially, fracturing the acetabulum, and consequently protruding into the pelvic cavity secondary to an impact to the lateral side of the greater trochanter. There is thus an invariable accompanying acetabular fracture.

Rarely, luxatio erecta of the hip joint may occur, whereby traumatic hip dislocation results in inferior dislocation of the femoral head and inversion of the femoral shaft.

Etiology

POSTERIOR DISLOCATION

The classic injury involves a passenger in a sudden deceleration motor vehicle accident where the knee is struck forcibly against the dashboard, pushing the hip joint out posteriorly. At the moment

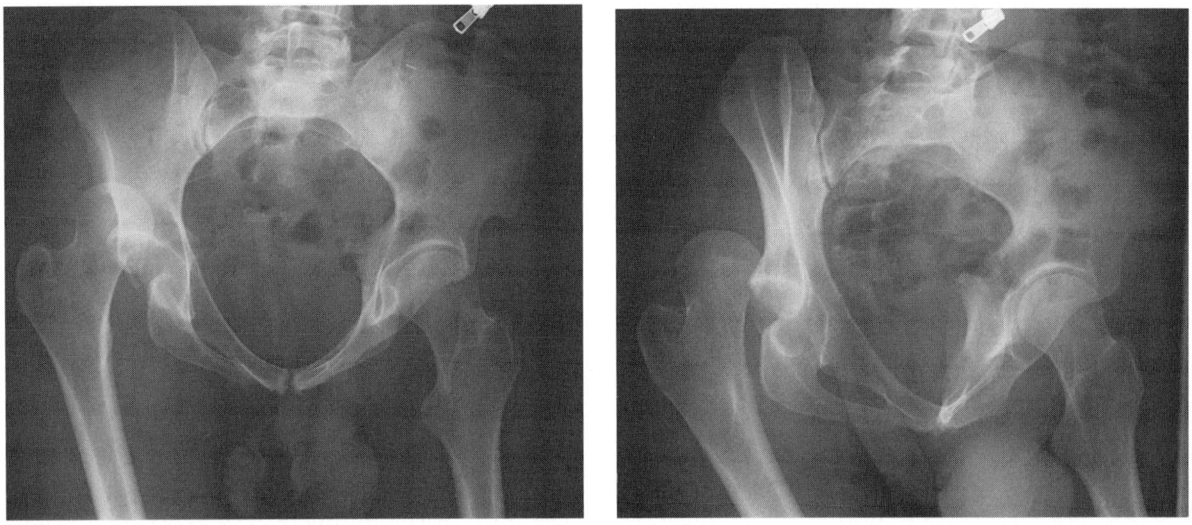

Figures 95D,95E An anteroposterior radiograph of the right hip (**95D**) shows clear dislocation of the right hip with superior displacement of the femoral head and femoral neck acetabular approximation. There is an associated comminuted fracture of the posterior acetabular margin and an associated fracture of the femoral head margin. Note the curvilinear density lateral to the femoral head. Although the above signs suggest a posterior direction of displacement, the subspinous location of the femoral head raises the possibility of an anterior dislocation. An additional Judet view (**95E**) was performed, confirming the direction of dislocation as posterior.

of impact, the affected leg is typically flexed and "crossed" over the midline. In this position, the femoral head is covered posteriorly only by capsule. The femoral head is driven posterolaterally and is maintained in a position superior to the level of the acetabulum by muscular contraction and spasm. The dislocation may occur on the job, for example, by a large weight landing on the back of a person leaning forward, whereby the femur remains stationary and the pelvis is pushed anteriorly.

ANTERIOR DISLOCATION

An anterior injury may occur from a direct blow on the posterior aspect of the abducted and externally rotated thigh, as may occur secondary to a fall from a height or an impact with the leg in this position (pointing laterally) during a high-energy contact sport.

CENTRAL ACETABULAR FRACTURE DISLOCATION

The typical mechanism is a blow to the lateral aspect of the hip, usually secondary to road traffic accidents, and occasionally following a fall on the side, usually from a considerable height.

TRANSIENT SUBLUXATION OR DISLOCATION WITH REDUCTION

When transient subluxation or dislocation with reduction has occurred, and there is no associated fracture, the pattern of associated muscle injury may be a useful secondary sign that such an injury has taken place.

In transient subluxation or dislocation, there may be mechanical disruption of the blood supply to the femoral head. Hemarthrosis may also contribute to vascular impairment. These patients are thus at increased risk of osteonecrosis, chondrolysis, and secondary osteoarthritis. The incidence of osteonecrosis increases with the delay in reduction of a dislocated hip.

Chondrolysis is manifest on plain films as loss of joint space, and both chondrolysis and osteonecrosis may be accurately detected with MRI.

Pathophysiology

The forces required to dislocate the hip are rarely generated during sporting activities, and hip dislocations are consequently unusual. Transient subluxation or dislocation with spontaneous reduction may occur in contact sports, however. They may be considered a muscle strain initially, and the subluxation may go unrecognized, particularly if there is not an associated acetabular rim fracture.

Clinical Findings

POSTERIOR DISLOCATION

The patient will complain of severe pain in the hip region and loss of motion. On examination, the typical deformity is that of flexion, adduction, and internal rotation with shortening of the affected limb, resulting in apposition of the sole of the affected foot with the instep of the contralateral foot. Evidence of injury to the knee may be seen (suggesting the mechanism of action), such as laceration, abrasion, or an accompanying fracture.

ANTERIOR DISLOCATION

The patient complains of severe pain and inability to move the hip. The typical deformity is flexion, abduction, and external rotation of the involved limb. The head of the femur may be palpable in the groin or in the vicinity of the anterior iliac spine.

CENTRAL ACETABULAR FRACTURE DISLOCATION

The patient experiences severe pain and loss of motion. There is no obvious deformity, although a hematoma and tenderness over the trochanter may be present. Attempts to move the hip are extremely painful.

Sciatic nerve injury is diagnosed by the inability of the patient to dorsiflex the foot and loss of sensation on the dorsum of the foot.

Complications

Complications arising with posterior dislocation and associated fractures are malunion after either conservative management or surgical fixation, with or without consequent osteoarthritis and avascular necrosis.

Other complications include the following:

- Osteochondral impaction fractures of the femoral head are present in as many as 63% of patients with posterior hip dislocation and in all patients with anterior dislocation.
- There may be associated femoral shaft and knee injuries.
- Avascular necrosis of the femoral head may be seen.
- Also seen is associated sciatic nerve injury (in up to 10% of cases), the incidence of which is limited by early reduction (15% if reduced within 8 hours, increasing to 50% if there is further delay in reduction).
- Rarely, if the time to relocation is prolonged, femoral vein and/or arterial thrombosis may occur.

ANTERIOR DISLOCATION

Fractures of the femoral head after anterior dislocation are characterized by a depression or "flattening" of the posterosuperior and lateral portion of the femoral head secondary to impaction at the time of dislocation.

Complications include

- Fractures of the anterior acetabular rim
- Additional fractures of the greater trochanter or the femoral neck
- Avascular necrosis of the femoral head (seen in 20 to 30% of cases)
- Posttraumatic osteoarthrosis
- Myositis ossificans

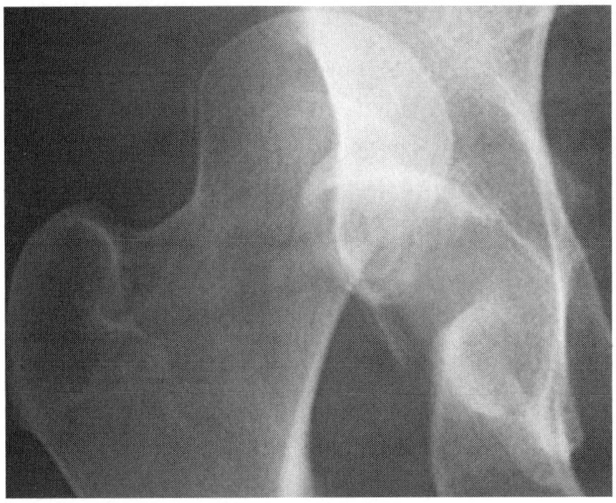

Figure 95F Enlarged view of **95D** shows more clearly the comminuted fracture of the posterior acetabular rim.

CENTRAL ACETABULAR FRACTURE DISLOCATION

Posttraumatic osteoarthrosis is almost universal after this injury, regardless of treatment, presumed to be as a result of the massive cartilaginous insult.

TRANSIENT SUBLUXATION OR DISLOCATION WITH REDUCTION

These patients are at increased risk of osteonecrosis, secondary to mechanical disruption of the blood supply to the femoral head during the subluxation/dislocation. The incidence of osteonecrosis increases with the delay in reduction of a dislocated hip. Hemarthrosis may also contribute to vascular impairment.

- Chondrolysis and consequent secondary osteoarthritis
- Associated muscle injury

Imaging Findings

RADIOGRAPHY

The principle signs of posterior dislocation are

- A dislocated hip
- Approximation of the femoral metaphysis to the acetabulum
- Deformity or posterior displacement of the fat plane anterior to the gluteus maximus
- A soft-tissue mass projecting behind the ischium

Oblique and coned-down radiographs aid considerably in the evaluation of the dislocated hip, particularly in the assessment of potentially obscure femoral head and acetabular injuries, which are frequently occult on the initial radiographs.

Because posterior dislocation of the hip produces superior displacement of the femoral head, inferoanterior dislocation is unlikely to be mistaken for a posterior dislocation on an anteroposterior radiograph of the pelvis. However, because of the shared superior displacement, the appearance of superoanterior dislocation on AP radiographs can be misleading, resulting in a misdiagnosis of a posterior dislocation. This misdiagnosis potentially results in failure of attempted closed reduction or, where an operative course is planned, in an incorrect surgical approach. In addition, recognition of an associated femoral head impaction fracture is crucial, as patients with this finding have a greater tendency to develop traumatic arthritis.

Chondrolysis is manifest on plain films as a loss of joint space.

COMPUTED TOMOGRAPHY

In the absence of penetrating trauma, intracapsular gas bubbles (representing intracapsular nitrogen bubbles resulting from the vacuum created by forcible distraction associated with dislocation) on CT are reliable indicators of recent hip dislocation (**Fig. 95B**) and may occasionally be the only objective finding. Gas bubbles are seen in as many as 81% of dislocated hips, including 92% of dislocations in patients scanned within 4 hours of admission. In one study, bubbles were present in 79% of reduced hip dislocations.

CT demonstrates an anterior cortical fracture of the femoral head (caused by impaction of the anterior femoral head against the posterior acetabular rim at the time of dislocation), not detected on plain radiographs, in up to 13% of cases.

This injury, which has been described as the Hill-Sachs lesion of the femur, is associated with fractures of the posterior acetabulum in 86% of cases.

ARTHROGRAPHY

Indications for arthrography include the following:

- Where a capsular tear is suspected as the cause of posttraumatic recurrent hip dislocation (a pseudobursa will be seen at the site of the capsular tear, which usually coincides with the direction of dislocation)
- Where an unsuccessful reduction of the hip joint is thought to be secondary to an internal joint derangement (although no intra-articular contrast was employed in the case depicted in **Fig. 95B**)

MAGNETIC RESONANCE IMAGING

Early signs of injuries after hip dislocation will be best detected using a combination of transaxial T1-, coronal T1-, and coronal T2-weighted (MPGR) sequences. Joint effusion/hemarthrosis is a universal finding.

Findings related to posterior dislocations include

- Isolated femoral head contusions (trabecular microfractures)
- Osteochondral defect
- Acetabular lip fractures
- Labral tear
- Intra-articular loose bodies
- Ligamentum teres entrapment
- Iliofemoral ligament injury
- Posterior fascial compartment injury

Findings related to anterior dislocations include

- Bony contusion
- Cortical fracture
- Labral tear
- Iliofemoral ligament injury

There are typical patterns of muscular compartment injuries depending on the direction of dislocation; that is, posterior dislocations give rise to posterior fascial compartment injury, whereas anterior dislocations give rise to anterior and medial fascial compartment injuries, with additional injuries to the gluteals.

MRI is the investigation of choice in demonstrating these injuries, the signs of which are most useful in the instance where the joint has spontaneously reduced after a transient subluxation/ dislocation, when the muscular injury is the only evidence that such a disruption has occurred. When transient subluxation or dislocation with reduction has occurred, and there is no associated fracture, the pattern of associated muscle injury may be a useful secondary sign that such an injury has taken place.

In transient subluxation or dislocation, avascular necrosis of the femoral head is a significant risk secondary to mechanical disruption of the blood supply to the femoral head and vascular impairment exacerbated by the presence of a hemarthrosis. MRI is the most sensitive investigation to detect the early changes of osteonecrosis.

Chondrolysis and osteochondral injuries are also best demonstrated by MRI.

In the later stages of investigation, evidence of secondary osteoarthritis may be present.

Treatment

POSTERIOR DISLOCATION

If there is no associated fracture,

- The femoral head should be relocated emergently to minimize the risk of avascular necrosis and sciatic nerve injury. The muscle bulk around the pelvic girdle and attendant spasm cannot usually be overcome without a general anesthetic to enable relocation.
- Relocation is followed by a 3-week period of immobilization using lower limb skin-traction with the hip in slight abduction, externally rotated and extended.
- Once there is painless motion at the hip, the patient is mobilized, and protected weight-bearing exercises are employed for 3 months.

Fracture Dislocation of the Femoral Head

If there is an associated fracture of the femoral head, studies have shown that ORIF provide greatest stability and minimize the incidence of posttraumatic osteoarthrosis.

Fracture dislocations of the femoral head are uncommon and are associated with a variable clinical outcome. In an attempt to stratify the injuries into distinct treatment groups, Pipkin (1957) classified femoral head fractures as

- *Type I* Femoral head fracture distal to the fovea
- *Type II* Femoral head fracture proximal to the fovea
- *Type III* Type I or II fracture associated with a femoral neck fracture
- *Type IV* Type I or II fracture associated with an acetabular rim fracture

As modified by Zehi et al in 1997, the classification system concentrates on the state of the femoral head alone:

- *Type I* Small fracture of the femoral head caudad to the fovea centralis (may be too small or too fragmented to be screw-fixated)
- *Type II* Larger fracture of the femoral head caudad to the fovea centralis
- *Type III* Large fracture of the femoral head proximal to the fovea centralis
- *Type IV* Comminuted fracture of the femoral head

Treatment options include

- Conservative/nonoperative treatment
- Excision of fracture fragments
- ORIF
- Arthroplasty
- Arthrodesis

Based on Zehi et al's modification, the following treatment stratification may be used:

- *Type 1* Excision of the fragment
- *Type II or III* Early accurate reduction with stable internal fixation
- *Type IV* Arthroplasty

Type II fractures are typically treated by ORIF via an anterior approach. Surgical dislocation is occasionally required to effect adequate fixation with countersunk 4.0-mm cancellous screws. After ORIF, patients are generally non–weight-bearing for 6 weeks postoperatively and progress to full weight bearing by 3 months.

Using this approach in type II fractures (the most common Pipkin fracture) results in a 92% clinical success rate.

ANTERIOR DISLOCATION

- As in posterior dislocation, the femoral head should be relocated emergently. Closed reduction is usually possible under general anesthesia, which, again, is followed by a period of immobilization using traction with the hip in slight abduction.

CENTRAL ACETABULAR FRACTURE DISLOCATION

Central acetabular fracture dislocations have been subclassified according to the pattern of the accompanying acetabular fracture:

- *Type 1* Intact acetabular roof with a large displaced fragment
- *Type 2* Completely disorganized acetabulum ("bag of bones")

Treatment is by type.

- *Type 1* Open reduction with internal fixation is usually possible.
- *Type 2* Anatomic reduction is usually not possible, and so the aim is to create a neoacetabulum by secondary intention using a conservative approach, that is, immobilization in traction followed by crutches for a period of 3 months.

Sciatic nerve injury is usually treated expectantly with a foot drop splint.

Prognosis

The incidence of sciatic nerve injury is said to be 15% if the dislocation is reduced within 8 hours but increases to 50% if there is further delay between reduction. Spontaneous recovery is usual unless the nerve is directly lacerated or is entrapped in fragments.

Avascular necrosis of the femoral head occurs in 20 to 30% of cases of anterior dislocation, the incidence dependent on the duration of dislocation prior to return to joint mobility.

Posttraumatic osteoarthrosis is invariable after a central acetabular fracture dislocation.

PEARLS

- If transient dislocation has occurred, in the presence of a femoral head impaction injury, the site of the femoral head injury permits the direction of the original dislocation to be inferred. Equally, when the direction of the original dislocation is known, the site of femoral head impaction can be predicted.
- In patients with posterior dislocation, the impaction occurs anteriorly in an arc between 11 and 1 o'clock.
- In those with anterior dislocation, osteochondral impaction occurs at the posterolateral aspect of the femoral head between 4 and 5 o'clock.
- When transient subluxation or dislocation with reduction has occurred, and there is no associated fracture, the pattern of associated muscle injury is a useful secondary sign suggesting that such an injury has taken place.

PITFALLS

- After closed reduction of a dislocated hip, a persistently widened hip joint indicates possible intra-articular osteochondral debris or retained femoral head fragments and should prompt further investigation via CT.
- A lateral view should always be attempted, as dislocation is frequently undetected by the initial AP radiograph performed as part of the routine trauma series.
- Ensure that a radiograph of the pelvis is performed if you diagnose a femoral shaft fracture to ensure a concomitant dislocation is not missed.
- Similarly, if a fracture of the acetabular rim (posterior or superior) is diagnosed, a dislocation must be presumed to have occurred, even if the joint is enlocated at initial radiography.

Suggested Readings

Glynn TP Jr, Kreipke DL, DeRosa GP. Computed tomography arthrography in traumatic hip dislocation: intra-articular and capsular findings. Skeletal Radiol 1989;18:29–31

Janzen DL, Munk PL, Connell DG, O'Brien PJ. Bilateral traumatic posterior hip dislocation: CT findings. Australas Radiol 1991;35:264–265

Laorr A, Greenspan A, Anderson MW, Moehring HD, McKinley T. Traumatic hip dislocation: early MRI findings. Skeletal Radiol 1995;24:239–245

Pipkin G. Treatment of grade IV fracture-dislocation of the hip. J Bone Joint Surg Am 1957;39-A(5):1027–1042

Tehranzadeh J, Vanarthos W, Pais MJ. Osteochondral impaction of the femoral head associated with hip dislocation: CT study in 35 patients. Am J Roentgenol 1990;155:1049–1052

Zehi K, Karray S, Litaiem T, Douik M. Fracture-luxation of the femur head. Acta Orthop Belg 1997;63:268–273

CASE 96

Hema N. Choudur, Anthony G. Ryan, and Peter L. Munk

Clinical Presentation

An elderly inpatient was sent for a chest radiograph after an awkward fall in the hospital.

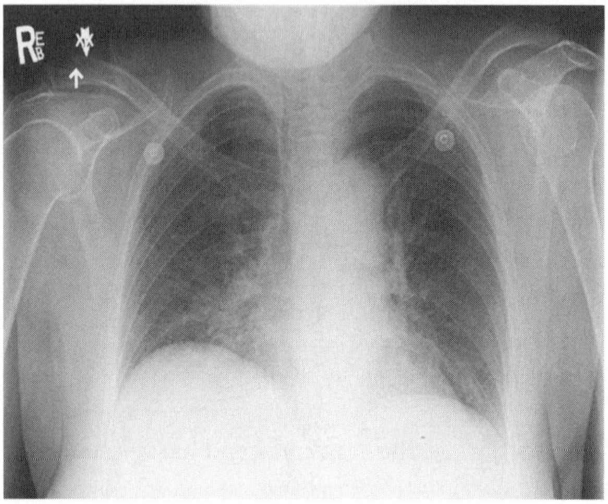

Figure 96A

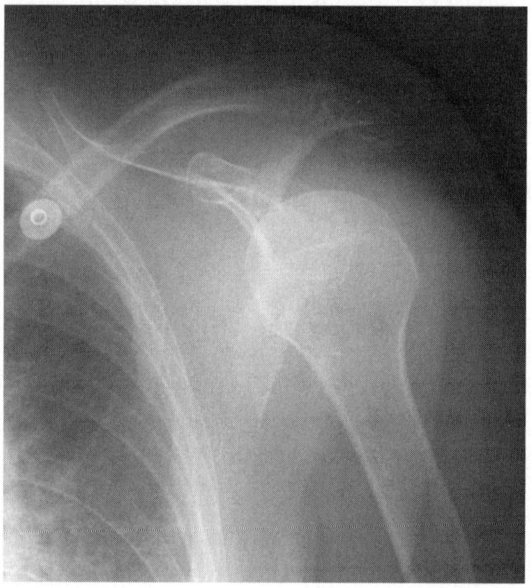

Figure 96B

Radiologic Findings

The chest radiograph (**Fig. 96A**), initially reported as showing no bone or joint abnormality, was reviewed, with the additional information that the patient complained of ongoing left shoulder pain. The radiograph shows the humeral head to be in a subcoracoid location. Further shoulder views (anteroposterior (AP), **Fig. 96B;** trans-scapular, **Fig. 96C**) confirm the subcoracoid, anterior location of the humeral head with respect to the glenoid.

Although both the postreduction AP (**Fig. 96D**) and axillary (**Fig. 96E**) views confirm relocation, the axillary view also demonstrates cortical discontinuity and a subchondral lucent line on the anterior aspect of the glenoid rim. Transaxial CT images (**Figs. 96F–96H**, from superior to inferior) demonstrate a minimally displaced fracture with a degree of fragmentation and a subchondral fracture line.

Diagnosis

Anterior dislocation of the left shoulder with a Bankart lesion.

Differential Diagnosis

None.

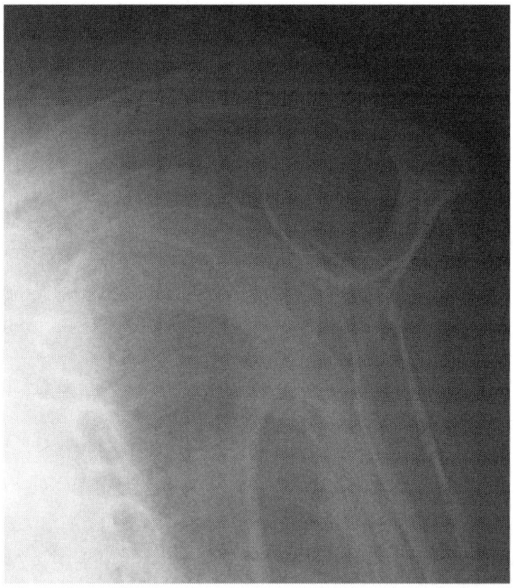

Figure 96C

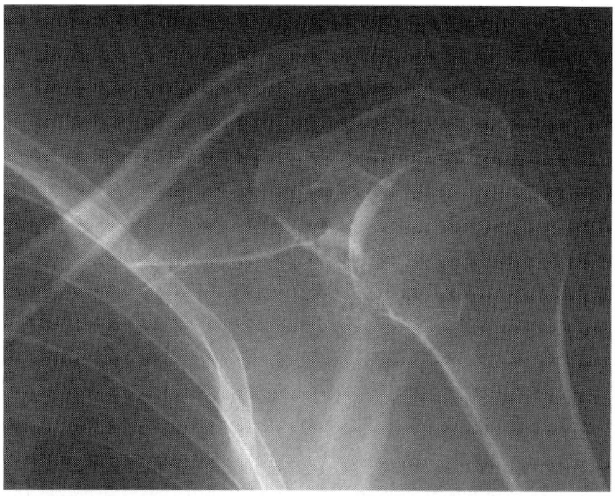

Figure 96D

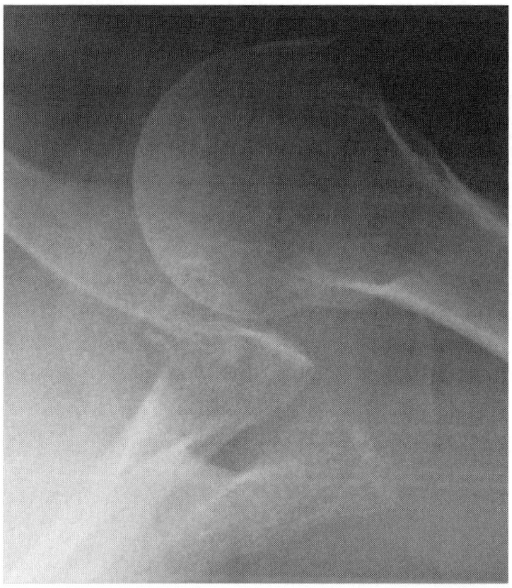

Figure 96E

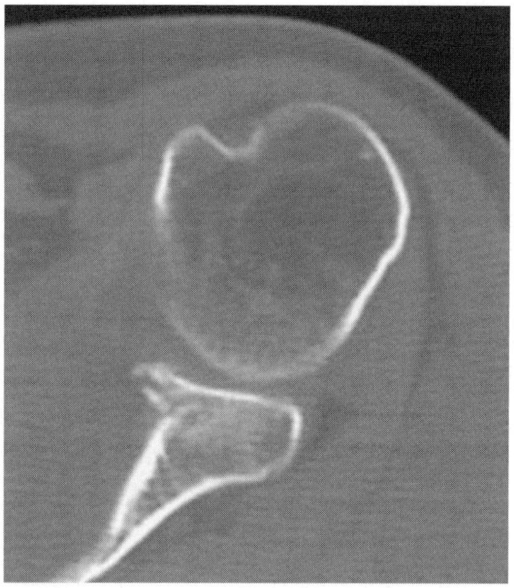

Figure 96F

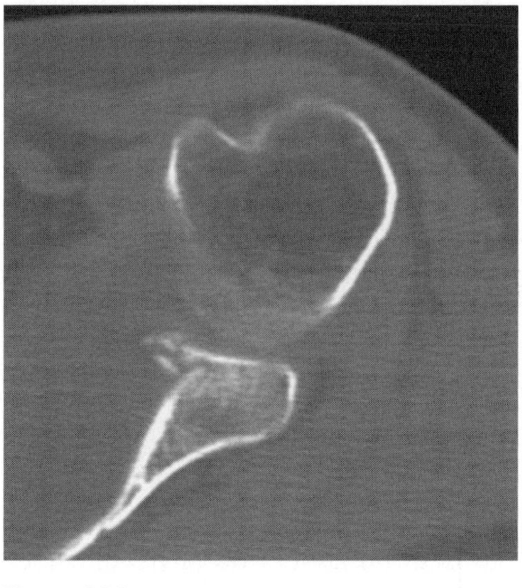

Figure 96G

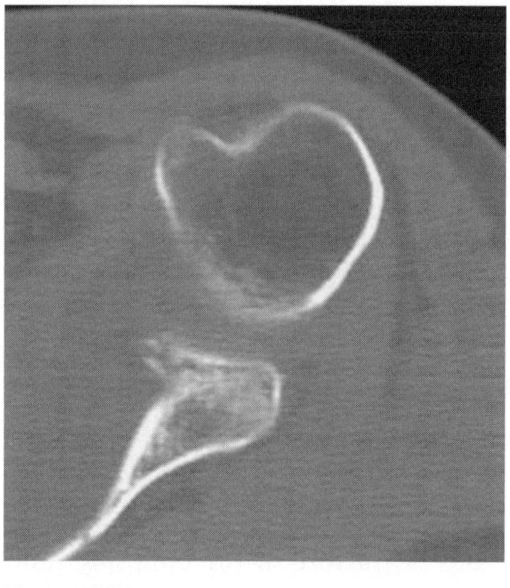

Figure 96H

Discussion

Background

The shoulder accounts for 50% of all joint dislocations. Traumatic anterior dislocations are the most common (90 to 98%), most of which are subcoracoid in location. Subglenoid, subclavicular, and, very rarely, intrathoracic dislocations may occur. Whereas labral tears following traumatic dislocation are more common in individuals younger than 40 years, rotator cuff tears are more frequent in older individuals.

Etiology

The vast majority of shoulder dislocations are traumatic, with several predisposing factors identified: a small or flat glenoid fossa, excessive anteversion or retroversion of the glenoid (a dysplastic glenoid is present in 13% of patients), weak rotator cuff muscles, neuromuscular disorders, or a redundant capsule result in a decrease in humeroglenoid stability. Also, laxity of ligaments as seen in Marfan or Ehlers-Danlos syndrome can result in nontraumatic dislocations, for example, after a sneeze or minimal motion.

Pathophysiology

Anterior dislocation is most commonly caused by forceful abduction and/or external rotation alone (in ~30% of cases); however, a direct blow to the posterior humerus, forced elevation and external rotation, or a fall onto an outstretched hand may also be causative.

Posterior glenohumeral dislocations are uncommon and account for ~2 to 10% of all shoulder dislocations. They can occur following a fall with the arm in adduction, internal rotation, and flexion, or following electroshock therapy and seizures. A direct blow to the anterior shoulder uncommonly can result in a posterior dislocation.

Inferior dislocations are rare and result from a hyperabduction force. Diagnosing inferior dislocations is crucial because of the high incidence of associated complications.

Superior dislocations are extremely rare and result from an extreme cephalad force to the adducted arm. Acromioclavicular injuries and fractures of the acromion, clavicle, and tuberosities are common attendants of such injuries.

Clinical Findings

In anterior dislocation, the patient presents with the arm in abduction and external rotation, with painful internal rotation. The humeral head can be palpated in front of the joint.

In posterior dislocation, the patient presents with the arm in adduction and internal rotation. The glenoid cavity is empty, and the coracoid is very prominent. The head may be seen prominently posteriorly.

In inferior dislocation (luxatio erecta), the patient presents with the arm in extreme abduction with the forearm held above the head—an Aunt Minnie of physical diagnosis.

Complications

- Bankart lesions (fractures of the glenoid rim secondary to impaction of the dislocating humeral head) occur in 80 to 90% of patients. These lesions may be purely bony, with a fracture of the anterior glenoid rim and an intact labrum.
- Hill-Sachs lesions (a fracture of the opposing humerus) are seen in about 70% of patients (see below). Loose bodies may result from this injury.

- Inferior glenoid labral tears occur in 50% of patients.
- Posterior glenoid labral tears occur in 11% of patients.
- Superior labrum anterior to posterior (SLAP) lesions are found in 8% of patients.
- Glenohumeral ligament insufficiency occurs in 50% of patients.
- Older patients are less likely to have a Bankart lesion and more likely to have a cuff tear, a greater tuberosity fracture, or an avulsion of the capsule and subscapularis from the lesser tuberosity. Younger patients have labral tears more frequently. Coracoid fractures can also occur.
- Partial or complete rotator cuff tears occur in about 10% of patients.
- Partial subscapularis tear occurs in 8% of patients.
- Biceps tendon lesions are found in 12% of patients.
- Brachial plexus injuries are in 11% of patients.
- Axillary nerve injuries occur in 8 to 10% of patients. In those suspected of having a brachial plexus injury, an angiogram (especially in the elderly) to rule out associated rupture of the axillary artery may be necessary. Pseudoaneurysms can occur in recurrent dislocations. Subclavian vein thrombosis can occur.
- Loose bodies are found in 5% of patients.

Radiologic Findings

RADIOGRAPHY

AP view (neutral/internal/external), trans-scapular Y, and axillary views are mandatory pre- and postreduction to confirm the presence and the direction and also to assess the postreduction location of the humeral head.

The axillary view clearly depicts glenohumeral subluxation or dislocation and anterior or posterior glenoid rim fractures. A standard axillary view is likely to be painful following an acute injury, as it requires 90 degrees of abduction; however, modified views avoiding excessive movement of the painful extremity are possible. The transverse axillary lateral requires the patient to abduct the arm only 10 to 30 degrees.

The scapular Y view is helpful for diagnosing dislocations and scapular fractures. This view, however, should not replace the axillary view because it does not show subtle subluxations of the glenohumeral joint or fractures of the glenoid rim.

In anterior dislocation, the humeral head located in the subcoracoid position raises the suspicion on the AP view (**Fig. 96A**), and is confirmed on the trans-scapular Y and axillary views.

Following reduction, fractures of the humerus, especially the greater trochanter, should be sought.

An associated impression of the anteroinferior glenoid rim on the posterolateral humeral head called the Hill-Sachs lesion is often visualized, more so in recurrent dislocations (**Figs. 96I–96L**). It is best seen in an AP view in internal rotation. A fracture of the anteroinferior glenoid rim may also occur, referred to as a Bankart lesion (**Figs. 96F–96H**).

In posterior dislocation, the axillary and trans-scapular views are far more contributory in diagnosing the posterior location of the humeral head with respect to the glenoid cavity.

The AP view may reveal a subtle increase in joint space between the anterior humeral margin and the inferior glenoid margin. Forty to 50% of such dislocations are overlooked on the initial evaluation, especially on the conventional AP-view radiographs.

The signs of a posterior dislocation on an AP view are

- The humeral head is fixed in internal rotation, resulting in overlapping of the humeral head and the glenoid margin.
- The distance between the articular surface of the humeral head and the inferior glenoid lip may be increased > 6 mm.

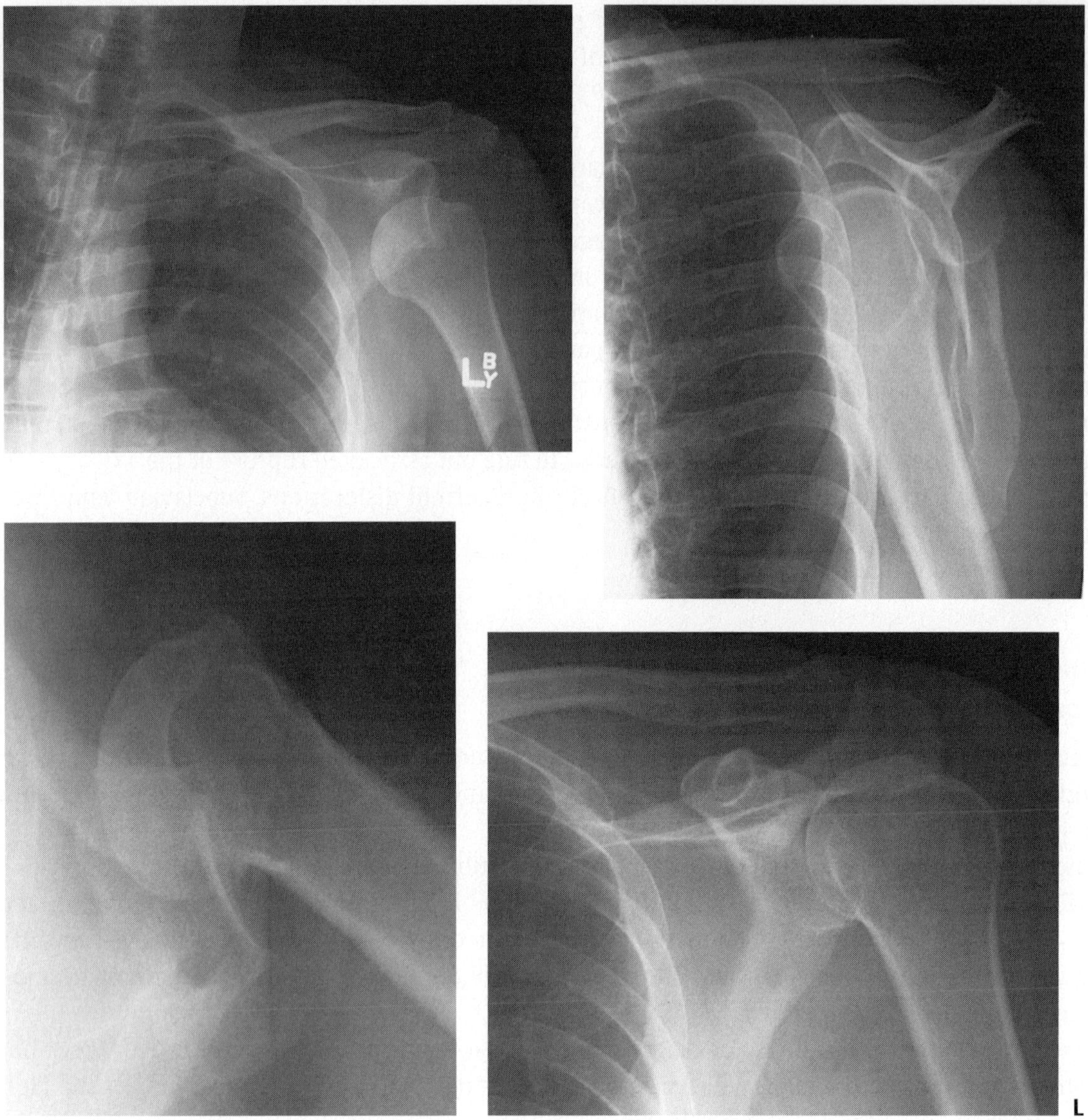

Figures 96I–96L AP (**96I**), trans-scapular (**96J**), and axial (**96K**) views show a clear anterior subcoracoid dislocation. **96L** Postreduction AP radiograph with the shoulder internally rotated shows a vertical line projected through the outer third of the humeral head, at the level of the tip of the acromion, typical of a Hill-Sachs lesion.

- A vacant glenoid cavity is seen.
- A vertical line (the "trough" line) may be seen in the medial aspect of the humeral head and indicates the presence of a compression fracture.
- There may be an associated fracture of the lesser tuberosity.

Inferior dislocation is least common and is best seen on the AP and trans-scapular Y views. It should be differentiated from pseudosubluxation, in which the presence of blood or effusion in the joint pushes the humeral head inferiorly. In the latter, follow-up radiographs reveal the restoration of normal glenohumeral articulation following resorption of the joint fluid/blood.

COMPUTED TOMOGRAPHY

CT with occasional reference to multiplanar reformats is often used to confirm a dislocation when the plain radiographs are ambiguous. The Hill-Sachs defect, Bankart lesion (**Figs. 96F–96H**), and other associated subtle fractures are clearly depicted on CT.

CT is sometimes necessary to confirm the presence of a posterior dislocation.

MAGNETIC RESONANCE ARTHROGRAPHY

MR arthrography using intra-articular gadolinium is the investigation of choice in the evaluation of recurrent shoulder dislocation where a soft-tissue defect is suspected. Labral defects or tears, capsulolabral separation, bicipital injuries, and ligamentous rupture are best evaluated by this modality.

Treatment

Closed reduction with sedation and analgesia are performed in an acute setting.

Conservative measures using a sling for 1 to 6 weeks are often successful, followed by rehabilitation. Modification of activity involving overhead work, manual labor, and high-risk sports helps to minimize recurrence.

Surgical treatment either by arthroscopy or open surgery may be indicated in recurrent dislocations, in those involved in sports, or due to inability to change work. Procedures are typically directed toward addressing capsular laxity, by an open capsular shift, arthroscopic capsular plication, thermal capsulorrhaphy, or rotator interval closure.

Prognosis

Nonathletes have a 30% recurrence risk with nonoperative treatment, whereas athletes have an 82% recurrence risk with nonoperative treatment.

Recurrence following the first dislocation depends on age, with a 100% recurrence rate reported below the age of 10 and between 0 and 25% above the age of 50.

PEARLS

- Posterior dislocations are the most difficult dislocation to diagnose on plain radiographs. They are only seen well on the axillary projection, which is the single best view and should be attempted in all cases. If the patient cannot be positioned for this view due to severe pain, a modified version of the axillary view or a CT scan are alternatives.
- Whereas labral tears following traumatic dislocation are more common in younger individuals (below 40), cuff tears are more frequent in older individuals. In addition, older patients are less likely to have a Bankart lesion and more likely to have a greater tuberosity fracture, an avulsion of the capsule and/or subscapularis from the lesser tuberosity. Thus, an MR arthrogram is less likely to be indicated in the older age group.
- Hill-Sachs lesions are best seen on AP views with the shoulder in internal rotation.

PITFALLS

- Although the trans-scapular Y view is useful in the diagnosis of dislocations and scapular fractures, it should not replace the axillary view, as the former does not show subtle subluxations of the glenohumeral joint or subtle fractures of the glenoid rim.
- In posterior dislocation, the AP view may reveal a subtle increase in joint space between the anterior humeral margin and the inferior glenoid margin; however, 40 to 50% of such dislocations are overlooked on the initial evaluation. The axillary and trans-scapular views are far more contributory in diagnosing the posterior location of the humeral head with respect to the glenoid cavity. A dislocation should never be excluded on the basis of a single projection.

- The least common direction of dislocation is the inferior dislocation, which is best seen on the AP and trans-scapular Y views. It should be differentiated from pseudosubluxation, in which the presence of blood or effusion in the joint pushes the humeral head inferiorly. In the latter, follow-up radiographs reveal the restoration of normal glenohumeral articulation following resorption of the joint fluid/blood.

Suggested Readings

Griffith JF, Antonio GE, Tong CW, Ming CK. Anterior shoulder dislocation: quantification of glenoid bone loss with CT. Am J Roentgenol 2003;180:1423–1430

Gumina S, Postacchini F. Anterior dislocation of the shoulder in elderly patients. J Bone Joint Surg Br 1997;79:540–543

Hall FM. MR arthrography of the posterior labrocapsular complex. Am J Roentgenol 2003;181:595

Yu JS, Ashman CJ, Jones G. The POLPSA lesion: MR imaging findings with arthroscopic correlation in patients with posterior instability. Skeletal Radiol 2002;31:396–399

CASE 97

Hema N. Choudur, Anthony G. Ryan, and Peter L. Munk

Clinical Presentation

This patient presented to the emergency department with pain and swelling around the elbow with limitation of movement following a fall on an outstretched hand.

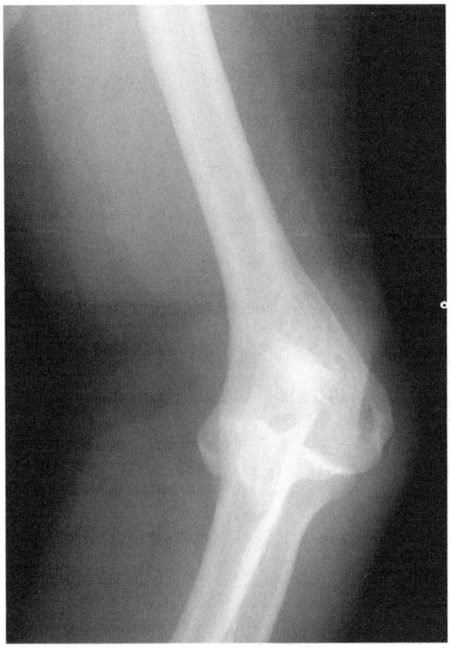

Figure 97A

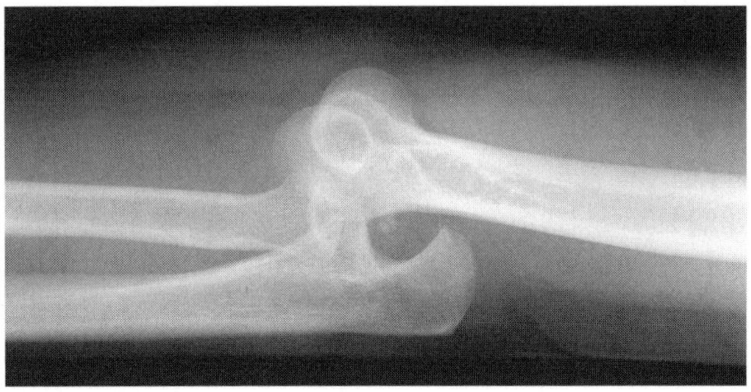

Figure 97B

Radiologic Findings

Anteroposterior (AP) and lateral views of the elbow (**Figs. 97A,97B**) were taken. The coranoid process of the ulna is disengaged from the trochlea, with the olecranon posteriorly dislocated. Note the small fracture of the coranoid process with soft-tissue swelling around the elbow joint.

Diagnosis

Posterior dislocation of the elbow.

Differential Diagnosis

- Radial head fracture
- Supracondylar fracture
- Medial epicondyle avulsion fracture and other fractures of the proximal forearm bones
- In children, nursemaid's elbow

Discussion

Background

In adults, elbow dislocations are quite common, occurring second in frequency to shoulder dislocations. In children and adolescents, supracondylar fractures are more common. The inherently stable elbow joint requires a fair degree of force to cause dislocation; therefore, bony fractures accompany dislocations in a third of the patients. Posterior dislocations of the elbow are the predominant type and account for 80 to 90% of all elbow dislocations. However, anterior, lateral, or divergent dislocations can occur.

Etiology

A fall on an outstretched hand with the elbow in extension results in posterior dislocation of the elbow. Coexisting shoulder, wrist, and distal radioulnar joint dislocations may occur.

Pathophysiology

The medial collateral ligament (MCL) is the main stabilizer of the elbow joint. It consists of an anterior oblique ligament and provides about 60% valgus stability, with the osseous articulation providing approximately 40% stability. The radial head is the most important secondary stabilizer. In simple dislocations, no fracture is present, but the capsule is ruptured.

Following the fall, the ligaments that stabilize the elbow joint, that is, the ulnar and lateral collateral ligaments, are severed, and the capsule is ruptured, with injury to the pronator/flexor origin and also to the brachialis origin. The coranoid process is disengaged from its articulation with the trochlea, causing the entire proximal ulna to dislocate posteriorly. Anterior dislocations can also occur, in which case a strong blow to the back of the flexed elbow is the cause, driving the olecranon anterior to the humerus.

The three intracapsular fat pads between the extensive synovia of the elbow and the joint capsule are no longer well seen.

It has also been observed that the patients who had dislocations had a shallower semilunar notch and a smaller coronoid process, seen in the lateral view, predisposing them to dislocations.

Clinical Findings

Pain and swelling around the elbow joint are the usual presentation. Reduced motion at the elbow joint may be elicited. The elbow is deformed, with the olecranon and epicondyles in one line at 90 degrees of elbow flexion, unlike the normal configuration, where the three structures form an equilateral triangle. Examiners should palpate for radial head fractures. On examination, the brachial pulse usually is normal with no sensory/motor deficits.

Complications

Brachial artery injury, median and ulnar nerve injuries, associated fractures and their complications, triceps avulsion in anterior dislocations, intra-articular bony fragments, and, in the later weeks, myositis ossificans are common complications. Valgus instability can occur in patients with MCL laxity. Posterolateral instability is another late complication, and surgical treatment is imperative.

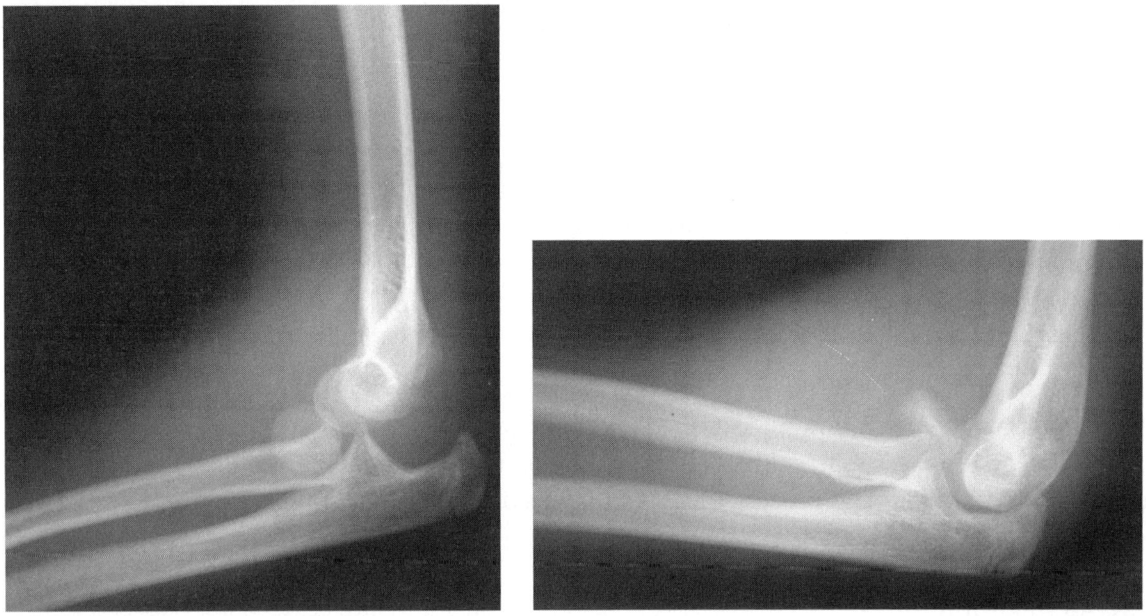

C D

Figures 97C,97D Radiographs show a posteriorly dislocated ulna with fracture of the radial head, before (**97C**) and after (**97D**) reduction.

Imaging Findings

RADIOGRAPHY

Standard AP and lateral views of the elbow joint reveal loss of normal congruity of the joint, with the olecranon dislocated posteriorly on the lateral view (**Fig. 97C**). Also, fractures of the coranoid process, olecranon, and radial head must be looked for carefully. There is discontinuity of the radio-capitellar line and overlap of the articular surfaces of the trochlea and ulna.

Postreduction radiographs are necessary for evaluating adequate reduction and also to assess for the presence of subtle fractures (**Fig. 97D**).

In anterior dislocation, the olecranon lies anterior to the humerus in the lateral view.

COMPUTED TOMOGRAPHY

CT is infrequently used to rule out an intra-articular fragment and to confirm subtle fractures.

MAGNETIC RESONANCE IMAGING

MRI is indicated to visualize the collateral ligament integrity, articular cartilage, capsule, neurovascular structures, and muscles around the elbow joint, usually prior to surgery.

Treatment

Simple dislocations are treated with reduction under local or general anesthesia, depending on the duration of injury; also, immobilization in a splint in 90 degrees of elbow flexion may be directed for 3 weeks, followed by rehabilitation. Early reduction is essential, because a delay may increase the risk of neurovascular compromise or damage to the articular cartilage. Vascular injury should be ruled out by angiography in the appropriate circumstances, such as loss of a palpable radial pulse.

Prognosis

Slight stiffness of the joint may persist for months after injury but usually does not affect function.

PEARL

- The presence of a peripheral pulse does not indicate the absence of a vascular injury, and in appropriate situations with severe dislocations, an angiogram is to be recommended.

PITFALLS

- Nerve injury to the median nerve is to be looked for carefully.
- A careful search for associated fractures on postreduction radiographs of elbow dislocations is mandated. Missed coronoid process fractures may lead to recurrent subluxation or dislocation.

Suggested Readings

Louis DS, Ricciardi JE, Spengler DM. Arterial injury: a complication of posterior elbow dislocation—a clinical and anatomical study. J Bone Joint Surg Am 1974;56:1631–1636

Olsen BS, Sojbjerg JO. The treatment of recurrent posterolateral instability of the elbow. J Bone Joint Surg Br 2003;85:342–346

Shearman CM, el-Khoury GY. Pitfalls in the radiologic evaluation of extremity trauma: Part I. The upper extremity. Am Fam Physician 1998;57:995–1002

CASE 98

Peter L. Munk and Anthony G. Ryan

Clinical Presentation

A 36-year-old man was involved in a motorcycle accident. The vehicle spun out of control, and he struck the ground on an outstretched wrist. The patient complained of severe pain and inability to move the wrist freely. On examination, the wrist was swollen and had limited passive motion.

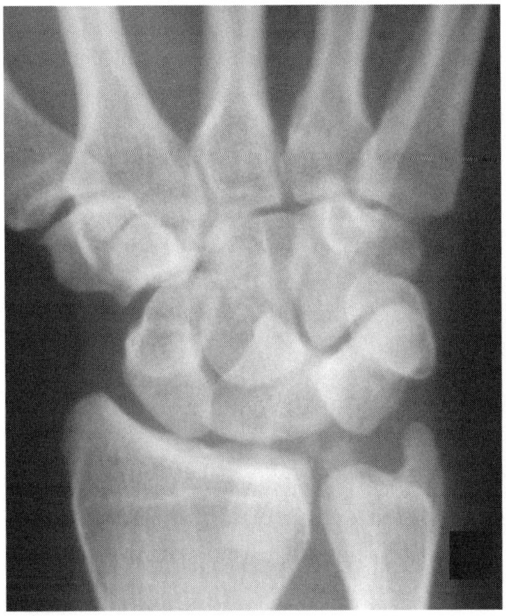

Figure 98A

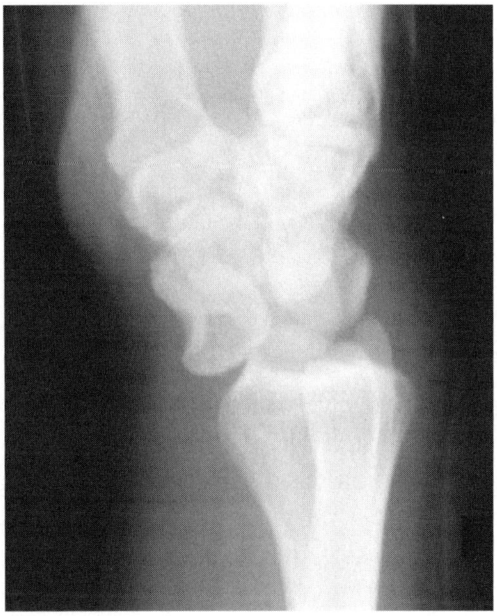

Figure 98B

Radiologic Findings

Radiographs of the wrist show several abnormalities. On the anteroposterior (AP) view, a markedly abnormal appearance of the proximal carpal row is observed (**Fig. 98A**). The normal carpal arcs of Gilula are disrupted, and the lunate has assumed a triangular, or "slice-of-pie," configuration. Examination of the lateral view reveals that the lunate has been displaced in the volar direction and is tilted anteriorly (**Fig. 98B**). No associated fractures are evident.

Diagnosis

Anterior dislocation of the lunate.

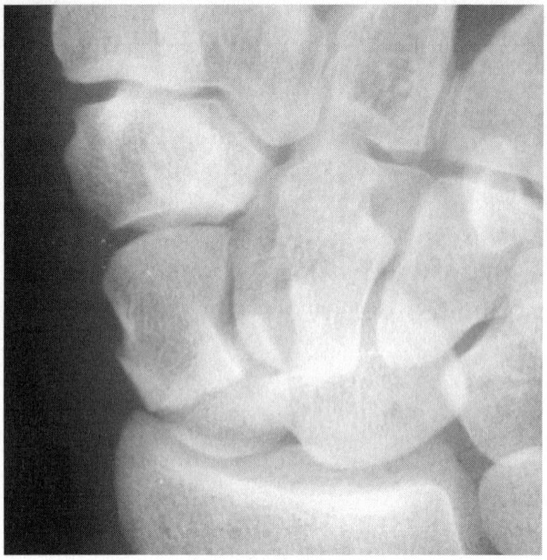

Figure 98C A focused oblique view of the scaphoid shows a transverse fracture through the waist of the scaphoid and a lunate dislocation, shown by the triangular shape assumed by the lunate. In addition, disruption of the first and second carpal arcs is evident.

Discussion

Background

Carpal dislocations can involve either multiple bones or, less frequently, a single bone, as in this case. They may occur in either the dorsal or the volar direction (in the case of several bones, the direction is designated depending on the displacement relative to the proximal carpal row). In this case, the isolated displacement of a single carpal bone is designated in the direction of its displacement. In most instances a clear history of trauma with the wrist held in dorsiflexion occurs. Rarely, a direct blow may cause the ejection of a carpal bone.

Not infrequently, fractures may be associated with lunate dislocation. These so-called perilunate fracture dislocations are more common than isolated lunate dislocations. The scaphoid is the most commonly fractured bone, although the capitate, distal radius, ulna, or triquetrum may be involved (**Fig. 98C**).

Complications

- Infrequently, tears of ligaments and other soft-tissue structures may cause these to become interposed within the proximal carpal row, impeding reduction.
- Only rarely is a fracture of the lunate detected.
- Surprisingly, avascular necrosis of the lunate is also an uncommon complication of this injury.

Imaging Findings

RADIOGRAPHY

Radiography is the most commonly used imaging modality. With lunate dislocation, the lunate is noted to have an abnormal configuration on the AP view, as indicated in this case. The carpal arcs (of Gilula) are very helpful in detection of this abnormality on AP radiographs. Displacement of the lunate disrupts the parallel nature of the cortical lines, which is normally apparent on this projection. The lateral view demonstrates abnormal placement relative to the longitudinal axis of the radius, frequently accompanied by volar tilting. The lunate no longer sits in the concavity of the distal radius.

COMPUTED TOMOGRAPHY

CT is helpful in evaluation of subtle fractures in adjacent bones that may not be appreciated on radiography.

MAGNETIC RESONANCE IMAGING

MRI shows associated ligamentous or cartilage abnormalities, if present.

Treatment

- In many instances, spontaneous reduction of a lunate dislocation occurs.
- In instances requiring reduction, traction and manipulation followed by prolonged immobilization are required.
- Operative reduction may be required if reduction is impeded by interposed soft tissues.
- Infrequently, tears of ligaments and other soft-tissue structures may cause these to become interposed within the proximal carpal row, impeding reduction.

PEARLS

- Gilula's arcs are described as follows:
  - *Arc I:* the proximal margins of the scaphoid, lunate, and triquetral bones
  - *Arc II:* the distal margins of the same bones
  - *Arc III:* the proximal margins of the capitate and hamate bones
- On the true lateral wrist radiograph, the radius, lunate, and capitate should be aligned.
- When the radius and capitate are aligned, but the lunate is displaced, the condition is called lunate dislocation. When the radius and lunate are aligned, but the capitate is malaligned with the lunate, it is described as perilunate dislocation of the wrist.

PITFALLS

- In normal subjects, disruption occurs in Gilula's arcs I and II, with the wrist held in ulnar and radial deviation; thus, if the wrist is not in true neutral on the AP views, injuries may be overcalled.
- The lateral view of the wrist should always be performed, as carpal dislocations are frequently evident only on this view.
- Care must be taken to avoid satisfaction of search when examining a wrist radiograph when one abnormality is detected, as multiple injuries may be present along the so-called zone of vulnerability: this zone is represented by a line corresponding to an inverted U passing through the radial styloid, the waist of the scaphoid, the proximal poles of the capitate and hamate, the triquetral, and the ulnar styloid.

Suggested Readings

Al-Ismail K, Torreggiani WC, Munk PL, Marchinkow LO, Lee MJ. Musculoskeletal case 17. Dislocation of the lunate bone. Can J Surg 2001;44:260–261,307–308

Gilula LA. Carpal injuries: analytic approach and case exercises. Am J Roentgenol 1979;133:503–517

Peh WC, Gilula LA. Normal disruption of carpal arcs. J Hand Surg [Am] 1996;21:561–566

Resnik CS, Gelberman RH, Resnick D. Transcaphoid, transcapitate, perilunate fracture dislocation (scaphocapitate syndrome). Skeletal Radiol 1983;9:192–196

CASE 99

Hema N. Choudur, Anthony G. Ryan, and Peter L. Munk

Clinical Presentation

A 56-year-old man presented with pain and decreased mobility of the left hip, status posthemiarthroplasty.

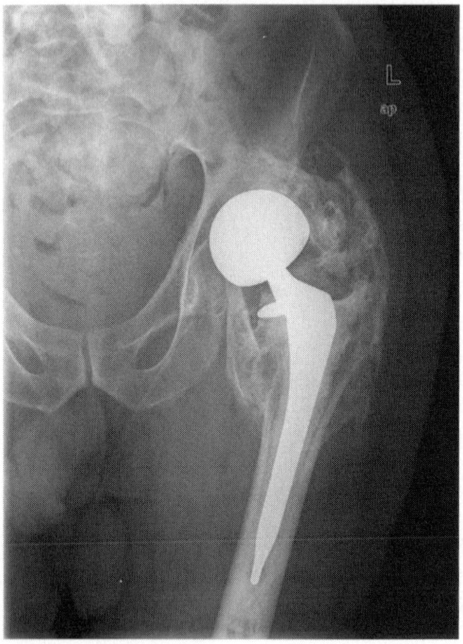

Figure 99A

Radiologic Findings

A conventional anteroposterior (AP) radiograph (**Fig. 99A**) of the left hip shows a left hemiarthroplasty with dense bony sheets and bars bridging the femoral shaft to the acetabular margins.

Diagnosis

Heterotopic ossification.

Differential Diagnosis

None.

Discussion

Heterotopic ossification is abnormal true bone formation in the extraskeletal soft tissues. It has various synonyms, including myositis ossificans, a term no longer recommended, as it suggests a primary inflammation of the muscle (which has been shown histologically not to be the case) and as the condition also affects tissues other than muscle, such as fascia and tendons. Thirty percent of cases are said to occur in subcutaneous fat. It frequently occurs in traumatized soft tissues (after surgery, after spinal cord/brain injury, and following burns) but can also occur under other conditions causing muscle paralysis, such as poliomyelitis.

Background

Postsurgical heterotopic ossification is one of the most common causes of extraskeletal soft-tissue ossification and is seen following hip arthroplasty in 8 to 70% of cases. The process begins within 1 week of surgery. Cartilage is laid down by the second week, with trabecular bone formation evident by about the fifth week. Mature bone is formed after 6 weeks. It may regress and even disappear. Sometimes, the process may progress or halt.

Clinical Findings

Initial pain and tenderness over the site of surgery may mimic cellulitis or a deep venous thrombosis (DVT). Later, an indurated hard mass becomes palpable. There are variable degrees of immobilization of the joint, depending on the amount of subsequent heterotopic bone formation.

Pathology

Trauma stimulates mesenchymal stem cells in the soft tissues, which then differentiate into osteoblasts, osteoid, and eventually heterotopic bone.

GROSS

Actual bone may be seen within the affected tissues.

MICROSCOPIC

Following trauma, spindle cell proliferation may be seen during the first week. By 7 to 10 days, primitive osteoid develops at the periphery. Woven bone and primitive cartilage are laid down by about the second week. Trabecular bone forms by 2 to 5 weeks. Peripheral mature lamellar bone and central immature bone are seen after 6 weeks.

Imaging Findings

RADIOGRAPHY

- Dense heterotopic ossification is noted at the affected site (e.g., surrounding an arthroplasty).
- The mineralization may follow the pattern of muscular fibers (**Figs. 99B,99C**)

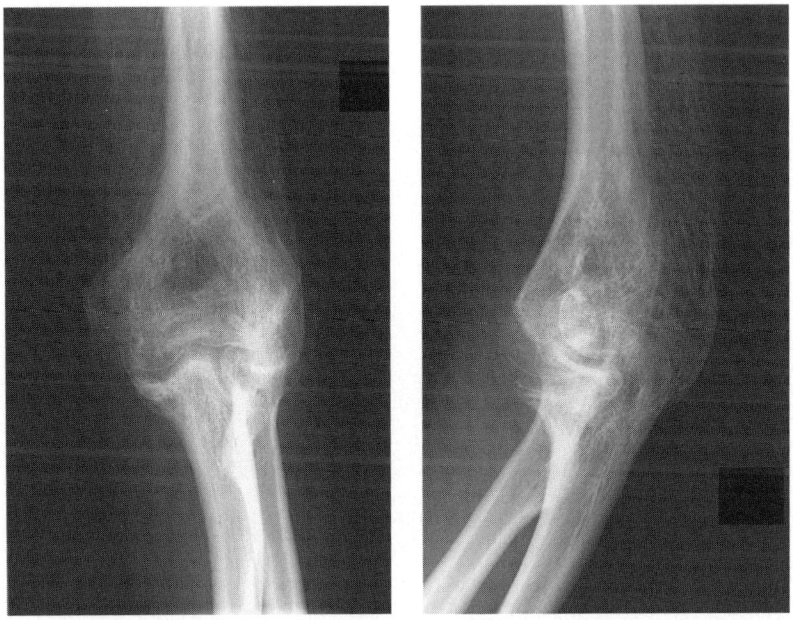

B C

Figures 99B,99C AP (**99B**) and lateral (**99C**) radiographs of the right elbow show posttraumatic heterotopic bone formation along the fibers of the triceps muscle.

- The extent is variable.
- When mature bone is present, a medullary cavity with a cortical margin may be clearly differentiated.
- The lesion is most dense at its periphery.
- Radiographs cannot detect mineralization during the first 2 weeks after trauma.

SCINTIGRAPHY

- Three-phase bone scan with technetium (Tc 99m) is the examination of choice for the earliest detection and assessment of maturity of a known lesion.
- First pass and blood pool imaging are abnormal in early heterotopic ossification due to hypervascularity. Early intervention is therefore possible even before the x-rays are positive.
- Increased soft-tissue uptake in the third phase of the bone scan is noted only when the osteoid formation occurs, permitting the assessment of maturity of the heterotopic bone (**Figs. 99D–99F**).

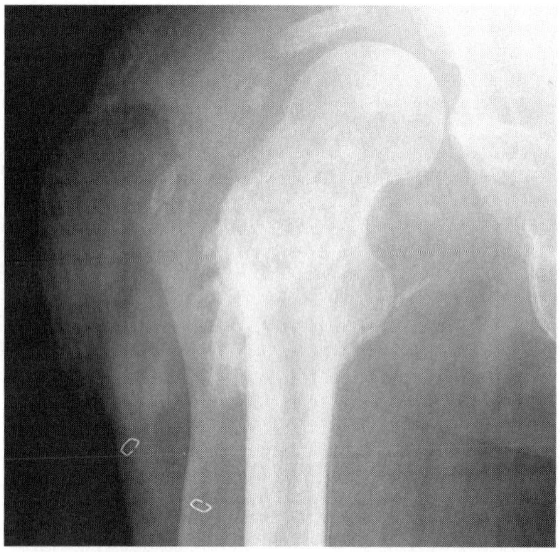

D

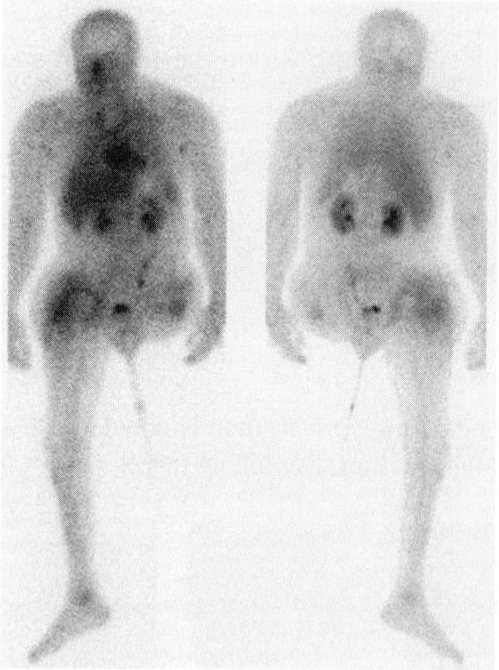

E

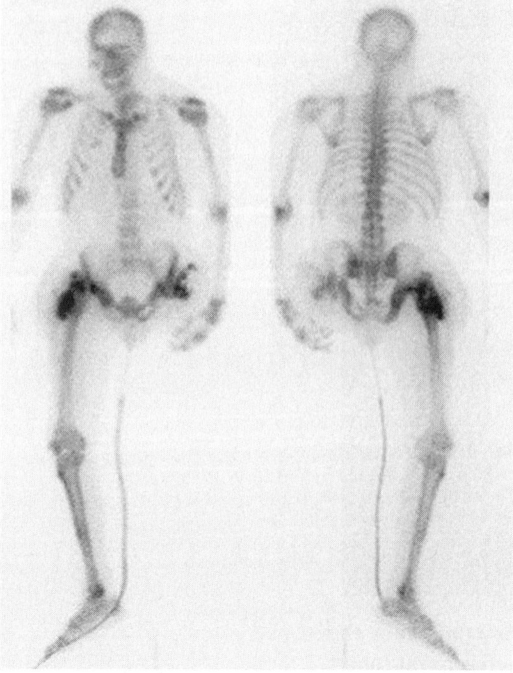

F

Figures 99D–99F Radiograph (**99D**) shows bone within the soft tissues of the right hip, suggestive of heterotopic ossification. Increased uptake of the radiotracer on all phases (blood pool **99E**, and static **99F**) of the three-phase bone scan confirms the presence of active osteoid.

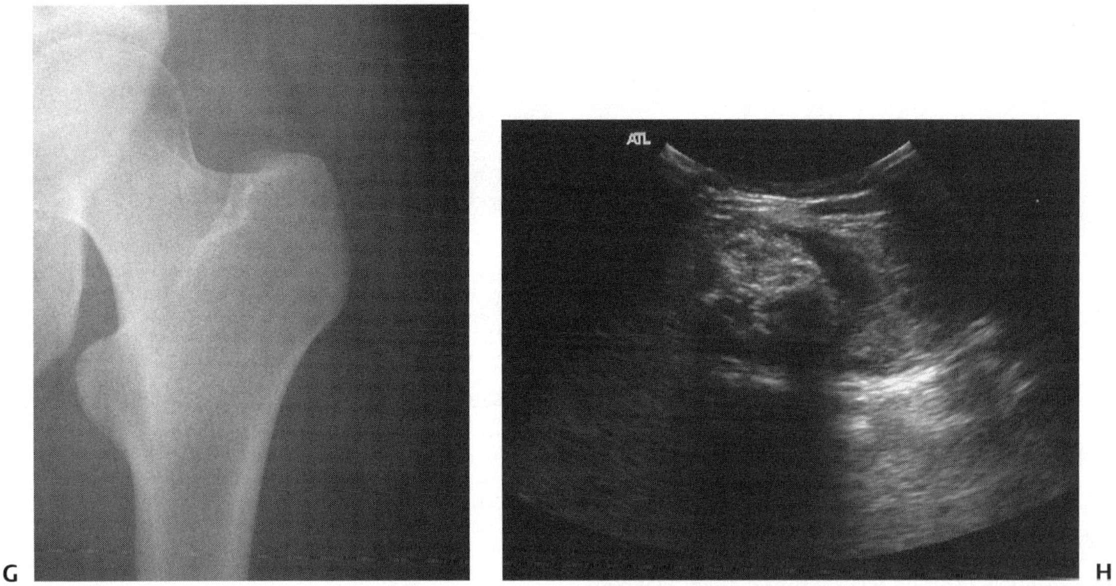

Figures 99G,99H Plain radiograph (**99G**) in a 20-year-old person after trauma shows faint calcifications within the proximal thigh (caudad to the greater trochanter). Corresponding ultrasound (**99H**) reveals a masslike appearance containing dense calcifications with marked acoustic shadowing.

- When the new bone is fully mature, osteoblastic activity ceases, and isotope uptake declines. It is in this inactive, fully mature stage (12 to 18 months) that any surgical débridement is performed, as otherwise the heterotopic ossification tends to recur.

ULTRASOUND

- Ultrasound can be useful in differentiating between DVT and heterotopic ossification, which have similar clinical presentations, that is, pain, tenderness, and induration.
- The findings that favor heterotopic ossification are
  - Disruption of normal lamellar skeletal muscle
  - A masslike pattern with peripheral echogenicity (**Figs. 99G,99H**)
  - Central hypoechogenicity
  - Once mineralized, echogenic sheets with acoustic shadowing may be demonstrable.

COMPUTED TOMOGRAPHY

- The earliest finding is an enlarged muscle belly containing foci of low attenuation.
- This is followed by demonstration of immature bone mineralization, which is evident prior to plain radiographs.

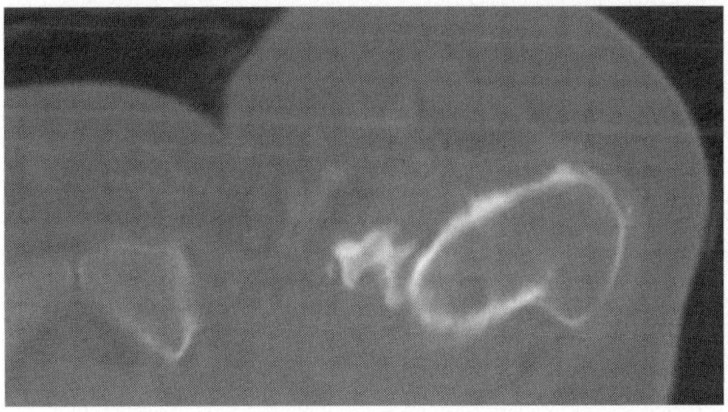

Figure 99I Mature heterotopic ossification is noted anterior to the left hip joint. Note the clearly differentiated cortex and medulla within the lesion.

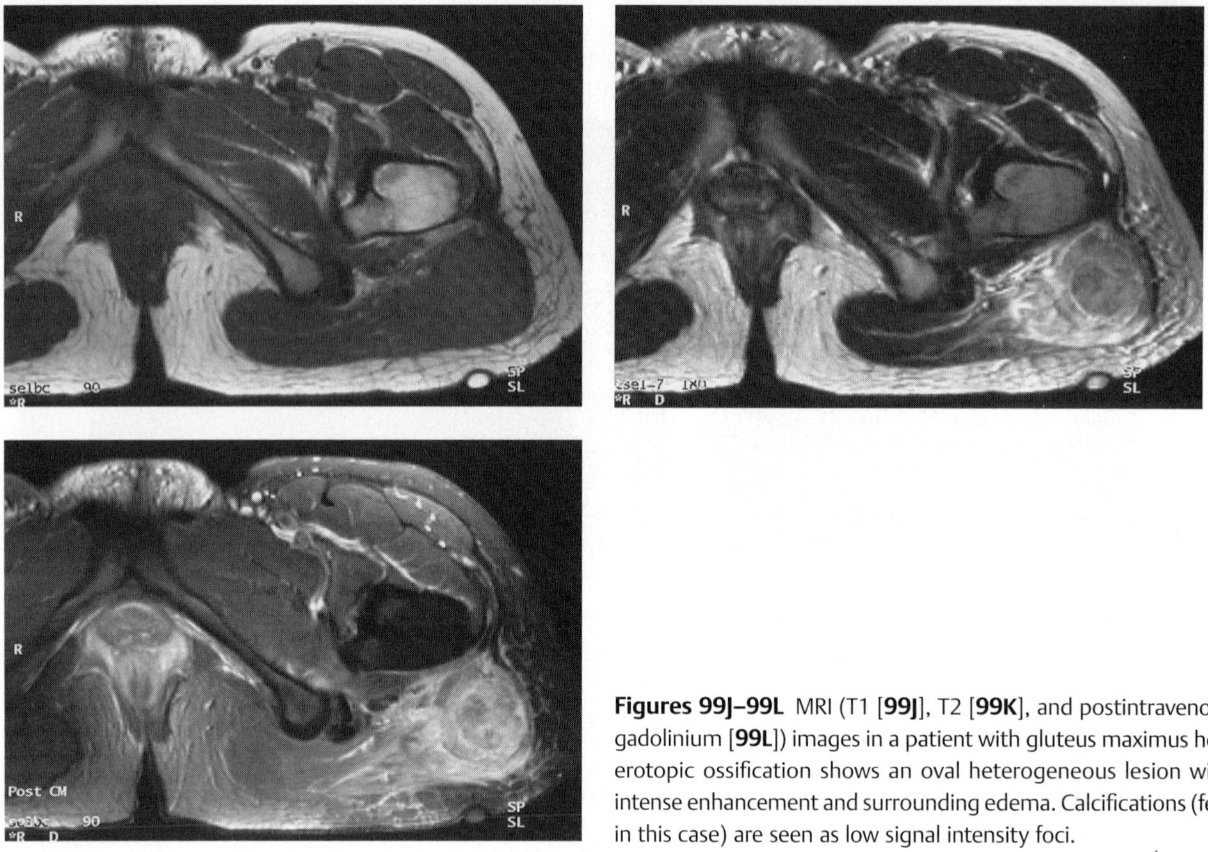

J K L

Figures 99J–99L MRI (T1 [**99J**], T2 [**99K**], and postintravenous gadolinium [**99L**]) images in a patient with gluteus maximus heterotopic ossification shows an oval heterogeneous lesion with intense enhancement and surrounding edema. Calcifications (few in this case) are seen as low signal intensity foci.

- On maturation, the peripheral cortex and central marrow are distinctly visualized (**Fig. 99I**).
- Inflammatory mass and soft-tissue neoplasm are potential pitfalls; however, the location of the densest calcification/ossification at the periphery favors heterotopic ossification.

MAGNETIC RESONANCE IMAGING

- In early heterotopic ossification, heterogeneous high T2-signal intensity with enlargement of the affected tissues may be seen with a low signal intensity rim.
- On administration of gadolinium, intense heterogeneous enhancement is seen (**Figs. 99J–99L**). This can be mistaken for a tumor, and biopsy may be performed to differentiate; however, this is fraught with danger, as the histological appearance of early heterotopic ossification mimics the appearance of sarcoma.
- In the later stages, a pattern of well-defined mature cortical bone (low-signal rim) and central heterogeneous high T2 signal is noted.

Treatment

- Depending on the degree and extent, the new bone may be resorbed with no treatment.
- A combination of external beam radiation and nonsteroidal anti-inflammatories (NSAIDs) (indomethacin and naproxen) has been used in the treatment of early heterotopic ossification formation, which has been shown to prevent lesion progression.
- Studies with oral etidronate in the treatment of early heterotopic ossification demonstrated on bone scan and ultrasound have shown favorable results.

- Surgical resection is indicated when the adjacent joint is immobilized by dense ossification; the results are variable, however. Such resection must be deferred until the fully mature stage (12 to 18 months), as prior to this, the heterotopic ossification is most likely to recur, sometimes with further progression.

Prognosis

- Indomethacin has been shown to reduce the risk of recurrence after resection.

PEARLS

- First pass and blood pool imaging are abnormal in early heterotopic ossification due to hypervascularity. Early intervention is therefore possible even before the x-rays are positive.
- On CT, the earliest finding is an enlarged muscle belly containing foci of low attenuation, followed by demonstration of immature bone mineralization, which is evident prior to its appearance on conventional radiographs.
- When the new bone is fully mature, osteoblastic activity ceases, and thus isotope uptake no longer occurs.

PITFALLS

- The early mineralization is not detectable on radiographs in the first 2 weeks after trauma.
- Heterotopic ossification may be mistaken for inflammatory mass/soft-tissue neoplasm; however, the location of the densest calcification/ossification at the periphery favors heterotopic ossification.
- If surgical débridement is performed prior to the fully mature stage, the heterotopic ossification tends to recur.

Suggested Reading

Bressler EL, Marn CS, Gore RM, Hendrix RW. Evaluation of ectopic bone by CT. Am J Roentgenol 1987;148:931–935

De Smet AA, Norris MA, Fisher DR. Magnetic resonance imaging of myositis ossificans: analysis of seven cases. Skeletal Radiol 1992;21:503–507

Kransdorf MJ, Meis JM, Jelinek JS. Myositis ossificans: MR appearance with radiologic-pathologic correlation. Am J Roentgenol 1991;157:1243–1248

Orzel JA, Rudd TG. Heterotopic bone formation: clinical, laboratory, and imaging correlation. J Nucl Med 1985;26:125–132

CASE 100

Peter L. Munk, Anthony G. Ryan, and Laurel O. Marchinkow

Clinical Presentation

A 5-year-old boy, having fallen from a chair, presented with pain, swelling, and reduced movement of his right arm.

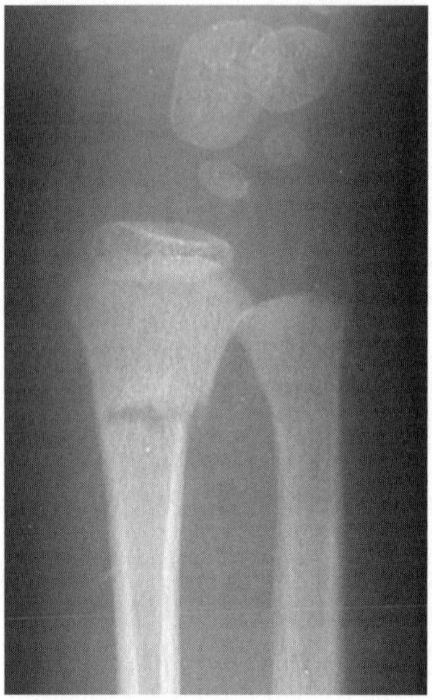

Figure 100A

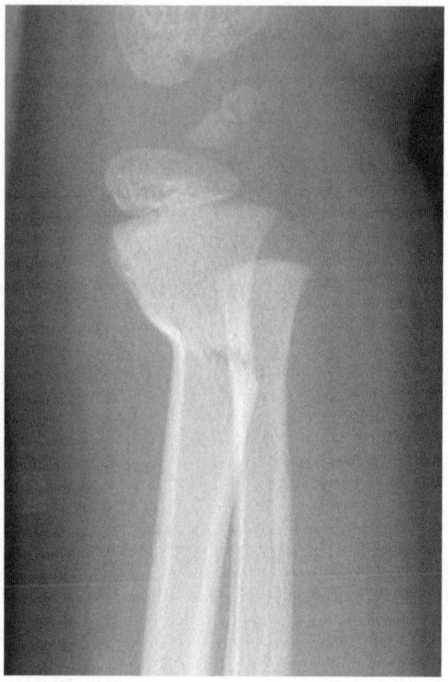

Figure 100B

Radiologic Findings

Anteroposterior (AP) (**Fig. 100A**) and lateral (**Fig. 100B**) images of the wrist show an incomplete fracture of the distal radius affecting the ulnar and volar aspects of the bone; however, the dorsal and radial aspects of the cortex are not breached.

Diagnosis

Greenstick fracture of the distal radius.

Differential Diagnosis

None.

Discussion

Background

The combination of Salter-Harris and greenstick fractures accounts for the vast majority of fractures seen in the pediatric population.

Etiology

- Trauma resulting in axial or "bending" forces accounts for greenstick fractures.
- Longitudinally oriented forces are frequently responsible for torus fractures; hence their alternative title "buckle" fractures.

Pathophysiology

The pediatric skeleton is far more plastic than the adult, frequently resulting in incomplete fractures due to the deformability of the immature bones. Several types of incomplete fractures are commonly encountered. Notable are two principal types of fractures that typically affect long bones, particularly in the upper extremity: greenstick and torus.

Clinical Findings

These fractures are essentially confined to the pediatric population, and a typical history of fall followed by immediate pain and swelling is usually given.

Complications

- Rarely, malunion
- Posttraumatic cortical defect at the site of the cortical break
- Even when fractures heal in a malaligned fashion, they are rarely refractured, given the propensity for the bones to realign with growth.

Imaging Findings

RADIOGRAPHY

Greenstick fracture

A greenstick fracture occurs due to a bending force on the bone, resulting in fracturing of the cortex on one side of the bone but not the other (**Fig. 100C**). The convex side of the stressed bone shows a radiolucent fracture line that does not extend to the concave side (**Figs. 100A,100B**). The most common sites for this are the midsections of the radius and ulna, the proximal diaphysis of the tibia, and the clavicle.

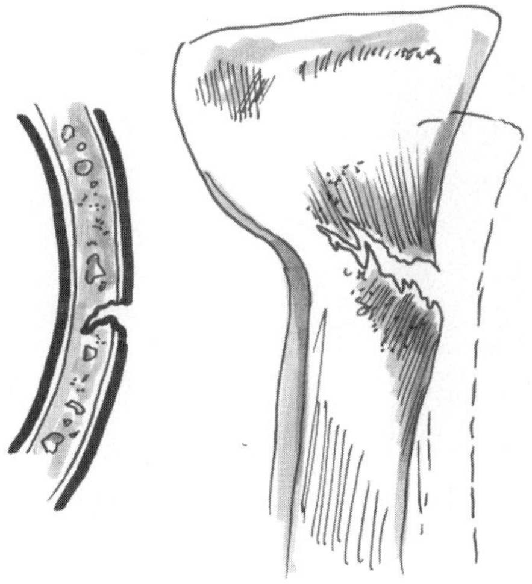

Figure 100C Diagrammatic representation of the nature of a greenstick fracture, the image on the left showing the bending forces involved, resulting in a fracture on the convex side of the bone with clear "bending" of the cortex of the concave side, but without actual cortical breach. The image on the right corresponds to the lateral radiograph of the reference case (**100B**).

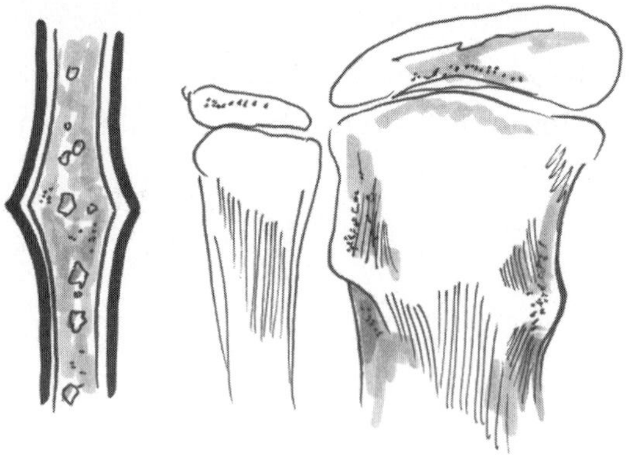

Figure 100D Diagrammatic representation of the nature of a torus fracture, the image on the left showing the longitudinal loading forces involved, resulting in "buckling" that affects the circumference of the affected bone. The image on the right corresponds to the AP radiograph of the torus reference case (**100E**).

Not unusually, one bone, such as the ulna, may have a complete fracture, whereas the adjacent bone, such as the radius, displays an incomplete fracture.

In the healing phase, areas of radiolucency are often seen at the fracture site, as are areas of heaped-up periosteal new bone. Late in the healing phase, the bone may gradually remodel, and it may be difficult to discern any trace of previous trauma.

Torus or buckle fracture

The torus or buckle fracture is a similar injury. In this case, the forces are usually inadequate to produce a frank breaching of the cortex. Instead, a wrinkle or buckle is noted in the cortex (**Figs. 100D–100F**). In this situation, a longitudinally oriented force is usually responsible.

The most common sites for these fractures are the metaphyses of long bones, particularly the radius and ulna. In the acute phase, the buckle may at times be quite subtle, or may be only visible on a single projection.

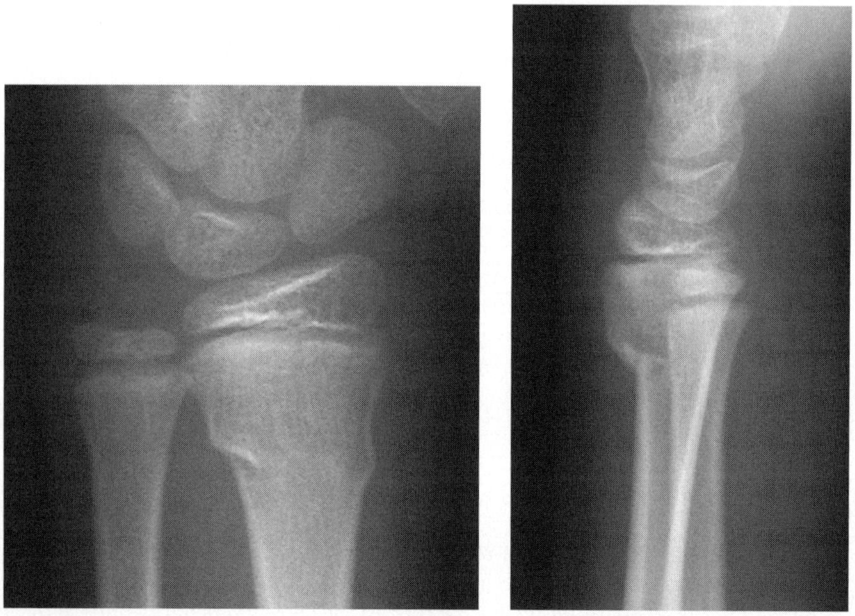

E F

Figures 100E,100F AP (**100E**) and lateral (**100F**) images of the wrist show a torus fracture of the distal radius, the "buckled" nature of the fracture particularly evident on the AP projection.

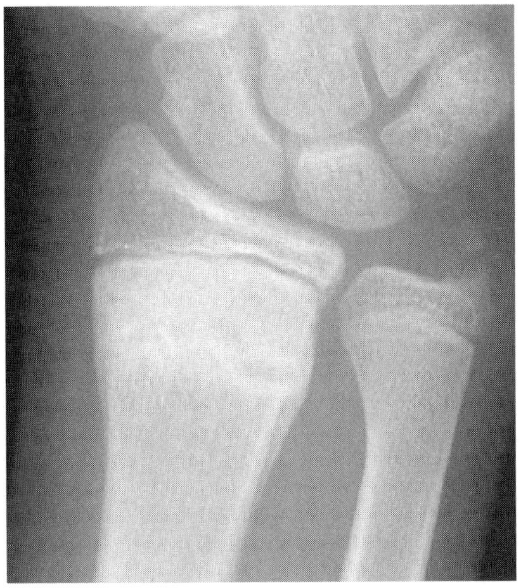

Figure 100G AP radiograph of a healing greenstick fracture of the distal radius shows bandlike areas of increased density, with dense periosteal new bone overlying the fracture site.

When doubt is present about the diagnosis, comparison with the contralateral extremity may be helpful, or a nuclear medicine bone scan can be obtained.

In the healing phase, bandlike areas of increased density are noted with dense periosteal new bone overlying the site of the fracture (**Fig. 100G**).

A variant of this fracture is the so-called bowing fracture, when the bone simply bends without producing any cortical deficiencies or irregularities (**Fig. 100H**). This is particularly frequent in the radius and ulna.

NUCLEAR MEDICINE SCAN

When doubt is present about the diagnosis, a nuclear medicine bone scan can be obtained.

COMPUTED TOMOGRAPHY/MAGNETIC RESONANCE IMAGING

Neither CT nor MRI is commonly employed in the evaluation of greenstick or torus fractures.

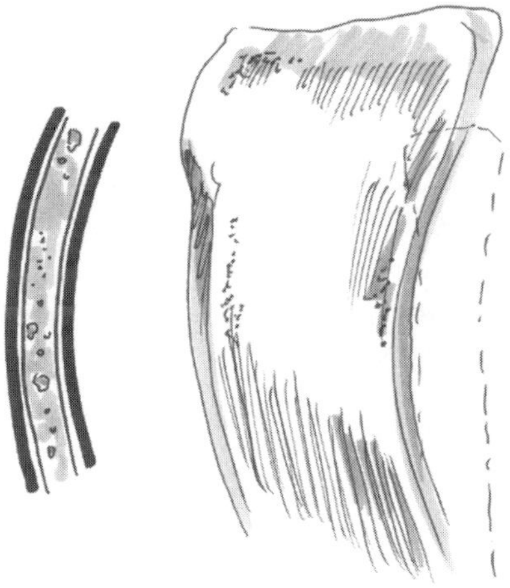

Figure 100H Diagrammatic representation of the nature of a "bowing" or "plastic" fracture, both images showing the bending forces involved, but without an actual cortical breach.

Treatment

Occasionally, “completion” of the fracture is required to correct angulation (if $>$ 15 degrees), followed by immobilization in a plaster cast.

Prognosis

As with the majority of pediatric injuries, the prognosis is excellent, with full recovery and return to function expected at 6 to 8 weeks for the upper limb and 10 to 12 weeks for the lower limb.

PEARLS

- Not only is the pediatric bone elastic, so too is the periosteum, which is, in addition, very thick in comparison to the adult’s.
- In greenstick fractures, the radiolucent fracture line is evident on the convex side of the stressed bone. The fracture line does not extend to the concave side.
- When doubt is present about the diagnosis, comparison with the contralateral extremity may be helpful, or a nuclear medicine bone scan can be obtained.

PITFALLS

- In the acute phase of a torus fracture, the buckle may be quite subtle; because there is little or no angulation, the fracture may be visible on a single projection only.
- Bowing fractures are frequently recognized only when the child attends a fracture clinic after an interval, at which time periosteal new bone may be evident.
- Bowing of one bone and a greenstick fracture of the other, for example, the radius or ulna, is a common occurrence. Failing to recognize the bowed bone in the presence of a greenstick fracture of the other rarely has significant consequences, as it is usually adequately treated by the immobilization of the greenstick fracture. If the bowed bone is significantly angled, however, it may need specific treatment.

Suggested Readings

Malghem J, Maldague B. Transient fatty cortical defects following fractures in children. Skeletal Radiol 1986;15:368–372

Noonan KJ, Price CT. Forearm and distal radius fractures in children. J Am Acad Orthop Surg 1998;6:146–156

Roach RT, Cassar-Pullicino V, Summers BN. Paediatric post-traumatic cortical defects of the distal radius. Pediatr Radiol 2002;32:333–339

CASE 101

Hema N. Choudur, Anthony G. Ryan, and Peter L. Munk

Clinical Presentation

A young man had had a motor vehicle accident several months prior to presenting. He had had a fracture of the right tibia, which had been casted; however, follow-up radiographs did not show any healing. Because there was severe pain at that site, an MRI was recommended to visualize any bony union and to exclude infection.

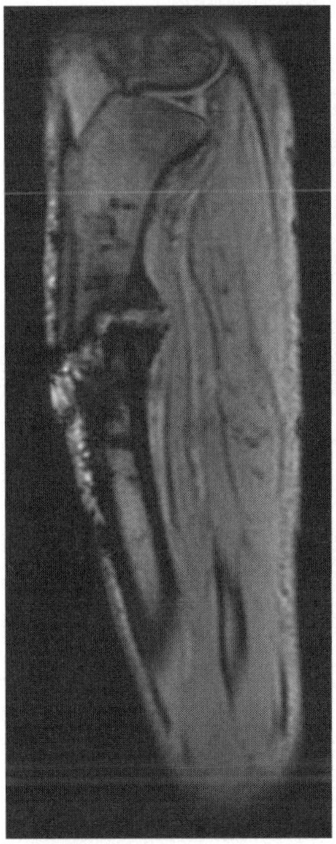

Figure 101A

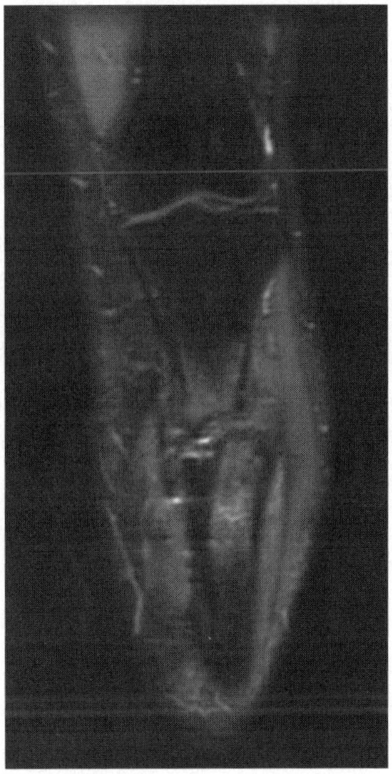

Figure 101B

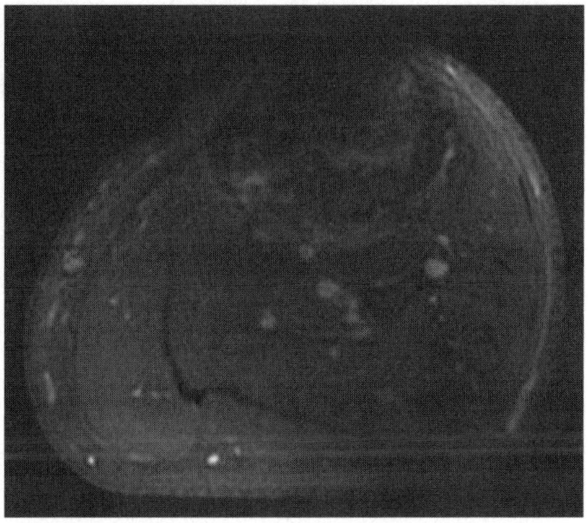

Figure 101C

Radiologic Findings

The MRI (**Fig. 101A**, sagittal MPGR; **Fig. 101B,** coronal FSTIR; and **Fig. 101C**, axial T1-weighted fat-saturated postgadolinium) reveals no osseous union between the fractured fragments. Although edema is evident in the adjacent marrow, there is no abnormal enhancement postgadolinium to suggest infection.

Diagnosis

Nonunion.

Differential Diagnosis

- Delayed union
- Malunion (**Figs. 101D** to **101G**)
- Infection

D 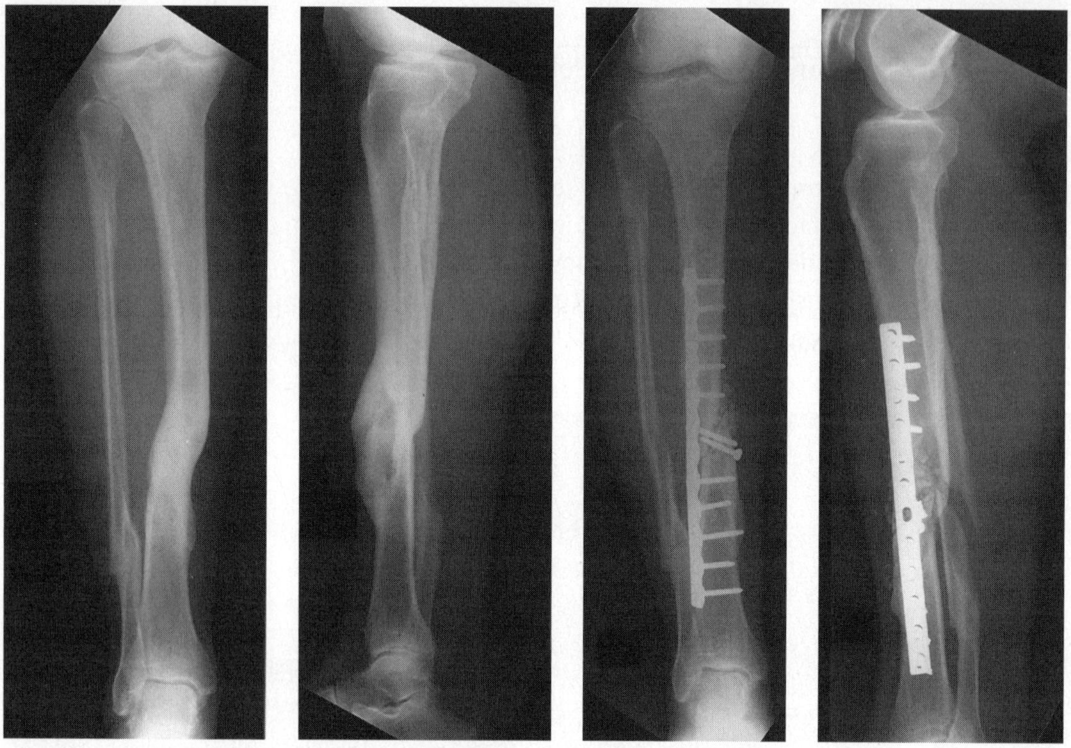 E–G

Figures 101D–101G AP (**101D**) and lateral (**101E**) views of the tibial fibula show marked angular deformity at the site of an old, healed fracture consistent with malunion. An osteotomy and plate fixation were required for correction as seen on the AP (**101F**) and lateral (**101G**) postoperative radiographs.

Discussion

The repair of a fracture is a continuous process, with the fracture tender and slightly mobile in the early stages becoming immobile and nontender in the later stages, noticeably seen on plain radiographs as bony fusion as against callus formation in the early stages.

A fracture is deemed nonunited when, given its maximum period of healing (which varies based on age, regional blood supply, location, and type of fracture), no osseous union is discernible on any of the imaging modalities.

Etiology

The etiology of nonunion is improper immobilization of the fracture, decreased blood supply, infection, intervening soft tissues, and inadequate mineralization of the adjacent bone. Fracture distraction and pathological fractures are other causes of nonunion.

Fractures of the upper limb heal faster than the lower, spiral better than transverse. In children, fractures heal faster than in adults. The most often encountered nonunions are in the tibia and femur, but those of the humerus, radius, ulna, and clavicle are also frequently seen.

Pathophysiology

There are three phases in fracture healing. In the inflammatory phase, there is interruption of the blood vessels and clot formation. In the reparative phase, organization of the blood clot occurs, with collagen fibers being laid with matrix formation and mineralization, seen as callus formation on radiographs. The last stage is that of remodeling, in which portions of the callus not needed for bony union are resorbed, and newer trabaculae are laid along the lines of stress. This stage lasts the longest.

The factors that delay or cause nonunion are extensive soft-tissue injury, comminution, decreased mineralization of the adjacent bone, involvement of the cortical versus cancellous bone (cancellous heals faster than cortical), improper immobilization, infection, pathological fractures, postradiation, avascular necrosis, intra-articular extension of fractures (synovial fluid causes clot lysis), older age of patients, and hormonal action, such as circulating steroids. Poor nutritional status and blood supply hinder bony fusion.

The occurrence of pseudoarthrosis or even fibrosis across the fracture is termed *nonunion*.

Clinical Findings

Pain and tenderness are common at the fracture site in delayed union. However, nonunion may be painlessly mobile. Nonunion is considered when a fracture has not united for 6 to 9 months.

Imaging Findings

RADIOGRAPHY

There is no definite osseous union. There may be mild callus formation or periosteal reaction. The fracture line is clearly visible, with the ends being sclerosed (**Figs. 101H,101I**).

Nonunions are called hypertrophic or atrophic (**Figs. 101H** and **101I**) based on the amount of callus formation.

H 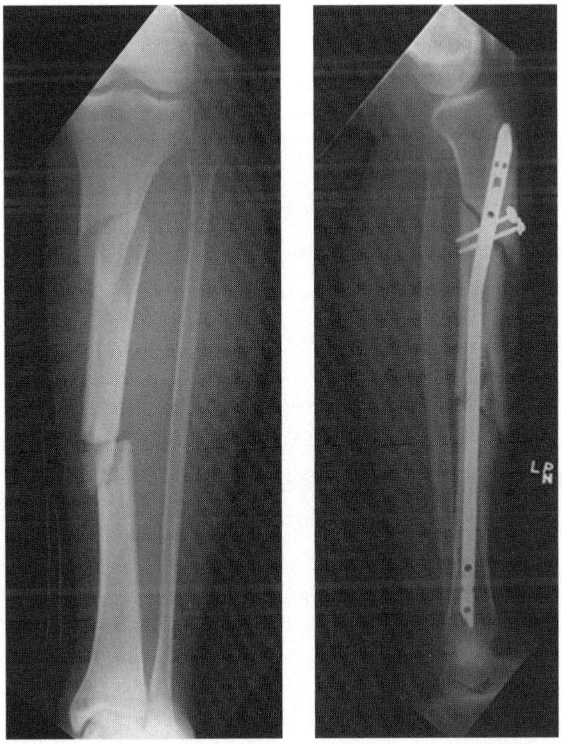 I

Figures 101H,101I AP (**101H**) and lateral (**101I**) views show atrophic nonunion 9 months after internal fixation of a tibial fracture. No callus is present at the fracture site.

COMPUTED TOMOGRAPHY

Bony union is shown well on CT in multiple planes with reformats. Further osteomyelitis and surrounding collections can be delineated on CT with intravenous contrast.

MAGNETIC RESONANCE IMAGING

Avascular necrosis, infection, and degree of bone union can be accurately evaluated by MRI.

Treatment

Asymptomatic fracture nonunions are treated only with splints, but some orthopedists use internal fixation and bone grafting.

- For hypertrophic nonunion, internal or external fixation is performed.
- For atrophic nonunion, bone grafting is the mode of management.

Prognosis

Salvage procedures are performed for painful nonunions. A variety of different procedures may be required, such as arthrodesis and soft-tissue interposition to create a painless pseudoarthrosis. Osteotomies, bone grafting, and arthroplasties result in favorable prognosis with some functional limitations.

PEARLS

In follow-up radiographs for fracture healing, the factors predictive of nonunion are

- Inadequate immobilization
- Improper reduction
- Avascular necrosis
- Demineralization of the bones
- Infection
- Loosening of prostheses or other fixation devices

PITFALL

- Fracture healing may be difficult to assess if follow-up films are obtained in different projections.

Suggested Readings

Morgan WJ, Breen TF, Coumas JM, Schulz LA. Role of magnetic resonance imaging in assessing factors affecting healing in scaphoid nonunions. Clin Orthop Relat Res 1997;336:240–246

Munk PL, Lee MJ. Gadolinium-enhanced MR imaging of scaphoid nonunions. Am J Roentgenol 2000;175:1184–1185

CASE 102

Hema N. Choudur, Anthony G. Ryan, and Peter L. Munk

Clinical Presentation

Following a motor vehicle accident, this patient presented to the emergency department with cervical instability and neck pain. No neurological compromise was noted.

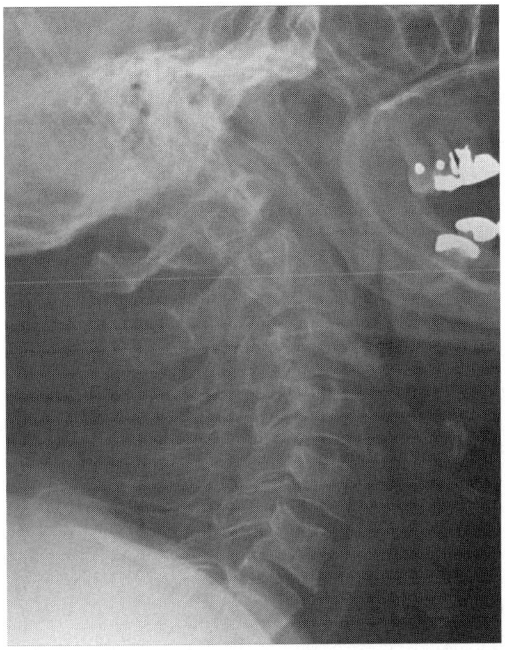

Figure 102A

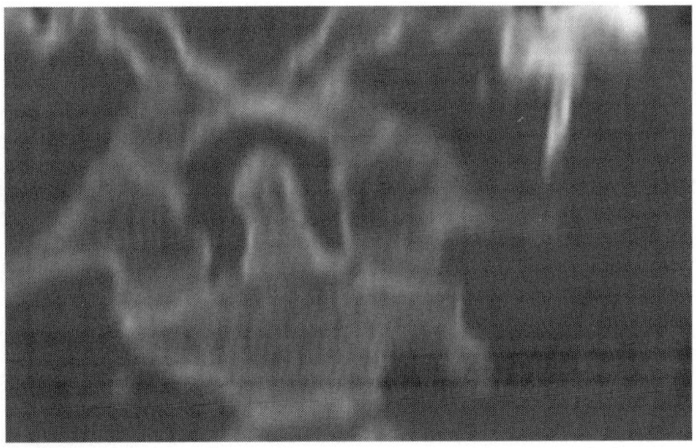

Figure 102B

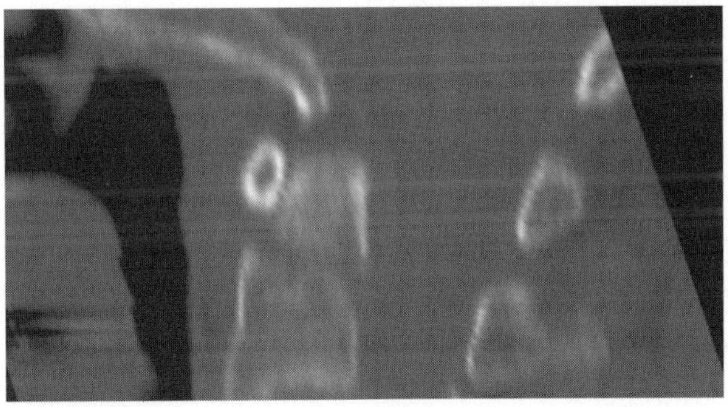

Figure 102C

Radiologic Findings

The initial lateral radiograph (**Fig. 102A**) reveals a faint lucency across the neck of the odontoid with suspicious narrowing of the atlantoaxial distance. A helical CT with reformats (**Fig. 102B,** coronal, and **Fig. 102C,** sagittal) clearly shows the transversely oriented, mildly displaced base of the odontoid fracture.

Diagnosis

Type 2 odontoid fracture with associated narrowing of the atlantoaxial interval.

Differential Diagnosis

None.

Discussion

Background

Odontoid fractures account for 1 to 2% of all spinal fractures and for 8 to 15% of all cervical spine fractures. Displaced odontoid fractures (15 to 85%) can result in neurological deficit and nonunion if not promptly and appropriately treated. Of cervical vertebral fractures, C2 fractures are the most common. These fractures can result in very sinister complications due to cord compression; therefore, their prompt recognition and treatment are imperative.

Etiology

Most of these fractures occur following blunt trauma to the neck and motor vehicle accidents. A flexion loading force is the most common etiology, with anterior displacement of the dens. An extension loading force with posterior displacement of the dens occurs in a minority of cases. A rotational force can also occur.

Pathophysiology

Following trauma to the dens, the bony break can be of three types:

- *Type 1* These fractures are very infrequent and involve the tip of the odontoid. They occur in 5% of cases. These avulsion injuries result in an obliquely oriented fracture. Associated tear of the apical and alar ligaments can occur with instability of the detached fragment.
- *Type 2* These fractures are the most frequent (60% of odontoid fractures), involving the base of the odontoid with or without displacement. Called body fracture, the fracture line passes above a horizontal line drawn through the upper border of the superior articular facets of the axis. These fractures result in severe complications, such as cord compression and respiratory distress as the atlas and occiput move as a unit. Identification of these fractures is therefore imperative. These fractures are also notorious for nonunion. Associated tear of the transverse ligament of the dens can occur and is well seen on MRI.
- *Type 3* Basilar fractures involve the body of the axis and occur below the line drawn through the superior articular facets of the axis. They heal well with immobilization. They are seen in 30% of odontoid fractures.

A vertical fracture through the dens has been described and is seen in 5% of odontoid fractures. Fracture site/stability was analyzed in particular by Roy-Camille, who published his own classification in 1973. The classification is based on the direction of the fracture line on lateral films and on a study of dynamic views. A fracture is considered to be unstable if it is displaced at presentation, or if, while originally undisplaced, it is found to be displaced on the dynamic views taken on or about day 10. The displacement will typically be in an anterior direction if the fracture line slopes forward. If the fracture line slopes backward, the displacement will normally be in a posterior direction. When the fracture line is horizontal, these fractures may displace either anteriorly or posteriorly. If associated with a wide interfragment gap and anterior and posterior comminution, it is termed a "bobby's helmet" fracture.

Clinical Findings

Patients usually present with a history of fall or blunt trauma or after a motor vehicle accident. They present to the emergency department with instability of the head. There is usually pain and decreased mobility of the neck, with the patient often holding his head in his hands.

Complications

In unstable fractures, neurological sequelae secondary to cord compression can occur and are most common in type 2 fractures with backward displacement. This can be assessed by plain radiographs to exclude displacement at the fracture site immediately after injury and with neutral and dynamic projections 10 days following an initially unstable fracture. The other complication is nonunion. The causes of nonunion are not due to interruption of blood supply and have been described as dependent on the direction of slope. The posteriorly directed slope is at the greatest risk for nonunion.

Imaging Findings

RADIOGRAPHY

There are different trauma protocols in different hospitals, but the standard anteroposterior and lateral views of the cervical spine are mandatory to look for atlantoaxial disruption and to screen for other cervical vertebral fractures. Although an open-mouth view is included as a routine projection in some hospitals, others opt for this view only when there is suspicion of an odontoid fracture. Fractures with purely lateral displacement are well seen on the open-mouth views and can be unstable if the alar ligaments are torn.

An optimally taken lateral view is the most useful projection, with dynamic views to ascertain atlantoaxial instability.

COMPUTED TOMOGRAPHY

A helical CT with reformats (as in our case) will detect even subtle fractures. Three-dimensional CT is considered most useful in evaluating odontoid fractures. The line of the fracture, its type, and atlantoaxial distance and stability, in addition to the amount of spinal canal compromise, are well depicted. At the level of the dens, the cord should occupy one third of the canal, the dens should occupy one third, and the remaining third is empty. Any variation in this division suggests pathology. In the absence of an MRI facility, a CT myelogram is sometimes useful to assess cord compression.

CT has shown a large number of asymmetrical fracture patterns in the coronal plane, with the fracture line extending from one side of the neck of the odontoid into the superior articular process of the axis on the other side. This pattern suggests a rotatory force and has an additional risk of instability, especially if the alar ligaments are no longer intact. CT can miss axial fractures, which are better visualized on plain radiographs. Also, the extent of subluxation and dislocation is better evaluated by plain radiographs. An asymmetrical fracture pattern resulting in fragment diastasis may be misjudged on the lateral view and is better evaluated by CT.

MAGNETIC RESONANCE IMAGING

The stability of the atlantoaxial joint and cord compression are best depicted by MRI. Subtle fractures are also visualized on inversion recovery sequences.

Treatment and Prognosis

The treatment varies depending on the type of fracture. The treatment provided would seek to reduce the fracture and to achieve perfect stability to prevent nonunion. If the radiographs taken at the time of injury do not reveal any instability, a repeat set of radiographs is called for in 10 days with dynamic views, and if the fracture is still stable, conservative treatment with a cast for 6 months is recommended. An initially unstable fracture or a fracture becoming unstable on day 10 is surgically treated.

- *Type 1* A cervical collar is usually sufficient for symptomatic relief.
- *Type 2* The treatment varies, depending on the slope stability of the fracture; surgical fixation can be C1–C2 wire fixation, spacer placement, spacer and wire fixation, anterior screw fixation, or posterior cervico-occipital fusion.
- *Type 3* Immobilization by cast

The neurological complications do not depend on the pattern or type of fragment displacement. In the literature, a mean displacement of ~13 mm produced neurological compromise. Traction has been reported to improve patients with displaced fractures. Anatomical reduction with halo traction or following surgery resulted in neurological recovery in a group of patients with neurological deficits.

Patients with cervicobrachial neuralgia tend to recover more rapidly and fully than those with quadriparesis.

PEARLS

- These fractures are often missed and result in neurological compromise and even death. Good-quality lateral and open-mouth views are mandatory, with dynamic views if necessary on the 10th day following injury.
- CT with reformats will detect subtle fractures and also help in analyzing three-dimensional stability, the level and direction of the fracture line, and rotation or translation of the fracture fragments.

PITFALL

- An axial fracture can be missed on CT and is best assessed on plain radiographs.

Suggested Readings

Acheson MB, Livingston RR, Richardson ML, Stimac GK. High-resolution CT scanning in the evaluation of cervical spine fractures: comparison with plain film examinations. Am J Roentgenol 1987;148:1179–1185

Blackmore CC. Evidence-based imaging evaluation of the cervical spine in trauma. Neuroimaging Clin N Am 2003;13:283–291

Crim JR, Moore K, Brodke D. Clearance of the cervical spine in multitrauma patients: the role of advanced imaging. Semin Ultrasound CT MR 2001;22:283–305

Roy-Camille R, Saillant G. Surgery of the cervical spine: osteosynthesis of the upper cervical spine. Nouv Presse Med 1972;1:2847–2849

CASE 103

Hema N. Choudur, Anthony G. Ryan, and Peter L. Munk

Clinical Findings

A middle-aged woman with known rheumatoid arthritis presented with sudden onset neck pain and instability. On examination, restricted motion of the neck was noted. No neurological deficit was present.

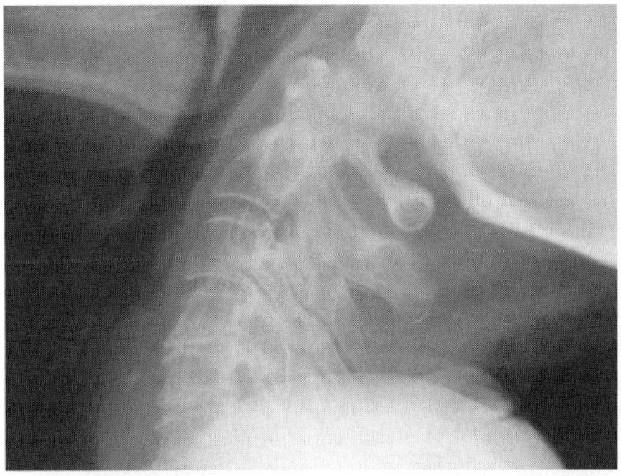

Figure 103A

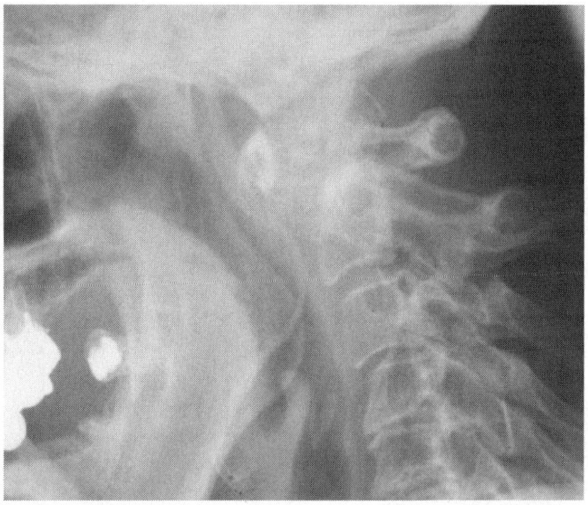

Figure 103B

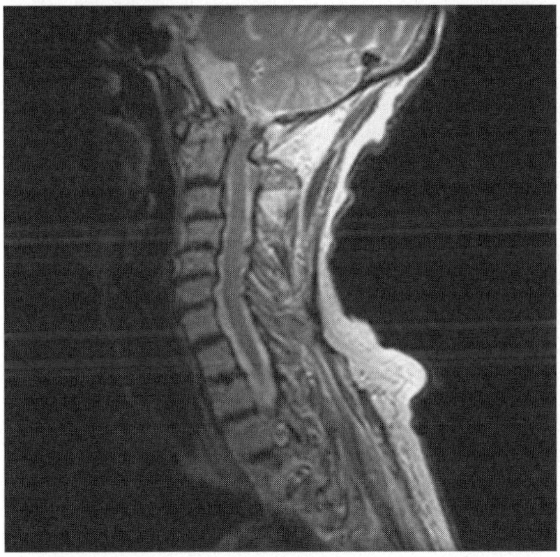

Figure 103C

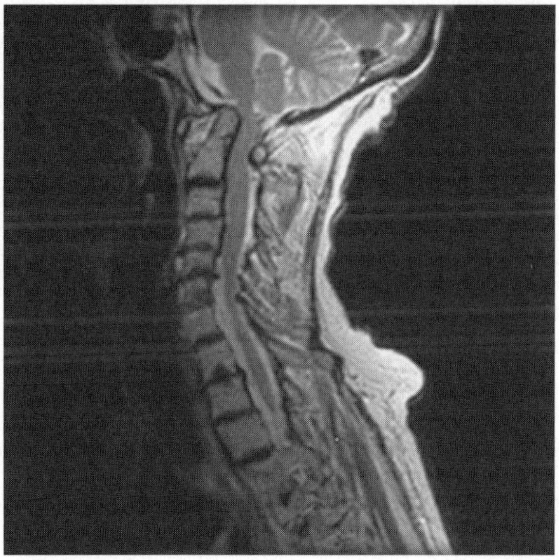

Figure 103D

Radiologic Findings

Initial cervical spine radiographs were unremarkable, but clinical instability indicated flexion and extension views. The extension view is unremarkable (**Fig. 103A**); however, increased distance between the posterior margin of the atlas and the anterior margin of the dens is evident on the flexion view (**Fig. 103B**), findings suggestive of atlantoaxial instability (AAI).

Subsequent MRI (**Figs. 103C–103E**, T2 and **Figs. 103F–103H**, T1 postgadolinium) reveals an avidly enhancing pannus eroding the anterior margin of the odontoid process on its left side. The spinal

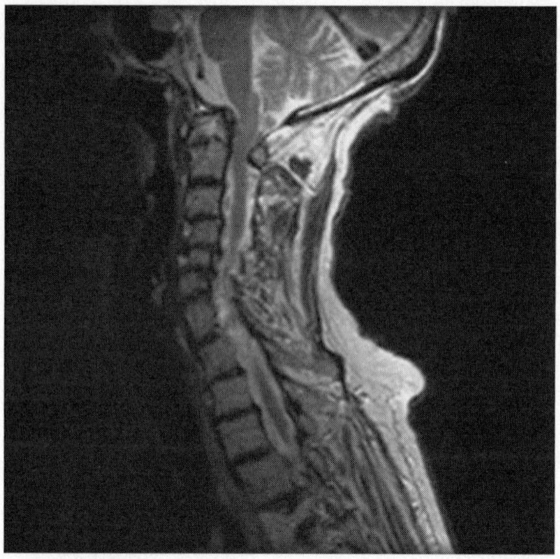

Figure 103E

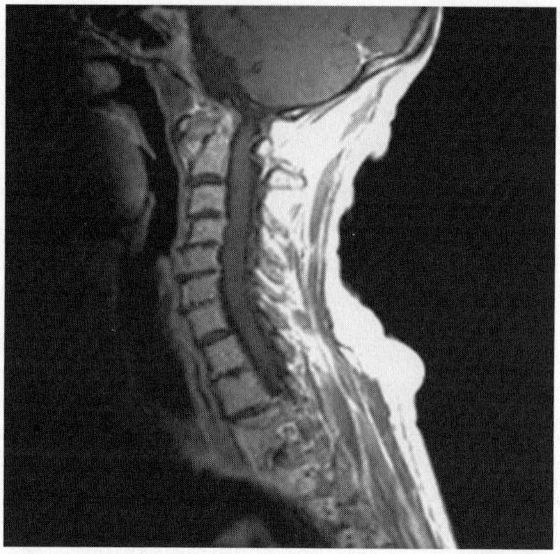

Figure 103F

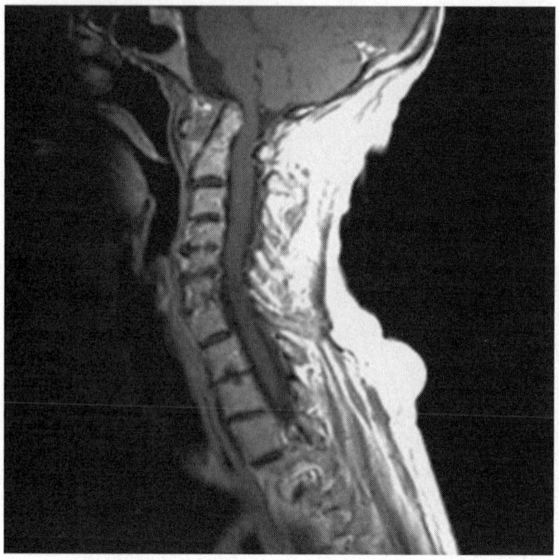

Figure 103G

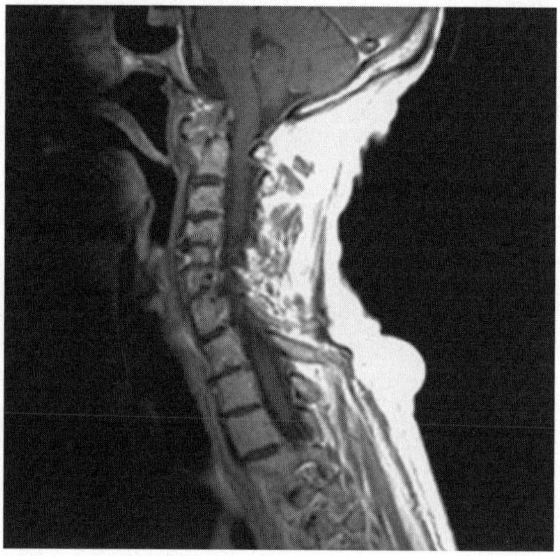

Figure 103H

cord is compressed posteriorly. Further cord impingement is evident inferiorly secondary to cervical spondylosis.

Diagnosis

AAI secondary to rheumatoid pannus.

Differential Diagnosis

- Traumatic AAI
- Ankylosing spondylitis

In the pediatric population, there are several potential causes of AAI:

- Children are more susceptible to AAI secondary to the steeper dens-facet angle and the rich vascular folds in the atlantoaxial and lateral atlantoaxial joint.

- Grisel's syndrome, in which respiratory infection traveling to the peridental venous plexus causes inflammation and subsequent laxity of the supporting ligaments
- Certain congenital conditions predispose, namely Down syndrome, Morquio's syndrome, and metabolic causes.

Discussion

Background

Excessive movement between C1–C2 may be either bony or ligamentous. A high index of clinical and radiologic suspicion is required, and although initial cervical radiographs may be unremarkable, suspected instability should be investigated further by dynamic cervical spine views or CT with reformats to demonstrate the instability.

The normal atlantoaxial distance (measured from the posterior margin of the anterior arch of the atlas to the anterior margin of the odontoid) is 3 mm in adults and 5 mm in children.

Movements at this joint include flexion-extension, rotation, and distraction. Atlantoaxial stability is primarily maintained by the transverse ligament and the facet capsules. The transverse ligament is the primary restraint for anteroposterior motion of the dens. The alar ligaments and the tectorial membrane prevent vertical translation of the atlas.

In cervical trauma, as many as 10% of patients show involvement of the atlantoaxial joint, the most common mechanism of action being forceful flexion with deceleration, as occurs when the head strikes the windshield in a motor vehicle accident.

In rheumatoid arthritis, the synovium and articular cartilage lining the transverse ligament and facet joints are involved. The inflammation and pannus can spread to the alar ligaments and can cause destruction of the subchondral bone and the dens (as is evident in the reference case). The instability is mainly in the anteroposterior plane and hence well demonstrated by flexion-extension views. Cervical spine involvement is seen in 30 to 80% of rheumatoid patients, the majority of whom are asymptomatic.

AAI may occur in association with many congenital syndromes including Down syndrome, congenital scoliosis, osteogenesis imperfecta, neurofibromatosis, Morquio's syndrome, Larsen's syndrome, pseudoachondroplasia, spondyloepiphyseal dysplasia congenita, chondrodysplasia punctata, metatropic dysplasia, and Kniest syndrome.

Laxity of the transverse ligament is the cause of AAI in Down syndrome. AAI is seen in 10 to 20% of asymptomatic and 1 to 2% of symptomatic Down syndrome patients. In Morquio's syndrome, the cause of AAI is hypoplasia or aplasia of the dens.

The bony causes of AAI include odontoid anomalies such as aplasia, hypoplasia, and os odontoideum. Atlanto-occipital fusion also predisposes a patient to the development of AAI. In spondyloepiphyseal dysplasia congenita, 40% of patients reveal AAI.

Pathological fractures of C1–C2 (e.g., metastatic deposits) can also result in AAI.

Clinical Findings

In children with known congenital syndromes, examination should be directed at detecting upper motor neuron signs.

Torticollis may be the presenting complaint of rotatory displacement. In those cases caused by infection, tenderness over the spine of the axis may be elicited and excessive motion to the side effected by the inciting infection.

Rheumatoid patients may present with occipital pain and on examination may show brainstem signs from basilar invagination, upper cranial nerve involvement, or myelopathy.

Complications

- Cervicomedullary compression
- Vertebral artery insufficiency due to the tortuous path of the artery at the atlantoaxial articulation

Imaging Findings

RADIOGRAPHY

- In a lateral view of the cervical spine in the neutral position, a distance > 4 to 5 mm is considered to be AAI.
- Occult AAI can be diagnosed on flexion-extension views, with a displacement of > 3.5 mm being significant.
- The posterior dental interval (from the posterior margin of the dens to the anterior margin of the posterior tubercle) will be correspondingly reduced, indicating the degree of secondary spinal canal stenosis.
- Prevertebral soft-tissue swelling secondary to traumatic hematoma or abscess formation is seen.
- An open-mouth odontoid view is useful to ascertain the central position of the dens. The lateral masses of C1 should overhang C2 in the horizontal plane by no more than 6.9 mm, as distances in excess of this likely indicate rupture of the transverse ligament.

COMPUTED TOMOGRAPHY

CT is useful in accurately measuring the atlantoaxial distance and also in assessing rotational displacement.

- *Type 1* Simple rotational displacement with the transverse ligament intact
- *Type 2* C1 on C2 anterior displacement < 5 mm with a tear of the transverse ligament. One facet acts as a pivot.
- *Type 3* C1 on C2 anterior displacement > 5 mm
- *Type 4* Posterior displacement of C1 on C2

Types 3 and 4 are unstable injuries.

MAGNETIC RESONANCE IMAGING

- MRI surpasses other modalities in the evaluation of soft tissues at the C1–C2 level
- Infections in particular are depicted clearly on the postgadolinium images.
- The size and location of the pannus in rheumatoid arthritis and the structures it involves are well visualized.
- Erosions and synovial inflammation in the facet joints and the status of the transverse ligament are also demonstrated clearly.

Treatment

Treatment involves stabilization of the cervical spine, protection of the spinal cord, and relief of neural compression.

ANTEROPOSTERIOR INSTABILITY

- Atlantoaxial distance > 4 mm is suggestive of a torn transverse ligament and needs surgical C1–C2 fixation.
- When the origin of the instability is bony, surgical correction is less likely to be successful.
- Cord compression > 60% does not respond to decompression; therefore, early detection is imperative.

In rheumatoid arthritis AAI, the indications for surgery are atlantoaxial distance > 8 mm on flexion-extension views; a posterior atlantodental interval ≤ 14 mm; subaxial subluxation > 3.5 mm; cord compression; or progressive neurologic deficit.

ROTATORY INSTABILITY

- Type 1 is treated with a brace.
- Type 2 is treated with a brace and watched for response. If it remains unstable, it is treated surgically. Those who present with a fixed deformity are also treated surgically.
- Types 3 and 4 are surgically treated with reduction and C1–C2 fixation.

Children with Down and other syndromes should be radiographically screened regularly, as should those with asymptomatic AAI.

Prognosis

The prognosis is good in those patients treated surgically for relief of pain (successful in ~95%) and myelopathy (successful in ~74%).

PEARLS

- In a lateral view of the cervical spine in the neutral position, a distance > 4 to 5 mm is considered AAI.
- Occult AAI can be diagnosed on flexion-extension views, with a displacement > 3.5 mm being significant.
- An open-mouth odontoid view is useful to ascertain the central position of the dens. The lateral masses of C1 should overhang C2 in the horizontal plane by no more than 6.9 mm, as distances in excess of this likely indicate rupture of the transverse ligament.

PITFALLS

- A normal lateral cervical spine radiograph does not exclude AAI, if the latter is suspected clinically, flexion and extension views should be performed.
- The dynamic nature of the instability means it may be missed on static CT of the cervical spine.

Suggested Readings

Larsson EM, Holtas S, Zygmunt S. Pre- and postoperative MR imaging of the craniocervical junction in rheumatoid arthritis. Am J Roentgenol 1989;152:561–566

Stein SM, Kirchner SG, Horev G, Hernanz-Schulman M. Atlanto-occipital subluxation in Down syndrome. Pediatr Radiol 1991;21:121–124

Vargas TM, Rybicki FJ, Ledbetter SM, MacKenzie JD. Atlantoaxial instability associated with an orthotopic os odontoideum: a multimodality imaging assessment. Emerg Radiol 2005;11:223–225

CASE 104

Hema N. Choudur, Anthony G. Ryan, and Peter L. Munk

Clinical Presentation

Following a diving injury in shallow waters, a young man was brought to the emergency department with quadriplegia.

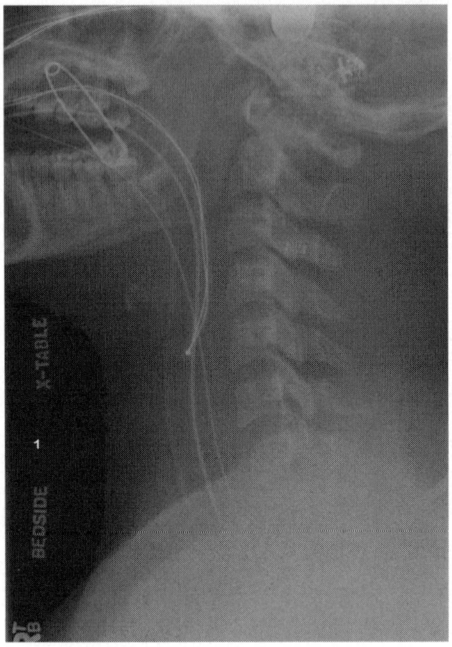

Figure 104A

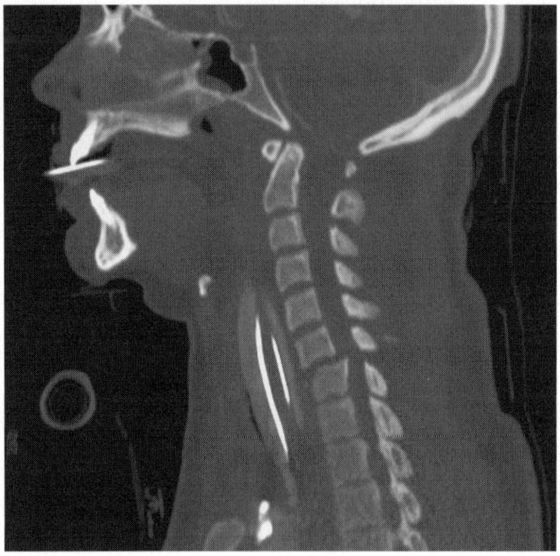

Figure 104B

Radiologic Findings

The lateral radiograph (**Fig. 104A**) reveals an anterosuperior C7 vertebral fracture with mild displacement of the fractured fragment. Also noted is the fracture of the superior articular process of the same vertebra.

Sagittal reformats from the subsequent CT (**Figs. 104B,104C**) show the C7 fracture fragment and C6 over C7 anterior subluxation causing spinal canal narrowing at the same level.

A T2-weighted sagittal image from the subsequent MRI (**Fig. 104D**) shows the C6 on C7 anterior subluxation with a tear of the posterior longitudinal ligament and buckling of the anterior longitudinal ligament. A hematoma interposed between the anterior longitudinal ligament and the vertebral body is evident. Clearly depicted is the transection of the cord at the same level, with post-traumatic high signal intensity within the cord above the level of injury.

A postfixation cervical spine lateral view (**Fig. 104E**) shows stabilization of the vertebrae at the level of the injury.

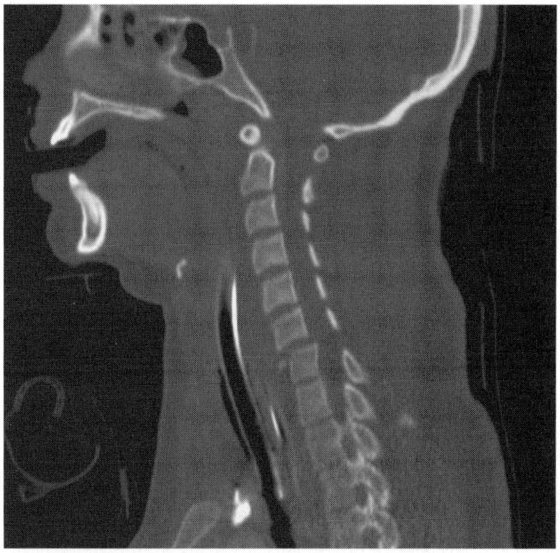

Figure 104C

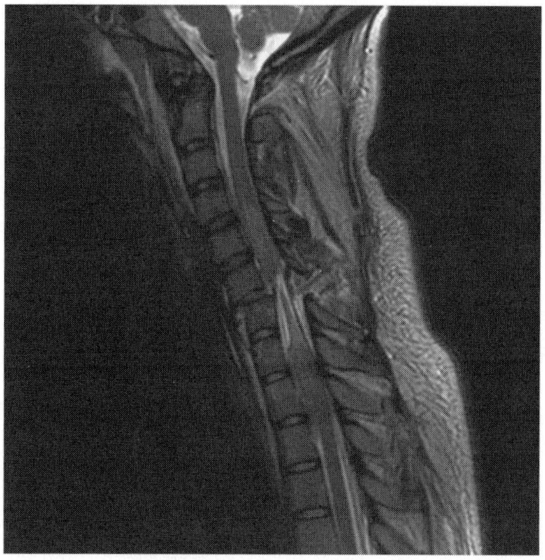

Figure 104D

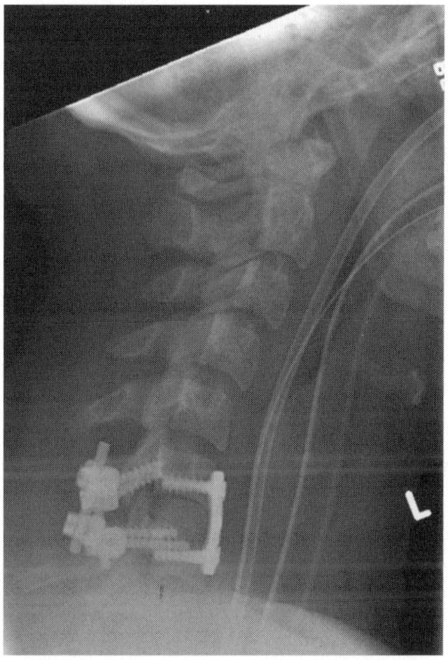

Figure 104E

Diagnosis

Flexion teardrop fracture with associated cord transection.

Differential Diagnosis

Wedge compression fractures are usually stable injuries. The posterior cortex is intact with no ligamentous injury.

Discussion

Background

These fractures were originally described by Schneider and Cann as “teardrop” fractures. Teardrop fractures represent 15% of traumatic cervical spine injuries. Injuries can be severe, with cord involvement

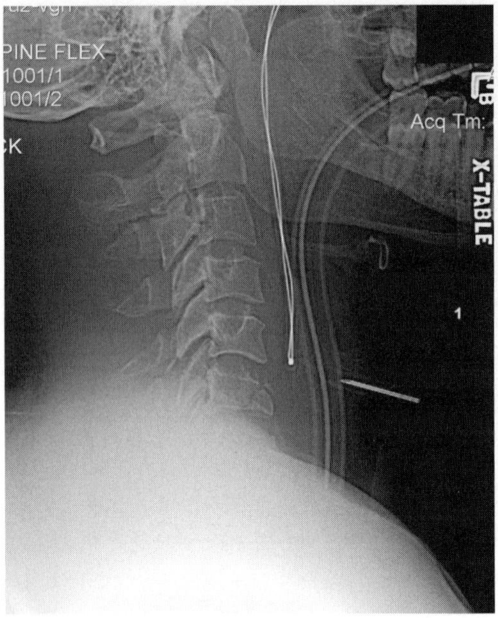

Figure 104F A plain radiograph lateral view shows an anteroinferior teardrop fracture. Note that the fracture fragment is vertically oriented (flexion teardrop), as opposed to a horizontally oriented fractured fragment in an extension teardrop fracture.

and quadriplegia in 60% of cases. These fractures are very unstable. The kyphosis can progress with neurologic deterioration. Stabilization is by operative means.

A common feature of teardrop fractures is a triangular teardrop fragment separated from the rest of the vertebral body. The most common is the anteroinferior portion (**Fig. 104F**) of the vertebral body; the second most common is the anterosuperior portion of the vertebral body.

Etiology

A hyperflexion injury results in an anteroinferior vertebral body fracture, described as a flexion teardrop fracture, and is more common in the lower cervical vertebrae. A hyperextension injury results in an extension teardrop fracture and is more common in the superior cervical vertebrae.

These fractures can result from a fall, diving, or a motor vehicle accident.

Pathophysiology

Following hyperflexion and compression, the apophyseal capsules are torn, with damage and narrowing of the inferior disk. The anterior longitudinal ligament is avulsed to varying degrees. The vertically fractured anteroinferior vertebral body fragment is dislocated to a varying degree and may lie on the vertebral body below or move further anteriorly. This injury is unstable due to disruption of the soft tissues binding the vertebral bodies together.

Two fracture patterns are associated with these fractures: an isolated fracture with no permanent neurologic sequelae and the three-part, two-plane fracture, in which there is an associated sagittal vertebral body fracture as well as fracture of the posterior neural arch. This latter pattern is almost always associated with permanent neurologic sequelae, specifically quadriplegia, as seen in our case.

In hyperextension injuries, the disrupting force involves the disk, the anterior longitudinal ligament, and the anteroinferior vertebral body. The posterior longitudinal ligament is separated from the adjoining vertebra and disk.

Clinical Findings

Clinical findings are variable, with some patients presenting with only neck pain and others with quadriplegia in flexion injuries. Extension injuries often reduce spontaneously and are difficult to diagnose.

Complications

Cord compression in flexion injuries is a grave complication and can result in permanent neurologic sequelae.

Imaging Findings

RADIOGRAPHY

The most characteristic feature of flexion teardrop fractures is the separation of the anteroinferior part of the affected vertebral body, usually C5, on the lateral view. The posterior fragment of the involved vertebra is displaced backward, with facet separation and backward displacement of the inferior facet, increase in the interspinous and interlaminar distances, and kyphotic deformity at the level of the fractured vertebra.

The column above the level of the fracture is posteriorly displaced. This injury is frequently associated with sagittal-body and laminar fractures and occurs predominantly at the C5 level.

Four types of flexion teardrop fractures are described: an occult form seen only on CT, teardrop fracture without displacement, teardrop fracture with mild to moderate displacement, and teardrop with posterior displacement and kyphosis $>$ 20 degrees. The last of the mentioned types results in neurologic sequelae such as quadriplegia.

Extension teardrop fractures

Extension teardrop fractures result from a hyperextension force causing impaction of the posterior elements and distraction of the anterior elements of the spinal column.

The most frequent radiologic feature is prevertebral soft-tissue swelling. This has been reported as the only plain radiographic sign of an extension injury. Other features include an increase in the height of the anterior disk space and fracture of the posterior spinal elements. The anterior longitudinal ligament and disk are torn. The posterior ligaments are usually intact.

The most severe form is the hyperextension fracture-dislocation. The lateral radiograph shows an avulsion fracture from the anteroinferior vertebral body. This “teardrop”-shaped fracture must be differentiated from a “flexion teardrop” fracture. In the extension injury, the teardrop fragment is usually longer horizontally than vertically. Characteristically, there is no kyphosis or posterior displacement of the vertebral body.

COMPUTED TOMOGRAPHY

Occult teardrop fractures are often incidentally recognized on CT and require no treatment. The size of the fractured fragment and the extent of displacement are seen on plain radiographs, but sometimes the sagittal component of the flexion teardrop fracture is only evident on CT. Because these fractures result in severe morbidity and mortality, CT should be recommended in clinically and radiographically suspicious cases. The extent of spinal canal narrowing can vary. The diameter of the spinal canal at the C5 level is on average ~17 mm but may be less than 14 mm in congenital/acquired stenosis. The diameter of the spinal cord at C5 is 10 mm. A posterior displacement $>$ 4 mm is associated with a high incidence of severe neurologic involvement. The extent of posterior displacement of the posterosuperior fragment and associated posterior neural element fractures are better evaluated on CT.

MAGNETIC RESONANCE IMAGING

The soft-tissue injury is clearly visualized on MRI, including the longitudinal ligaments, disk, prevertebral soft tissues, and the state of the cord itself.

Treatment

In flexion injuries with an undisplaced small fragment, only conservative treatment is required, with halo immobilization. But displaced fragments need surgical removal with anterior or posterior vertebral body stabilization. The aim of surgery would be to stabilize the spinal canal and the cord, often performed as an emergency procedure.

Extension injuries are usually managed conservatively.

Prognosis

The neurologic sequelae are usually permanent in those presenting with quadriplegia and progressive kyphosis in spite of emergency surgical treatment. Those with a lesser degree of neurologic involvement may improve following rapid surgical management.

PEARL

- CT/MRI is mandatory in suspicious cases to evaluate the components of the injury.

PITFALL

- The danger lies in missing a sagittal fracture of the three-component flexion injury on plain radiographs in an acute setting.

Suggested Readings

Green JD, Harle TS, Harris JH Jr. Anterior subluxation of the cervical spine: hyperflexion sprain. Am J Neuroradiol 1981;2:243–250

Kim KS, Chen HH, Russell EJ, Rogers LF. Flexion teardrop fracture of the cervical spine: radiographic characteristics. Am J Roentgenol 1989;152:319–326

Lee C, Kim KS, Rogers LF. Triangular cervical vertebral body fractures: diagnostic significance. Am J Roentgenol 1982;138:1123–1132

Torg JS, Pavlov H, O'Neill MJ, et al. The axial load teardrop fracture: a biomechanical, clinical and roentgenographic analysis. J Sports Med 1991;19:355–364

CASE 105

Hema N. Choudur, Anthony G. Ryan, and Peter L. Munk

Clinical Presentation

Two cases presented to the emergency department following motor vehicle accidents. The first, a C3 paraplegic, sustained an injury when his car crashed down a 300-m embankment (**Figs. 105A–105M**); the second was a windshield impact injury (**Figs. 105N–105S**).

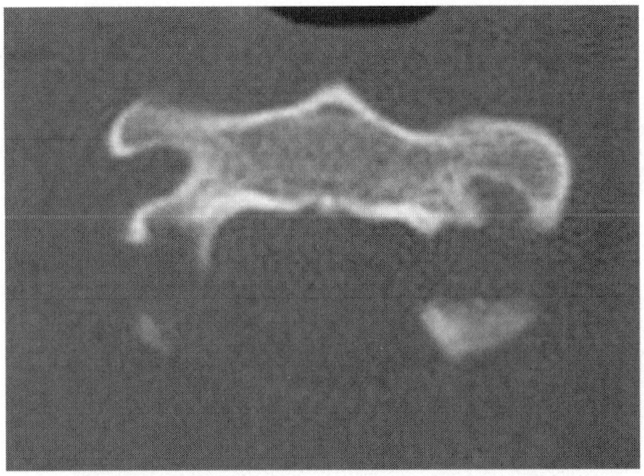

Figure 105A

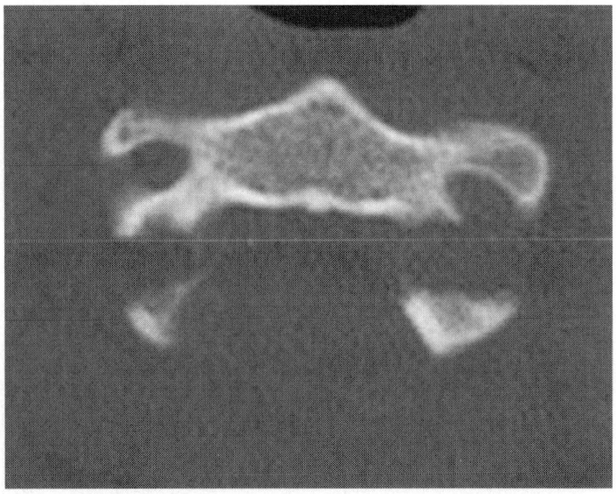

Figure 105B

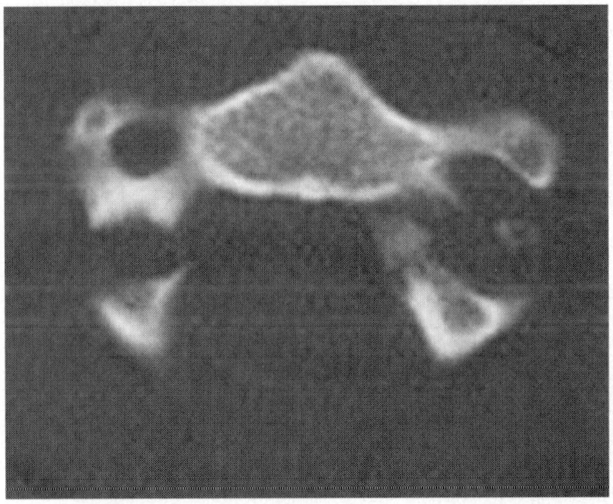

Figure 105C

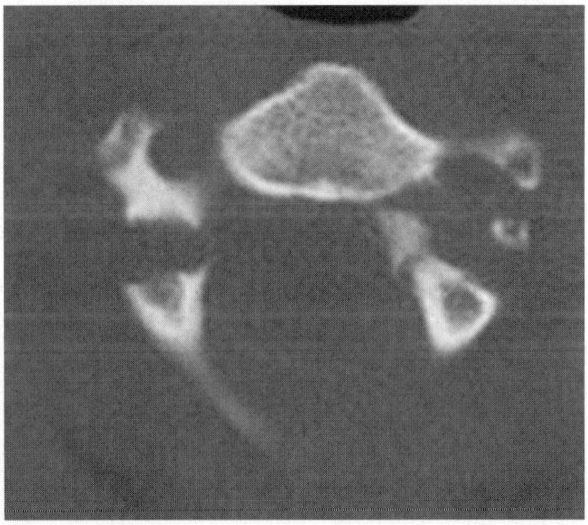

Figure 105D

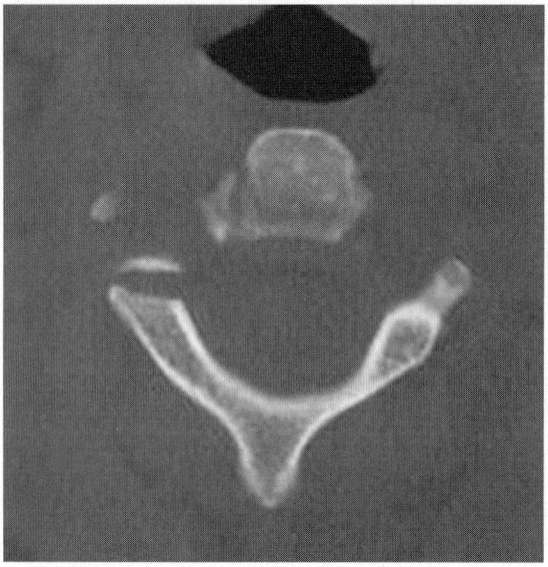

Figure 105E

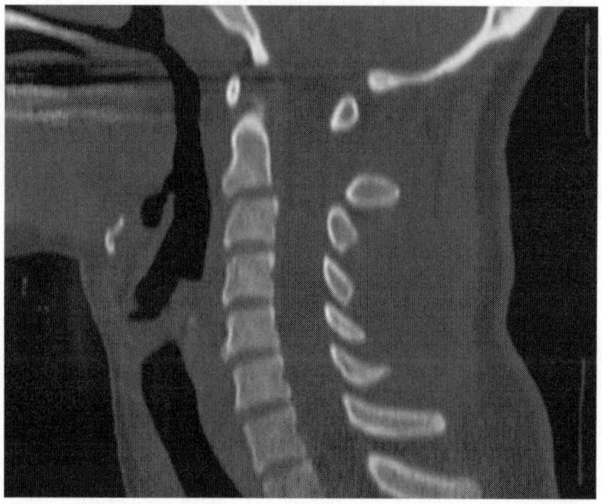

Figure 105F

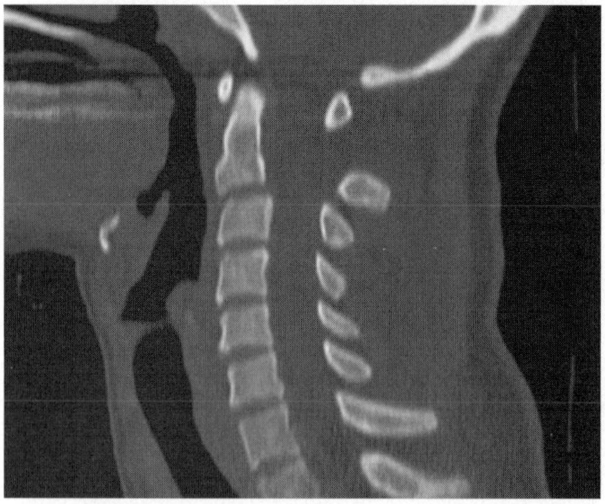

Figure 105G

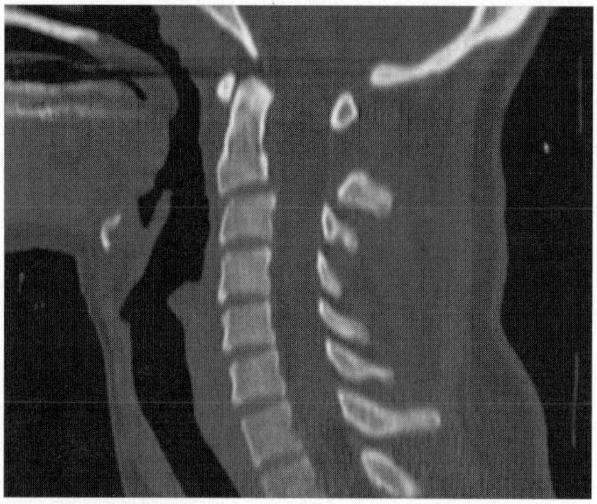

Figure 105H

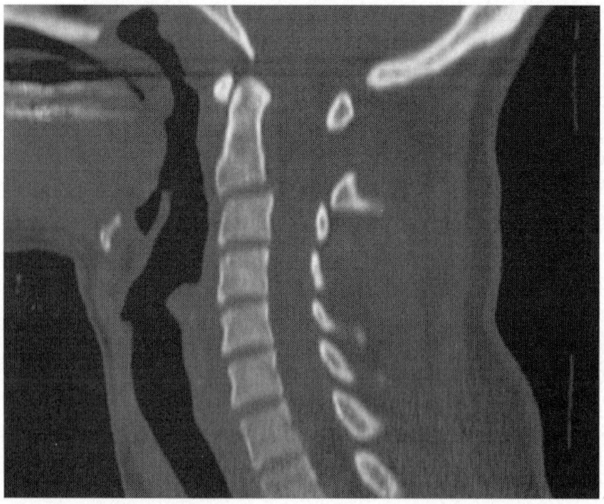

Figure 105I

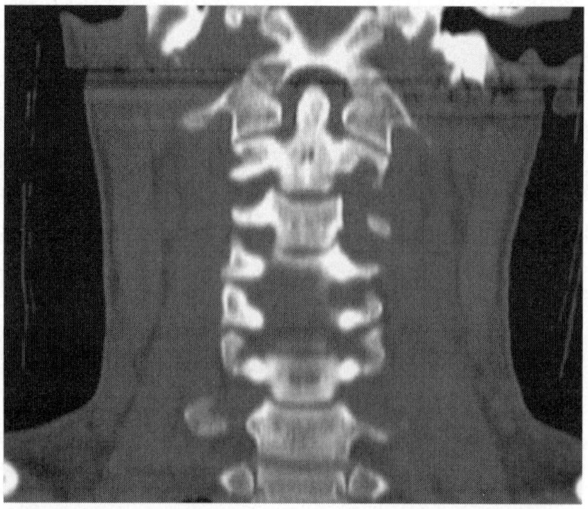

Figure 105J

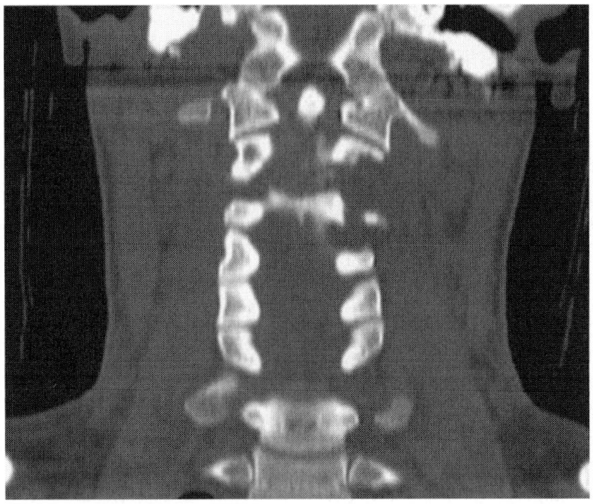

Figure 105K

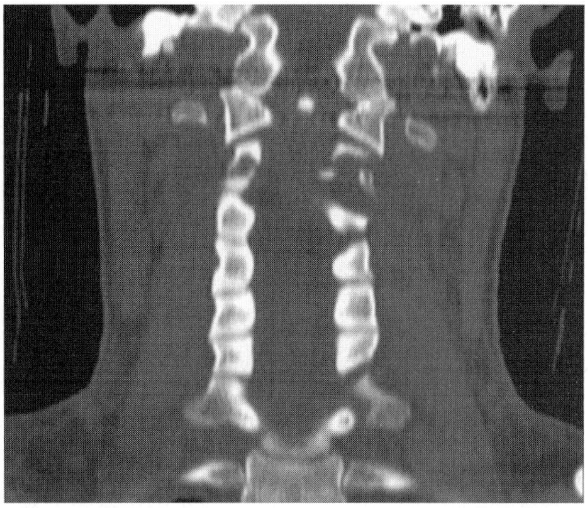

Figure 105L

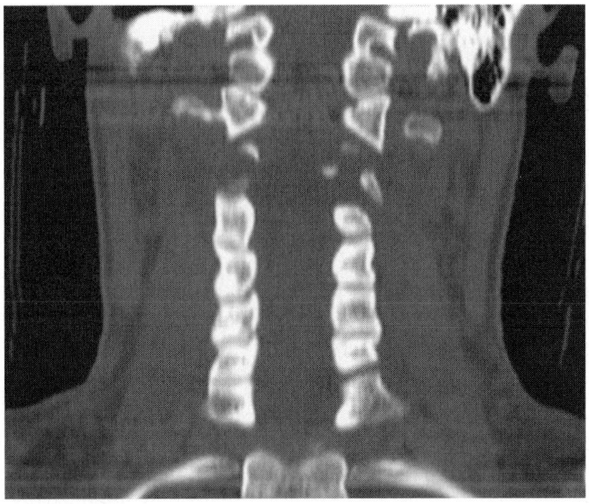

Figure 105M

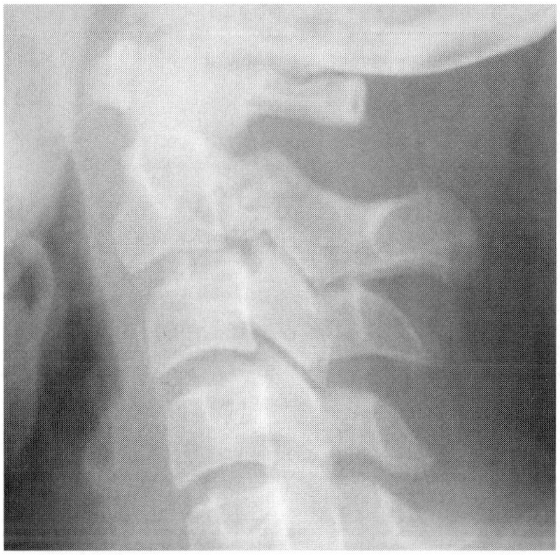

Figure 105N

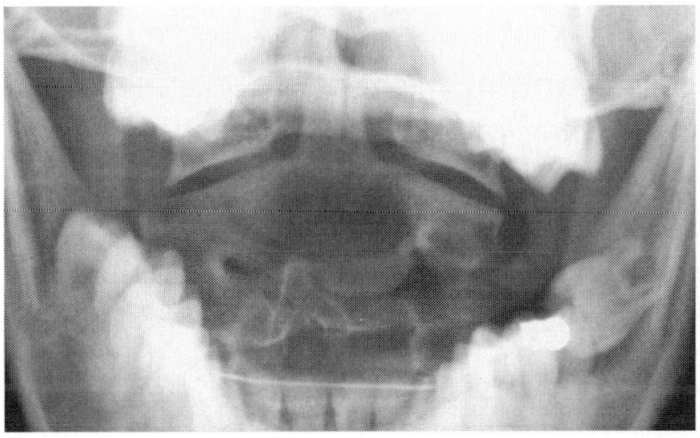

Figure 105O

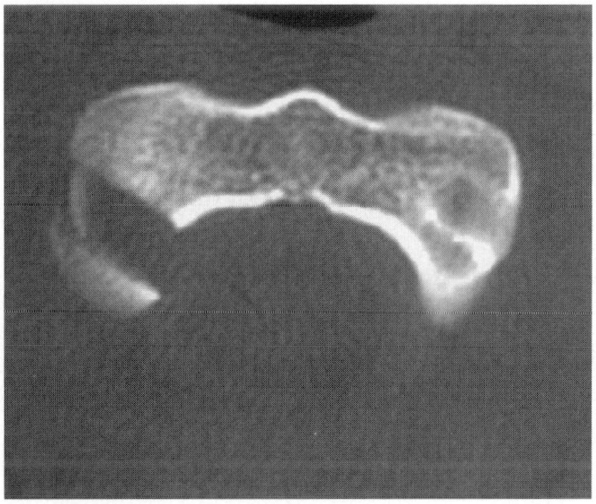

Figure 105P

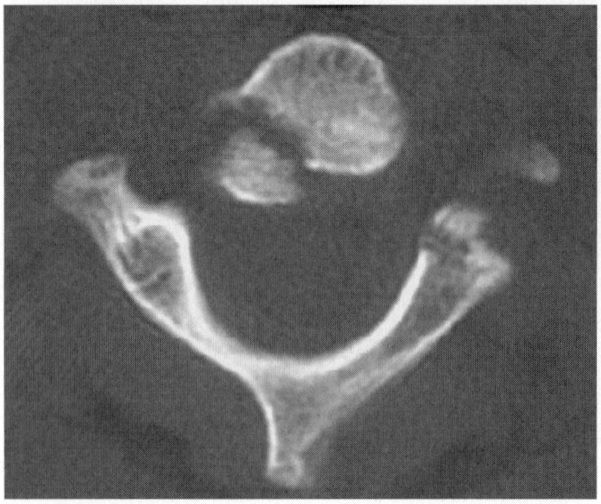

Figure 105Q

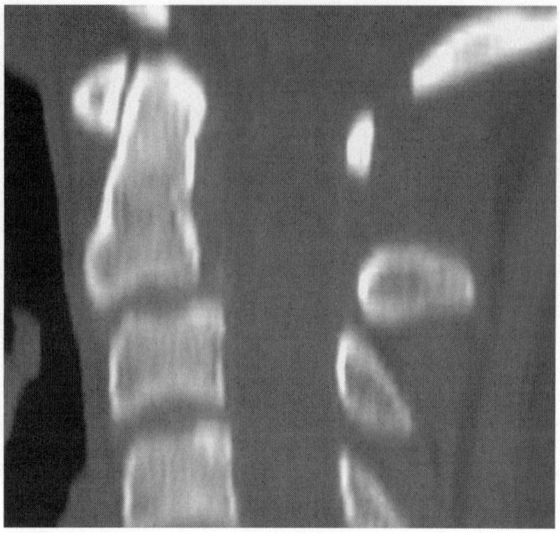

Figure 105R

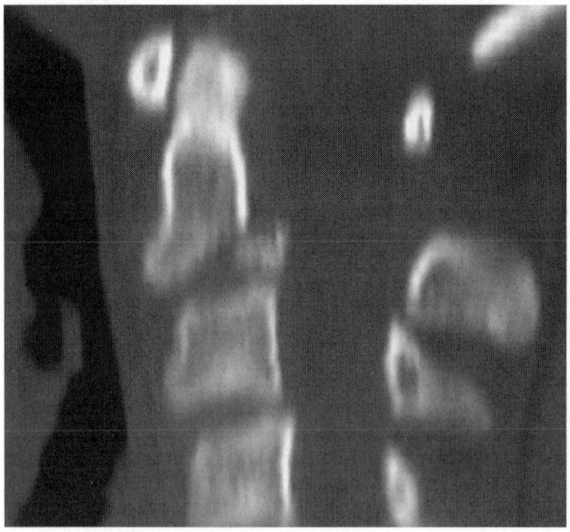

Figure 105S

Radiologic Findings

Case 1

Axial 1 mm CT slices (**Figs. 105A–105E**) with sagittal (**Figs. 105F–105I**) and coronal (**Figs. 105J–105M**) reformats show a comminuted fracture of the C2 left pedicle involving the posterior transverse foramen. The largest fragment is displaced posteromedially by 7 mm, with extension into the posterior transverse foramen. Mild effacement of the thecal sac is evident.

A linear fracture through the right pedicle is noted with a 6 mm posterior displacement. Two mm C2 over C3 anterolisthesis is seen. The posterior spinolaminar line is disrupted, and the spinous process of C2 is displaced posteriorly. CT angiography was negative for vertebral artery involvement.

Case 2

Lateral view of the spine (**Fig. 105N**), open-mouth view (**Fig. 105O**), and CT axial slices (**Figs. 105P,105Q**) with sagittal reformats (**Figs. 105R,105S**) reveal a fracture passing obliquely through the right lateral mass, with anterior subluxation < 3 mm.

Diagnosis

- *Case 1* Type 2 bipedicular hangman's fracture.
- *Case 2* Type 1 hangman's fracture.

A diagnosis of C2 traumatic spondylolisthesis was made in both cases with an unstable fracture in each.

Differential Diagnosis

None.

Discussion

Background

Schneider in 1964 called C2 fractures "hangman's" fractures, as they were similar to those seen in judicial hangings. This fracture is classically a C2 bilateral pedicle fracture with distraction of the C2–C3 disk, as well as ligamentous disruption between C2 and C3, which explains the listhesis at this level.

However, because most of these fractures are seen following motor vehicle accidents, the term *traumatic spondylolisthesis* is more frequently used. This term was coined by Garber in 1964. The varying degrees of disk and ligamentous disruption make it different from the typical hangman's fracture.

Etiology

The distraction is primarily due to a hyperextension force with an axial loading and with varying degrees of lateral flexion. Some of these injuries are fatal.

Pathophysiology

In a motor vehicle accident, when the head strikes the windshield, the C2 pedicles are cleaved, with acute distraction of the C2–C3 binding structures, such as the disk and the posterior and anterior longitudinal ligaments. The force causes subluxation of C2 over C3 to varying degrees.

One third of these patients have additional cervical injuries, but fortunately, the bilateral pedicular fractures cause decompression of the spinal canal; therefore, spinal cord compression is seldom seen.

Clinical Findings

Neck instability and pain following a motor vehicle accident is the most common history.

Imaging Findings

RADIOGRAPHY

The lateral view of the cervical spine typically reveals an oblique lucency across the C2 pedicle and posterior neural arch. Furthermore, the C2 vertebral body is seen anteriorly subluxated on C3 (spondylolisthesis) to varying degrees. The posterior spinolaminar line is disrupted, and there could be widening of the interspinous distance. The open-mouth view reveals the line of fracture running through the pedicles and lateral masses.

The injuries have been classified based on the degree of anterior displacement of C2 on C3 and the degree of stability:

Type 1 injury

Less than 3 mm of anterior subluxation of C2 on C3 is seen. The anterior and posterior longitudinal ligaments are intact, with a well-preserved intervening disk. The injury is considered stable. Associated injuries of the C1 posterior neural arch, odontoid fractures, and C1 lateral mass fractures may be present.

The mechanism of this injury is hyperextension with an axial load. It is seen in 26% of such injuries.

Type 2 injury

This type of injury is more common (56%) and is unstable. It results from a flexion force with axial loading following the hyperextension injury with axial loading. There is a tear of the posterior longitudinal ligament and a part of the C2–C3 disk with mild injury of the anterior longitudinal ligament. This is secondary to the flexion force.

Plain radiographs and lateral views reveal anterior displacement with angulation.

An associated injury is a C3 compression fracture.

Type 2A injury

Seen infrequently in 6% of cases, there is no anterior displacement of C2 over C3, but there is severe angulation. This injury is secondary to a greater degree of flexion force. The C2 pedicles are fractured and distracted, with gross damage to the disk and mild injury of the anterior longitudinal ligament.

Type 3 injury

Seen in ~9% of the fractures, there is severe displacement of C2 over C3 with gross angulation. The injury is due to flexion with axial compression. Not only is there a fracture of the pedicles bilaterally, but the facets are unilaterally or bilaterally dislocated. Varying degrees of anterior and posterior longitudinal ligament injury occur. This fracture results in severe neurologic sequelae.

Plain radiographs detect the subluxation better than CT. Sometimes additional oblique views are taken to delineate the line of the fracture.

COMPUTED TOMOGRAPHY

CT is used to confirm a suspicious fracture, delineate its extent/side, and also visualize it in the axial plane. The amount of comminution and displacement of the fractured fragments are assessed. Vertebral artery involvement is evaluated on CT angiography postintravenous contrast studies.

MAGNETIC RESONANCE IMAGING

MRI is not mandatory to make the diagnosis, but it clearly shows the subluxation/dislocation. MRI also helps to characterize the ligamentous tear (anterior/posterior longitudinal) disk and neural involvement. Therefore, it is indicated when considering accurate classification for subsequent management and prognosis.

Treatment

Methods for treatment of traumatic spondylolisthesis of the axis are currently a topic of dispute. The decisive factor for therapy is whether the injury is stable or unstable. When instability is present, anterior C2–C3 fixation with plate osteosynthesis is the method of choice. Stable injuries are treated by the application of a halo vest or Philadelphia collar.

Type 1 injury

- Usually treated with a collar or halo

Type 2 injury

- Traction in extension/external fixation for a week, followed by halo immobilization for 12 weeks if there is < 3- to 4-mm subluxation and slight angulation (10 degrees)
- Weighted extension traction for 6 weeks, followed by a halo immobilization, or an anterior plating or transpedicular screw fixation.

Type 2A injury

- Closed reduction in extension and compression under fluoroscopy, followed by a halo immobilization, or surgical management using an anterior plating or a transpedicular screw

Type 3 injury

Surgical treatment is mandatory if the fracture line extends to the dislocated facet, or just posterior to it, making the fracture unstable. A lateral mass plate, interspinous wire, or oblique wire will stabilize the vertebrae. The pedicle fractures are then treated with a transpedicular screw or halo immobilization.

Complications

Nonunion and malunion are fairly uncommon. Spinal cord injury is not a usual complication but can occur with type 3 fractures. Vertebral artery injury occurs in as many as 25% of cases.

PEARL

- Subluxations are clearly depicted on plain radiographs, facet dislocation on CT, and soft-tissue, disk, and neural injury on MRI.

PITFALL

- Poor-quality lateral views may miss subtle fractures, and a CT scan is suggested in such cases.

Suggested Readings

Daffner RH, Brown RR, Goldberg AL. A new classification for cervical vertebral injuries: influence of CT. Skeletal Radiol 2000;29:125–132

Garber JN. Abnormalities of the atlas and axis vertebrae: congenital and traumatic. J Bone Joint Surg Am 1964;46:1782–1791

Moch AL, Schweitzer ME, Parker L. Prevertebral soft tissue swelling following trauma: usefulness following tube placement. Skeletal Radiol 2000;29:340–345

Schneider RC, Livingston KE, Cave AJ, et al. "Hangman's fracture" of the cervical spine. J Neurosurg 1965;22:141–154

Williams JP III, Baker DH, Miller WA. CT appearance of congenital defect resembling the hangman's fracture. Pediatr Radiol 1999;29:549–550

CASE 106

Hema N. Choudur, Anthony G. Ryan, and Peter L. Munk

Clinical Presentation

This patient presented with multiple injuries following a motor vehicle accident. No neurologic deficit was noted.

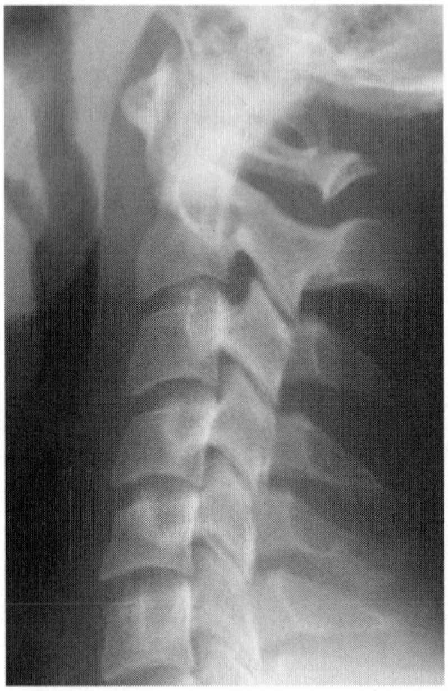

Figure 106A

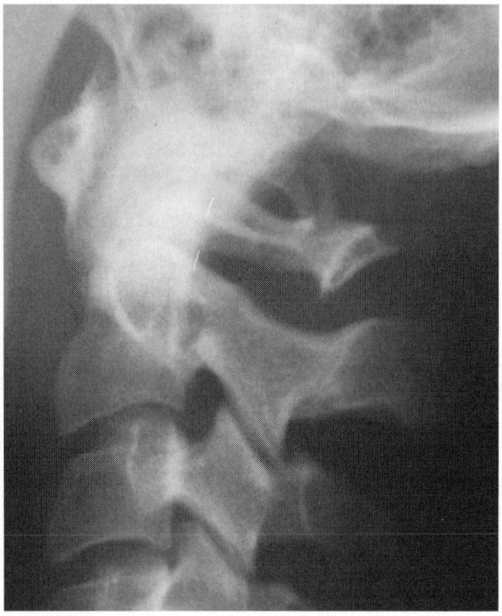

Figure 106B

Radiologic Findings

A fracture of the posterior arch of C1 is evident on the lateral views (**Figs. 106A** and **106B** [enlargement]). Displacement of the lateral masses of the atlas is evident on the C1–C2 open-mouth view (**Fig. 106C,** open mouth). The CT images (**Fig. 106D,** axial; **Fig. 106E,** sagittal reformat; **Fig. 106F,** coronal reformat) reveal bilateral anterior and right posterior arch C1 fractures with suspicious discontinuity of the transverse ligament and displacement of the lateral masses by 7 mm.

Diagnosis

Jefferson's fracture.

Differential Diagnosis

None.

Discussion

Background

Burst fractures of the atlas were originally described as four-part fractures by Jefferson in 1920. However, a review of the literature, radiographs, and CT studies indicates that the majority are two-

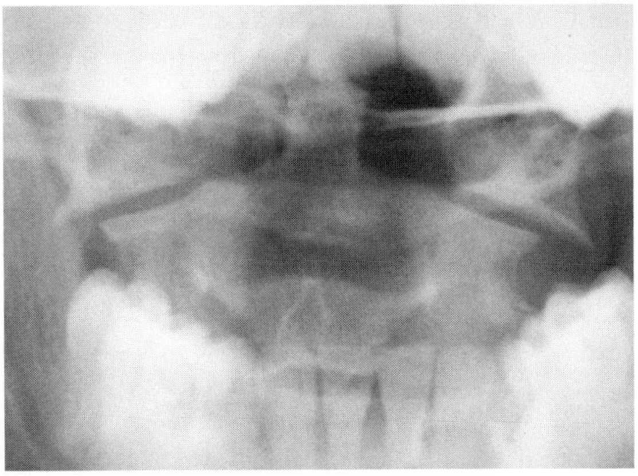

Figure 106C

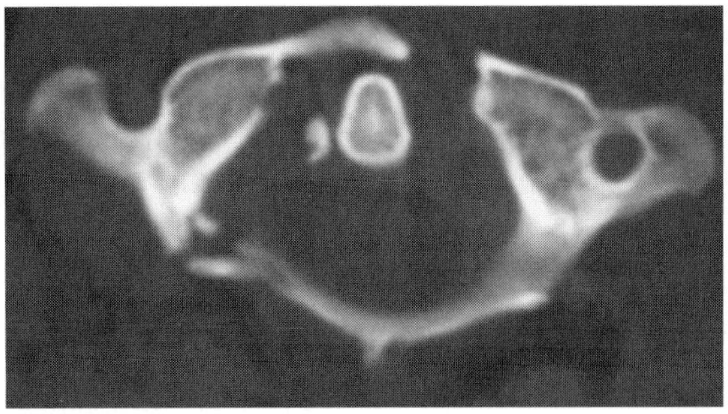

Figure 106D

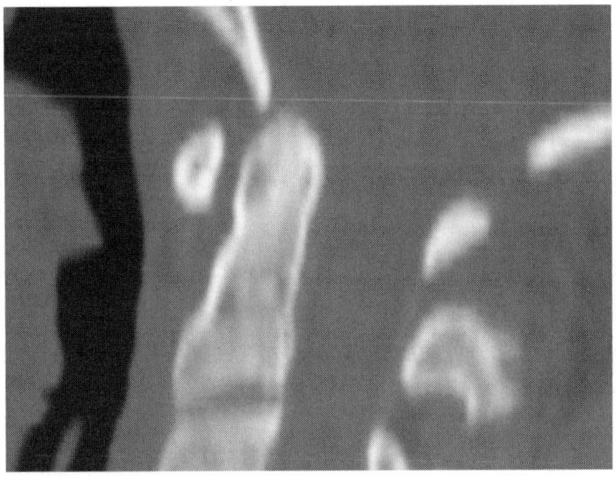

Figure 106E

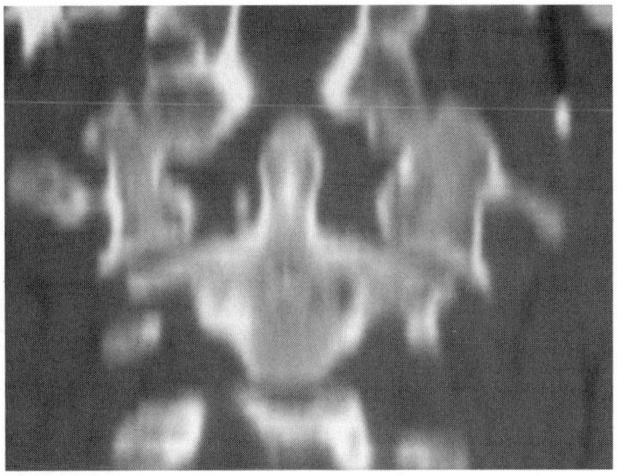

Figure 106F

part fractures. An axial force produces these fractures, which may be stable or unstable. Any suspicion on plain radiographs is confirmed with CT. The management varies depending on the stability of the fracture. Most cause no neurologic sequelae.

Fractures of the first cervical vertebra (C1) account for 7% of all acute cervical spine fractures. Isolated atlas fractures are most commonly bilateral or multiple fractures through the C1 ring. Frequently (in 44% of cases), the atlas is fractured in combination with the axis.

Etiology

An axial loading force, like a diving injury, causes the atlas to break, with splaying of the fracture fragments. In the classical Jefferson's fracture, it is striking that there is no fracture of the atlas, which may be due to simple symmetric compressive force. Flexion, extension, oblique flexion, and extension with axial tilting are the various mechanisms involved in variants of Jefferson's fractures.

Pathophysiology

The disrupting force results in a break of the arch of the atlas at one or more sites. Classical Jefferson's fracture is bilateral anterior and posterior arch fractures with lateral displacement of the lateral masses. This may result in a tear of the transverse ligament when it is classified as an unstable fracture. Sometimes, only the anterior or the posterior arches may be fractured unilaterally or bilaterally, or an oblique fracture through the anterior arch on one side and the posterior arch on the other can occur, called Jefferson's variants. Usually the spinal cord escapes unscathed, but in unstable fractures, the associated atlantoaxial instability calls for immediate operative management.

Associated injuries are odontoid fractures, atlantoaxial instability, atlantoaxial rotatory fixation (presenting with torticollis), occipital condylar fractures, and lower cervical spine injuries.

Imaging Findings

RADIOGRAPHY

The open-mouth anteroposterior view is the single most useful radiograph when the lateral masses are displaced from the superior articular facets of the axis. The Jefferson or burst fracture of the atlas is frequently overlooked on plain radiographs. This is because neurological deficit is usually absent and physical findings are nonspecific. In addition, diagnosis of this fracture is unusual on the lateral radiograph of the cervical spine. Increase in the retropharyngeal soft-tissue space is valuable both as an indication of upper cervical spine trauma and in distinguishing a Jefferson fracture from the more common fracture of the posterior arch of the atlas. The fracture line is noted in the lateral view as a lucency, the extent of which is variable and involves the anterior and posterior arches bilaterally in the classical Jefferson type. However, unilateral and only single-arch fractures may also occur. These variations are better evaluated on CT axial slices with reformats in three planes.

A careful note of associated fractures of the cervical vertebrae, especially fractures of the odontoid (type 2), is imperative, as these may require urgent management.

COMPUTED TOMOGRAPHY

Most trauma centers now rely on CT in an acute setting and with good reason, as atlas fractures are often missed on plain radiographs. Moreover, the type and extent of the fracture lines are better evaluated on axial CT slices (no more than 3 mm thick) with reformats and three-dimensional reconstruction.

If the displacement of the lateral masses is 2 to 7 mm, conservative treatment is sufficient. If the displacement is > 7 mm, operative treatment is required.

The fracture is termed stable if the transverse ligament is intact. If it is torn, it is termed unstable.

Jefferson's variants

The Jefferson's variants are evaluated better on CT. They can occur as unilateral arch fractures, bilateral anterior or bilateral posterior arch fractures, or unilateral or bilateral lateral mass fractures. In anterior bony ring disruption, the posterior longitudinal ligament can be torn (flexion injury), allowing C1–C2 subluxation to occur. Although all the fractures are potentially unstable, subluxation may not be evident on lateral radiographs. In one study, these Jefferson's variants were associated with transverse ligament tears. Three of the 11 patients studied were quadriplegic, and two died as a result of their spinal cord injury. These unstable atlas fractures were similar to the classical Jefferson's fracture in appearance and mechanism, except that they had fewer than four breaks in the atlas ring and were associated with severe neurologic injury and lower level spine injuries. The pattern of bilateral anterior arch fractures was associated more often with neurologic injury. Because of these differences, they are referred to as Jefferson's variant fractures to distinguish them from the classical Jefferson's fracture and to emphasize the seriousness of this injury.

Associated fractures of the odontoid, the type and the degree of atlantoaxial instability, and integrity of the occipital condyles are better evaluated on axial high-resolution CT and coronal reconstruction.

Nonunion and pseudoarthrosis can be accurately visualized on CT.

MAGNETIC RESONANCE IMAGING

Subtle fractures of the atlas can be visualized on MRI. The T1 sequences reveal a hypointense fracture line, and the T2 and inversion recovery sequences may reveal surrounding edema. Also, atlantoaxial instability is well demonstrated. The transverse ligament, the posterior longitudinal ligament, and associated odontoid injuries are visualized in addition to the state of the spinal cord.

Complications

- Nonunion
- Pseudoarthrosis
- Associated occipital condyle fracture is rare and can be missed during medical evaluation and on plain radiographs. This fracture can be associated with cranial nerve injuries (31%), the hypoglossal nerve being the most frequently involved.
- Vertebral artery occlusion can be diagnosed by contrast-enhanced CT.
- Basilar invagination has been reported secondary to atlas fractures.

Treatment

The stability of a burst fracture of the atlas (Jefferson's fracture) should be determined to decide upon the appropriate treatment. Stable Jefferson's fractures are treated conservatively. Patients with fractures with displacement of 2 to 7 mm are treated with immobilization in a halo vest; however, those with serious ligamentous disruption need surgical fusion as a preferential form of initial treatment.

Unstable fractures need immediate operative treatment. Unstable fractures include those with a rupture of the transverse ligament and those in which union has been incomplete despite treatment. An occiput-to-C2 or atlantoaxial arthrodesis may be indicated. Primary C1–C2 transfacet and transarticular screw fixations have been the described as useful alternative treatments for unstable Jefferson's fractures.

However, in some studies, patients who had fractures with severe spreading of the lateral masses (> 7 mm) were treated with reduction of the lateral masses by axial traction until healing of the arch had occurred. They reported no atlantoaxial instability in any patient at follow-up.

Prognosis

Most patients with isolated classic Jefferson's fractures recover without neurologic sequelae. However, the variants and associated injuries causing atlantoaxial instability can result in cord damage.

PEARL

- Subtle alterations such as prevertebral soft-tissue swelling should be regarded as highly suspicious for fracture. A careful search pattern that surveys all the visible anatomical structures must be evolved, and in all questionable cases or high-risk fracture patients with an apparently negative plain radiograph, a CT scan should be advised.

PITFALL

- Causes of false-negative interpretation may be osteoporosis, suboptimal film quality, and overlapping bone structures. For medicolegal purposes, these possibilities should be indicated on the x-ray report. If painful symptoms persist, a CT exam is advised.

Suggested Readings

Chambers AA, Gaskill MF. Midline anterior atlas clefts: CT findings. J Comput Assist Tomogr 1992;16:868–870

Lee C, Woodring JH. Unstable Jefferson variant atlas fractures: an unrecognized cervical injury. Am J Neuroradiol 1991;12:1105–1110

Torreggiani WC, Keogh C, Al-Ismail K, Marchinkow LO, Munk PL. Musculoskeletal case 20: Jefferson fracture (C1 burst fracture). Can J Surg 2002;45:16,65–66

CASE 107

Hema N. Choudur, Anthony G. Ryan, and Peter L. Munk

Clinical Presentation

A 28-year-old man presented with acute pain and tenderness in the posteroinferior neck following an episode of shoveling snow. No focal swelling was noted on clinical examination, but there was slight restriction in neck movements.

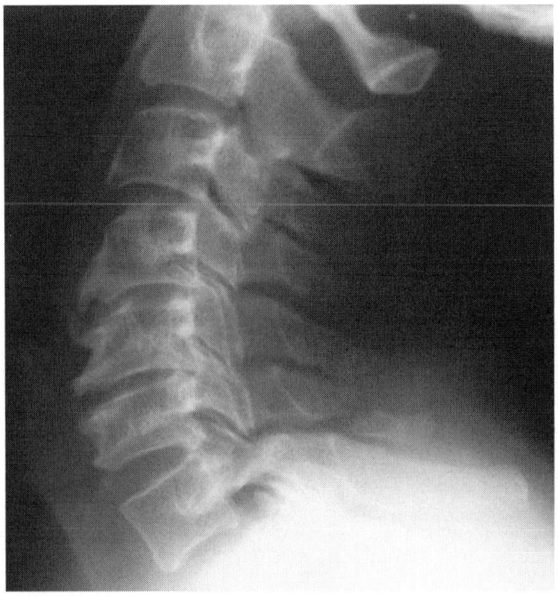

Figure 107A

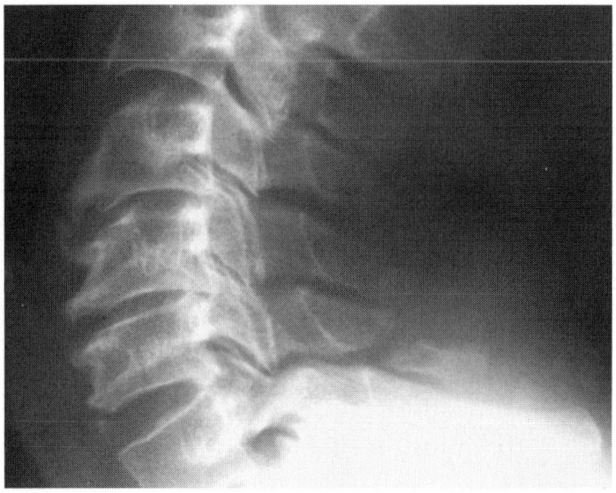

Figure 107B

Radiologic Findings

Lateral views of the cervical spine (**Figs. 107A,107B**) show an oblique fracture through the C7 spinous process.

Diagnosis

Clay shoveler's fracture.

Differential Diagnosis

None.

Discussion

Background

This stable cervical injury is incidentally seen on many cervical spine radiographs and occurs in the lower cervical spinous processes, usually C7.

Etiology

Hyperflexion of the cervical spine causes C3–T3 spinous process fractures. The term *clay-shoveler's fracture* was first used in the 19th century to describe injuries suffered by Australian clay shovelers. The tug injuries, avulsions of the supraspinous ligaments, occurred as the workers tossed shovelfuls of heavy, sticky clay over their shoulders. Currently, the fracture is seen in weight lifters and other atheletes and is occasionally the result of blunt trauma.

Pathophysiology

The injury is stable. The mechanism is an avulsion of the supraspinous ligament with an underlying bony fragment during powerful hyperflexion.

Imaging Findings

RADIOGRAPHY

Plain radiographs characteristically reveal a vertical or oblique fracture of the C6–T1 spinous processes. On the anteroposterior view, a double spinous process is seen due to displacement of the fracture.

COMPUTED TOMOGRAPHY

Subtle fractures, not evident on radiographs, may become apparent on CT, particularly in patients with muscular shoulders and inadequate visualization of the cervicothoracic junction.

Treatment

- Because the injury is stable, immobilization is sufficient and results in good healing.

Prognosis

- This is the most common and, fortunately, the safest of fractures of the cervical spine, with an excellent prognosis.

PEARLS

- Considering the diagnosis is a key factor, because all other features of the radiographs are likely to be normal, and a systematic search must be undertaken to detect subtle injuries.
- A particular instance of clay-shoveler's fracture may occur in adolescents: Schmitt's disease involves avulsion of the ossification process of the tip of the spinous process.

PITFALLS

- Disruption of the spinolaminar line, or "spinolaminar breach," as described by Helms et al, occurs in spinous process fractures complicated by extension through the lamina into the spinal canal. These injuries are potentially unstable, as the posterior ligamentous complex may be disrupted. The key to distinguishing these injuries from a simple clay-shoveler's fracture is that, in the latter, the spinolaminar line should be intact. Any clinical evidence of instability should be pursued by flexion extension views in the first instance.

- A proportion of clay-shoveler's fractures is missed on radiographs but may become apparent subsequently on CT, particularly in patients with overlapping soft tissues, such as muscular shoulders, and inadequate visualization of the cervicothoracic junction.

Acknowledgment

Radiographs courtesy of Dr. Dick Daffner, Allegheny General Hospital, Pittsburgh, PA.

Suggested Readings

Cancelmo JJ Jr. Clay shoveler's fracture: a helpful diagnostic sign. Am J Roentgenol Radium Ther Nucl Med 1972;115:540–543

Lin JT, Lee JL, Lee ST. Evaluation of occult cervical spine fractures on radiographs and CT. Emerg Radiol 2003;10:128–134

Matar LD, Helms CA, Richardson WJ. "Spinolaminar breach": an important sign in cervical spinous process fractures. Skeletal Radiol 2000;29:75–80

Nuber GW, Schafer MF. Clay shovelers' injuries: a report of two injuries sustained from football. Am J Sports Med 1987;15:182–183

Weston WJ. Clay shoveler's disease in adolescents (Schmitt's disease): a report of two cases. Br J Radiol 1957;30:378–380

CASE 108

Hema N. Choudur, Anthony G. Ryan, and Peter L. Munk

Clinical Presentation

A 29-year-old man presented to the emergency department with back pain following a motor vehicle accident. He had been wearing a lap-only seat belt at the time of the accident. No neurologic deficit was elicited. Clinical exam revealed posterior tenderness, hematoma, and interspinous widening but with no kyphosis.

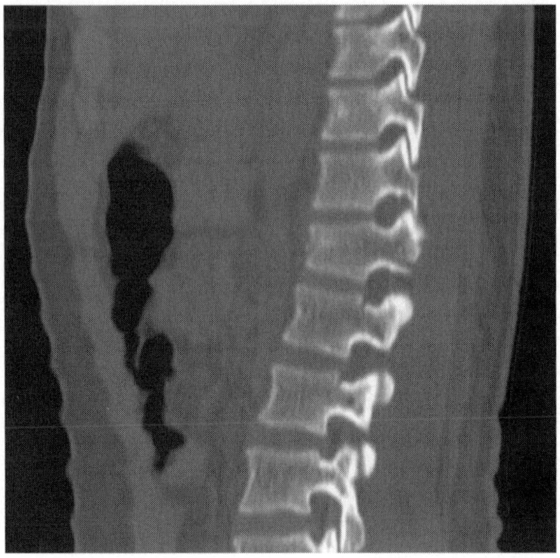

Figure 108A

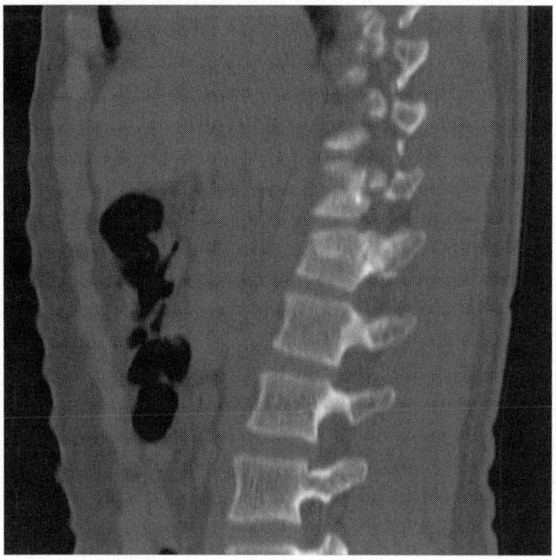

Figure 108B

Radiologic Findings

Plain radiographs (not shown) suggested a transverse fracture involving the L1 vertebral body, laminae, pedicles, and spinous process with no vertebral body displacement.

CT with sagittal and coronal reformats (**Figs. 108A,108B** sagittal; **Figs. 108C,108D** coronal) confirmed a transverse fracture of the L1 vertebral body extending through all the posterior elements. No spinal canal compromise was evident.

A postfixation radiograph (**Fig. 108E**) demonstrates successful fixation of the fracture. The patient made a full recovery.

Diagnosis

Chance fracture.

Differential Diagnosis

Similar fractures can occur in ankylosing spondylitis, where displacement is frequently seen. These fractures heal well, but sometimes fibrous union and pseudoarthrosis can occur. Other stigmata of ankylosing spondylitis are usually evident.

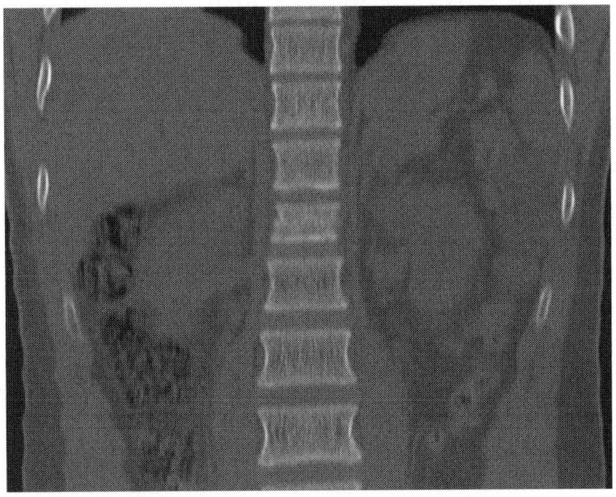

Figure 108C

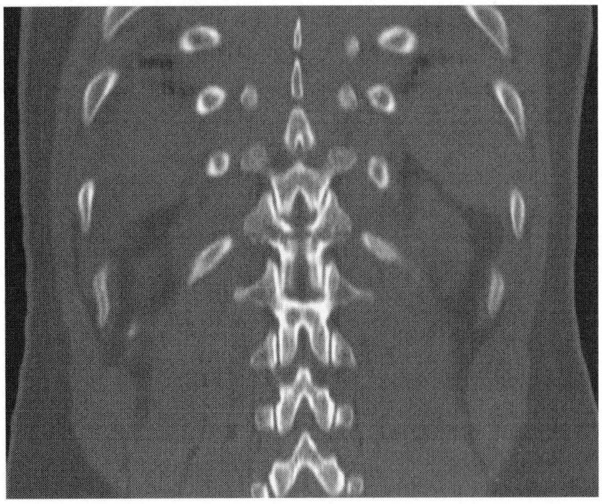

Figure 108D

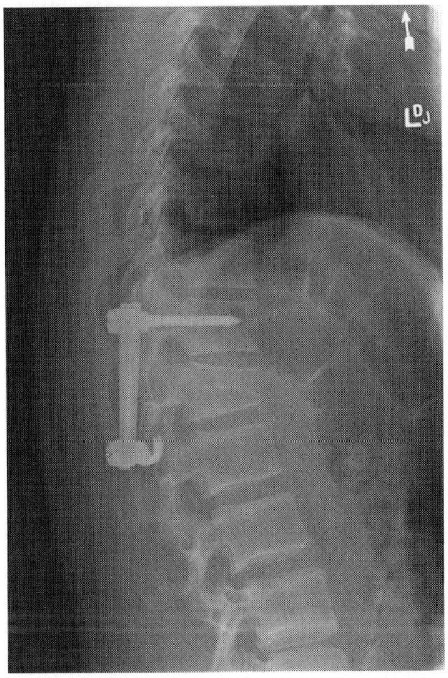

Figure 108E

Discussion

Background

First described by Chance, a British radiologist, in 1948, these fractures most often result from a seatbelt injury.

Etiology

The hyperflexion-distraction injury that occurs following a sudden deceleration in a motor vehicle accident causes four different types of injury:

1. A horizontal fracture through the spinous process, pedicles, transverse processes, and vertebral bodies, which is seen in older patients with more brittle bones. The posterior ligamentous complex remains essentially intact, other than the supraspinous ligament. This has been termed a *fulcrum fracture.*

2. A ligamentous and disk injury, causing a disruption of the posterior spinous ligaments, articular facets, and intervertebral disks without associated bony avulsion. These injuries tend to occur more commonly in younger patients with more resilient spines. They may be clinically unstable and require internal fixation.
3. A bony, ligamentous, and disk injury resulting in a transverse fracture of the posterior elements with or without extension to the posterosuperior or posteroinferior aspect of the vertebral body. This is the classic Chance fracture.
4. Smith fracture is one in which the superior articular processes and a small posterior fragment of the vertebral body are included with the arch fracture. The spinous process is intact, but the interspinous and supraspinous ligaments are torn.

Pathophysiology

The thoracic spine above T11 is very stable by virtue of its narrow disk spaces, frontally directed facets, and articulation with the ribs. By comparison, the 11th and 12th thoracic vertebrae with their floating ribs and oblique facets are less stable.

The absence of ribs and the larger disk spaces render the lumbar spine more mobile. In a hyperflexion injury, the whole lumbar spine bends acutely, with a concomitant fracture through the lower thoracic and upper lumbar vertebrae (T11–L2). In children, midlumbar fractures occur, as the axis of flexion is slightly lower.

The injury causes a tear or break of the posterior and anterior vertebrae and/or ligaments/disks. Typically, no spinal canal narrowing occurs.

Complications

- Unstable spine conus and/or cauda equina
- Contusion of the conus and/or cauda equina

The incidence of neurologic sequelae in association with seat-belt injuries is 15%.

Imaging Findings

RADIOGRAPHY

The three "columns" of the spine are as follows:

- The anterior vertebral body, its disk, and the anterior longitudinal ligament
- The posterior half of the vertebral body, its disk, and the posterior longitudinal ligament
- The posterior neural arch and its ligaments

In a classic Chance fracture, all three bony columns are cleaved in a transverse plane, with sparing of the ligaments. Such fracture is quite accurately determined on anteroposterior (AP) and lateral conventional radiographs using the following signs:

- The open pedicle sign: a lucency on the medial aspects of the pedicles
- A "vacant" or "empty" appearance of the vertebral body on the AP film, as the posterior elements are no longer projected through the vertebral body
- A break or discontinuity in the cortex of the pedicles or spinous process on the AP view
- Horizontal fractures, though transverse processes should raise suspicion of other fractures
- Increased height of the posterior vertebral body or the disk space on the lateral view
- Decreased anterior vertebral body height

- Jumped facets and interspinous widening

COMPUTED TOMOGRAPHY

- CT with reformats (as in the reference case) demonstrates the fracture line and its extent as well as the presence or absence of spinal canal compromise.
- A paraspinal hematoma is a frequent accompaniment and is well demonstrated on CT.

MAGNETIC RESONANCE IMAGING

- MRI is infrequently performed for Chance fractures unless there is neurologic deficit at the level of the conus/cauda equina. When performed, it clearly delineates any accompanying ligamentous and or discal injury.

Treatment

- These fractures are usually reduced by external manipulation and immobilization in hyperextension and heal without any sequelae. Some residual back pain may persist.
- In a minority of patients (polytrauma and obese), operative fixation by posterior spinal fusion and autologous bone grafts are necessary to stabilize the vertebra.
- Untreated cases may progress to kyphosis and constant back pain.
- Contusion of the conus and/or cauda equina is the only rare presenting complication. Fifteen percent of seat-belt injuries result in neurologic sequelae.

Prognosis

- Most cases heal adequately without residual complications. Rarely, backache persists.

PEARLS

- In motor vehicle accidents and falls, a careful look for anterior abdominal wall ecchymosis and plain radiographic assessment of the dorsolumbar spine are warranted, even if there is only backache at the outset, as a Chance fracture may be missed and, if untreated, progress to kyphosis. Prompt reduction with appropriate treatment results in a good outcome.
- Chance fractures are associated with significant intra-abdominal injuries in 30 to 50% of cases; such injuries should be looked for, especially when CT is performed.
- A "vacant" or "empty" appearance of the vertebral body on the AP film is a useful sign for detecting Chance fractures, as the posterior elements are no longer projected through the vertebral body.

PITFALLS

- Similar fractures can occur in ankylosing spondylitis, where displacement is frequently seen. These fractures heal well, but sometimes fibrous union and pseudoarthrosis can occur. Other stigmata of ankylosing spondylitis are usually in evidence.
- In adults, the classic site of fracture is between T11 and L2. In children, the fracture should be looked for at a lower level (midlumbar), as the axis of flexion is slightly lower.
- In the presence of neurologic deficit, MRI is indicated, as CT will miss conus and cauda equina contusion.

Suggested Readings

Chance GQ. Note on a flexion fracture of the spine. Br J Radiol 1948;21:452–453

Eismont FJ. Flexion-distraction injuries of the thoracic and lumbar spine. In: Spine Trauma. Philadelphia, PA: WB Saunders; 1998:402–414

Reid AB, Letts RM, Black GB. Pediatric Chance fractures: association with intra-abdominal injuries and seatbelt use. J Trauma 1990;30:384–391

Rogers LF. The roentgenographic appearance of transverse or chance fractures of the spine: the seat belt fracture. Am J Roentgenol Radium Ther Nucl Med 1971;111:844–849

Smith WS, Kaufer H. Patterns and mechanisms of lumbar injuries associated with lap seat belts. J Bone Joint Surg Am 1969;51:239–254

CASE 109

Hema N. Choudur, Anthony G. Ryan, and Peter L. Munk

Clinical Presentation

An elderly woman complained of long-standing back pain with no history of trauma. On questioning, she admitted having widespread bony pain.

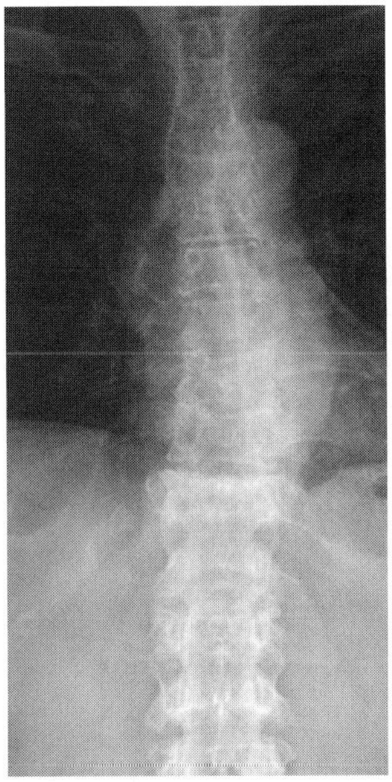

Figure 109A

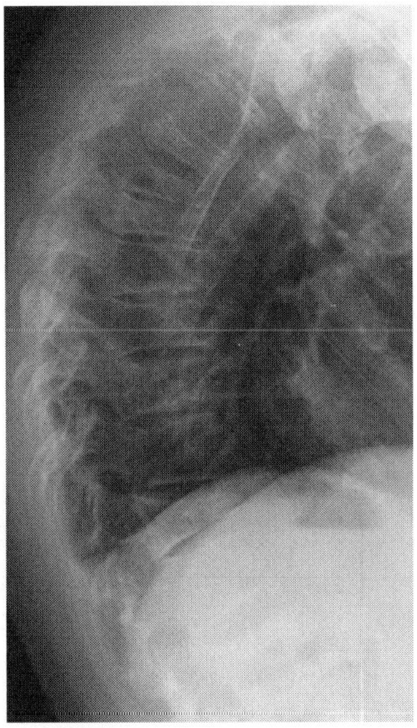

Figure 109B

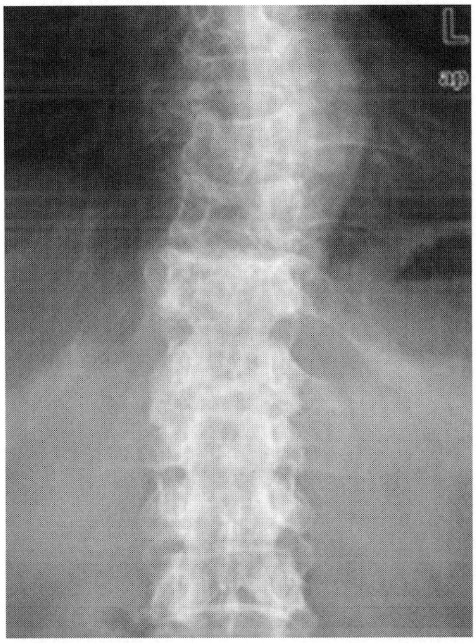

Figure 109C

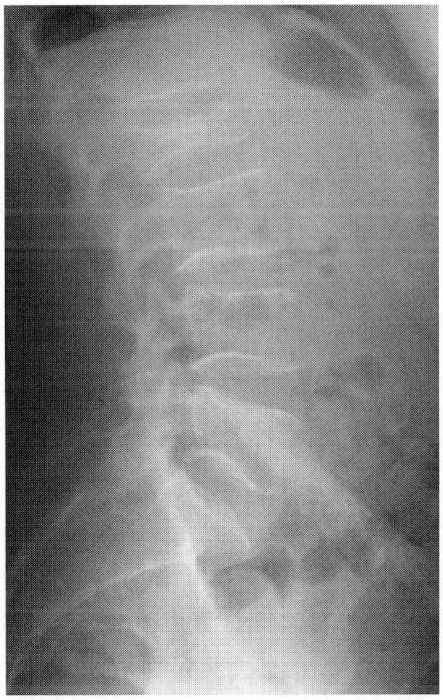

Figure 109D

Radiologic Findings

Plain radiographs of the dorsal and lumbar spine anteroposterior (AP) and lateral views (**Figs. 109A–109D**), show mid-dorsal and L2 compression fractures with no paravertebral soft tissue and normal adjacent disk spaces. There was a generalized decrease in bone density.

Diagnosis

Compression fractures.

Differential Diagnosis

- The differential diagnosis for osteoporotic compression fractures includes osteomalacia, multiple myeloma, hyperparathyroidism, and Paget's disease.
- Fractures may be secondary to malignancy, hemangioma, or infection.
- Chance fractures and burst fractures may have the same plain radiographic appearances as a traumatic compression fracture, and a CT scan may be necessary to differentiate them.

Discussion

Background

The most common cause of compression fracture is osteoporosis. These fractures can occur without trauma and remain silent. Progressive kyphosis may be the only indication of a compressed vertebra. Some patients have intense pain at the site of the vertebral compression fracture. Most commonly, these patients are treated conservatively; however, in a significant proportion, back pain persists, and the prolonged immobilization places them at risk for complications, such as pneumonia, urosepsis, and deep venous thrombosis. These patients may now be treated with vertebroplasty or kyphoplasty, which alleviates the pain and permits return to full mobilization in over 80% of cases.

Etiology

Most nontraumatic compression fractures are osteoporotic. One third are seen in the lumbar vertebrae, a third in the thoracolumbar vertebrae, and a third in the thoracic vertebrae. Seventy-five percent of women older than 65 years with scoliosis have at least one osteoporotic wedge fracture. Other causes include trauma, malignancy, infection, and hemangiomas. Traumatic fractures are frequent in the dorsolumbar junction.

Pathophysiology

Most of these fractures occur in the dorsolumbar region or in the lower lumbar vertebrae. The classification is based on the three-column anatomical theories of Dennis. If more than two columns are involved, then the fracture is rendered unstable.

The wedge compression of the anterior column results in a stable injury with either the superior, inferior, or both end plates being fractured. Sometimes, the anterior end plate is fractured and bows forward. This injury follows an axial compressive force with mild flexion of the spine at the time of injury. The middle column is intact. These fractures are called wedge compression fractures. If they occur paracentrally, they are called lateral wedge compression fractures.

Burst fractures result from high impact axial force with compression of the anterior, middle, and posterior columns. These fractures are unstable, and the spinal canal compromise depends on the extent of the compression, the resulting deformity, and the displacement of the fractured fragments.

Clinical Findings

Pain and tenderness at the site of the fracture, progressive kyphosis, and scoliosis are the common clinical findings in the absence of trauma.

Complications

Complications include immediate or delayed neurologic manifestations and progressive kyphosis.

Imaging Findings

RADIOGRAPHY

In the lateral view of the spine, the anterior height of the vertebral body is diminished, and the posterior height remains normal. No anterior or posterior translation of the vertebral body is evident. The degree of anterior compression should be no more than 40% with respect to the posterior vertebral body height, in which case a burst fracture is to be considered. In burst fractures, the lateral x-ray may show a decreased height of the entire vertebral body. On the AP view, an increase in the interpedicular space may indicate an unstable fracture.

COMPUTED TOMOGRAPHY

Good visualization of the vertebral body elements is possible on CT to rule out a Chance fracture or a burst fracture. CT also accurately shows the spinal canal and the amount of neural compromise, and it delineates the exact extent of the fracture. All patients with wedge fractures with more than 50% loss of height should have a CT scan to rule out middle column and burst fractures. The disadvantage of axial CT is its inability to detect subtle horizontally oriented fractures and minimal compression fractures, which is overcome by frontal and sagittal reformats.

MAGNETIC RESONANCE IMAGING

MRI is indicated only if the patient has neurologic deficit, radicular symptoms, or signs of infection or malignancy.

Treatment

Conservative, nonoperative treatment consists of pain relief, bracing, and rehabilitation. It remains the standard for compression fractures, with most of the patients being treated symptomatically with a short period of bed rest until the pain has diminished. Early ambulation is encouraged in a hyperextension orthosis, with continuing treatment for osteoporosis. Axial loading is discouraged for about 3 months. Periodic radiographic monitoring of the fracture is important, as some fractures worsen in a couple of months and may require surgical stabilization.

Nonoperative treatment with hyperextension orthosis is initially considered for some unstable fractures, those that result in compression of more than 50% of the vertebral body height, an angulation $>$ 20 degrees of the thoracolumbar spine, multiple adjacent wedge compression fractures, and involvement of more than two columns. However, if the spine develops progressive kyphosis and pain persists, operative methods are indicated in the form of anterior or posterior vertebral body stabilization.

Immediate surgery is indicated in those patients with neurologic deficit following a traumatic fracture and in those with a radiologically unstable injury. Radiographic instability is seen in those cases with severe ligamentous disruption, with canal compromise to an extent that neurologic symptoms occur, and when translation of the vertebrae is seen on dynamic views.

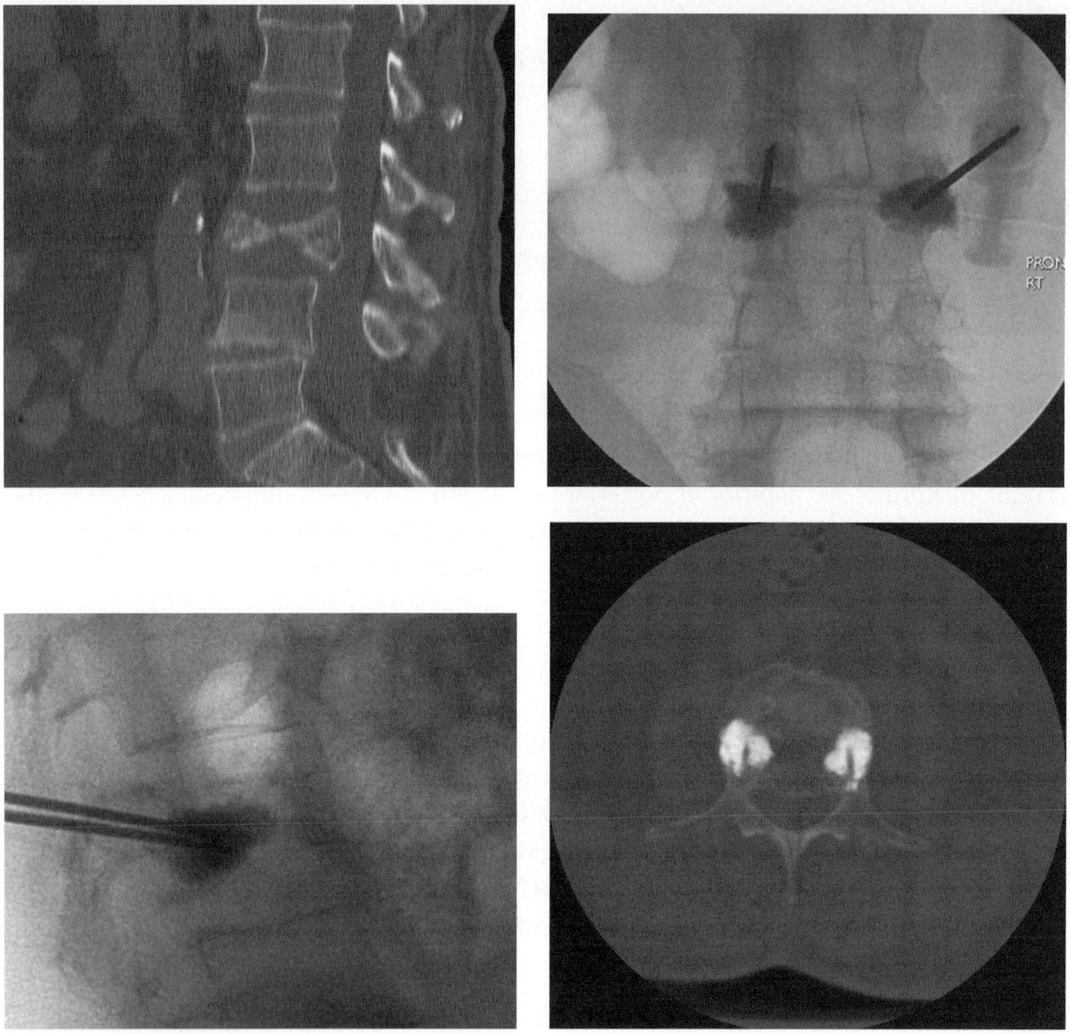

E F G H

Figures 109E–109H Preprocedural CT (reformat) (**109E**) clearly demonstrates a marked osteopenotic compression fracture of L3. Intraprocedural fluorscopy (**109F** [AP], **109G** [lateral]) demonstrates two transpedicular needles in situ during active injection. Postprocedural transaxial CT (**109H**) demonstrates two intravertebral cement deposits. The needle tracks are clearly visible within the cement.

Percutaneous vertebroplasty (**Figs. 109E–109H**) and kyphoplasty are recent advances to alleviate pain and increase the inherent vertebral body strength. Most reports in the literature consider pain from osteoporotic compression fractures, hemangiomas, and malignancy unresponsive to conservative measures as suitable indications.

Surgical intervention is sought to remove a fragment causing spinal compromise and to stabilize an unstable spine, using, appropriately, an anterior or posterior approach.

Prognosis

The prognosis is excellent for those with a mild degree of wedge compression. Those with persistent pain respond well to vertebroplasty with continuing treatment for osteoporosis. It is only the traumatic/burst fractures with neurologic sequelae that have long-term complications.

PEARL

- A CT assessment is sometimes necessary for an innocent-looking wedge compression fracture that may actually represent a burst or Chance fracture.

PITFALL

- Progressive kyphosis in an initial mild compression wedge fracture is often missed due to lack of periodic radiographic follow-up.

Suggested Readings

Dunnagan SA, Knox MF, Deaton CW. Osteoporotic compression fracture with persistent pain: treatment with percutaneous vertebroplasty. J Ark Med Soc 1999;96:258–259

Harrington KD. Vertebral compression fractures: differentiation between benign and malignant causes. Iowa Orthop J 1993;13:85–96

Von Feldt JM. Managing osteoporotic fractures: minimizing pain and disability. Rev Rhum Engl Ed 1997;64(6 Suppl):78S–80S

CASE 110

Anthony G. Ryan and Peter L. Munk

Clinical Presentation

A 65-year-old man with painful hands and feet came to our institution. The request form read, "erosive arthropathy?"

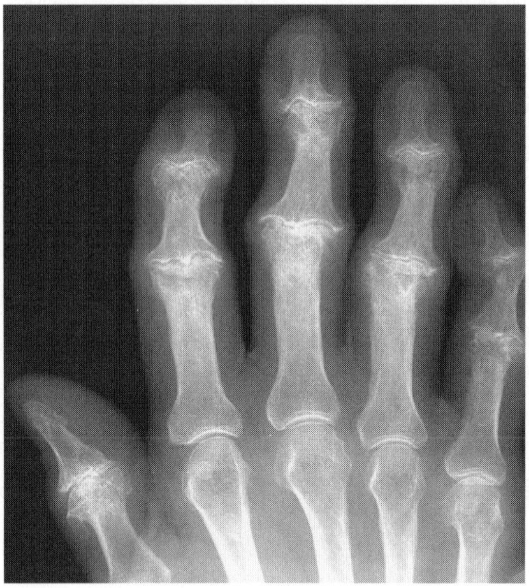

Figure 110A

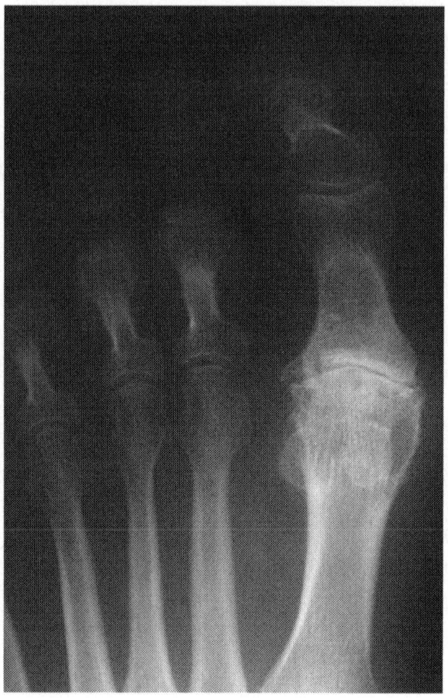

Figure 110B

Radiologic Findings

An anteroposterior (AP) radiograph of the hand (**Fig. 110A**) shows marked joint space loss, articular surface irregularity, subchondral sclerosis and cyst formation, and marginal osteophyte formation at the proximal interphalangeal (PIP) and distal interphalangeal (DIP) joints of the second to fifth digits and of the interphalangeal joint of the thumb. No erosions are evident.

An AP radiograph of the foot (**Fig. 110B**) shows the same changes to be present in the metatarsophalangeal (MTP) joint of the great toe.

Diagnosis

Osteoarthritis.

Differential Diagnosis

Erosive osteoarthritis.

Discussion

Background

Osteoarthritis is a group of conditions encompassing a primary abnormality of joints lined by hyaline cartilage and also reflecting a common final pathway of degenerative changes and attempted repair. It represents the most common arthropathy, its prevalence increasing with age.

Etiology

Primary osteoarthritis represents an intrinsic abnormality of articular cartilage with no superimposed associated joint disease. In this condition, spontaneous degeneration of the joint occurs without a preexisting disorder, such as trauma, and can manifest itself early in life.

More commonly, secondary osteoarthritis is encountered, and it is this disease process that is most frequently encountered as individuals age or after a joint is traumatized. Obesity also significantly increases the likelihood that osteoarthritis will develop, particularly in the lower extremities.

A variety of other diseases, such as acromegaly, Wilson's disease, intra-articular hemorrhage, and chronic neurologic conditions, may contribute to the development of this process.

Pathophysiology

Fundamentally, osteoarthritis represents failure of maintenance of cartilage integrity with degeneration of cartilage and reparative bone formation. In most instances, the process is noninflammatory. Typically, the disease process is slowly progressive, although severe trauma may significantly accelerate its development.

Repetitive minor stress is felt to play a crucial role in the development of osteoarthritis. This presumably results in low-grade damage to the cartilage preventing normal absorption and transmission of stress through a joint. This subsequently results in trabecular fracturing as well as cartilage erosion.

Cartilage itself has a limited capacity for healing. Subchondral trabeculae, however, may undergo osteoblastic repair, producing increased stiffness in the bone, thereby requiring overlying cartilage to absorb more of the stress, which in turn results in increasing damage. This downward spiral eventually leads to development of frank osteoarthritis.

Clinical Findings

Patients are typically middle-aged or older. There may be a history of trauma to the joint, especially in those patients presenting at an early age. The increasing prevalence of obesity is associated with an increasing incidence of osteoarthritis, particularly in the lower extremities. A history of other predisposing conditions may be elicited, for example, prior avascular necrosis of the femoral head, acromegaly, Wilson's disease, intra-articular hemorrhage, and chronic neurologic conditions.

Erosive osteoarthritis is characterized by an abrupt onset of painful joints, with morning stiffness and occasional throbbing paresthesias of the fingertips.

Complications

- Joint pain
- Loss of joint function
- Bone necrosis
- Joint ankylosis

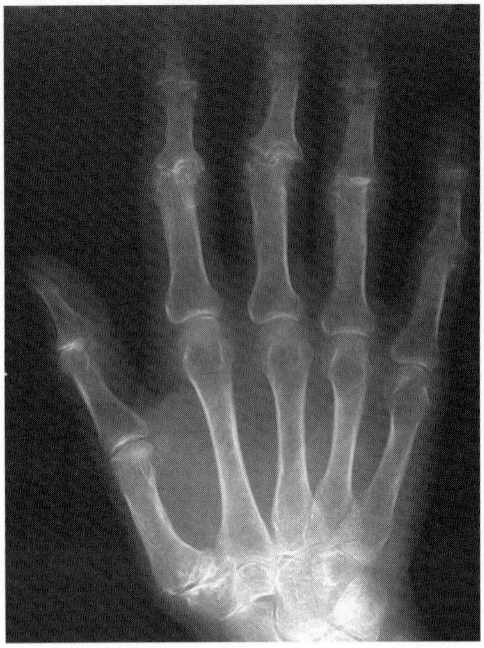

Figure 110C AP radiograph of the hand shows the characteristic "gull-wing pattern" of erosive arthritis affecting the PIP joints and, to a lesser extent, the DIP joints. Ankylosis of the fifth PIP is present. The inflammatory component of the condition is evinced by the central erosions present.

Pathology

GROSS

Failure of maintenance of cartilage integrity leads to degeneration and erosion of cartilage.

Subchondral trabecular fracturing and reparative bone formation or bone resorption lead to "cyst" formation (not true cysts, as they do not have a cellular lining).

MICROSCOPIC

Although the process tends not to be inflammatory, there may be evidence of synovitis, which, in the case of erosive arthritis, is severe and proliferative. The latter may be indistinguishable from rheumatoid arthritis, exhibiting subchondral granulation tissue, lymphocytic aggregation, plasma cell infiltration, and subsynovial fibrosis.

Imaging Findings

RADIOGRAPHY

- The cardinal radiographic findings in osteoarthritis include joint space narrowing, marginal osteophyte formation, subchondral sclerosis, and development of subarticular cysts (geodes), which may contain granulation tissue and/or gas and fluid.
- Joint effusions may also be present, and in classic osteoarthritis, a minimal amount of inflammatory response with synovial hypertrophy can often be demonstrated.
- Debris within the joint from damaged cartilage, abraded bone, and broken osteophytes can often be demonstrated. This debris may often be manifested as loose bodies or "joint mice."
- An important subset of osteoarthritis is erosive osteoarthritis. In this condition, the inflammatory component of the disease is more prominent. This disease is found far more frequently in postmenopausal women (12:1, female:male) and classically affects the interphalangeal joints of the hands (**Fig. 110C**). The DIPs are affected before the PIPs. Other joints, such as the hip and knee, are also commonly affected. The arthropathy tends to be symmetrical. An extensive destructive

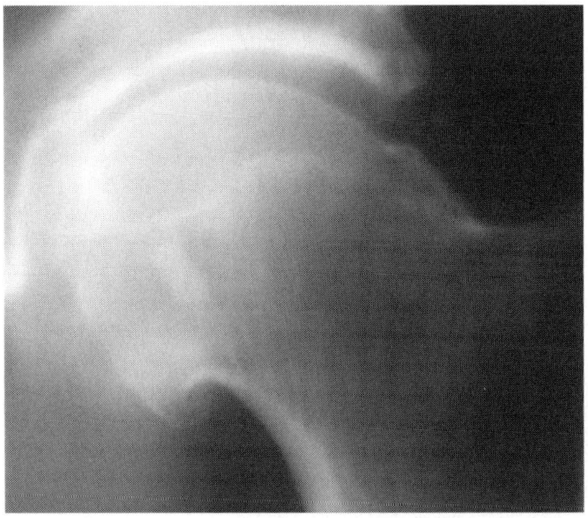
D

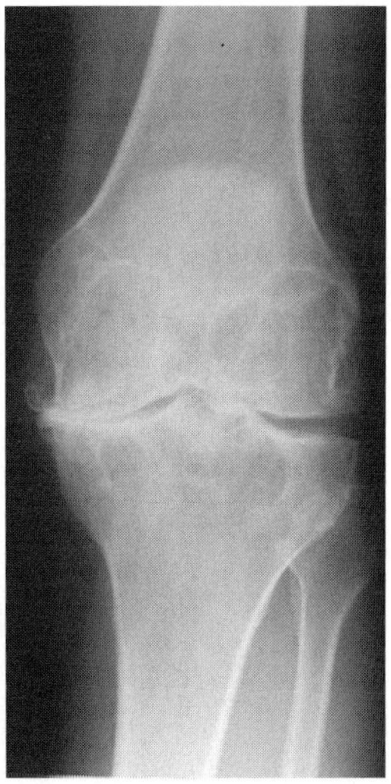
E

Figures 110D,110E Coned view of the hip joint shows changes consistent with early osteoarthrosis, namely, minimal joint space loss, subchondral sclerosis and cyst formation, and marginal osteophyte formation. **110E** Marked osteoarthritis of the knee causes loss of the medial compartment joint space, prominent subchondral sclerosis and marginal osteophyte formation, and marked geode formation in both medial and lateral compartments.

erosive component with very prominent osteophytes around the joints can be observed, and the disease tends to be more rapidly progressive than classic osteoarthritis. Deformities are common, such as subluxation, contractures, and Heberden's (DIP) and Bouchard's (PIP) nodes. Ankylosis and opera-glass digits may occur in severe cases, the former occurring in as many as 15% of cases.

- Any joint may be affected by osteoarthritis, although weight-bearing joints such as the hips and knees are particularly prone (**Figs. 110D,110E**), as are joints frequently undergoing stress or strain (interphalangeal joints, first carpometacarpal joint). See **Figs. 110F** and **110G**.
- Joints that have been traumatized or that have undergone extensive cartilage damage from other causes, such as infection (**Fig. 110H**), also may develop changes that may be severe.
- Joints that undergo abnormal nonphysiologic stresses due to malalignment will inevitably develop osteoarthritis. Examples of this include Legg-Calvé-Perthes disease, congenital hip dislocation, and patients who previously had rickets. This is in line with the rule of thumb that osteoarthritis occurs in normal joints when abnormal forces are applied or in abnormal joints when normal forces are applied.
- As the disease progresses, the articular surfaces become increasingly abnormal due to eburnation of bone on bone, and bone necrosis may occur. Collapse of the articular surfaces can also be encountered, and, rarely, joint ankylosis may develop.

COMPUTED TOMOGRAPHY

- CT demonstrates many of the findings of osteoarthritis, including osteophyte formation, joint space narrowing (**Fig. 110I**), and the presence of loose bodies within the joint (**Fig. 110J**). Subchondral cysts are also well visualized (**Fig. 110K**).

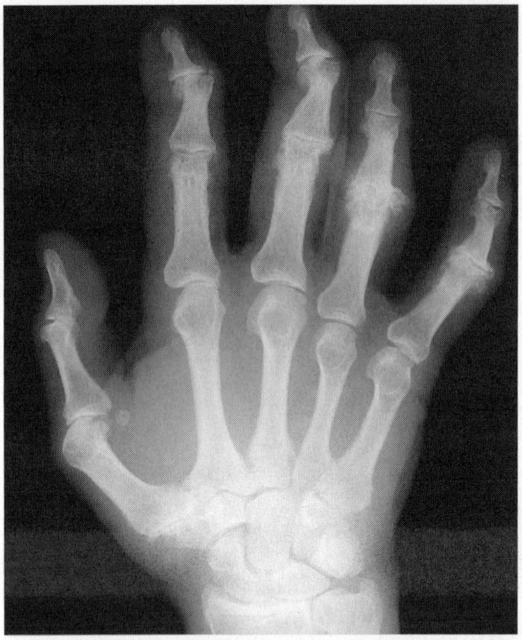

F

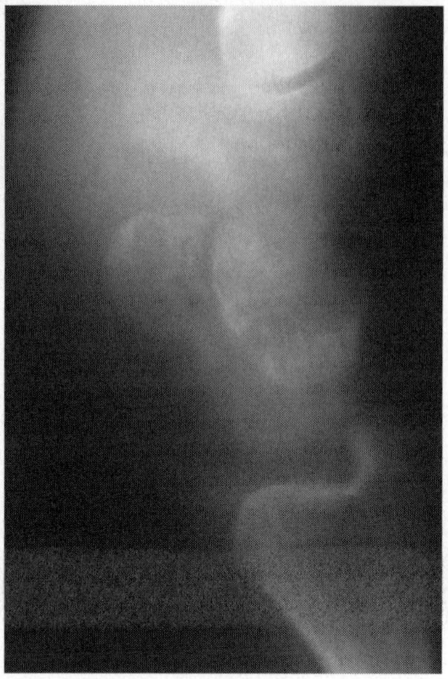

G

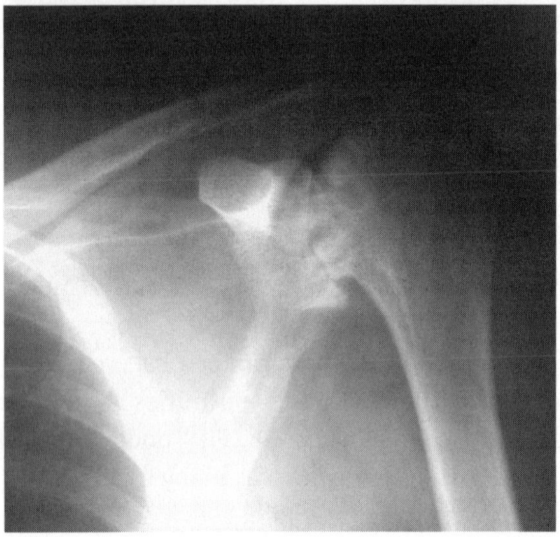

H

Figures 110F–110H AP radiograph of the hand shows moderately advanced osteoarthritis of the PIP joints and, to a lesser degree, the DIP joints. Note the prominent hypertrophic osteophytes arising from the margins of the PIP joint of the ring finger. **110G** Osteoarthritis of the triquetral-pisiform articulation, although not frequently described, is seen reasonably often. An unusual association exists between osteoarthritis of this joint and primary biliary cirrhosis. **110H** Severe osteoarthritis of the shoulder is seen after septic arthritis. Marked joint space loss, subchondral sclerosis, and geode formation are present. Minimal osteophyte formation is evident at the inferior margin of the humeral head articular surface.

- The detection of loose bodies and the evaluation of cartilage in the joint can be enhanced by using arthrography either with dilute contrast or gases (air, CO_2).

MAGNETIC RESONANCE IMAGING

- With MRI, the morphologic changes of the joint are usually well demonstrated. Surrounding soft-tissue structures such as ligaments and menisci often become damaged secondarily and are shown to advantage.

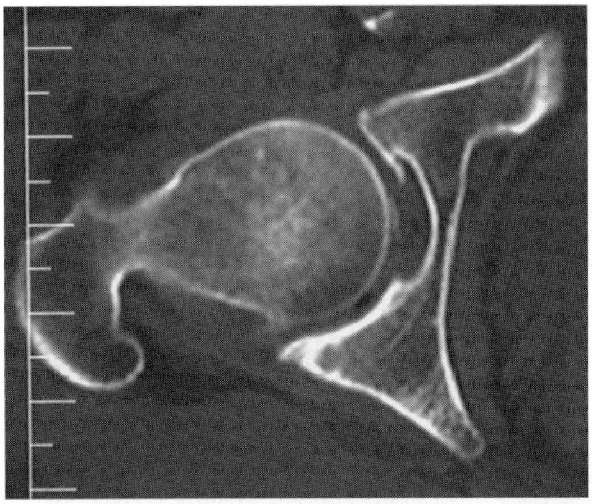

I

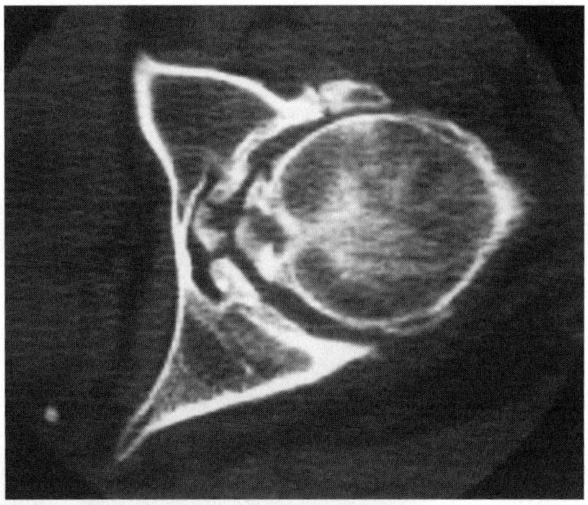

J

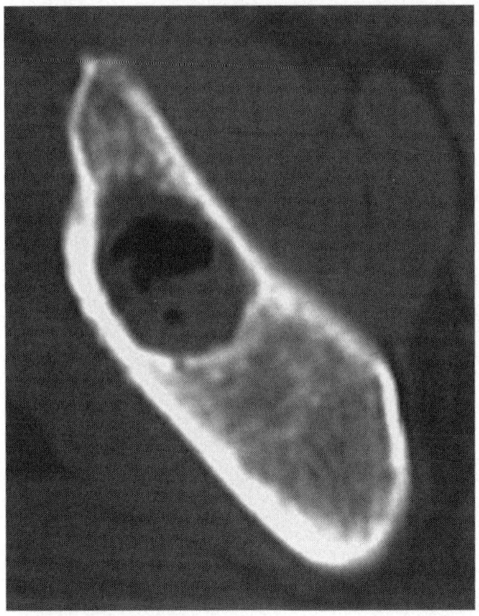

K

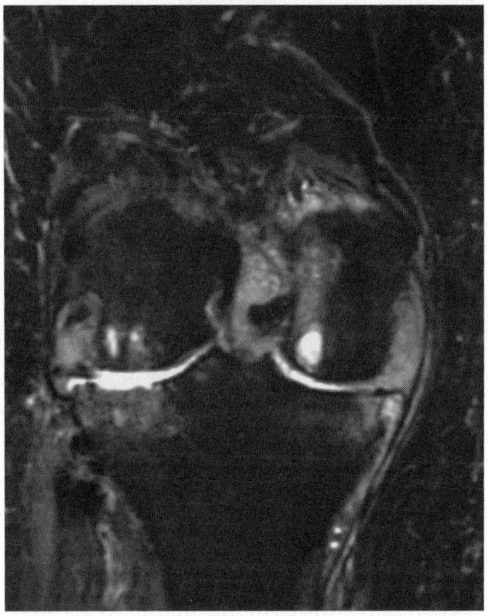

L

Figures 110I–110L Early evidence of osteoarthritis on a transaxial CT image shows minimal subchondral sclerosis on the acetabular aspect of the joint (posteriorly) and corresponding early osteophyte formation on the femoral head. A tiny bubble of nitrogen is evident within the joint. **110J** Transaxial CT shows advanced osteoarthritic changes with prominent loose body formation secondary to osteophyte fracture and fragmentation of denuded subchondral bone. **110K** Transaxial CT image cephalad to the acetabular roof in which a giant geode is present. Copious gas is evident within the geode cavity. **110L** Coronal STIR shows high signal intensity within subchondral bone (tibial and femoral condyles especially) consistent with edema. A small joint effusion is present. Note that the lateral tibial condyle in particular is denuded of cartilage and that the cortical margin is discontinuous. Cyst formation is evident in both femoral condyles.

- Subchondral bone may demonstrate abnormal increased signal intensity due to a combination of edema and granulation tissue (**Fig. 110L**). This may develop over time into fibrosis or sclerosis, represented by low signal on all sequences (**Figs. 110M,110N**).
- MRI is useful in demonstrating the integrity of cartilage, particularly if fat-saturated spoiled GRASS (Gradient Recalled Acquisition in Steady State) sequences are employed (**Fig. 110O**). These sequences are especially useful in the evaluation of early changes before they become clearly manifest on radiography.

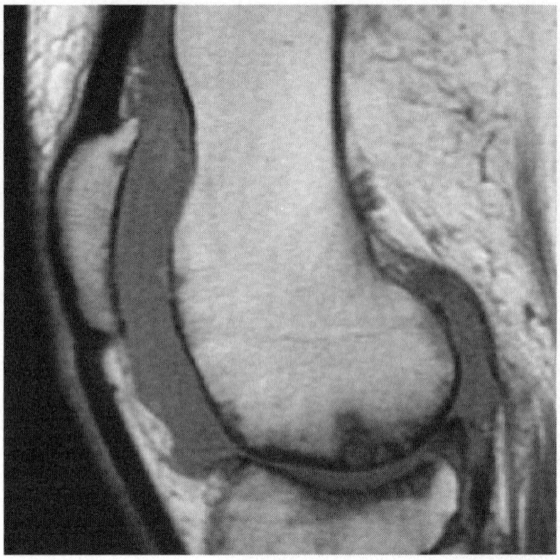

M

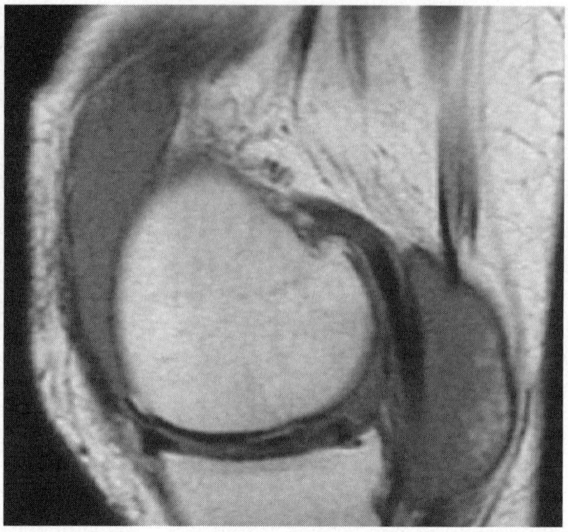

N

Figures 110M,110N 110M A sagittal T1-weighted image of the knee shows almost complete absence of cartilage, with marked low signal intensity in the femoral and tibial subchondral bone consistent with sclerosis and a round cyst of intensity more closely related to the moderate joint effusion present. **110N** An ajacent slice to **110M** shows cartilaginous thinning, osteophyte formation, and the posterior aspect of the joint effusion, seen to contain multiple higher signal loose bodies ("joint mice") in the dependent portion of the capsule.

Treatment

Conservative measures include the following:

- Joint support using canes, for example, may provide symptomatic relief.
- Physiotherapy to strengthen adjacent musculature may help to prevent rapid deterioration.
- Nonsteroidal anti-inflammatory drugs, although less effective than in the inflammatory arthropathies, may provide considerable relief.
- Steroids may be helpful in erosive osteoarthritis, or more aggressive immunosuppression with methotrexate and gold.

Surgical options include the following:

- Osteotomy produces realignment of a joint, redirecting the forces through less affected cartilage, which can relieve pain and buy time prior to joint replacement.
- Synovectomy may be required in the erosive variant.
- Arthroplasty
- Implant placement (**Fig. 110P**)

Prognosis

Arthroplasty provides reliable and durable relief of pain and can restore considerable function.

PEARLS

- The detection of loose bodies and the evaluation of cartilage in the joint can be enhanced by using arthrography either with dilute contrast or gases (air, CO_2).

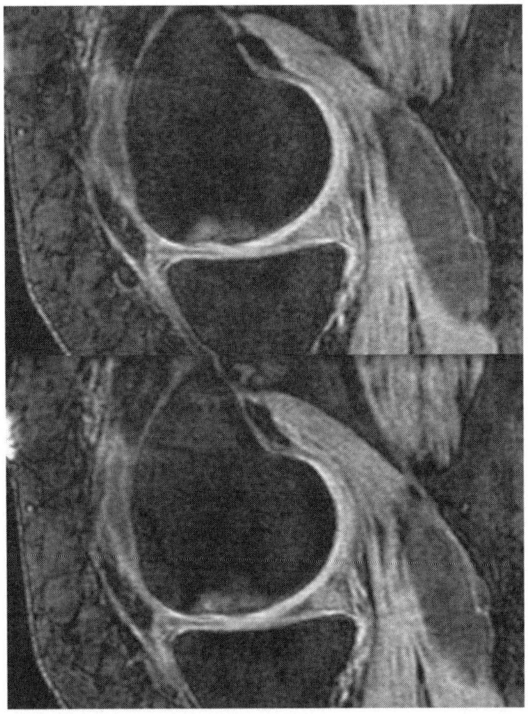

O

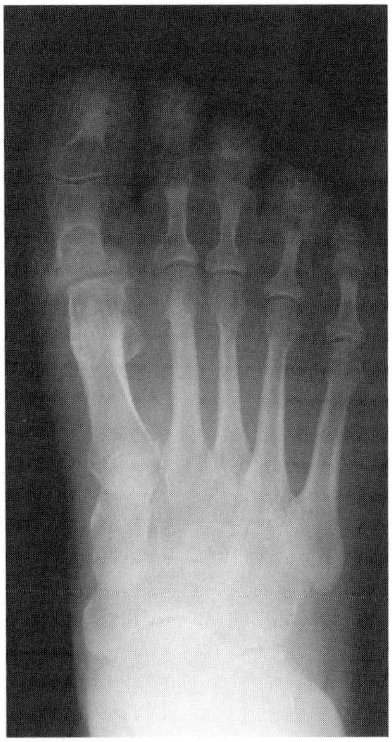

P

Figures 110O,110P 110O Adjacent slices from thin-section slice spoiled GRASS shows early focal cartilaginous thinning and altered intracartilaginous signal change. Focal high signal intensity within the subjacent subchondral bone represents edema. **110P** AP radiograph of the foot demonstrating replacement of the base of the first phalanx with a silicone placement as part of reconstruction of painful rigid valgus of the first metatarsophalangeal joint.

- In erosive osteoarthritis, an extensive destructive component with very prominent osteophytes around the joints can be observed, and the disease tends to be more rapidly progressive than classic osteoarthritis.
- MRI is useful in demonstrating the integrity of cartilage, particularly if fat-saturated spoiled GRASS sequences are employed. These sequences are particularly useful in the evaluation of early changes before they become clearly manifest on radiography.

PITFALLS

- Radiographic change tends to be a poor predictor of osteoarthritis in the interphalangeal joints compared with the hip, knee, and carpometacarpal joints.
- Osteoarthritis preferentially affects the medial compartment of the knee in 75% of cases; if the arthropathy present affects all compartments, one should consider crystal deposition disease or an inflammatory arthropathy.
- In the hip, as the joint space narrows, the femoral head tends to migrate on a superolateral direction in the majority of cases (60%); if the femoral head migration is axial, one should consider crystal deposition or an inflammatory arthropathy.

Suggested Readings

Altman RD, Hochberg M, Murphy WA Jr, Wolfe F, Lequesne M. Atlas of individual radiographic features in osteoarthritis. Osteoarthritis Cartilage 1995;3 Suppl A:3–70

Bancroft LW, Peterson JJ, Kransdorf MJ. Cysts, geodes and erosions. Radiol Clin North Am 2004;42:73–87

Greenspan A. Erosive osteoarthritis. Semin Musculoskelet Radiol 2003;7:155–159

Gupta KB, Duryea J, Weissman BN. Radiographic evaluation of osteoarthritis. Radiol Clin North Am 2004;42:11–41

Karachalios T, Zibis A, Papanagiotou P, et al. MR imaging findings in early osteoarthritis of the knee. Eur J Radiol 2004;50:225–230

CASE 111

Peter L. Munk and Anthony G. Ryan

Clinical Presentation

A 56-year-old woman presented with chronically painful and stiff hands and wrists. The stiffness was maximal on rising and improved slightly after an hour or so. Marked soft-tissue swelling was evident on examination of the dorsum of the right wrist and around the left second and third metacarpophalangeal (MCP) joints.

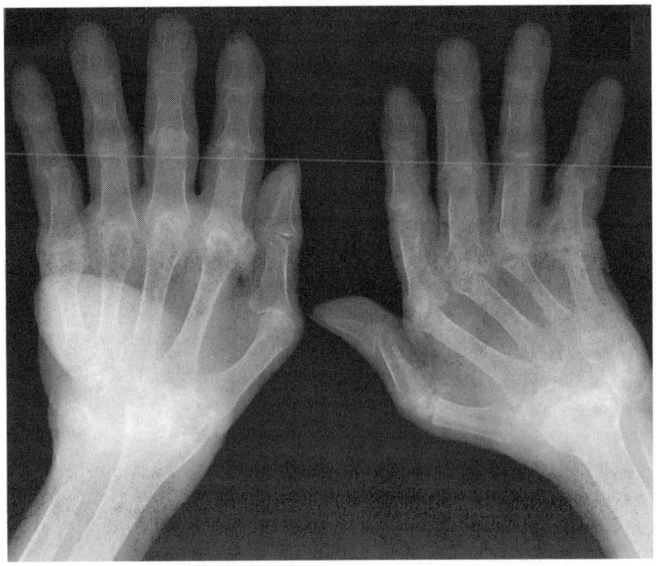

Figure 111A

Radiologic Findings

Radiograph of both hands (**Fig. 111A**) shows tapering absence of both distal ulnae and almost complete absence of the carpal bones of each wrist. The radius appears to articulate directly with the metacarpals bilaterally.

Almost complete erosion of the metacarpal heads resulting in ulnar deviation and partial subluxation of the MCP joints is evident on the left. Less advanced erosive change at the MCP joints is evident on the right. Further erosive changes are evident at the heads of the proximal phalanges, giving rise to subluxation of the proximal interphalangeal (PIP) joints bilaterally.

Massive soft-tissue swelling is evident projected through the ulnar aspect of the dorsum of the hand on the right. Less prominent soft-tissue swelling is evident over the second and third MCPs on the right and further soft-tissue swelling overlying the second to fourth MCPs on the left. The bones are diffusely osteopenic.

Diagnosis

Severe advanced rheumatoid arthritis.

Differential Diagnosis

- Inflammatory arthropathy
- Seronegative arthropathy, for example, psoriatic arthropathy
- Neuropathic arthropathy

Discussion

Background

Rheumatoid arthritis and juvenile rheumatoid arthritis appear to be two distinctly separate diseases, although there may be some cases that occur in children that more closely resemble the adult form.

Etiology

The etiology of rheumatoid arthritis remains controversial. Autoimmune phenomena have often been used to explain this disease process, although others advocate that a close relationship with an infectious agent may exist. An increased incidence of rheumatoid arthritis has been demonstrated in patients with human leukocyte antigen (HLA) DR4. An increased incidence postpartum has been identified.

Pathophysiology

RHEUMATOID ARTHRITIS

A diffuse inflammatory synovitis results in inflammatory cells and macrophages replacing normal synovial tissue, occasionally replacing the complete synovial membrane. The infiltrated/abnormal "synovium" is often referred to as pannus, which is typically highly vascular and can become markedly hypertrophic, filling the joint completely with very little of the joint space occupied by fluid.

Pannus is also aggressively destructive, in part by preventing synovial fluid from nourishing cartilage, and also by the release of a variety of lysosomal enzymes that destroy cartilage and adjacent soft tissues and can even result in extensive osseous destruction.

As the disease continues to progress, and more and more pannus is elaborated, narrowing of the joint space occurs, especially as pannus extends across the joint, destroying cartilage as it goes. It is also at this stage that the first osseous erosions begin to occur, especially at the edges of articular cartilage; this is particularly well observed in the hands and feet.

Patients may develop accompanying periarticular osteopenia, both from the hyperemia associated with the disease and from disuse secondary to pain. Cysts may form below joint surfaces and may be invaded by pannus, which at times can be very destructive and migrate for long distances along the medullary space.

A common feature, especially in the hands and feet, is malalignment, caused by soft-tissue changes resulting in the rupture of tendons and the destruction of ligaments, as well as by loss of bone due to erosion. All of these changes may be found in any joint of the body, including the spine and the large articulating joints, as well as the small joints of the hands and feet.

Ligamentous insufficiency, particularly in the spine, may be best demonstrated using flexion and extension views. This is commonly done to determine the integrity of the atlantoaxial articulation.

In the later stages, fibrosis may become increasingly dominant and may contribute to fibrous ankylosis in the later stages of the disease.

JUVENILE RHEUMATOID ARTHRITIS

Typically, an intense synovitis is present, and erosions of the cartilage resemble those seen in adults. Unlike in adults, osseous ankylosis is often encountered. Early closure of the growth plate and growth arrest can be observed.

Clinical Findings

RHEUMATOID ARTHRITIS

The adult form of rheumatoid arthritis is one of the more common arthropathies and is the most common of the inflammatory arthritides. It is a complex systemic disease with multiple manifestations that may affect any organ system. Women are affected appreciably more often than men. In general, patients will present between the ages of 25 and 55.

The clinical criteria used in making the diagnosis include

1. Morning stiffness in and around joints lasting for at least an hour before improving maximally
2. Soft-tissue swelling of three or more joint areas as observed by a physician
3. Swelling of the PIP, MCP, or wrist joints
4. Symmetric swelling
5. Rheumatoid nodules
6. Presence of rheumatoid factor
7. Radiographic erosions, periarticular osteopenia, or both affecting hand, wrist, or both joints

Although not all patients will show all of the above features, to make the diagnosis, patients must demonstrate the first four and usually one or more of the last three.

The most typical presentation is of a gradual onset polyarthritis. The most commonly involved joints are in the fingers and toes, although other major joints, particularly the knee and ankle, are frequently affected. Any synovial joint may be affected, including the temporomandibular joint and synovial spine articulations.

In general, joint findings are symmetric, particularly in the periphery; this is often a useful differentiating feature. More centrally along the spinal axis and sacroiliac joints, the symmetry may not be quite as striking.

In the spine, the area of principal concern usually centers on the C1–C2 articulation, as erosion of the structures at this site may lead to cord compression, with catastrophic outcomes.

Not only joints but also bursa and tendon sheaths may be affected.

Occasionally, patients will also demonstrate subcutaneous nodules, which may be widespread. Generally, less than a quarter of patients demonstrate this manifestation.

Patients may also manifest generalized systemic symptoms, such as fatigue, anorexia, weight loss, and muscular pain and stiffness.

JUVENILE RHEUMATOID ARTHRITIS

This is sometimes eponymously called Still's disease. Patients frequently present with rashes, lymphadenopathy, fever, increased white cell count, and splenomegaly, and may be rheumatoid factor-negative. As in adults, females are at least twice as frequently affected as males. The age of onset is younger than 18 years in almost all instances.

Early in the disease, joints may not show any swelling, but they may be painful. Patients initially may present with a single abnormal joint, which can become increasingly generalized with time. As the disease progresses, joint swelling is more pronounced and is accompanied by loss of motion and soft-tissue contractures.

The knees, hips, and ankles are most frequently affected, although it is not unusual for the hands and feet to be involved. When the latter are involved, the distribution tends to be symmetric, as in the adult form.

Complications

RHEUMATOID ARTHRITIS

- Ruptured tendons
- Septic arthritis
- Joint rupture leading to Baker's cysts
- In the spine, the area of principal concern usually centers on the C1–C2 articulation, as erosion of the structures at this site may lead to cord compression with catastrophic outcomes, for example, paralysis and sudden death.
- Amyloidosis

JUVENILE RHEUMATOID ARTHRITIS

- Loss of motion and soft-tissue contractures

Pathology

GROSS

Rheumatoid arthritis

The joint may fill completely with tissue, with very little of the joint being occupied by fluid. This tissue is also aggressively destructive, in part by preventing synovial fluid from nourishing cartilage, and also by the release of a variety of different enzymes from the lysosomes which destroy cartilage, adjacent soft tissues, and can even result in extensive osseous destruction.

In the later stages fibrosis may become increasingly dominant and may contribute to fibrous ankylosis in the late stages of the disease.

Even when synovectomy is performed, a new synovial membrane will regenerate which may also go on to show changes of rheumatoid arthritis. The abnormal "synovium" is often referred to as a pannus.

Juvenile rheumatoid arthritis

Cartilaginous erosions resemble those seen in adults. Unlike in adults, osseous ankylosis is often encountered. Early closure of the growth plate and growth arrest can be observed.

MICROSCOPIC

Rheumatoid arthritis

A diffuse inflammatory synovitis that secondarily involves adjacent cartilaginous and osseous structures as well as soft tissues is encountered with this disease. Normal synovial tissue becomes replaced by inflammatory cells and macrophages. This may result in complete replacement of the entire synovial membrane. This tissue is typically highly vascular and can become markedly hypertrophic with a villous appearance.

Juvenile rheumatoid arthritis

An intense synovitis typically is present, and erosions of the cartilage resemble those seen in adults.

Imaging Findings

RADIOGRAPHY

Rheumatoid arthritis

- Almost invariably, early in the course of the disease, joints are radiographically unremarkable.

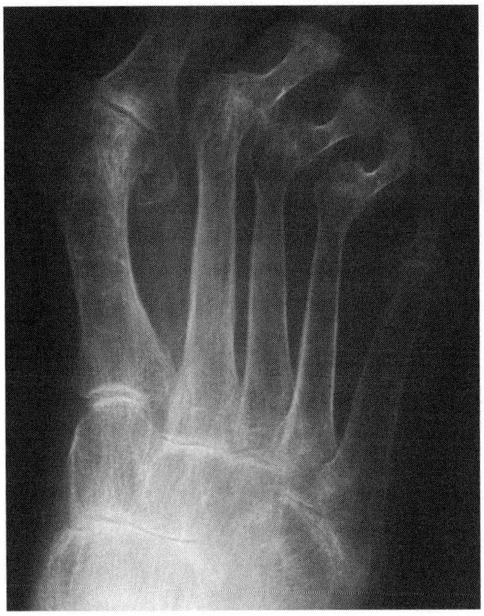

Figure 111B Anteroposterior (AP) radiograph of the foot shows diffuse osteopenia, erosions, marked loss of joint space, and fibular deviation of the metatarsophalangeal joints.

- Symmetric, fusiform soft-tissue swelling can be observed, particularly in the hands and feet.
- As the disease progresses and more pannus is elaborated, uniform joint space narrowing occurs, especially as pannus extends across the joint, destroying cartilage as it goes.
- It is also at this stage that the first osseous erosions begin to occur, especially at the edges of articular cartilage, where the bone is relatively unprotected. This is particularly well observed in the hands and feet. In the wrist, the ulnar styloid and the pisotriquetral articulation are affected at an early stage.
- Patients may develop accompanying periarticular osteopenia both from the hyperemia associated with this disease and from disuse secondary to pain.
- Synovial cysts may form below joint surfaces (**Fig. 111A**) and may be invaded by pannus, which at times can be very destructive and can migrate for long distances along the medullary space.
- A common feature, especially in the hands and feet, is malalignment, caused by soft-tissue changes resulting in the rupture of tendons and the destruction of ligaments, as well as by loss of bone due to erosion. An ulnar "drift" is the typical result.
- All of these changes may be found in any joint of the body, including the spine and the large articulating joints, as well as the small joints of the hands and feet (**Fig. 111B**). The feet are affected in addition to the hands in 80 to 90% of patients, preceding the hand signs in 10 to 20%.
- In the knee, the joint space loss is universal, in contradistinction to osteoarthritis, which affects the medial compartment to a greater extent. In the hip (affected in 50% of patients), the loss of joint space leads to axial and medial migration of the femoral head.
- No reactive bone formation
- The cervical spine is affected in 60 to 80% of patients, and all the synovial joints in relation to the vertebral body may be affected, that is, the apophyseal joints and the joints of Luschka. Spinous process erosions occasionally may be seen.

Factors identified as having increased risk of cord compression in rheumatoid arthritis are the following:

- Anterior atlantodental interval (AADI) > 9 mm (> 3 mm defines atlantoaxial subluxation). The AADI is measured from the posteroinferior margin of the anterior arch to the anterior surface of the odontoid.

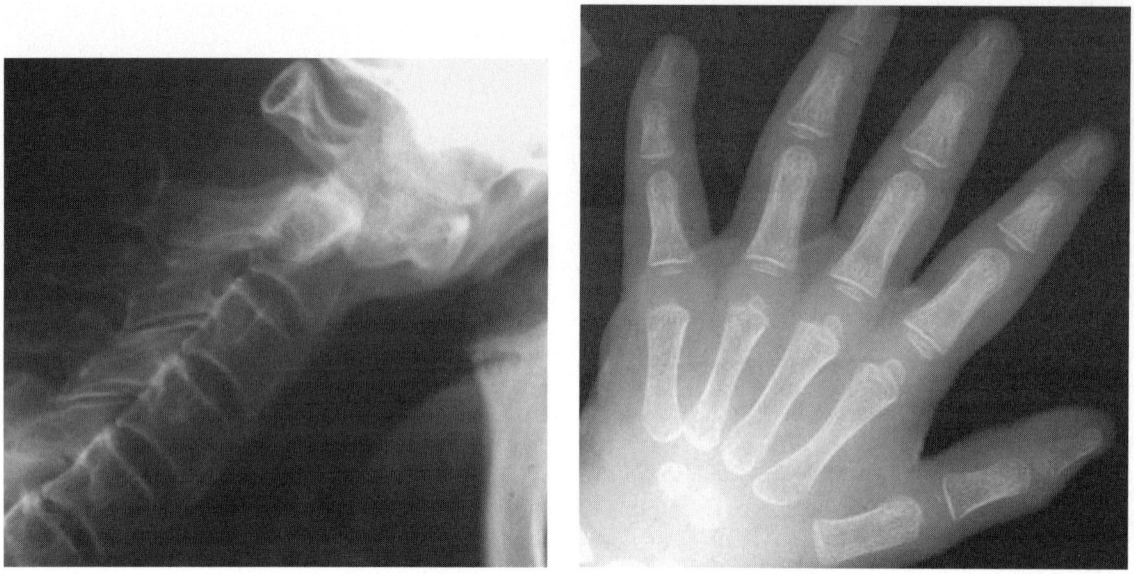

C D

Figures 111C,111D 111C Lateral cervical spine radiograph shows pronounced erosion of the odontoid and associated atlantoaxial subluxation. Note the markedly increased anterior atlantodental interval and the decreased posterior atlantodental interval. **111D** AP radiograph of the hand of a child with juvenile rheumatoid arthritis shows soft-tissue swelling centered on the metacarpophalangeal and proximal interphalangeal joints, with associated periosteal new bone formation evident along the shafts of the second to fourth proximal phalanges.

- Basilar invagination, particularly in association with atlantoaxial subluxation
- Subaxial canal diameter < 14 mm
- Subluxations occur in 43 to 86% of cases, and as many as 61% of rheumatoid patients undergoing hip or knee replacement have cervical instability. The ligamentous insufficiency secondary to erosion of the transverse and alar ligaments may be best demonstrated initially using flexion and extension views, to determine the integrity of the atlantoaxial articulation (**Fig. 111C**), as neutral radiographs will miss up to 48% of atlantoaxial subluxations.

Juvenile rheumatoid arthritis

- As in the adult form, soft-tissue swelling may be a prominent feature early in the disease, with accompanying joint effusions and periarticular osteoporosis.
- Several features, however, are encountered in juvenile rheumatoid arthritis that are not usually encountered in the adult form, particularly the formation of periosteal new bone near the sites of the affected joint (**Fig. 111D**).
- Ankylosis of joints is far more common than in adults, and although this may be fibrous, osseous ankylosis is not unusual. Ankylosis may often occur in the spine in the apophyseal joints.
- Because the skeleton is still growing, growth disturbances may create significant clinical problems, including hyperemia, leading to overgrowth in some instances.
- Osteoporosis is often a far more striking feature of this disease than in adults, who often will develop osteoporosis for other reasons.

ULTRASOUND

- Although ultrasound may identify synovial hypertrophy and erosions, bony abnormalities are frequently missed.

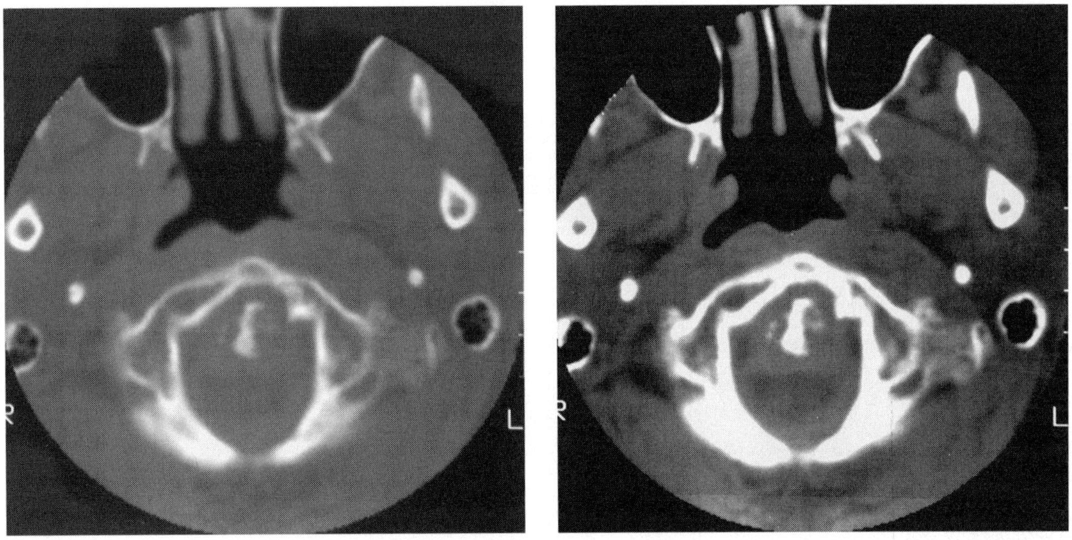

E F

Figures 111E Transaxial CT slice at the level of the odontoid peg shows considerable osseous erosion. **111F** The same CT slice displayed on soft-tissue windows demonstrating significant pannus surrounding the peg.

- Power Doppler has been shown to correlate well with dynamic MRI, especially when ultrasound contrast agents were employed.
- Ultrasound is very time-consuming when multiple joints are involved.
- Ultrasound is ideal in the diagnosis of Baker's cysts and tenosynovitis. In the latter, ultrasound-guided injection of tendon sheaths may be particularly useful.

COMPUTED TOMOGRAPHY

- CT is helpful in demonstrating the extent of osseous erosion by pannus as well as narrowing of joints. An excellent example of the former would be at the atlantoaxial articulation, where pannus may completely erode the odontoid (**Figs. 111E,111F**) and in severe cases be sufficiently extensive to compress the spinal cord.
- Infusion of intravenous contrast often will permit good delineation of the abnormal soft tissue frequently associated with this disease.

MAGNETIC RESONANCE IMAGING

- In recent years, MRI has come to play an important role in the assessment of patients with rheumatoid arthritis, as it is better able to show the soft-tissue changes than radiography. In addition, the greater sensitivity of MRI allows earlier detection and commencement of disease-modifying therapies before significant disability becomes established. In a comparative study, MRI demonstrated bone erosions of the humeral head in 96% of cases, compared with 92% on ultrasound, 77% on CT, and 73% on conventional radiography.
- Often the osseous erosion and invasion of the marrow space can be demonstrated on MRI (**Figs. 111F,111G**), although crisp cortical detail is better provided by CT.
- Pannus is typically of low signal on T1-weighted images (unless hemorrhage has occurred) and may be low or bright on T2-weighted sequences.
- Pannus enhances intensely with the administration of intravenous gadolinium (**Figs. 111H–111M**), some studies indicating that enhancement rates correlate with the aggressiveness of the disease on dynamic MRI. Active synovitis is best demonstrated on T1-weighted fat-saturated images after intravenous gadolinium.

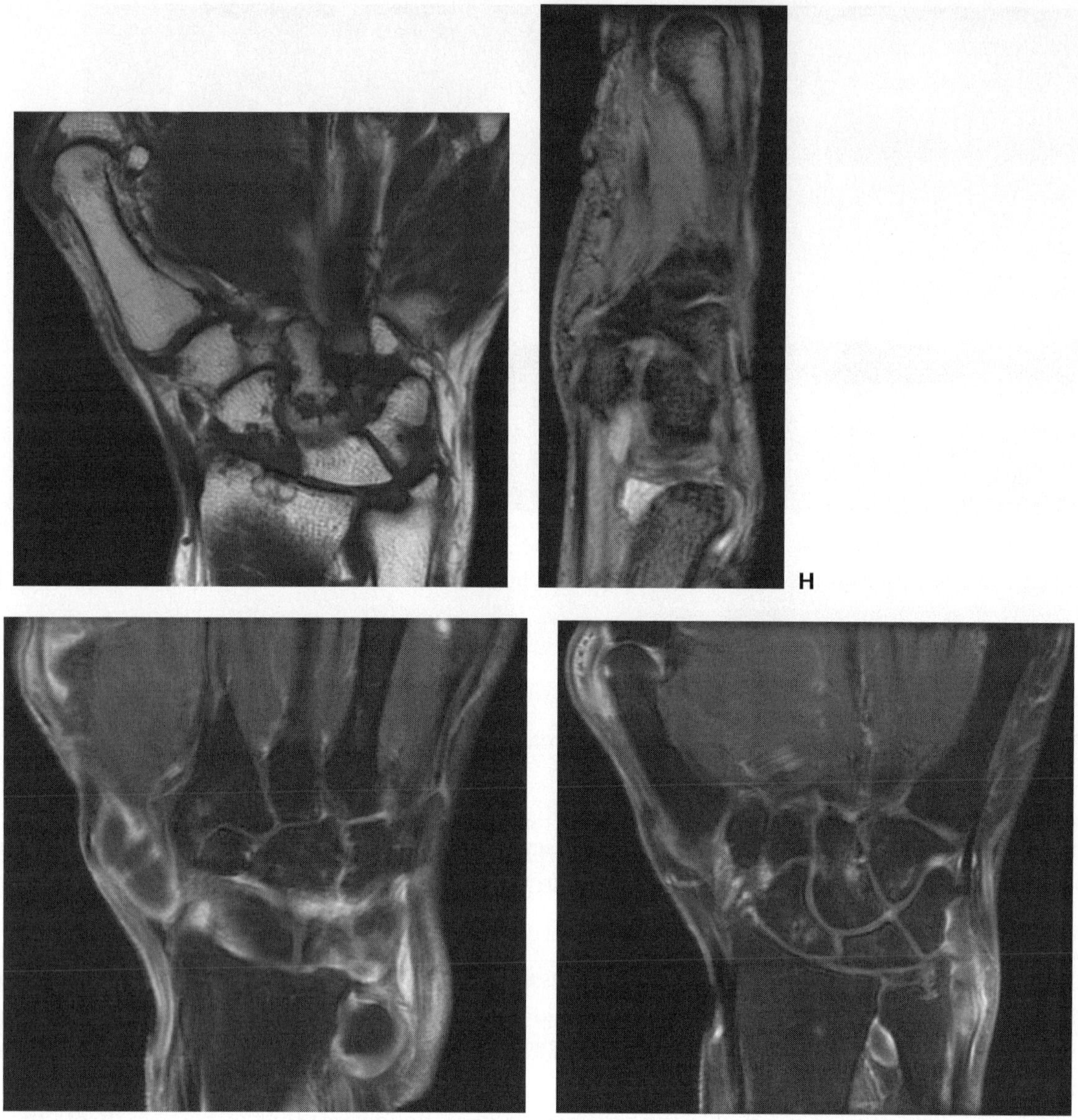

G H I J

Figures 111G–111J Coronal T1-weighted image shows multiple osseous erosions, joint space loss, and low-signal pannus throughout the carpus and affecting the first carpometacarpal and metacarpophalangeal joints. **111H** Sagittal MPGR image shows high signal intensity fluid (effusion) around the head of the ulna and erosions at the pisotriquetral articulation. **111I** and **111J** Adjacent coronal T1-weighted fat-saturated images after intravenous gadolinium show enhancement at the sites of osseous erosion in the pannus in relation to the neck of the ulna and within the tendon sheaths of the extensor pollicis longus and extensor carpi ulnaris, as well as swelling and signal abnormality within the substance of the latter.

- Gadolinium enhancement aids in differentiating between the presence of pannus and fluid within a joint, as the fluid will not enhance, although it should be cautioned that gadolinium will slowly seep into the joint fluid after several minutes, making differentiation between the two more difficult.
- A remarkable feature of this disease on MRI is that, in spite of the marked distention of joints and bursae, at times relatively little of the volume is occupied by synovial fluid. Recognizing this prevents the frequently futile attempts to aspirate synovial fluid from such joints.
- MRI is also extremely helpful in demonstrating tenosynovitis and the integrity of tendons, which can often be compromised by invasion of pannus (**Figs. 111H–111M**).

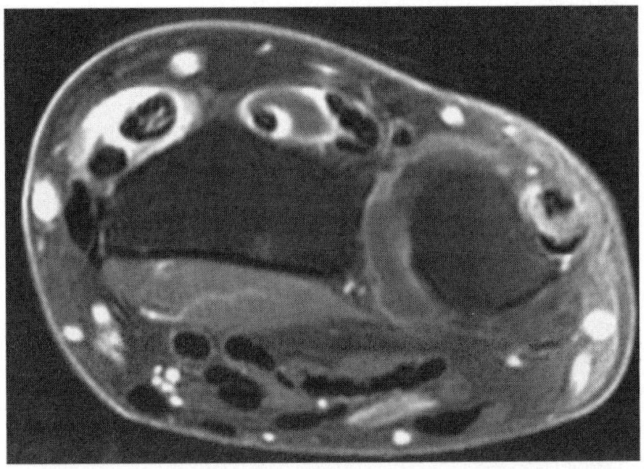
K

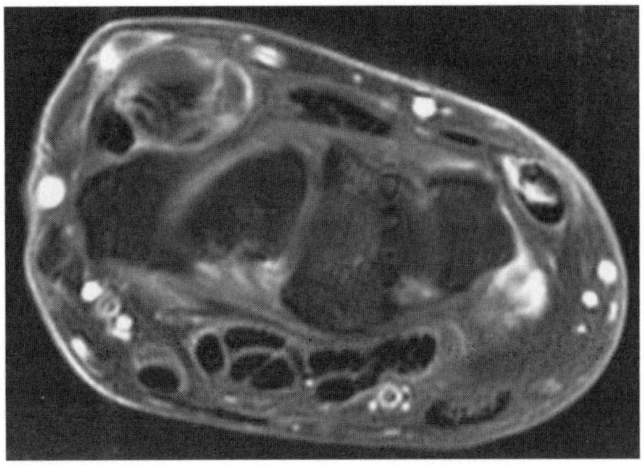
L

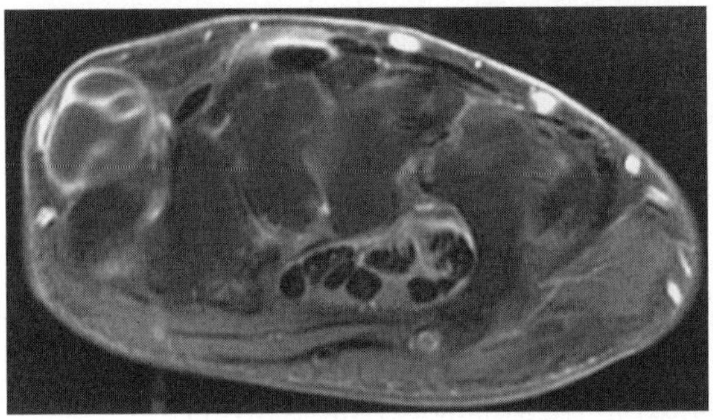
M

Figures 111K–111M (same patient as in **111I,111J**) Adjacent transaxial fat-saturated T1-weighted images after intravenous gadolinium at the levels of the ulnar neck (**111K**), radioscaphoid articulation (**111L**), and distal carpal row (**111M**), respectively, show enhancing pannus between the radius and ulna, distal radioulnar joint effusion, marked swelling, and increased intrasubstance signal in the extensor carpi ulnaris and extensor pollicis longus tendons and discontinuity of the latter. There is an "empty sheath" sign and marked associated tendon sheath enhancement at the level of the distal carpal row. This is consistent with acute active rheumatoid arthritis with tenosynovitis and partial tear of the extensor carpi ulnaris and complete tear of the extensor pollicis longus.

- MRI is also useful in demonstrating abnormal bursae, which often will expand to many times their normal volume.
- MRI is particularly helpful in the assessment of patients who require surgery, as it shows the full soft-tissue and intramedullary involvement of the disease due to the aggressively expanding pannus. An excellent example of this would be at the atlantoaxial articulation, where pannus may be sufficiently extensive to compress the spinal cord.
- Not infrequently, rheumatoid patients will also demonstrate the presence of Baker's cysts, which may rupture; all of this can also be well demonstrated with CT and ultrasound, although MRI frequently will show the extent of the inflammation more precisely.
- Experimental studies have shown a significant correlation between total synovial volume and the subsequent development of bone erosions.

Treatment

RHEUMATOID ARTHRITIS

Conservative

- Nonsteroidal anti-inflammatory drugs (NSAIDs)
- Steroids (systemic and intra-articular)
- Immunosuppressants (penicillamine, gold, azathioprine, methotrexate)
- Physical therapy and rehabilitation
- Orthotics

Surgery

Surgery is indicated for joints whose function is severely limited. Disability may arise from subluxation or from the mechanical impairment secondary to cartilage destruction and joint space fibrosis.

- Synovectomy and tendon transfer can contribute where articular cartilage is intact.
- Bone excision, for example, the head of the ulna and the metatarsal heads, is appropriate for pain relief and increased range of motion.
- Arthrodesis or arthroplasty is indicated in cases of severe cartilage destruction and joint fibrosis. The hip, knee, MCP, and elbow joints are all usefully replaced, whereas the wrist and interphalangeal joints tend to do better with fusion.
- Anterior atlantodental interval > 9 mm is taken as an indication for cervical stabilization, given the significantly increased risk of spontaneous cord compression.

JUVENILE RHEUMATOID ARTHRITIS

- NSAIDs
- Gold and penicillamine used less often
- Steroids avoided to prevent growth problems
- Joint support and deformity protection (rest, splinting, physical therapy)

Prognosis

RHEUMATOID ARTHRITIS

Even when synovectomy is performed, a new synovial membrane will regenerate, which may also go on to show changes of rheumatoid arthritis.

Disease progression may occur despite all therapies, at which time treatment becomes primarily symptomatic.

JUVENILE RHEUMATOID ARTHRITIS

Spontaneous remissions are expected in up to 85% before the age of 20.

PEARLS

- Several features are encountered in juvenile rheumatoid arthritis that are not usually encountered in the adult form, particularly the formation of periosteal new bone near the sites of the affected joint.
- Similarly, ankylosis of joints is far more common in the juvenile form than in adults, and although this may be fibrous, osseous ankylosis is not unusual. Ankylosis may also occur in the spine in the apophyseal joints.
- Active synovitis is best demonstrated on T1-weighted fat-saturated images after intravenous gadolinium.

PITFALLS

- Gadolinium enhancement aids in differentiating between the presence of pannus and fluid within a joint, as the latter will not enhance, although it should be cautioned that gadolinium will slowly seep into the joint fluid after several minutes, making differentiation between the two more difficult.
- The odontoid process enhances normally after intravenous gadolinium and so caution must be exercised in diagnosing disease at this site.
- A remarkable feature of this disease on MRI is that, in spite of the marked distention of joints and bursae, at times relatively little of the volume is occupied by synovial fluid. Recognizing this prevents the frequently futile attempts to aspirate synovial fluid from such joints.

Suggested Readings

Azouz EM. Arthritis in children: conventional and advanced imaging. Semin Musculoskelet Radiol 2003;7:95–102

Castor WR, Miller JD, Russell AS, Chiu PL, Grace M, Hanson J. Computed tomography of the craniocervical junction in rheumatoid arthritis. J Comput Assist Tomogr 1983;7:31–36

Castro S, Verstraete K, Mielants H, Vanderstraeten G, de Reuck J, Veys EM. Cervical spine involvement in rheumatoid arthritis: a clinical, neurological and radiological evaluation. Clin Exp Rheumatol 1994;12:369–374

Peterfy CG. Is there a role for extremity magnetic resonance imaging in routine clinical management of rheumatoid arthritis? J Rheumatol 2004;31:640–644

Roche CJ, Eyes BE, Whitehouse GH. The rheumatoid cervical spine: signs of instability on plain cervical radiographs. Clin Radiol 2002;57:241–249

Tehranzadeh J, Ashikyan O, Dascalos J. Advanced imaging of early rheumatoid arthritis. Radiol Clin North Am 2004;42:89–107

Wakefield RJ, Conaghan PG, Jarrett S, Emery P. Noninvasive techniques for assessing skeletal changes in inflammatory arthritis: imaging technique. Curr Opin Rheumatol 2004;16:435–442

CASE 112

Peter L. Munk and Anthony G. Ryan

Clinical Presentation

A 41-year-old man with a skin rash presented with painful feet.

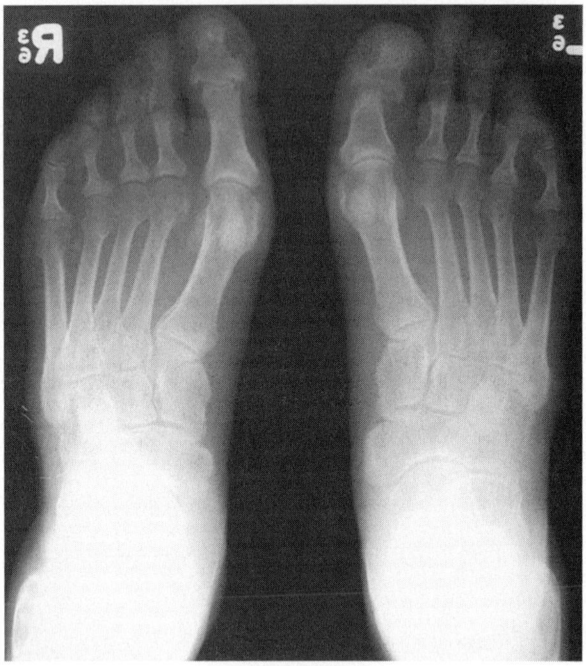

Figure 112A

Radiologic Findings

A radiograph of the feet (**Fig. 112A**) shows bilateral erosion of the head of the first metatarsal, worse on the left where the head is almost completely destroyed. Corresponding but less florid erosion is present on the distal aspect of this joint, producing a characteristic deformity.

Diagnosis

Psoriatic arthropathy, demonstrating "pencil-in-cup" deformity of the left first interphalangeal joint.

Differential Diagnosis

- Reactive arthritis (Reiter's disease)
- Rheumatoid arthritis
- Gout

Discussion

Background

Psoriatic arthritis combines many features of rheumatoid arthritis, in which synovial inflammation predominates, and ankylosing spondylitis, in which ligamentous inflammation predominates.

Psoriatic arthritis is most often associated with the classically recognized skin manifestations. In a distinct minority of patients, arthritic changes may appear before skin changes.

Etiology

Psoriatic arthritis is of unknown etiology, although human leukocyte antigen (HLA) B27 levels are increased in 20% of patients with peripheral arthritis and 50% of patients with axial arthritis. An infectious etiology has been proposed.

Pathophysiology

Psoriatic anthropathy is characterized by a profound synovitis of unknown etiology but which is associated with dysregulated angiogenesis and the presence of increased concentrations of an inflammatory serine protease.

Clinical Findings

Psoriatic arthropathy most commonly affects patients between the ages of 20 and 40 years. Arthritis is said to occur in 5 to 8% of patients with psoriasis. Although there is an equal sex distribution, spine and distal interphalangeal disease is more common in men, whereas a symmetric polyarthritis is more common in women.

The arthropathy precedes the characteristic rash in 10% of patients; in the majority (75%), the rash is present first.

The distal interphalangeal joints of the fingers and feet are often affected; however, unlike in rheumatoid arthritis, joint involvement is frequently asymmetric.

Patients report painful swollen joints. Soft-tissue swelling around the affected joints compounds the joint swelling secondary to the frequently present effusions. Joints may be stiff and immobile if bony ankylosis has occurred.

Lower back pain and diminished back flexion may be present secondary to sacroiliac or spinal involvement.

Stages of Disease

A spectrum of clinical severity exists. Most patients demonstrate a monoarticular pattern or an asymmetric oligoarticular pattern.

Other patients have a more extensive involvement of their joints, which at times can closely mimic rheumatoid arthritis; however, rheumatoid factor is negative.

A polyarthritis affects primarily the distal interphalangeal joints. A spondylarthritis closely mimics ankylosing spondylosis.

In some patients, the process may become extremely mutilating and destructive, affecting multiple joints in the hands and feet; this is known as arthritis mutilans. When this occurs, the proximal interphalangeal (PIP) and distal interphalangeal (DIP) joints telescope, resulting in loose skin and soft tissue of the affected digits. In this condition, the clinician is able to move the digits in and out longitudinally, giving rise to the characteristic description of an opera-glass digit (main en lorgnette).

Complications

- Devastating atlantoaxial subluxation may occur, resulting in cord compression and quadriplegia.

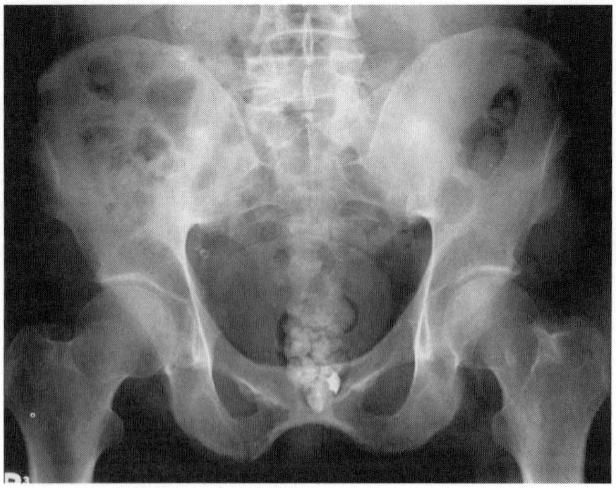

Figure 112B Anteroposterior radiograph of the pelvis shows asymmetric sacroiliitis as evinced by absence of the right sacroiliac joint space secondary to bony ankylosis and associated adjacent sclerosis. Similar but less florid changes are evident on the left.

Pathology

GROSS

Cartilaginous erosion and destruction of subchondral bone may occur to varying degrees, depending on the severity of the disease. Enthesopathy may also occur.

MICROSCOPIC

Patients demonstrate extensive synovitis, which can closely resemble that of rheumatoid arthritis. Vascular changes have been identified in both the skin condition and arthropathy.

Imaging Findings

RADIOGRAPHY

- Unlike in rheumatoid arthritis, joint involvement is frequently asymmetric.
- In the hands and feet, fusiform soft-tissue swelling is typical, giving rise to "sausage" digits.
- The DIP joints of the fingers and feet are most often affected, with pronounced loss of joint space. There may be extensive destruction of the phalangeal tufts with or without involvement of the DIP joint surfaces; tuft destruction is usually associated with marked nail changes.
- Erosions are seen to be marginal in the majority of cases. In advanced cases, the erosions progress to involve the entire articular surface, producing a so-called pencil-in-cup deformity. This may further progress to frank bony ankylosis, particularly in the interphalangeal joints.
- Periosteal new bone is occasionally also noted accompanying these findings, not only in the phalanges but also at the inferior surface of the calcaneus and at tendon and ligamentous insertions.
- Joint effusions are often present.
- Osteopenia is not a feature.
- The sacroiliac joints are affected (**Fig. 112B**) in 30 to 50% of cases. The involvement is usually asymmetric and affects the iliac aspect to a greater extent than the sacral aspect.
- Spinal involvement is frequently present, manifested as bulky syndesmophytes, which classically arise from the midbody of the vertebra rather than more marginally, as seen in ankylosing spondylitis. Radiographic evidence of severe spondylitis in psoriasis is said to correlate strongly and specifically with HLA B27 positivity.

- Atlantoaxial subluxation can be encountered in these patients.

ULTRASOUND

The periosteal reaction, tendon edema, and tendon calcifications associated with enthesopathy may be visible using high-resolution transducers.

COMPUTED TOMOGRAPHY

- CT can demonstrate elegantly early erosive changes in the sacroiliac joints, such as erosions and reactive sclerosis.

MAGNETIC RESONANCE IMAGING

- MRI findings are nonspecific, demonstrating loss of cartilage, joint effusion with extensive synovitis, marrow edema, and subchondral erosions. The appearance may be difficult to differentiate from that of rheumatoid arthritis. T2-weighted and STIR sequences are most helpful in the identification of subtle marrow edema.
- MRI is more sensitive than radiographs in the detection of early erosions, with periarticular high signal representing the earliest indication of inflammation.
- The appearances of sacroiliitis are, again, nonspecific, but include focal or wavy low signal intensity in cartilage on T1-weighted images, with corresponding high signal intensity on T2-weighted images.
- Joint sclerosis may be evident as low signal intensity on both T1- and T2-weighted images.
- Gadolinium enhancement increases the sensitivity of the examination in the detection of early inflammation.

Treatment

- Those with mild cases may be managed successfully with simple analgesia, for example, acetaminophen.
- Those with more moderate disease require nonsteroidal anti-inflammatory drugs.
- Severe progressive cases may require immunosuppressives such as azathioprine. Gold may also be effective.
- Newer biologic agents are showing promise against the disease, for example, tumor necrosis factor (TNF)-α antagonists.
- Reconstructive surgery or implants occasionally may be required.

Prognosis

- The prognosis mirrors the severity of the disease. Successful treatment of the skin disease does not necessarily modify the state of the arthropathy.

PEARLS

- Although there is an equal sex distribution, spine and distal interphalangeal disease is more common in men, whereas a symmetric polyarthritis is more common in women.
- Unlike in rheumatoid arthritis, involvement of joints is frequently asymmetric.
- Juxta-articular osteoporosis is not a feature, allowing one to differentiate this condition from its close relation, reactive arthritis (Reiter's syndrome).

PITFALLS

- MRI findings are nonspecific, demonstrating loss of cartilage and joint effusion with synovitis. The appearance may be difficult to differentiate from that of rheumatoid arthritis.
- Periostitis in the absence of joint findings suggests reactive arthritis (Reiter's syndrome) over psoriasis.
- Although the "mouse-ear" appearance (periosteal new bone proliferation in association with marginal erosions) may suggest osteoarthritic osteophytes at first glance, recognizing the presence of the underlying erosion enables one to make the correct diagnosis.

Suggested Readings

Frediani B, Falsetti P, Storri L, et al. Quadricepital tendon enthesitis in psoriatic arthritis and rheumatoid arthritis: ultrasound examinations and clinical correlations. J Rheumatol 2001;28:2566–2568

Gladman DD. Psoriatic arthritis. Rheum Dis Clin North Am 1998;24:829–844

Klecker RJ, Weissman BN. Imaging features of psoriatic arthritis and Reiter's syndrome. Semin Musculoskelet Radiol 2003;7:115–126

Yu W, Feng F, Dion E, Yang H, Jiang M, Genant HK. Comparison of radiography, computed tomography and magnetic resonance imaging in the detection of sacroiliitis accompanying ankylosing spondylitis. Skeletal Radiol 1998;27:311–320

CASE 113

Anthony G. Ryan and Peter L. Munk

Clinical Presentation

A 25-year-old man presented with an acute exacerbation of a recurrently painful heel.

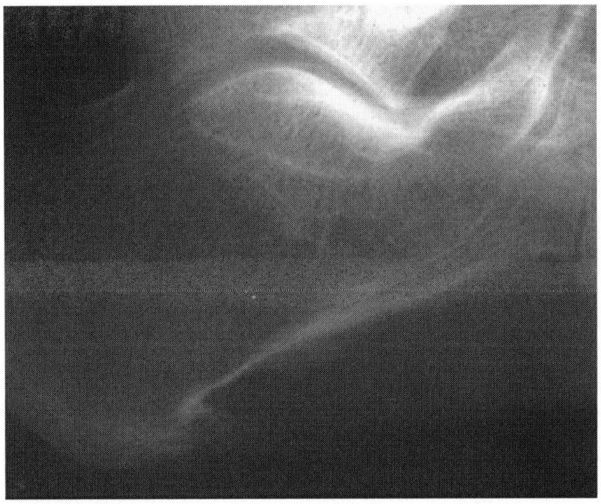

Figure 113A

Radiologic Findings

A lateral radiograph of the heel (**Fig. 113A**) shows a calcaneal spur and a periosteal reaction along the inferior aspect of the calcaneus.

Diagnosis

Reactive arthritis (Reiter's disease).

Differential Diagnosis

- Other seronegative spondyloarthropathies, such as psoriatic or ankylosing spondylitis
- Rheumatoid arthritis

Discussion

Background

The seronegative spondyloarthropathies consist of ankylosing spondylitis, psoriatic arthritis, reactive arthritis (Reiter's syndrome), enteropathic spondylitis, and undifferentiated spondyloarthropathy, all of which share common clinical and radiographic features with characteristic involvement of the sacroiliac joints, the spine, and the peripheral joints.

The criteria for diagnosing one of the inflammatory spondyloarthropathies are spine pain or synovitis plus one of the following:

- Family history
- Psoriasis/inflammatory bowel disease
- Urethritis/cervicitis/diarrhea within 1 month
- Buttock pain
- Enthesopathy
- Sacroiliitis

All of the above typically affect young adults. If a seronegative spondyloarthropathy presents in patients under the age of 16, it is referred to as "juvenile."

Previously known as Reiter's syndrome, the condition is now more correctly called reactive arthritis and is clearly identified as one of the spondyloarthritis group of diseases.

When the typical arthritis is accompanied by urethritis and conjunctivitis, the term ***Reiter's syndrome*** still properly applies, with circinate balanitis (30%), buccal ulcerations, and a dermatitis (keratogenic blennorrhagia) as frequent additional findings.

Etiology

It appears that at least two factors are necessary for the development of reactive arthritis: an initiating infectious agent and a genetic predisposition. The infectious agent is most commonly a gram-negative bacterium with lipopolysaccharide as an integral component of its outer membrane, contracted via either a sexually transmitted urethritis or a dysentery. Chlamydia has recently been identified as a potential organism.

The prevalence of the human leukocyte antigen (HLA) B27 in Reiter's arthritis is quoted as between 63 and 93%. Conversely, the prevalence of spondyloarthropathies in a given population correlates directly with the prevalence of the HLA-B27 antigen. The presence of HLA-B27 strongly predisposes individuals to the development of reactive arthritis after an enteric or genitourinary infection. The disease is more severe in patients who are HLA-positive and tends to pursue a more aggressive and chronically relapsing course.

Pathophysiology

HLA-B27 appears to modulate the interaction between reactive arthritis–triggering bacteria and immune cells by a mechanism unrelated to the antigen presentation function of HLA-B27.

Molecular mimicry, the phenomenon of protein products from dissimilar genes sharing similar structures eliciting an immune response to both self and microbial proteins, has been proposed as a potential mechanism by which infections trigger autoimmune diseases. The molecules identified to demonstrate most consistent mimicry are chlamydial heat shock proteins 60, the deoxyribonucleic acid (DNA) primase of *Chlamydia trachomatis*, and chlamydial OmcB proteins, thus potentially implicating this organism in the initiation and maintenance of reactive arthritis.

In addition, elevated levels of tumor necrosis factor-α (TNF-α) have been identified in the synovium of patients with reactive and undifferentiated arthritis, implicating TNF-α in the pathogenesis of these disorders.

Clinical Findings

Patients (the vast majority male, in their third and fourth decades) typically present with a triad of symptoms, namely, painful joints, painful eyes, and painful urination, reflecting underlying arthritis, conjunctivitis, and urethritis. There is a frequent history of a recent infection, either sexually transmitted or a diarrheal illness (*Shigella, Salmonella, Yersinia,* or enteric *Campylobacter*).

The arthritis is typically mono- or pauciarticular, asymmetric, and involves lower extremity peripheral joints predominantly.

Enthesitis is the term given to inflammation at the site of ligamentous attachment to bone and is a frequent attendant of reactive arthritis. Reflecting this, heel pain is present in 26 to 50% of cases and may affect the region of the Achilles' insertion or the plantar surface of the calcaneus, which may be visibly or palpably swollen on examination.

Dactylitis and tenosynovitis are frequently present early on in as many as 17% of patients. Less commonly, patients may present with inflammatory spinal pain, sacroiliitis, chest wall pain, lesions of the lung apices, and aortic incompetence together with conduction disturbances. All of these may also occur in isolation.

When the arthritis is isolated and oligoarticular, particularly in the presence of a urethritis, it must be differentiated from gonococcal arthritis by aspiration.

In reactive arthritis, joint aspiration reveals a turbid yellow fluid.

The erythrocyte sedimentation rate is typically raised acutely.

There is an association between patients with human immunodeficiency virus (HIV) infection and with seronegative arthritis, of whom ~54% have Reiter's syndrome. The arthropathy precedes the acquired immunodeficiency syndrome in 64% of patients with stage IV HIV infection. These patients are indistinguishable radiographically from patients with typical seronegative disorders; however, there is a predominance of lower extremity abnormalities in patients with HIV.

Reactive arthritis, like psoriatic arthritis, differs from ankylosing spondylitis in its inconstant involvement of the spine and greater involvement of peripheral joints.

Reactive arthritis differs from psoriatic arthritis in its predominant involvement of the lower limbs, particularly the feet, with relative sparing of the hands and wrists.

Complications

- Gastric ulcer and hemorrhage
- Aortic incompetence
- Heart block
- Amyloidosis
- Hydronephrosis
- Optic neuritis
- Retinitis
- Pericarditis
- Valvulitis
- Peripheral neuritis
- Pleurisy
- Pneumonitis
- Purpura
- Thrombophlebitis

Pathology

GROSS

- Hypertrophic new bone formation at entheses and in a periarticular distribution

MICROSCOPIC

- Synovitis, chondritis, and enthesitis predominantly
- Synovial fluid is inflammatory, with a high polymorphonuclear white cell count, but is usually sterile.

Imaging Findings

RADIOGRAPHY

- Although Reiter's syndrome has nonspecific radiographic findings, the diagnosis may be made based on recognition of the characteristic morphologic changes and distribution. Synovial and cartilaginous joints are affected, as are entheses. Distal appendicular involvement is characteristic, with the small joints of the foot (40 to 55% of cases, particularly involving the interphalangeal and metatarsophalangeal joints), the ankle (30 to 50% of cases), and the knee most frequently affected. The symphysis pubis and manubriosternal joint are uncommonly involved.
- The typical findings are of concomitant erosions and bony spurs, but only in advanced phases.
- Although osteoporosis may be present acutely, it is not chronically; thus, normal mineralization aids in differentiating Reiter's syndrome from rheumatoid arthritis. The distribution of arthritis also differs from that seen in classic rheumatoid arthritis, with asymmetry and involvement of the distal interphalangeal joints more common in psoriatic disease and Reiter's syndrome.
- Ill-defined bony periarticular erosions that progress centrally, with florid adjacent linear or fluffy bony proliferation (proliferative erosions), are typical. Uniform joint space loss is typical.
- Periostitis may occur without evidence of synovitis and tends to occur along the shafts of small bones (metatarsals and phalanges), the malleoli, and the distal femur. Acutely, the new bone formation is typically irregular with indistinct margins, becoming more distinct as the initial inflammation subsides.
- There is typically superficial resorption of the cortical surface underlying the insertions of ligaments and tendons and beneath bursae, with concomitant periosteal reaction and subchondral sclerosis and eburnation; these findings are typically seen at the ischial tuberosities and the greater femoral trochanter.
- Calcaneal abnormalities are documented in 25 to 50% of patients, particularly plantar and posterior erosions, hyperostosis, and enthesophytes. Radiographic changes, that is, irregular calcaneal spurs (at the insertion of the plantar fascia), and periostitis in the region of the heel are typically present only in chronic cases and are conspicuous by their absence in the acute onset. Soft-tissue edema along the plantar surface of the calcaneus is said to be an early sign.
- Despite the prevalence of calcaneal disease, posterior calcaneal enthesophytes are actually more common in psoriatic and ankylosing spondylitis.

Axial involvement

- Axial involvement is usually a late finding, and when present, the radiographic changes are indistinguishable from those of psoriatic arthritis.

Sacroiliac joints

- Sacroiliitis is more common with recurrences and in the presence of chronic disease, eventually occurring in 50% of all cases. Bilaterally asymmetric erosions and repair, with findings more evident on the iliac side of the joint, are presumably due to the thinner cartilaginous covering when compared with the sacral side.
- Erosions and periarticular osteoporosis contribute to pseudowidening of the joint acutely; however, bony proliferation occurs quickly, resulting in sclerosis, and may progress eventually to ankylosis, although the latter is much less common than in ankylosing spondylitis.

- The superior fibrous portion may be prominently affected in addition to the caudad synovial portion, demonstrating blurring and eburnation of both sides of the joint.
- Paravertebral ossifications have a typical appearance: they are nonmarginal, bulky, unilateral at a given level, asymmetric, and tend to spare the anterior surface of the spine. The cervical spine is often spared.

Soft tissues

- Effusions, periarticular edema, bursitis, and tendinitis are common, producing soft-tissue swelling.
- Achilles' tendinitis is evident as thickening ($>$ 8 mm) on a lateral ankle radiograph and obliteration of adjacent fat planes.
- Retrocalcaneal bursitis is evinced by a radiodense opacity displacing Kager's fat pad.

ULTRASOUND

- Enthesopathy is identified as swelling of entheses and peritendinous soft tissues.
- Achilles' and patellar tendons may be obviously thickened and hypoechoic when acutely inflamed.
- Distended bursae may be demonstrated to good effect.
- Dactylitis producing '"sausage"' digits may be demonstrated on ultrasound to be due to flexor tenosynovitis.

COMPUTED TOMOGRAPHY

- CT has greater sensitivity than radiographs for the early erosive signs of sacroiliitis.

RADIONUCLIDE IMAGING

- Increased technetium Tc 99m pyrophosphate uptake is demonstrated in the region of the heel, for example, in the sub-Achilles' bursa and the joints of the forefoot, thought to be secondary to the increased blood flow and avid binding to immature collagen and articular cartilage. This may aid in the recognition of synovitis before radiographic evidence develops.

MAGNETIC RESONANCE IMAGING

- Subchondral edema is best demonstrated on T2-weighted fat-saturated or STIR sequences.

Sacroiliitis

- Direct imaging of changes in the synovium, articular cartilage, and subchondral bone is the most sensitive and specific for sacroiliitis and other changes in the axial skeleton.
- MRI shows the inflammation of the bone adjacent to the insertion of entheses as well as the soft-tissue changes.
- Dactylitis is another typical manifestation of seronegative spondyloarthropathies.

Treatment

As in any arthritis, the goals of treatment are to

- Suppress and control synovitis
- Preserve joint function

Conservative measures include

- Physical therapy
- Splinting in the acute phase (compare case 111)
- Aspirate joints to relieve tension and slow chondrolysis

Medications include aspirin and other nonsteroidal anti-inflammatory drugs (e.g., indomethacin). Also recommended are immunosuppressants, such as

- Systemic or intra-articular steroids
- Sulphasalazine, methotrexate, azathioprine, or pamidronate
- Tumor necrosis factor (TNF) blockers have been demonstrated to relieve symptoms and signs and retard radiographic progression of both peripheral arthritis and enthesitis as well as spinal disease, which often has been refractory to other agents.

Prognosis

- Early recognition and appropriate treatment can help to limit disability.
- The acute arthritis usually resolves in several months; however, 50% of patients are expected to develop recurrences of arthritis, iritis, or spondylitis.
- Recurrent synovitis is the most common recurrence, typically resulting in a recurrent knee effusion.
- Interestingly, recurrences are usually not associated with progressive joint destruction.
- A high serum interleukin-2R level at baseline is a predictor of remission in patients with acute reactive arthritis.

PEARLS

- Reiter's syndrome, like psoriatic arthritis, differs from ankylosing spondylitis in its inconstant involvement of the spine and greater involvement of peripheral joints. It differs from psoriatic arthritis in its predominant involvement of the lower limbs, particularly the feet, with relative sparing of the hands and wrists.
- The axial skeletal changes of psoriatic arthritis and Reiter's syndrome are often indistinguishable.
- Distal appendicular involvement is characteristic of psoriatic arthritis and Reiter's syndrome.
- Proliferative erosions and enthesitis, periostitis, and normal mineralization aid in differentiating Reiter's syndrome from rheumatoid arthritis.
- The distribution of arthritis also differs from that seen in classic rheumatoid arthritis, with asymmetry and involvement of the distal interphalangeal joints more common in psoriatic disease and Reiter's syndrome.

PITFALLS

- Despite the prevalence of calcaneal disease, posterior calcaneal enthesophytes are actually more common in psoriatic and ankylosing spondylitis.
- Reiter's syndrome may be differentiated from psoriatic arthritis by the presence of periostitis without joint findings, less ankylosis of interphalangeal joints, greater involvement of the metatarsophalangeal than interphalangeal joints, and the predominance of lower extremity involvement.
- Proliferative erosions and enthesitis, periostitis, and normal mineralization aid in differentiating Reiter's syndrome from rheumatoid arthritis. The distribution of arthritis also differs from that seen in classic rheumatoid arthritis, with asymmetry and involvement of the distal interphalangeal joints more common in Reiter's syndrome.

Suggested Readings

Flagg SD, Meador R, Hsia E, Kitumnuaypong T, Schumacher HR. Jr. Decreased pain and synovial inflammation after etanercept therapy in patients with reactive and undifferentiated arthritis: an open-label trial. Arthritis Rheum 2005;53(4):613–617

Klecker RJ, Weissman BN. Imaging features of psoriatic arthritis and Reiter's syndrome. Semin Musculoskelet Radiol 2003;7(2):115–126

Rosenberg ZS, Norman A, Solomon G. Arthritis associated with HIV infection: radiographic manifestations. Radiology 1989;173:171–176

Schumacher TM, Genant HK, Kellet MJ, Mall JC, Fye KH. HLA-B27 associated arthropathies. Radiology 1978;126:289–297

Sholkoff SD, Glickman MG, Steinbach HL. Roentgenology of Reiter's syndrome. Radiology 1970;97: 497–503

CASE 114

Peter L. Munk and Anthony G. Ryan

Clinical Presentation

A 53-year-old man with bilateral ankle pain and a hard swelling overlying the anterior aspect of the left ankle came to our institution.

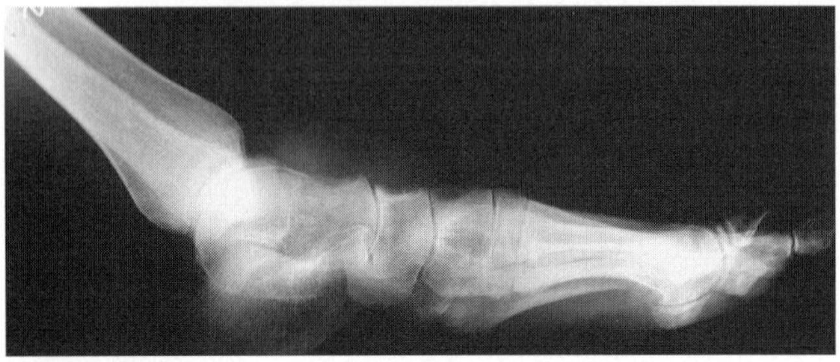

Figure 114A

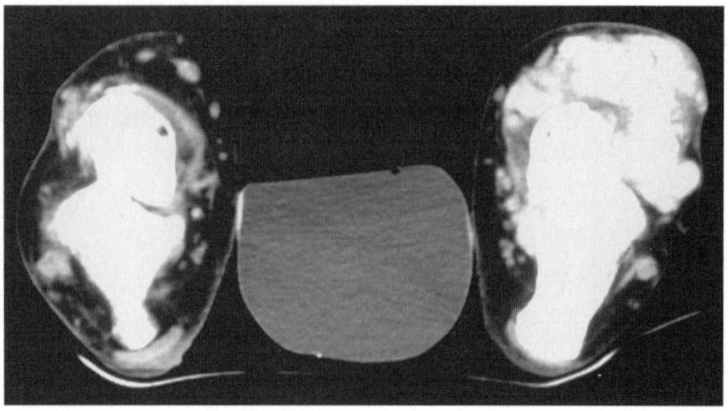

Figure 114B

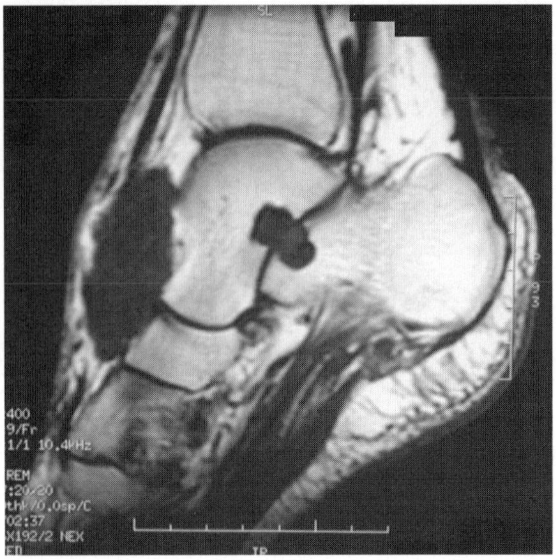

Figure 114C

Radiologic Findings

A lateral plain film of the left ankle (**Fig. 114A**) shows a dense soft-tissue mass anterior to the tarsus in association with surface erosions of the talus and navicular. A corresponding CT of both feet (**Fig. 114B**) shows widespread hyperattenuating deposits within the soft tissues anterior to the tarsus on the left.

A sagittal T1-weighted image of the left ankle (**Fig. 114C**) shows marked low signal intensity within the soft-tissue mass and also within the sinus tarsi (the normal high signal of sinus tarsi fat is absent). The cortical erosions are also demonstrated to good effect.

Diagnosis

Gouty tophus with erosions of underlying bones.

Differential Diagnosis

The combination of findings on radiographs, CT, and MRI is essentially pathognomonic of tophaceous gout.

Discussion

Background

Gout is a metabolic disease associated with increased serum uric acid levels (hyperuricemia) and attacks of acute, painful arthritis. Hyperuricemia by itself does not constitute gout. Typically, patients have had hyperuricemia for 10 to 12 years that is inadequately or not treated before the initial episode of gouty arthritis occurs.

Etiology

Gout is a metabolic disease associated with increased serum uric acid levels (hyperuricemia) and associated with intra- and periarticular deposition of monosodium urate crystals. Primary or idiopathic gout appears to be transmitted as an autosomal dominant process, with low penetrance in females. The vast majority of cases are idiopathic, although occasionally patients with inherited metabolic defects may develop gout, as might patients with malignancies producing marked nucleic acid turnover, such as leukemia.

Caucasians appear to be more frequently afflicted than other racial groups, except for the Maori, where the prevalence among males reaches 10%.

Pathophysiology

Urates are produced in the metabolism of purine nucleic acid, and either overproduction or undersecretion results in hyperuricemia. Symptoms occur with attacks of joint pain inflammation secondary to deposits of the urates in articular, periarticular, and tenosynovial soft tissues.

Joints appear to be affected more than other tissues because of the lower solubility of urates in synovial fluid than plasma, and the lower temperature of peripheral joints further diminishes their solubility.

Clinical Findings

The majority of these patients are middle-aged males. The most common site for an initial attack is the first metatarsophalangeal joint (podagra), although many other joints are commonly afflicted, such as the knee, elbow, wrist, and the small joints of the hands and feet. There is usually a sudden onset of severe pain centered on the joint that is associated with swelling, erythema, marked tenderness, and loss of function. The shoulder and spine are less frequently affected than most other sites.

Although the initial clinical episode affects a single joint, as the disease progresses, multiple joints typically become affected. Symptoms occur with attacks of joint pain and inflammation secondary to deposits of the urates in articular, periarticular, and tenosynovial soft tissues. Once attacks occur, they last several days to weeks without treatment, and the joint becomes swollen, red, markedly tender, and difficult to move.

Tophi are nontender, hard deposits most frequently occurring in the hands and feet, as well as in the extensor surface of the elbows, although they may present at any site. They may present occasionally as soft-tissue masses in patients who are otherwise asymptomatic.

Stages of Disease

Five clinical stages are described:

- Asymptomatic hyperuricemia
- Acute gouty arthritis
- Interval phase
- Recurrent arthritis
- Chronic tophaceous gout

Complications

- Joint pain
- Calcified bone infarcts are not infrequently associated with gout.

Pathology

GROSS

- Juxta-articular erosions

MICROSCOPIC

- In ongoing cases, an acute synovitis secondary to monosodium urate deposits is evident with a chronic granulomatous reaction.

Imaging Findings

RADIOGRAPHY

- The classic finding is that of periarticular erosions with well-defined overhanging margins (**Fig. 114D**); radiographic findings are not normally seen in the early symptomatic stages of the disease, but erosions gradually progress if the patient is inadequately or not treated (**Fig. 114E**).
- The erosions can extend into the joint and eventually coalesce, producing progressive destruction of the articular margins (**Fig. 114E**). The joint space is typically preserved until late, however.
- The most common site for an initial attack is the first metatarsophalangeal joint (in 90%), described clinically as podagra, although many other joints are commonly afflicted, such as the knee, elbow (**Fig. 114F**), wrist, and the small joints of the hands and feet. The shoulder and spine are less frequently affected than most other sites.
- Although the initial clinical episode affects a single joint, as the disease progresses, multiple joints typically become affected. The resultant polyarthropathy is asymmetric.
- Tophi are typically evident as dense soft-tissue masses adjacent to a joint or in the line of a tendon. Focal calcifications may or may not be seen.
- Olecranon bursitis may be evident as prominent soft-tissue swelling overlying the olecranon (**Fig. 114F**).
- Calcified bone infarcts are not infrequently associated with gout.

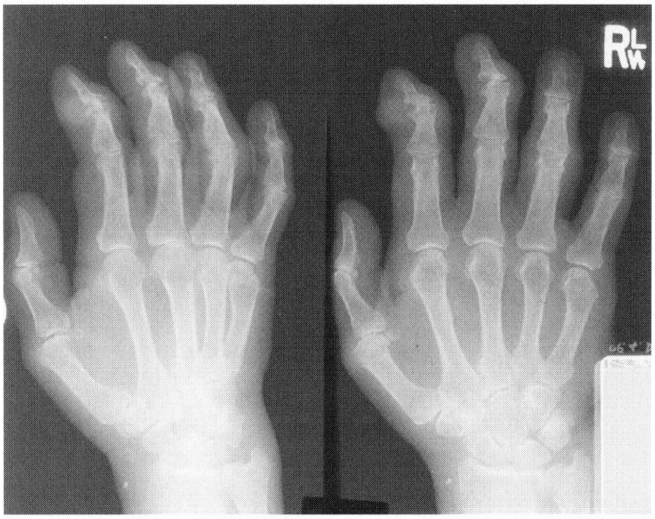

Figure 114D Anteroposterior and oblique radiographs of the right hand in a 58-year-old male with pain and clinical swelling of the distal interphalangeal joints (thought initially to be osteoarthrosis). Well-defined erosions with overhanging edges affecting the digits of the second and third fingers are seen with associated dense swelling in the adjacent soft tissues consistent with tophi. Further dense swelling is evident in relation to the fourth proximal interphalangeal joints.

COMPUTED TOMOGRAPHY

- CT better defines the periarticular erosions and the calcifications encountered in advanced-stage lesions.
- Calcified bone infarcts are clearly seen on CT.

MAGNETIC RESONANCE IMAGING

- Collection of urate in the soft tissue is known as a tophus, which is typically surrounded by an intense vascular reaction. These can, at times, reach considerable size, produce erosion of the underlying bone, and may demonstrate focal calcification.

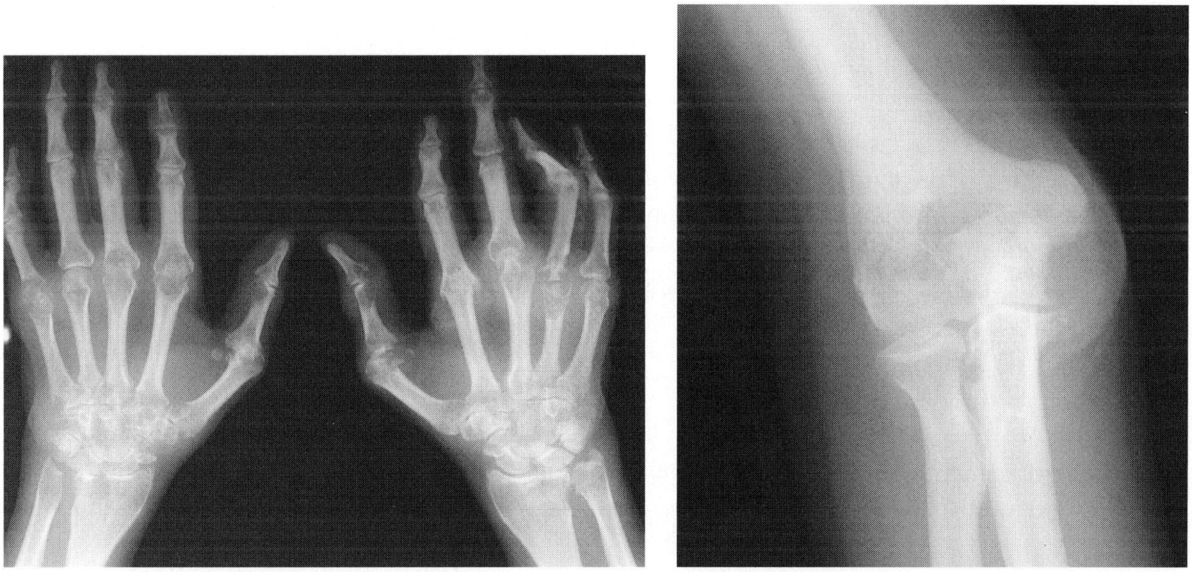

E F

Figures 114E,114F **114E** Bilateral hand radiograph showing severe changes associated with untreated gout in a stoic 47-year-old woman. There are florid erosions affecting many of the metacarpal phalangeal and interphalangeal (IP) joints bilaterally and the carpus on the right, producing gross destruction of many of the affected bones and articulations. The appearances raise the differential of rheumatoid arthritis; however, the less advanced erosions, such as the thumb IP joints and distal interphalangeal joints of the left third digit show the typical juxta-articular, well-defined erosions with overhanging edges. **114F** Elbow radiograph shows a well-defined juxta-articular erosion of the radial aspect of the ulnar coronoid and prominent soft-tissue swelling, the latter reflecting the presence of an olecranon bursitis.

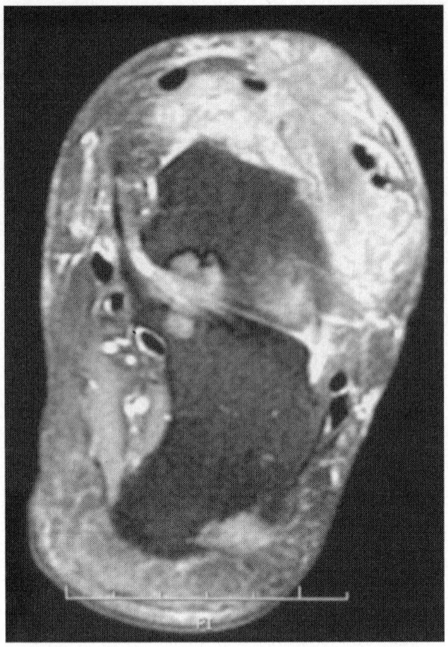

Figure 114G T1-weighted fat-saturated postintravenous gadolinium image of the patient in the reference case (**114A** to **114C**) shows intense enhancement of the tophus anterior to the talus. Marrow edema is present in the posterior talus adjacent to the calcaneal articulation.

- MRI also demonstrates these features, and if intravenous contrast is utilized, the intensely vascular nature of any tophi that are present is strikingly evident (**Fig. 114G**). Bone marrow edema in the surrounding osseous structures can also be appreciated.
- Calcified bone infarcts may be evident.

Treatment

Acute attacks respond promptly to anti-inflammatory drugs, for example, indomethacin. Thereafter, it is vital to reduce the circulating hyperuricemia by the administration of allopurinol to prevent recurrent attacks, but not until 4 weeks after the acute event has settled, as it can precipitate an acute gout attack.

Prognosis

- If untreated, an acute attack of gout usually settles over the course of 2 to 3 weeks.
- If untreated, attacks recur, increasing in frequency and intensity.

PEARLS

- The classic finding is juxta-articular erosions with well-defined overhanging margins, the latter sometimes referred to as the "shelf" sign.
- When the disease involves multiple joints, the polyarthropathy is typically asymmetric.
- Tophi are intensely vascular and thus will enhance vividly on MRI.

PITFALLS

- Radiographic findings are not normally seen in the early symptomatic stages of the disease, but erosions gradually progress if the patient is inadequately or not treated.
- The clinical presentation may be so sudden and the attending erythema so conspicuous that the working diagnosis may initially be that of septic arthritis. Aspiration of the joint in such cases should thus be sent for biochemical analysis for crystals, in addition to the standard Gram's stain and culture and sensitivity. Often, only a miniscule amount of fluid is required on a slide for the recognition of the birefringent monosodium urate crystals.
- Because radiographic findings are not normally seen in the early symptomatic stages of the disease, one must keep a high index of suspicion for the condition in the appropriate clinical setting.

Suggested Readings

Bloch C, Hermann G, Yu T-F. A radiologic reevaluation of gout: a study of 2,000 patients. Am J Roentgenol 1980;134:781–787

Chaoui A, Garcia J, Kurt AM. Gouty tophus simulating soft tissue tumor in a heart transplant recipient. Skeletal Radiol 1997;26:626–628

Martel W. The overhanging margin of bone: a roentgenologic manifestation of gout. Radiology 1968;91:755–756

Yu JS, Chung C, Recht M, Dailiana T, Jurdi R. MR imaging of tophaceous gout. Am J Roentgenol 1997;168:523–527

CASE 115

Anthony G. Ryan and Peter L. Munk

Clinical Presentation

A 33-year-old man presented with chronic back pain.

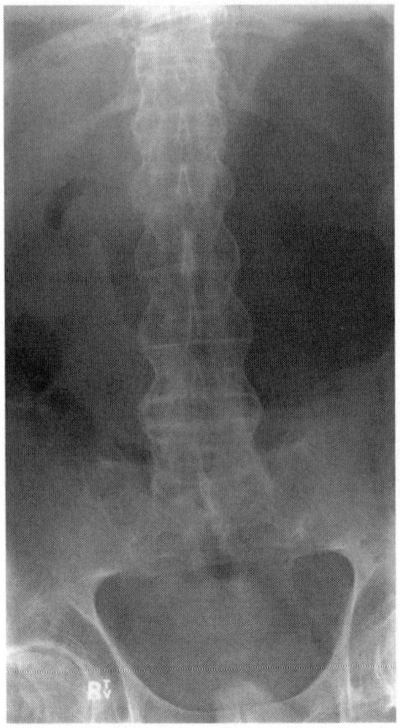

Figure 115A

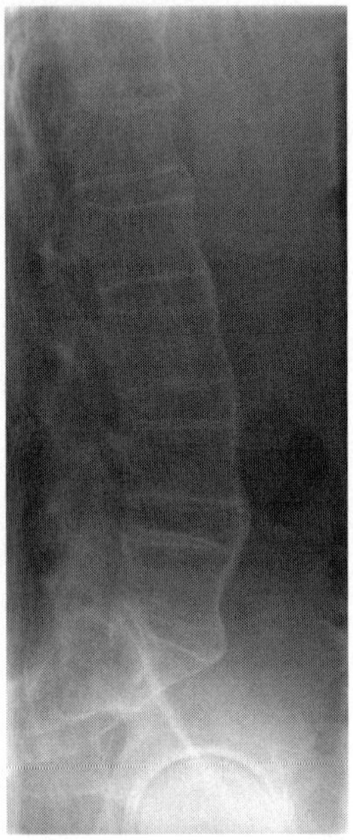

Figure 115B

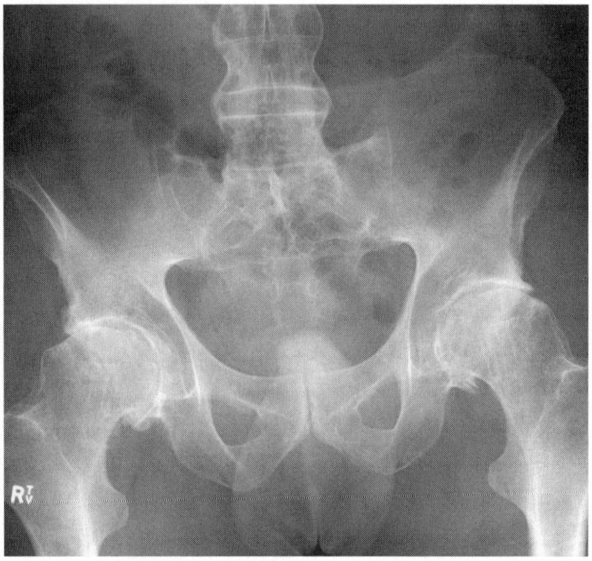

Figure 115C

Radiologic Findings

Anteroposterior (AP) (**Fig. 115A**) and lateral (**Fig. 115B**) radiographs of the lumbar spine show bilaterally symmetric fine bridging syndesmophytes throughout the visualized spine. An AP radiograph of the pelvis (**Fig. 115C**) shows symmetric absence and complete bony fusion of the sacroiliac joints, with bilaterally symmetric hip joint space narrowing, axial migration of the femoral heads, erosions, and subchondral sclerosis.

Diagnosis

Ankylosing spondylitis.

Differential Diagnosis

Other seronegative arthropathies, especially enteropathic arthropathy, are differential diagnoses. The bilateral symmetry and bridging nature of the syndesmophytes make the other seronegative spondyloarthropathies (psoriatic arthritis and reactive arthritis) less likely. Syndesmophytosis and the degree of osseous fusion at the sacroiliac joints make rheumatoid arthritis very unlikely.

Discussion

Background

The seronegative spondyloarthropathies consist of ankylosing spondylitis, psoriatic arthritis, reactive arthritis (Reiter's disease), enteropathic spondylitis, and undifferentiated spondyloarthropathy, all of which share common clinical and radiographic features, with characteristic involvement of the sacroiliac joints, spine, and peripheral joints.

The spondyloarthritides affect synovial and cartilaginous joints (including the intervertebral disks and their junctions with adjacent vertebral bodies) and entheses. Ankylosing spondylitis is seen as the prototype of the spondyloarthritides, but it may also be viewed as a potential end point of any one of the spondyloarthritides.

The criteria for diagnosing one of the inflammatory spondyloarthropathies are spine pain or synovitis plus one of the following:

- Family history
- Psoriasis/inflammatory bowel disease
- Urethritis/cervicitis/diarrhea within 1 month
- Buttock pain
- Enthesopathy
- Sacroiliitis

Sacroiliitis in the presence of appropriate clinical symptoms is said to be diagnostic for ankylosing spondylitis, although the presence of typically inflammatory back pain plus at least two other typical features of spondyloarthropathy (e.g., enthesitis and uveitis) is highly predictive of early ankylosing spondylitis.

Etiology

The etiology of ankylosing spondylitis remains unknown; however, it is presumed to relate to an as yet unidentified chronic intracellular infectious agent, or agents, initiating a series of autoimmune phenomena in susceptible hosts. Unlike reactive arthritis (Reiter's syndrome), no specific microbe has been identified in ankylosing spondylitis, although cross-reactivity has been demonstrated between *Klebsiella* and human leukocyte antigen (HLA) B27.

The chief host susceptibility is related to the presence of the major histocompatibility complex HLA-B27 allele, for which over 90% of patients with ankylosing spondylosis are positive, compared with a maximum of 8% in the nonaffected population. Although the incidence of ankylosing spondylosis in the general population is ~0.01%, the incidence in patients with HLA-B27 positivity is 20%.

Pathophysiology

The condition is characterized by pathological processes of bone and soft-tissue inflammation affecting bone (osteitis), synovial joints (synovitis), cartilage (chondritis), discovertebral junction (spondylodiskitis), and entheses (enthesitis), with bony repair and ossification occurring consecutively and occasionally concurrently.

Two theories currently dominate the potential origin of arthritogenic peptides: an immunological theory, incriminating a cross-reaction between self-proteins (e.g., host proteoglycans) and bacterial peptides via molecular mimicry (HLA-B27 itself possibly serving as an autoantigen), and a microbiological theory, which proposes that latent bacteria residing within macrophagic or dendritic cells undergo reactivation through a process facilitated by (possibly faulty secondary to misfolding) the HLA-B27 molecule, resulting in impaired intracellular killing of bacteria.

The actual mechanism is likely to be a combination of the two, a complex interplay between genetic factors, including HLA-B27, and environmental factors.

In the infectious theory, infected cells migrate from mucous membranes (e.g., inflamed intestine leading to an impaired gut–blood barrier) to the target tissues, particularly the bone marrow located near entheses, and, via HLA-mediated agents, produce inflammatory cellular and cytokine (tumor necrosis factor-α and interleukin-10) infiltrates, which in turn cause acute local inflammation. The intracellular bacteria may, at a later stage, undergo transient reactivation to cause recurrent inflammation and contribute to ongoing chronic inflammatory response.

Clinical Findings

The disease typically starts between 15 and 35 years of age and affects men between three and five times as often as women. It is rare in people of African or Japanese descent but common in people with innate high levels of HLA-B27, such as the Haida Indians of British Columbia, in whom the highest prevalence of ankylosing spondylitis (4.5%) has been reported (50% of the population is HLA-B27–positive).

Ankylosing spondylitis is characterized by an insidious onset of low back pain and stiffness, the latter worse in the morning. The pain is typically inflammatory in nature; that is, it disturbs sleep, is worse in the morning, and is relieved by exercise.

The back pain is most commonly due to sacroiliitis, with pain in the buttocks radiating to the legs a typical feature. Occasionally, there is evidence of plantar fasciitis on presentation. Later in the course of the disease, new onset of mechanical back pain is suspicious for superimposed fracture.

On examination, there is loss of lumbar lordosis and increased kyphosis, with a variable limitation of spinal flexion and reduced inspiratory chest excursion. Pelvic and chest wall tenderness is frequently demonstrable. Enthesopathy is manifest by periarticular tenderness.

The manner of presentation and course tend to be different in females, who present at an older age, have a higher incidence of initial and subsequent peripheral joint disease, a higher incidence of cervical spine disease, and a milder, less progressive disease course. The appendicular involvement is more apparent clinically than radiographically.

A juvenile form is also recognized in which symptoms develop before the age of 17; the most common presentation is with lower limb appendicular (asymmetric, oligoarticular), rather than axial, joint involvement. In these patients, the course tends to be progressive.

The erythrocyte sedimentation rate and C-reactive protein level are typically raised on presentation in all forms.

Extraskeletal manifestations include the following:

- Iritis in 20%, occurring more commonly with peripheral arthropathy
- Uveitis
- Apical pulmonary fibrosis, in which 1% develop cavitation. This may be indistinguishable from tuberculosis initially; however, the skeletal changes are usually advanced by the time of diagnosis, making the origin of the pulmonary changes more obvious.
- Ascending aortitis, aortic incompetence, conduction defects, and pericarditis
- Amyloidosis
- Inflammatory bowel disease

Complications

VERTEBRAL FRACTURES

These patients are more susceptible to vertebral fractures secondary to the loss of spinal flexibility and increased bone fragility. The addition of diffuse paraspinal ossification, ossified facet joints, and

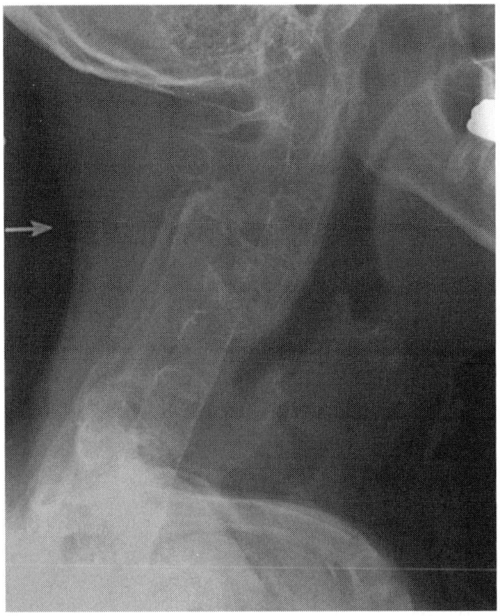

Figure 115D Lateral radiograph of the cervical spine in a woman complaining of severe neck pain, having bumped her head on a sink when bending down, demonstrating a transdiscal fracture dislocation involving the posterior elements, probably representing "completion" of a stress fracture. Neurologic recovery occurred slowly after reduction and fixation. Cervical spine fractures are three times more common in patients with ankylosing spondylitis compared with the population at large.

inflammatory osteitis creates a fused, brittle spine. Even minor trauma can produce an unstable injury as a result of disruption of the ossified supporting ligaments.

There are three recognized vertebral fracture patterns:

- Simple vertebral compression fractures osteoporosis-related; occur early in the course before ankylosis, typically resulting in a stable kyphosis
- Transversely oriented shear fractures acute fractures of the ankylosed spine that usually traverse the disk space, continue through the posterior elements, and invariably disrupt the ossified supporting ligaments (**Fig. 115D**). In the latter injury, all three columns of the spine are involved, resulting in unstable fractures potentially accompanied by dislocation and neurologic injury.
- Stress fractures associated with pseudoarthrosis (cf. Andersson lesion below); do not usually occur before 10 to 12 years of disease

CAUDA EQUINA SYNDROME

The exact cause of the cauda equina syndrome has not yet been determined, but it may be due to demyelination, postirradiation ischemia, or compression from spinal arachnoiditis. Clinically, patients will complain of cutaneous sensory impairment of the lower limbs and perineum with sphincter disturbances. Motor impairment occurs less frequently, and associated pain is an inconstant feature. Saccular dilatation of the caudal dural sac and dorsal arachnoid diverticulae that erode the lamina and spinous processes are characteristic myelographic and CT findings. Dorsal arachnoid diverticulae occur in the lumbar spine with erosion of posterior elements.

MUSCULAR ATROPHY

The paraspinal and psoas muscles are frequently affected secondary to gross ankylosis of the hip joints and the spine.

Pathology

GROSS

Erosion, reactive hyperostosis, and eburnation of affected bone are identified. Fibrous or bony ankylosis of the joints is seen.

MICROSCOPIC

The pathological hallmark of the disease is acute and chronic inflammation leading to osteitis, chondritis, synovitis, spondylodiskitis, and enthesitis, with bony repair and ossification occurring consecutively and concurrently. Endochondral ossification across the joints leads to eventual bony ankylosis.

Effusions, when present, are sterile.

Imaging Findings

RADIOGRAPHY

As the name of the disease suggests, ankylosis is the radiographic hallmark, principally affecting the sacroiliac joints and spine, with less frequent involvement of the pubic symphysis, hips, shoulders, knees, hands, feet, and sternoclavicular, acromioclavicular, sternomanubrial, and temporomandibular joints. Structural damage is an important end point in the assessment of ankylosing spondylitis.

Axial skeleton

Axial skeletal disorders identified on radiogaphy include sacroiliitis, pubic symphysis erosions, enthesitis, and spinal irregularities.

Sacroiliac disease

Sacroiliitis is regarded as a sine qua non of the diagnosis of ankylosing spondylitis in the majority of existing criteria (e.g., the modified New York criteria), but the disease is usually not evident until 8 years into its course.

- Sacroiliitis may be unilateral and asymmetric initially, becoming bilaterally symmetric as the disease progresses. Both the synovial and ligamentous portions are affected.
- Blurring of articular margins followed by irregular joint space widening secondary to cartilaginous destruction and subchondral erosions is the typical pattern.
- These erosions and the reactive patchy sclerosis predominate on the iliac side of the joint, thought to be secondary to the thinner covering of cartilage found on the iliac side. The sclerosis fades somewhat as the joint space narrows and progresses to first fibrous, then bony, ankylosis (**Fig. 115C**).

Pubic symphysis

- The pubic symphysis demonstrates erosions (**Fig. 115E**) with or without sclerosis and ankylosis in 16 to 23% of patients.

Entheses

- Peripheral enthesitis gives rise to erosions and periostitic whiskering at the site of ligamentous and tendinous insertions in advanced cases; the ischial tuberosity (**Fig. 115E**), iliac crest, ischiopubic rami, greater femoral trochanter, and external protuberance of the calcaneus are most frequently affected.

The spine is involved initially in 60 to 70% of cases. The zone of involvement ascends from the lumbar to the cervical spine (the latter said to be more common in women). Women are more likely to have cervical spine and sacroiliac joint involvement, with sparing of the intervening segments and frequent and severe osteitis pubis. Joint ankylosis and adjacent syndesmophytes occur at the same levels. Sacroiliac changes tend to be synchronous with the spine signs.

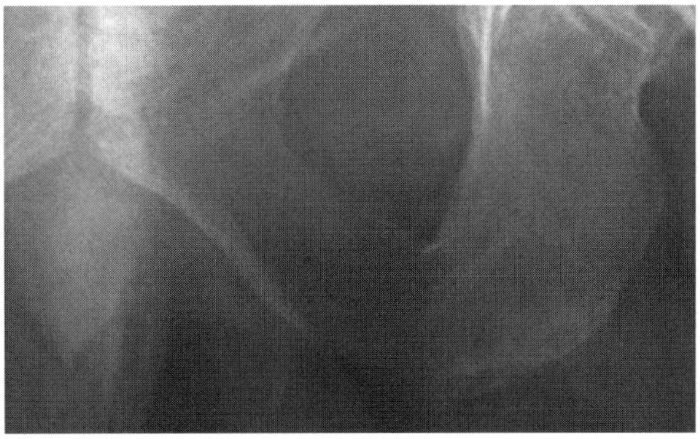

Figure 115E Focused view of the pubic symphysis and ischium shows focal erosions on both, with greater reactive sclerosis in evidence at the symphysis.

- Other spinal abnormalities found on radiography are disk calcification (central, eccentric, circular, or linear intradiscal collections) and vertebral body and discovertebral junction lesions (Romanus and Andersson).
  - The characteristic Romanus lesion of the vertebral bodies comprises "squared" vertebral bodies with shiny corners. Subchondral erosions, secondary to subchondral osteitis at the site of anulus fibrosus and anterior longitudinal ligament insertion, " shave" the top and bottom margins (as seen on a lateral radiograph) back to the level of the concavity of the body, resulting in a straight anterior margin and the characteristic vertebral body "squaring."
  - The "shiny corners" reflect the reactive sclerosis in response to the osteitis; hence the alternative name for the Romanus lesion of spondylitis anterior. Additional "squaring" may be effected by "filling in" behind the anterior longitudinal ligament due to ossification of the latter or reactive new bone formation on the anterior surface of the vertebral body.
  - The findings in diffuse spondylodiskitis (in comparison to the focal, anterior spondylitis of the Romanus lesion) are collectively termed the Andersson lesion and include herniation of disk material into the vertebral body secondary to weakening induced by intense destructive subchondral osteitis underlying the vertebral end plate, usually evinced by narrowing of the disk space, and a marginated defect in the adjacent vertebral bodies surrounded by a wide area of reactive sclerosis.
  - A further manifestation of the Andersson lesion (diffuse spondylodiskitis) arises secondary to a transdiscal stress fracture (usually at the thoracolumbar junction and including posterior element fractures), followed by fibrous nonunion and a resultant pseudoarthrosis. Continuing motion at the pseudoarthrosis leads to proliferation of the fibrous callus, resulting in frank destruction of the adjacent vertebral bodies. These lesions are usually evinced by widening of the apparent radiolucent disk space secondary to the vertebral end plate destruction and a zone of reactive sclerosis.

Other classic findings on radiography are the following:

- Marginal syndesmophytes, thin vertical spicules bridging the vertebral bodies secondary to ossification of the outer fibers of the anulus fibrosus
- The "dagger" sign, a descriptive term for a single longitudinal, radiodense line running centrally on the spine on an AP view that arises from ossification of the supraspinous and interspinous ligaments

- The term *trolley track sign*, seen on an AP view, is applied when the central line of the dagger sign is joined by the addition of two parallel, more lateral lines resulting from bilateral ossification of the apophyseal joints.
- The so-called bamboo spine typical of the condition arises from the undulating contour along the margins of the vertebral bodies and disk spaces secondary to the presence of syndesmophytes and ligamentous and joint calcification/ossification.
- The apophyseal, costotransverse, and costovertebral joints may all be affected, with hazy erosions and subchondral sclerosis progressing to ankylosis.
- Asymmetric erosions of laminar and spinous processes in the lumbar spine
- Kyphosis
- Osteoporosis develops in long-standing cases and may be severe, including biconcave deformities of multiple vertebral bodies.
- Posterior longitudinal ligament and ligamentum flavum calcification and ossification are unusual manifestations.

When a fracture occurs in the cervical spine (**Fig. 115D**), concomitant epidural hematoma (seen to occur more frequently in patients with ankylosing spondylitis) can reduce the spinal canal caliber, disastrously leading to dramatic neurologic sequelae.

The presence of osteopenia and deformity makes minimally displaced fractures difficult to detect; one must specifically analyze each radiograph for disk space widening and discontinuity of the ossified paraspinal ligaments. New back pain in patients with ankylosing spondylitis or other diseases with paraspinal ossification should be assumed to be caused by fracture until proven otherwise, especially later in the course, as intrinsic pain tends to recede as the spine fuses.

Cord impingement may arise secondary to hypertrophic bone or ossified ligaments or retropulsed bone fragments.

Appendicular skeleton

Ankylosing spondylitis in the appendicular skeleton, as identified on radiography, is initially involved in 10 to 20%, and eventually in 50%, of cases. It tends to be mild and transient, with asymmetric involvement of a few joints being typical. On radiography, the ankylosis is similar to rheumatoid arthritis, but the peripheral synovitis is less severe and more discrete. Subchondral sclerosis and chondral ossification lead to bony ankylosis, the latter typically occurring in adults with rheumatoid arthritis in the wrist and ankle.

Disorders identified on radiography are seen in the hip; the metacarpophalangeal (MCP), proximal interphalangeal (PIP), and distal interphalangeal (DIP) joints; and the calcaneus/Achilles' tendon.

The hip (**Fig. 115F**) is the most commonly affected nonaxial joint. On radiography, disorders seen include

- Bilateral symmetric involvement
- Axial narrowing
- Collar of osteophytes
- Ankylosis (occurs more commonly in younger affected patients)
- Acetabular protrusio

MCP, PIP, and DIP joint abnormalities found in 10 to 30% of cases include

- Exuberant osseous proliferation
- Osteoporosis, joint space narrowing, and erosions (however, the deformities tend to be less severe than in rheumatoid arthritis)

Calcaneus/Achilles' tendon disorders are also seen.

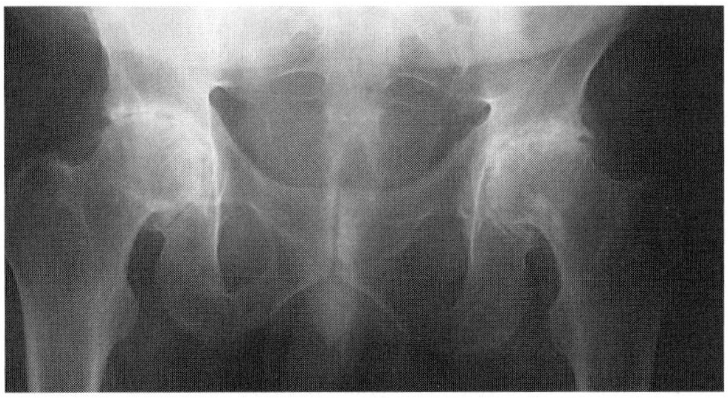

Figure 115F AP radiograph of the pelvis shows typical ankylosing spondylitis affecting the hips resulting in loss of joint space, axial migration of the femoral head, prominent erosions and reactive sclerosis, and a collar of osteophytes bilaterally. The pubic symphysis and both ischial tuberosities are also involved (same patient as **115E**).

- Achilles' tendinitis is evinced by a thickened tendon on a lateral radiograph (> 8 mm).
- Retrocalcaneal bursitis obliterates the normal radiolucency, usually seen extending at least 2 mm below the level of the superior surface of the calcaneus anterior to the distal Achilles' tendon.

ULTRASOUND

- Bursal fluid collections are easily demonstrated.
- Peritendinous soft tissues and entheses' swelling may be seen.

COMPUTED TOMOGRAPHY

- Although several studies have demonstrated the promise of multidetector CT in detecting spinal fractures in ankylosing spondylitis, transaxial CT has diagnostic limitations because of the typically transverse fracture planc. Multiplanar reconstructions are likely to resolve the issue, particularly when thin sections are performed at acquisition.
- Atrophy of the posterior spinal muscles and the psoas muscle is related to gross ankylosis and consequent lack of motion.
- In cases with suspicious, but not diagnostic, abnormalities on plain films (grade 1 of the New York criteria) CT permits the diagnosis of sacroilitis because it shows a higher degree of sensitivity for early osseous erosions.
- CT may demonstrate spinal stenosis and ligamentous discontinuity, especially when the ligaments are calcified/ossified.

MAGNETIC RESONANCE IMAGING

At any location, early and acute active inflammation is best demonstrated by use of fluid-sensitive sequences (T2-weighted fat-saturated or STIR) with or without the use of intravenous (IV) gadolinium-DTPA (diethylenetriamine penta-acetic acid).

Sacroiliitis

- MRI is superior to CT in the early diagnosis of sacroiliitis, as it can detect the cartilaginous and subchondral abnormalities that precede bony changes. Fat-suppressed T1-weighted and FSE T2-weighted images demonstrate the normal cortical surface as a smoothly continuous low-signal line on both, facilitating the detection of subtle erosions.
- The sacral and iliac cartilages are frequently divided by a small cavity, represented on T1-weighted images as a line of very low intensity.
- On T1-weighted images with fat saturation, normal articular cartilage is intermediate to high signal intensity; it is homogeneously low or intermediate on T2-weighted images.

- Volume averaging at the junction of the cephalad ligamentous and caudal synovial joints should not be mistaken for erosion.
- The earliest evidence of sacroiliitis appears to be subchondral edema, reflecting the underlying osteitis, which is most marked anteriorly on the iliac side and appears as low T1-weighted and high T2-weighted signal with prominent enhancement postgadolinium on T1-weighted fat-saturated images.
- Loss of cartilage is evinced by loss of uniformity on both T1- and T2-weighted images, with some high signal evident on T2-weighted images. Erosions appear as increased cortical signal intensity on both T1- and T2-weighted images, with cortical, and occasional subchondral, discontinuity. Erosions are typically accompanied by cartilage loss and subchondral edema.

Three types of subchondral changes on MRI are described in relation to the sacroiliac joint:

- *Type I:* Low on T1, high on T2, reflecting acute inflammatory edema
- *Type II:* Low on both T1 and T2, reflecting sclerosis; may be seen crossing the joint as either fibrous or osseous tissue
- *Type III:* Fat intensity on all sequences; thought to reflect ongoing or subacute inflammation

The degree of subchondral enhancement on dynamic post-IV gadolinium MRI has been demonstrated to correlate closely to the degree of inflammation and the severity of symptoms. Where there is complete bony ankylosis, continuous marrow signal across the joint is evident. Involvement of the pubic symphysis produces similar MRI appearances, with the edema most marked anteriorly.

Spinal irregularities

- Inflammatory lesions of the spine, such as spondylitis and spondylodiskitis, can be visualized early by MRI. The facility with which MRI demonstrates the presence and degree of inflammation is now in use as an important outcome measure in clinical trials.
- Ligamentous ossification typically demonstrates low-signal linearity on all sequences.

Vertebral osteitis (spondylitis)

- Typical inflammatory signal is returned at the corners of the vertebrae, that is, low on T1- and high on T2-weighted images. If severe, the edema may be evident diffusely throughout the vertebral body. Contrast enhancement is typical at these sites, best demonstrated on a T1-weighted fat-saturated sequence.
- Low signal on both T1- and T2-weighted images suggests sclerosis.
- When syndesmophytes are evident radiographically, high signal intensity has been demonstrated on both T1 and T2, without contrast enhancement at the site of vertebral body corners, representing yellow marrow accumulation in the healing phase of enthesitis.
- Disk space signal is generally normal during the phase of vertebral osteitis.

Spondylodiskitis

The inflammatory subtype of the Andersson lesion demonstrates high intradiscal signal and high signal within the adjacent vertebral body on T2-weighted images surrounded by a sclerotic low-signal rim.

The noninflammatory subtype (secondary to pseudoarthrosis) is characterized by low signal intensity on T1- and heterogeneous high signal on T2-weighted images, the latter thought to reflect low-signal fibrous tissue and high-signal vascularized edematous tissue. These findings are also typically seen in the posterior elements.

The lack of a paravertebral mass and an epidural component helps to differentiate these lesions from infectious diskitis.

Fractures

- Fracture lines are low on T1- and high on T2-weighted images.
- Stress fractures may demonstrate low signal on both T1- and T2-weighted images if the diagnosis is delayed secondary to fibrous union.
- Epidural hematomas may be evident as long, tapered extradural masses.
- Other complications, such as cord contusion and transection, are easily seen.

Disk abnormalities

- Discal calcification is seen as increased signal intensity on T1; the larger the size of the calcium crystals, the greater the signal intensity.

Treatment

PHYSICAL THERAPY

An exercise program helps to relieve symptoms, maintain movement, and prevent deformity.

NONSTEROIDAL ANTI-INFLAMMATORY DRUGS (NSAIDs)

Indomethacin relieves night pain and morning stiffness, although it does not modify the disease. In refractory cases, steroids and sulphasalazine are used with mixed results.

IMMUNOSUPPRESSANTS

Azathioprine is effective for the peripheral disease but not the axial. Penicillamine and gold are not effective.

NEWER AGENTS

Infliximab and etanercept are tumor necrosis factor-α antagonists that have been shown to produce an apparently durable reduction in spinal inflammation (often refractory to other agents). It is thought, however, that this class of drugs serves only to suspend the disease process, which is likely to proceed when the medications are withdrawn.

Antibiotic therapy directed against the putative agents thus far has not modified the disease process, thought in part to be due to antibiotics' inability to fully eradicate the responsible intracellular bacteria.

SURGERY

Spine

In general, two major circumstances pertain with respect to surgery on the spine in ankylosing spondylosis:

- Elective correction of kyphosis and emergency reduction of acute fractures
- Correction of thoracolumbar kyphosis

A meta-analysis of surgery for fixed thoracolumbar kyphosis revealed that 52% of cases had opening wedge osteotomy, 29% had polysegmental wedge osteotomies, and 18% had closing wedge osteotomy.

The mean age at the time of operation was 41 years, with a male:female ratio of 7.5:1. The average correction achieved ranged from 37 to 40 degrees, with open wedge and polysegmental wedge osteotomies most successful.

The perioperative mortality was 4%, usually secondary to pulmonary, cardiac, or intestinal complications. Neurologic complications were reported in all techniques, including permanent paraplegia.

Emergency reduction of acute fractures

Prompt reduction and stabilization, typically with posterior fusion and instrumentation, significantly improves the prognosis for those with neurologic injuries.

Periphery

- Hip replacement is usually required for patients younger than age 50; 70% of patients will require bilateral replacements.
- After total hip replacement, hypertrophic new bone formation may be prominent (expected in 10%), with occasional recurrent ankylosis.

Prognosis

- The overall tendency is for symptoms to improve with age, but ankylosing spondylitis seldom resolves completely. Twenty percent of patients progress to significant disability, in whom progressive limitation of spinal movement occurs over the course of a few years.
- Early proximal appendicular joint involvement is a poor prognostic sign.
- The earlier the disease starts, the more severe it tends to be. Hip disease is more likely when the disease starts in the teenage years; however, if the disease starts after age 22, hip replacement is rarely required.
- With current treatments, the severe kyphoses seen previously can usually be prevented.
- In women, the course of the disease is less severe.
- In contrast to rheumatoid arthritis, no remission occurs in pregnancy; however, the condition does not deteriorate.
- Death secondary to the disease occurs as a result of cervical spine fracture, aortitis, or, rarely, amyloidosis.

PEARLS

- Ankylosing spondylitis predominates in the axial skeleton in men, where it eventually leads to fusion of the vertebrae and sacroiliac joints. In women, the disease tends to affect the appendicular skeleton to a greater extent. Women are also more likely to have cervical spine and sacroiliac joint involvement with sparing of the intervening segments and frequent and severe osteitis pubis.
- In ankylosing spondylosis, the erosions and sclerosis seen in relation to sacroiliitis predominate on the iliac side of the joint. Although osteitis condensans ilii also affects the iliac side of the sacroiliac joint, it does not affect the sacral side and is not associated with erosive change in the joint.
- The radiographic features of degenerative disease of the sacroiliac joint (occurring in middle-aged and elderly patients) simulate those of ankylosing spondylitis. These include interosseous space narrowing, subchondral sclerosis, and osteophytosis. Anterior bridging osteophytes can mimic ankylosis on an AP radiograph. The sclerosis that occurs in degenerative disease tends to be focal and most common on the superior and inferior margins of the articular cavity, in contrast to that seen in ankylosing spondylitis, which is more diffuse and more dominant on the iliac side of the joint.
- Subchondral sclerosis and chondral ossification lead to bony ankylosis, the latter occurring typically in adults with rheumatoid arthritis in the wrist and ankle.

PITFALLS

- Because of the transverse fracture plane frequently seen in the spine, transaxial CT has potential diagnostic limitations; thus, multiplanar reformats should be obtained in every case. In problem cases, MRI and radionuclide scintigraphy may be required.
- The axial skeletal changes of ankylosing spondylitis and enteropathic arthropathy are often indistinguishable.
- The presence of osteopenia and deformity make minimally displaced fractures difficult to detect; one must specifically analyze each radiograph for disk space widening and discontinuity of the ossified paraspinal ligaments. New back pain in patients with ankylosing spondylitis should be presumed to be caused by fracture until proven otherwise.
- Transdiscal pseudoarthroses seen in ankylosing spondylitis may mimic infectious spondylitis. CT and MRI may help to resolve the issue, as, in infection, there is usually widely increased discal signal on T2-weighted images, whereas in ankylosing spondylitis, the typical lack of paravertebral mass or an epidural component mitigates against infection. Distinction is not always possible on imaging alone, however, and aspiration biopsy is occasionally required.

Suggested Readings

Braunstein EM, Martel W, Moidel R. Ankylosing spondylitis in men and women: a clinical and radiographic comparison. Radiology 1982;144:91–94

Karasick D, Schweitzer ME, Abidi NA, Cotler JM. Fractures of the vertebrae with spinal cord injuries in patients with ankylosing spondylitis: imaging findings. Am J Roentgenol 1995;165:1205–1208

Levine DS, Forbat SM, Saifuddin A. MRI of the axial skeletal manifestations of ankylosing spondylitis. Clin Radiol 2004;59:400–413

Resnick D. Patterns of peripheral joint disease in ankylosing spondylitis. Radiology 1974;110:523–532

Vinson EN, Major NM. MR imaging of ankylosing spondylitis. Semin Musculoskelet Radiol 2003;7:103–113

van der Linden S, Valkenburg HA, Cats A. Arthritis evaluation of diagnostic criteria for ankylosing spondylitis: a proposal for modification of the New York criteria. Rheum 1984;27:361–368

CASE 116

Hema N. Choudur, Anthony G. Ryan, and Peter L. Munk

Clinical Presentation

As a child, the young woman in this case suffered from an attack of rheumatic fever. Subsequently, she developed mitral stenosis and had a mitral valve replacement. She also developed progressive painless deformity of the hands and feet. On clinical examination, the deformities were reducible with mild compressive pressure on a flat surface. No associated tenderness was elicited.

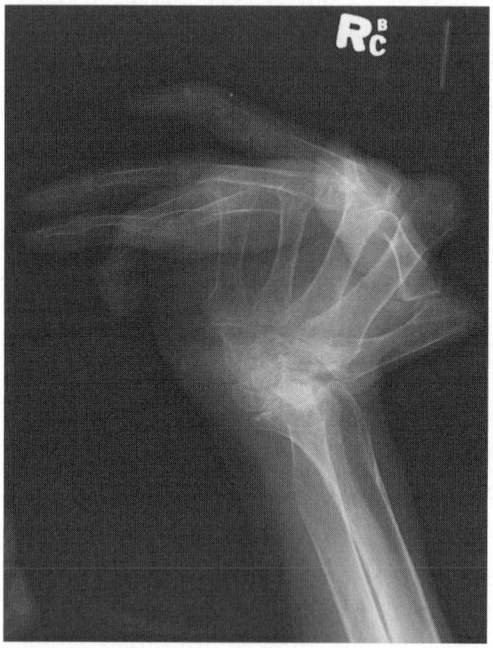

Figure 116A

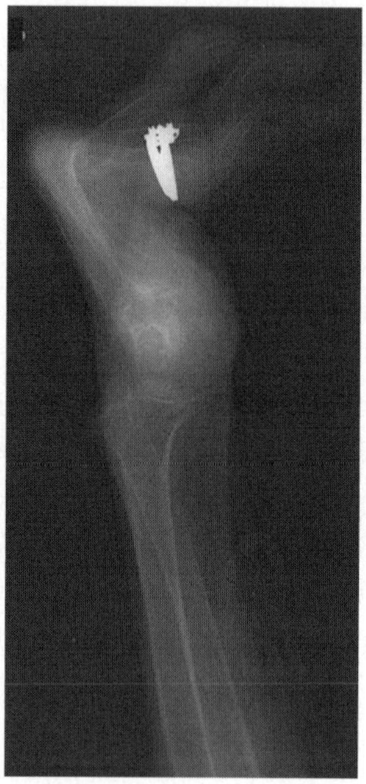

Figure 116B

Radiologic Findings

Radiographs of the hands and feet (**Figs. 116A–116F**) demonstrate a nonerosive arthropathy of both hands, seen as flexion deformities of the metacarpophalangeal joints with associated ulnar deviation. Hyperextension of the second to fifth proximal interphalangeal joints with flexion deformity of the second and fifth distal interphalangeal joints is also present. No erosions, periarticular osteopenia, or soft-tissue swelling is evident. Similar findings are present in the feet.

Diagnosis

Jaccoud's nonerosive arthropathy.

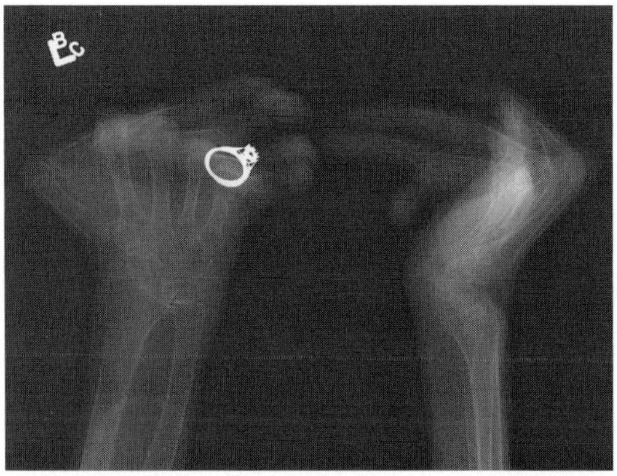

Figure 116C

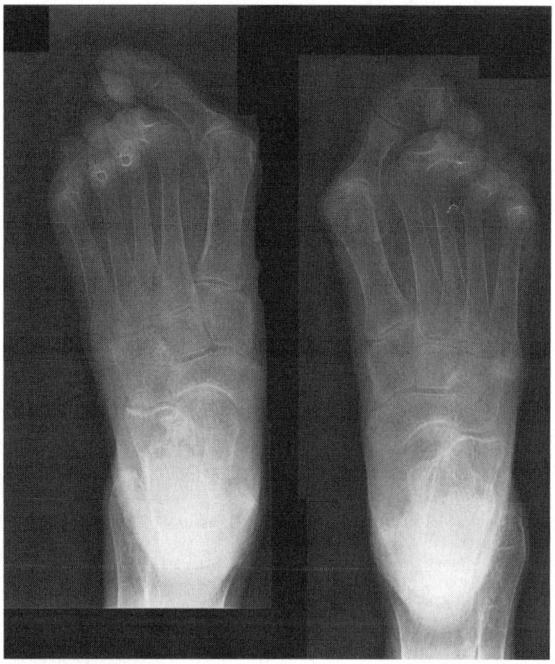

Figure 116D

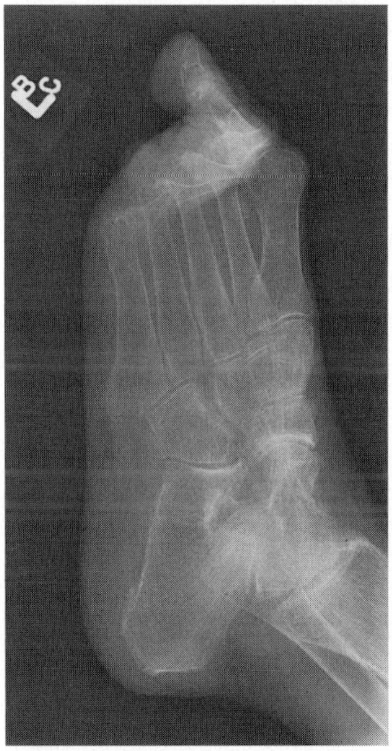

Figure 116E

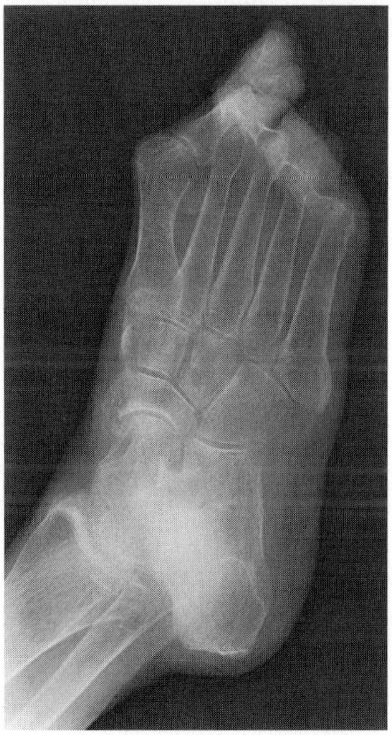

Figure 116F

Differential Diagnosis

On clinical examination, this characteristic deformity may be found in the collagen vascular diseases, especially systemic lupus erythematosus (SLE).

It is very rare that similar radiologic findings may be seen in rheumatoid arthritis, ankylosing spondylitis, or Ehlers-Danlos syndrome.

Discussion

Background

The first described case was in 1867, when Jaccoud described the chronic deforming arthropathy in a person with rheumatic fever and recurring polyarthritis. Later, similar nondeforming arthropathy was noted in other arthritides, especially SLE. There have been case reports of a similar arthropathy and radiologic findings in scleroderma, dermatomyositis, psoriasis, inflammatory bowel disease, mycosis fungoides, and even malignancy.

Etiology

During the recurrent attacks of polyarthritis following rheumatic fever, the capsule around the small joints of the hands becomes fibrotic and thickened, with contractures of the adjacent tendons, resulting in deformity of the hands.

Pathophysiology

Characteristically, the capsule of the small joints of the hands is inflamed in the first attack of rheumatic fever, with associated soft-tissue nodules, smaller than seen in rheumatoid arthritis. During the subsequent attacks of arthritis, the capsule thickens and becomes fibrotic. Rarely, secondary pressure hook erosions occur on the volar and radial aspects of the metacarpophalangeal joints.

The contracted tendons are displaced into the intermetacarpophalangeal spaces, resulting in deformities. In the chronic arthropathy, the synovium is not involved, clearly differentiating it from rheumatoid arthritis with its characteristic marginal erosions.

The most commonly described distribution is in both hands, but, not uncommonly, the feet may be affected. Hallux valgus with widening and flattening of the forefeet has been described, which was not seen in our case.

Clinical Findings

Delayed detection of this arthropathy is frequent, as there is no associated functional impairment. The absence of pain and tenderness is characteristic, as is the correctable deformity. A previous history of rheumatic fever is elicited in some parts of the world; however, in western populations, this deforming arthropathy occurs in association with collagen vascular disease, seen in 50% of the cases of SLE (**Figs. 116G,116H**).

Typically, ulnar deviation of the hands with flexion deformity at the metacarpophalangeal joints, especially the fourth and fifth, with hyperextension of the interphalangeal joints, is seen. The reversibility of the deformity is characteristic.

In the feet, fibular deviation and subluxation of the metatarsophalangeal joints are most frequently seen in the first and second toes. Shoulder instability can also be encountered. Diminution of the articular cartilage may be related either to disuse atrophy or to pressure of the apposing bones in subluxated joints.

Stages of Disease

Recurrent attacks of acute rheumatic fever with an inflammatory polyarthritis are followed by a slowly deforming painless arthropathy. Whereas the polyarthritis that occurs with rheumatic fever

G 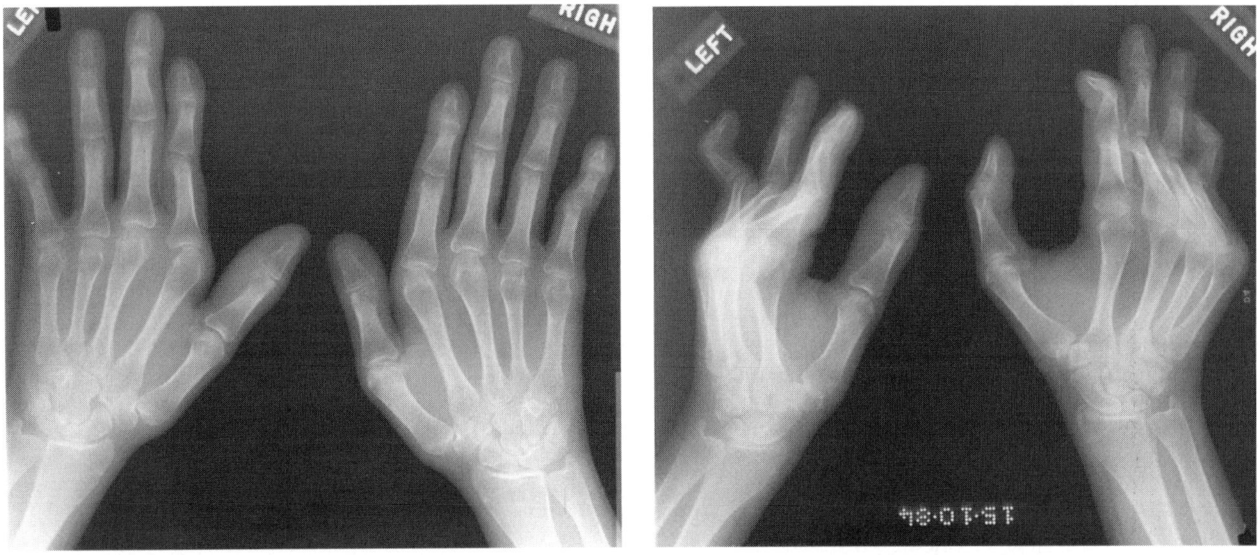 H

Figures 116G,116H Radiographs showing painless nonerosive deforming arthropathy of both hands of a patient known to have SLE.

involves the synovium and occurs in the large joints, such as the knees and ankles, chronic arthropathy involves the small joints of the hands and feet and spares the synovium.

Complications

Long-standing arthropathy with flexion contractures may be disabling.

Imaging Findings

RADIOGRAPHY

Standardized anteroposterior (AP) and oblique views are sufficient to diagnose this entity with a carefully taken history and laboratory work-up.

The ulnar deviation of the second to fifth fingers is well depicted on radiographs. Mild pressure on the fingers in the AP view corrects the deformity, including the flexion deformity of the fingers. No erosions or joint space narrowing is noted, unlike in rheumatoid arthritis. Rarely, hooklike erosions are noted on the radial and volar aspects of the metacarpal heads, but these tend to be away from the joint space, again differentiating Jaccoud's arthropathy from rheumatoid arthritis.

Periarticular osteopenia is often a feature, but no soft-tissue swelling is noted.

COMPUTED TOMOGRAPHY AND SONOGRAPHY

CT and sonography have a limited role to play. However, the absence of tenosynovitis/joint synovitis/erosions can be visualized using a dedicated high-frequency probe.

MAGNETIC RESONANCE IMAGING

Although there are many studies in the literature regarding the use of MRI to diagnose activity of the pannus in rheumatoid arthritis, its progression, extent of erosions, and joint involvement, there is a lesser role in the diagnosis of Jaccoud's arthropathy.

Treatment

The deformities are classified so that appropriate surgical treatment can be determined. Joint stabilization with realignment of the extensor tendons to center over the metacarpophalangeal joints yields good results in early deformities. In more severe cases, either Swanson implants are used, or metacarpal shortening osteotomy is performed.

Prognosis

The disease is slowly progressive, with flexion contractures developing secondary to the long-standing deformities, resulting in functional impairment.

PEARL

- Nonerosive, painless, deforming, correctable arthropathy with a previous history of rheumatic fever or associated with collagen vascular disease is the characteristic feature of this disease.

PITFALL

- The deformity may not be apparent on AP views, as the alignment may be corrected while positioning the patient.

Suggested Readings

Murphy WA, Staple TW. Jaccoud's arthropathy reviewed. Am J Roentgenol Radium Ther Nucl Med 1973;118:300–307

Pastershank SP, Resnick D. "Hook" erosions in Jaccoud's arthropathy. J Can Assoc Radiol 1980;31: 174–175

Scutellari PN, Orzincolo C, Franceschini F, Stabellini R, Govoni M, Trotta F. Radiological picture of the hand and foot in systemic lupus erythematosus. Radiol Med (Torino) 1987;74:498–503

CASE 117

Anthony G. Ryan and Peter L. Munk

Clinical Presentation

A 43-year-old man presented with stiffness and diminished range of motion in his shoulder and right elbow but no pain. He was status 1 year post–motor vehicle accident, at which time he experienced a whiplash injury to the cervical spine but could recall no injury to his upper limbs.

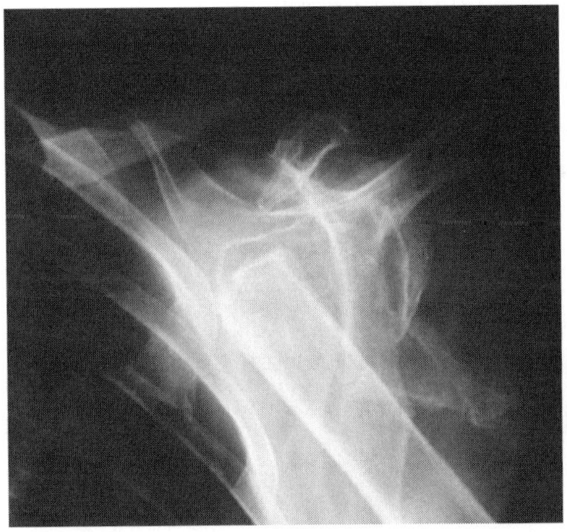

Figure 117A

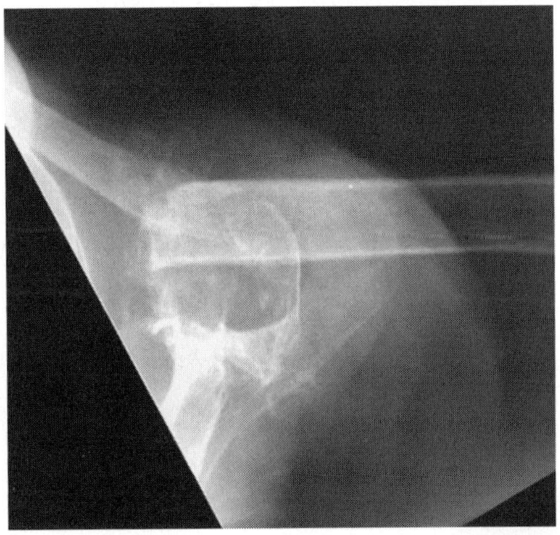

Figure 117B

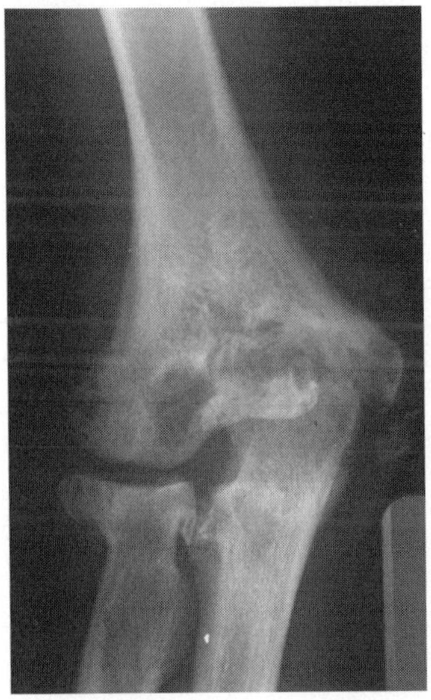

Figure 117C

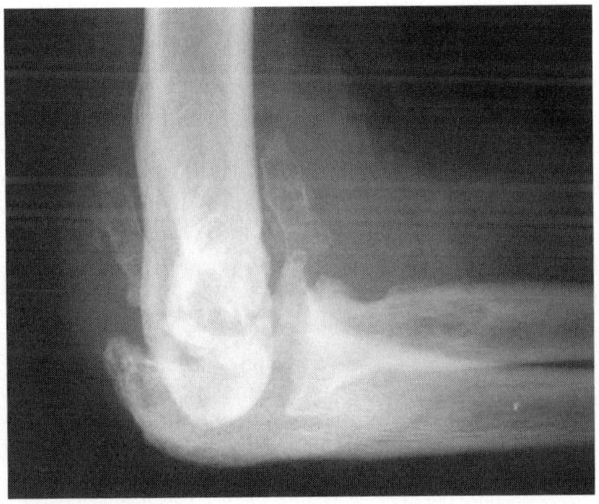

Figure 117D

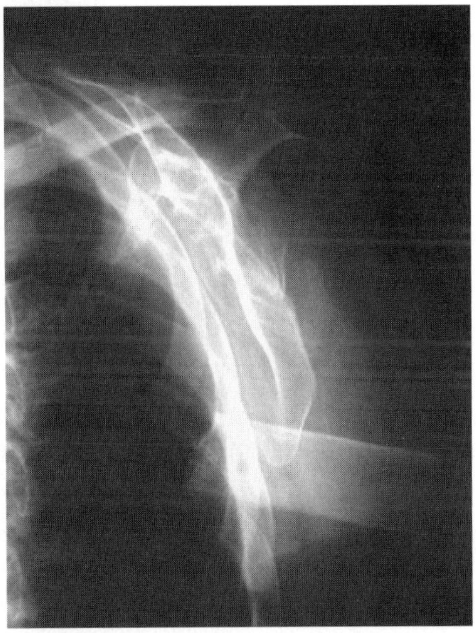

Figure 117E

Radiologic Findings

An anteroposterior (AP) radiograph of the left shoulder (**Fig. 117A**) shows no discernible humeral head, a very sharp margin to the end of the proximal humerus, and ossific fragments projected within the confines of the shoulder joint capsule, including a crescentic radiodensity projected lateral to the proximal humerus. The axial view (**Fig. 117B**) shows the proximal margin of the extant humerus, immediately anterior to which is a faint, round ossific density and through which is projected an ossific "ghost" of the humeral head, both fragments representing the remainder of the humeral head.

AP (**Fig. 117C**) and lateral (**Fig. 117D**) radiographs of the right elbow demonstrate multiple well-defined erosions of the capitellum, radial head, coronoid process, olecranon, and destructive erosion of the trochlea. The lateral radiograph in particular demonstrates a dense effusion and multiple large ossific fragments anterior and posterior to the joint.

Further investigations were performed, and a presumptive diagnosis was reached. The left arm was placed in a U-slab for 2 weeks, and a further radiograph of the shoulder was obtained (**Fig. 117E**), which shows further displacement of the humeral shaft and residual, but less prominent, ossific fragments within the shoulder capsule.

Diagnosis

Neuropathic (Charcot) joint secondary to acquired posttraumatic cervical syrinx (demonstrated on concurrent MRI)

Differential Diagnosis

- Calcium pyrophosphate dihydrate deposition disease
- Milwaukee shoulder (hydroscyapatite crystal arthropathy)
- Septic arthritis

Discussion

Background

Neuropathic arthropathy is a progressive, degenerative arthropathy secondary to an underlying neuropathy. Any condition that leads to loss of sensation in a joint impedes both pain perception and proprioception, resulting in severely altered biomechanics (particularly in weight-bearing joints). This lack of feedback prevents patients from protecting themselves by discontinuing the damaging activity, resulting in repeated traumatic injury.

Etiology

There are two major causes of a denervated joint, congenital and acquired.

CONGENITAL

- Myelomeningocele
- Congenital indifference/insensitivity to pain

ACQUIRED

Central neuropathy

- Trauma: brain, spinal cord injury (**Fig. 117F**)
- Syringomyelia (shoulder)

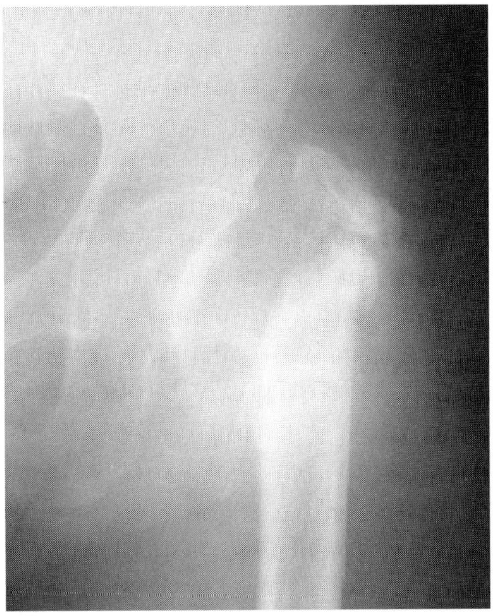

Figure 117F AP radiograph of the left hip in a quadriplegic patient receiving in-bed physiotherapy. Crepitus heard on passive mobilization prompted the radiograph, which reveals almost complete destruction of the femoral head, disarticulation of the hip joint, and large intra-articular bony fragments.

- Neurosyphilis/tabes dorsalis (the condition in which Charcot originally described the joint abnormalities); usually affects the knee
- Spinal cord tumors/infection

Peripheral neuropathy

- Diabetes mellitus (most common overall cause, affecting between 5 and 10% of diabetics), usually affecting the foot
- Leprosy
- Peripheral nerve injury
- Chronic alcoholism

Iatrogenic

- Chronic pain relief medications
- Repeated intra-articular steroid injections

Other, less common causes

- Scleroderma, Raynaud's disease, Ehler-Danlos syndrome
- Rheumatoid arthritis, psoriasis
- Amyloid infiltration of nerves, adrenal hypercorticism
- Klippel-Trénaunay-Weber syndrome
- Trauma, with or without infection, for example, after fractures and dislocations

Pathophysiology

Repeated trauma leads eventually to a neuropathic arthropathy characterized by fibrillation, degeneration, and eventual erosion of the articular cartilage. These changes are compounded by the attendant sympathetic dysfunction, which produces local hyperemia and consequent bone resorption. Because of the repeated trauma, the supporting structures of the joint become strained and eventually lax, compounding the propensity to subluxation and dislocation.

The distribution of the neuropathy provides a clue as to the possible etiology. The pattern of arthropathy mirrors the dysfunction in the sensory pathway, which may have a central or more peripheral origin (e.g., the peripheral neuropathy of a diabetic as opposed to the central cord defect of a syrinx).

Clinical Findings

The affected joint is usually painless but is swollen and warm on examination. Pain is said to be a reasonable indicator of the presence of infection.

The white cell count and erythrocyte sedimentation rate are typically normal unless there is concomitant infection.

In seeking to prevent the condition in diabetics, frequent sensory testing, especially in the presence of a lower limb injury, should be performed.

In the pediatric population, in addition to Charcot joints, the presence of a neuropathy predisposes the lower limbs to other typical injuries, namely

- Fractures of the metaphysis and diaphysis of long bones
- Epiphyseal separation
- Soft-tissue ulceration

The clinician must have a high index of suspicion for a Charcot joint in the presence of predisposing conditions (e.g., myelomeningocele or congenital indifference to pain), and localized soft-tissue swelling, warmth, or hyperemia near a joint should be investigated promptly with radiographs of the joints and adjacent bones, as severe structural deformities can develop rapidly in the absence of a timely diagnosis.

Stages of Disease

ATROPHIC PHASE

In the early phase of injury, there is a typical hyperemic response, resulting in an influx of osteoclasts and macrophages to the joint, resulting in destruction and resorption of bone and cartilage. The initial cartilage loss puts the articular surface at risk for further trauma, resulting in progressive joint destruction.

HYPERTROPHIC, REPARATIVE PHASE

This occurs in approximately 60% of cases, resulting in sclerosis around the joint.

Complications

- Progressive joint destruction and disarticulation
- Structural foot deformities
- Foot ulceration
- Osteomyelitis
- Threatened limb

In patients with spinal cord lesions, Charcot joints in the spine below the level of injury may give rise to headaches and sweating associated with sitting up and bed transfers secondary to autonomic dysreflexia, which is expected to respond to prolonged bed rest.

Pathology

GROSS

Fibrillation, degeneration, and eventual erosion of the articular cartilage may be seen. Erosion, eburnation, fragmentation, and frank destruction of the underlying bone may occur.

MICROSCOPIC

The initial, atrophic phase is characterized by a typical hyperemic response accompanied by an influx of osteoclasts and macrophages, resulting in bone and cartilaginous resorption. These changes are compounded by the attendant sympathetic dysfunction, which in turn exacerbates the local hyperemia. A pronounced synovitis may be present secondary to the resultant intra-articular debris.

The hypertrophic, reparative phase is characterized by osteoblastic influx, resulting in osseous sclerosis.

Imaging Findings

RADIOGRAPHY

There are two distinct patterns of appearance, depending on the phase of the process: hypertrophic (20%) and atrophic (40%). The most frequent presentation is a combination of the two (40%).

Whatever the pattern, the common features are joint space narrowing and joint instability leading to subluxation or dislocation. There is almost invariably a prominent, persistent joint effusion. The bone density is usually normal or of increased density.

In the atrophic stage there is resorption of the (eburnated) articular bone. In the hypertrophic stage, there is, in addition,

- Marked fragmentation of articular bone and prominent reactive bone formation
- Calcifications that may be visible in the soft tissues

Despite the presence of hyperemia, it is a rule of thumb that juxta-articular osteoporosis is not present unless there is superimposed infection.

The typical radiographic findings are summarized by the mnemonic “6Ds”:

- Destruction
- Dislocation
- Debris (fragmentation and heteropic new bone formation)
- Density
- Disorganization
- Distension

The combination of the first three “Ds” is quite specific for a neuropathic joint.

Rapid progression is typical. Where bony destruction has occurred, the margin of the remnant is characteristically sharp.

COMPUTED TOMOGRAPHY

- Bony changes are seen elegantly (**Figs. 117G–117I**).

MAGNETIC RESONANCE IMAGING

MRI is the investigation of choice in the assessment of the neuropathic joint and its potential complications (particularly in the diabetic patient, where infection is a frequent complication), such as

- Osteomyelitis
- Abscess
- Septic arthritis
- Tenosynovitis

A distinctive pattern for neuroarthropathy in the absence of infection has been identified, namely low signal intensity on T1- and T2-weighted images within the bone marrow space adjacent to the involved joint. Similarly, in the hypertrophic phase, osteosclerosis produces low signal intensity on both T1- and T2-weighted images.

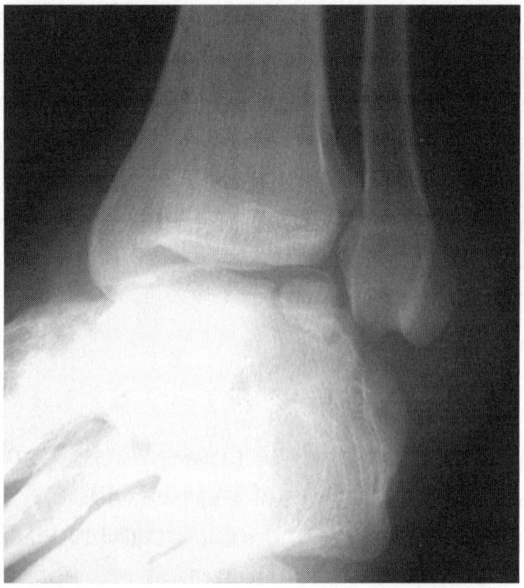

G

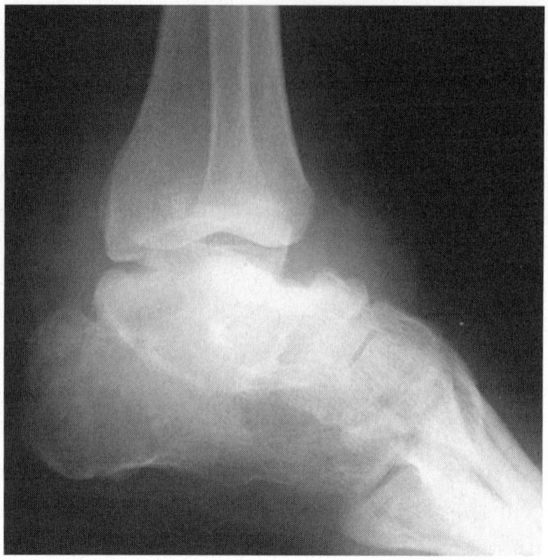

H

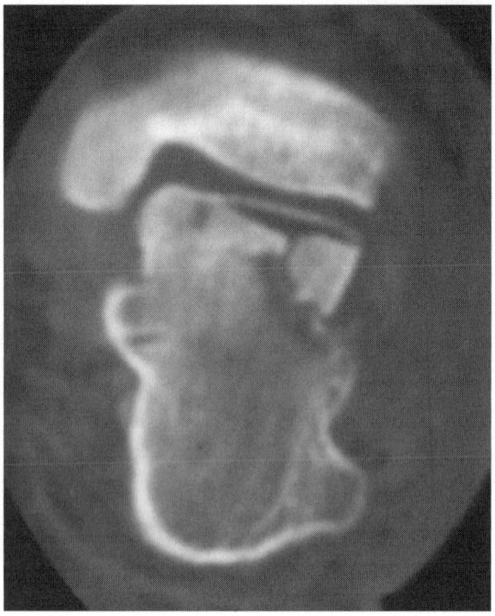

I

Figures 117G–117I AP (**117G**) and lateral (**117H**) radiographs of the left ankle in a chronic alcoholic show a dense effusion, loss of congruity of the ankle mortise, and a fracture of the talar dome associated with subchondral lucency, fragmentation, and collapse. **117I** Coronal reconstruction from CT of the same ankle as in **117G** elegantly demonstrates all the above findings, the subchondral collapse and imminent further collapse clarified when compared with the radiograph. The sclerosis on both sides of the mortise is clearly evident, again, more so than on the corresponding radiographs.

When the spine is involved, as it is in 6 to 21% of cases, the same features as described above are seen in the intervertebral and facet joints, with resultant lysis, sclerosis, large osteophyte formation, and eventual scoliosis. Prominent disk space destruction is typical.

Treatment

The treatment for Charcot joint seeks to prevent various complications, such as skin lesions, infections, and delayed union. In the pediatric population, immobilization of the limb generally leads to prompt healing of fractures and epiphyseal separation.

Total knee arthroplasty is performed in a proportion of patients with end-stage neuropathic arthropathy; however, surgery tends to be complex, being more similar to revision than primary arthroplasty, reflecting the diminished bone stock and altered biovascular milieu. Strict adherence to the revision arthroplasty principles of limb alignment restoration, reinforcement of bony defects by bone grafting or augmented prostheses, ligamentous balancing, and selection of appropriate constrained prostheses are required for a favorable outcome. In one study, extensive bone fragmentation and bone defects were present in 95% of cases, necessitating the use of metal wedge augments, autologous bone grafting, and bone allografts. In the same study, ligamentous instability indicated the use of long-stem components and rotating hinge prostheses in a significant proportion of cases.

External fixation of foot and ankle deformities has been utilized for reconstruction and stabilization of both infected and noninfected Charcot deformities of the foot and ankle, permitting early weight-bearing and postoperative foot adjustment or manipulation if necessary. The proponents of external fixation argue in its favor despite the challenges of the Charcot foot, for example, osteoporosis, osteomyelitis, poor wound healing, and poor compliance.

Prognosis

Untreated, neuropathic joints can lead to severe disability, particularly in the lower limb, where limited mobility or immobility can result in attendant complications (e.g., pneumonia, urosepsis, and deep venous thrombosis).

As above, in appropriately selected patients, total knee arthroplasty leads to a significant reduction in pain and improvement in range of motion and other measures of function. Even in initially successful arthroplasties, however, this group of patients frequently experiences complications relating to the procedure, requiring reoperation for prosthetic fracture, aseptic loosening, instability, and deep infection at a higher rate than standard primary arthroplasty.

PEARLS

- Juxta-articular osteoporosis is not present unless there is superimposed infection.
- In seeking to confirm or refute the presence of infection within a neuropathic joint, multicentric involvement supports a diagnosis of infection.
- Similarly, a distinctive pattern for noninfected neuroarthropathy has been described on MRI, namely low signal intensity on T1- and T2-weighted images within the bone marrow space adjacent to the involved joint.
- The etiology of the diseased joint can usually be discerned from the location of the joint affected, for example:
  - *Feet:* diabetes, alcoholism
  - *Foot and ankle:* diabetes, myelomeningocele
  - *Knee, ankle, foot:* congenital insensitivity to pain
  - *Lumbar spine and knee:* tabes
  - *Shoulder:* syringomyelia

PITFALLS

- Despite the presence of hyperemia, juxta-articular osteoporosis is not present unless there is superimposed infection.
- Charcot joints of the spine should be considered in patients with spinal cord lesions who develop autonomic dysreflexia.
- The clinician must have a high index of suspicion for a Charcot joint in the presence of predisposing conditions (e.g., myelomeningocele or congenital indifference to pain), and localized soft-tissue swelling, warmth, or hyperemia near a joint should be investigated promptly with radiographs of the joints and adjacent bones, as severe structural deformities can develop rapidly in the absence of a timely diagnosis.

Suggested Readings

Beltran J, Campanini DS, Knight C, McCalla M. The diabetic foot: magnetic resonance imaging evaluation. Skeletal Radiol 1990;19:37–41

Browne RF, Murphy SM, Torreggiani WC, Munk PL. Musculoskeletal case 29: neuropathic shoulder secondary to syringomyelia. Can J Surg 2003;46:300,309–310

Cooper PS. Application of external fixators for management of Charcot deformities of the foot and ankle. Foot Ankle Clin 2002;7:207–254

Lee L, Blume PA, Sumpio B. Charcot joint disease in diabetes mellitus. Ann Vasc Surg 2003;117:571–580

Parvizi J, Marrs J, Morrey BF. Total knee arthroplasty for neuropathic (Charcot) joints. Clin Orthop Relat Res 2003;416:145–150

Schneider R, Goldman AB, Bohne WH. Neuropathic injuries to the lower extremities in children. Radiology 1978;128:713–718

CASE 118

Peter L. Munk and Anthony G. Ryan

Clinical Presentation

A 70-year-old woman presented with complaints of diffuse pain throughout her right upper limb, with more focal pain at the wrist and shoulder. On examination, soft-tissue swelling was evident on the dorsum of the hand.

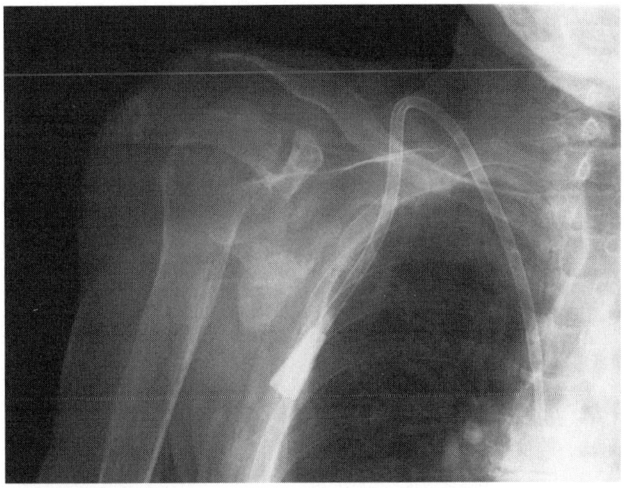

Figure 118A

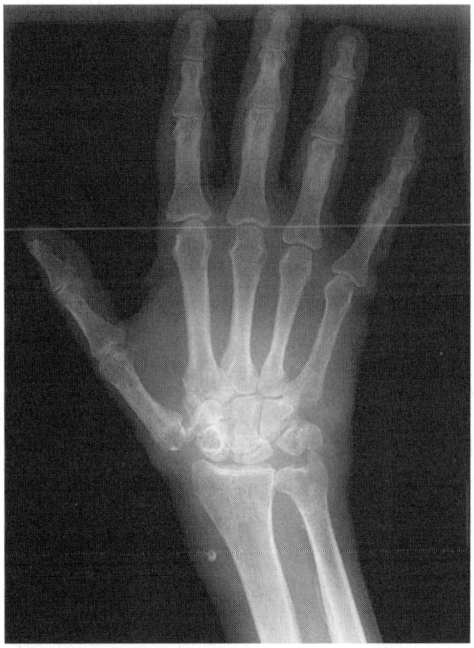

Figure 118B

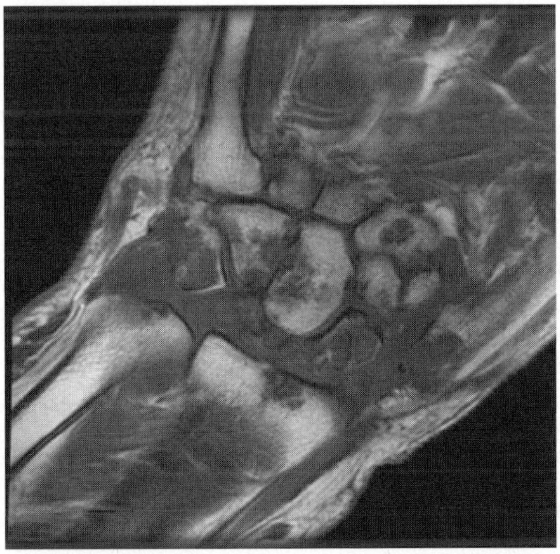

Figure 118C

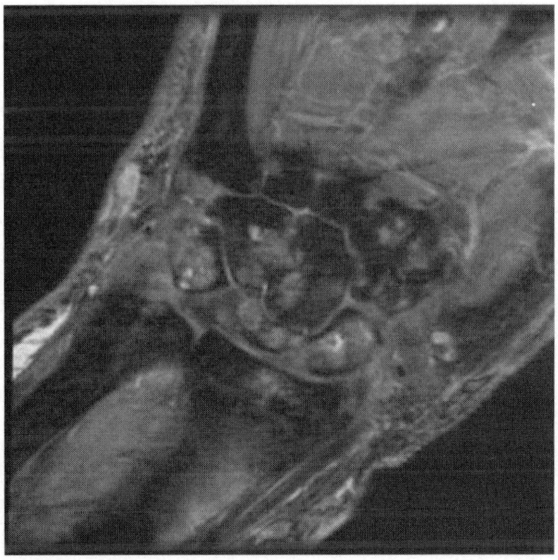

Figure 118D

Radiologic Findings

An anteroposterior (AP) shoulder radiograph (**Fig. 118A**) shows a right internal jugular hemodialysis catheter in situ. There is diffuse osteoporosis. The clavicle is discontinuous laterally, the inferior portion of which is tapered. The lateral portion is projected anterior to the head of the humerus, which is deformed and subluxated in relation to the glenoid fossa.

An AP radiograph of the right hand and wrist (**Fig. 118B**) shows diffuse soft-tissue swelling overlying the dorsum of the hand and distal wrist. Multiple erosions are evident, for example, at the base of the fifth metacarpal and distal ulna, as is deformity of the proximal carpal row bones and trapezium, the latter associated with subluxation of the first carpometacarpal joint. Calcification is evident within the ulnar artery, as is a phlebolith in a previous fistula site on the radial aspect of the wrist. Cystic change is evident at the base of the fifth metacarpal.

A coronal T1-weighted image (**Fig. 118C**) shows low signal intensity material essentially filling the joint space and eroding into the carpal bones, almost replacing some of the latter, particularly the proximal carpal row. Only a very small portion of the trapezium remains. Erosions secondary to the encroaching material are evident within the distal radius and ulna, as well as at the base of the second metacarpal.

A corresponding postgadolinium image (**Fig. 118D**) shows that the eroding material enhances moderately.

Diagnosis

Dialysis-induced amyloid arthropathy.

Differential Diagnosis

- Septic arthritis
- Infectious arthritis
- Secondary hyperparathyroidism

Discussion

Background

Despite the widespread use of renal transplantation, a larger number of patients are currently undergoing hemodialysis than at any other time in history. These patients often will develop arthritic and periarthritic changes. Many of these changes are due to osteodystrophy and secondary hyperparathyroidism, both of which are dealt with separately in other chapters.

Many of the changes are, however, due to deposition of amyloid.

Etiology

Beta$_2$-microglobulin is a protein polysaccharide (frequently consisting of immunoglobulin light chains) that, the presence of a normally functioning glomerulus, is freely filtered from serum.

In patients without glomerular function, this protein accumulates in serum and frequently reaches levels 40 to 50 times that normally encountered. This is not reduced by hemodialysis, as the cellulose-based hemodialysis membranes cannot filter beta$_2$-microglobulin. This results in a tendency to systemic deposition via the capillaries of a variety of different tissues.

In addition to chronic renal failure and hemodialysis, amyloid deposition occurs in myeloma, medullary carcinoma of the thyroid, rheumatoid arthritis, and chronic sepsis.

Pathophysiology

The polymerization and subsequent deposition of beta$_2$-microglobulin associated with amyloidosis appears to affect principally the musculoskeletal system. Amyloid deposition within joints and tenosynovium is particularly common, with a predilection for the wrist. This protein is also deposited in many other joints, often leading to arthralgia and, with progression, frank arthropathy.

Clinical Findings

The patient is typically receiving hemodialysis and presents with diffuse or focal pain within the affected limb or joint. Rubbery periarticular soft-tissue swelling and loss of function within the joint are the typical presentations of a patient with amyloid arthropathy. One of the first manifestations in many individuals is the development of carpal tunnel syndrome due to deposition within the wrist joints and tendon sheaths.

Stages of Disease

There are three distinct musculoskeletal manifestations that may or may not occur synchronously:

- Deposition around the tendons of the carpal tunnel, leading to carpal tunnel syndrome (affecting 2 to 30% of hemodialysis patients)
- Osseous and intra-articular deposition
- Spinal deposition, leading to a destructive spondyloarthropathy

Complications

- Carpal tunnel syndrome and other nerve entrapment disorders secondary to deposition within the wrist joints and tendon sheaths
- Arthralgia
- Arthropathies
- Bone erosion due to deposition within the periarticular soft tissues and synovial membranes
- Deposition within bone itself, resulting in cystic change and, at times, pathologic fracture
- Spondyloarthropathy

Pathology

GROSS

Amyloid is a pink amorphous, acellular material. The deposits may be seen not only within joints, tenosynovium, and bone but also in smooth muscle and the heart, tongue, nerves, kidneys, skin, and submandibular glands.

MICROSCOPIC

Beta$_2$-microglobulin is an eosinophilic material that stains with Congo red, producing a characteristic fibrillar appearance under polarized microscopy and the use of immunoperoxidase. Its deposition in tissues is centered on capillaries and larger vessel endothelium, leading in some cases to vascular occlusion, ischemic changes, and eventually infarction. There is little or no evidence of an inflammatory response, despite the proposed role of complement activation in its formation.

Imaging Findings

RADIOGRAPHY

- Erosions into bone due to deposition within the periarticular soft tissues and synovial membranes can be encountered, as well as deposition within bone itself, resulting in focal medullary lesions with endosteal scalloping and leading to cystic change and, at times, pathologic fractures. Amyloid deposition occurs most commonly in the carpus, particularly the scaphoid, lunate, and capitate, and less frequently in the humeral head, the patella, and around the hip.
- Erosive changes may be seen in any joint. Large (hip, knee, and shoulder) and small joints can be affected, although generally only a few joints are symptomatic at any given time.
- In the appendicular skeleton, subluxation of the humeral (**Fig. 118A**) and femoral heads may be present.
- Osteoporosis (**Fig. 118A**)
- At times, amyloid may present as periarticular masses due to extensive focal deposition within the soft tissues.
- In the spine, peridiscal erosive changes (**Fig. 118E**) have been well described, occurring in as many as 15% of patients on chronic hemodialysis, although these are frequently asymptomatic until the process is far advanced. The cervical and lumbar spines are most frequently affected. The typical appearances include erosions with accompanying sclerosis, vertebral body compression, disk space narrowing, and facet joint involvement leading to subluxation. The lack of osteophytes

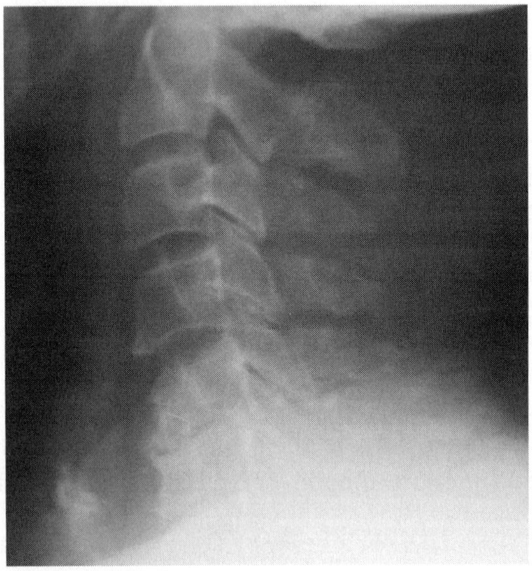
E

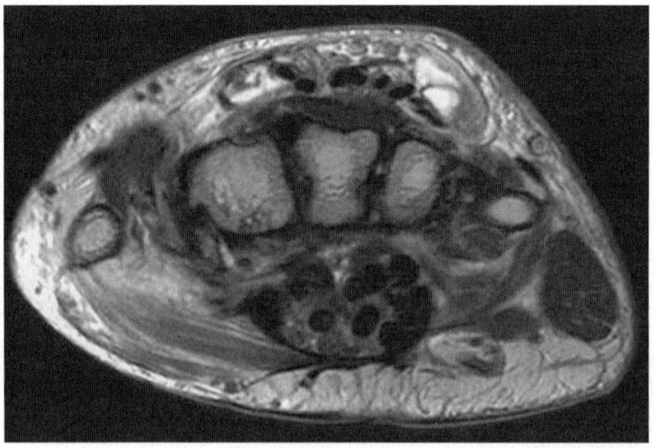
F

Figures 118E,118F **118E** Lateral cervical spine in the same patient demonstrates minimal peridiscal erosive changes in relation to the C5–C6 disk space, which is correspondingly reduced in height. **118F** Axial T2-weighted image in a different patient complaining of symptoms suggestive of carpal tunnel syndrome shows thickened flexor tendons and intermediate signal intensity material surrounding them within the carpal tunnel. Amyloid arthropathy was confirmed histologically at tunnel release.

helps to differentiate amyloid arthropathy from simple degeneration. In one third of patients, the progression of the changes may be so rapid as to simulate infection.

MAGNETIC RESONANCE IMAGING

- With MRI, amyloid will typically be seen as low signal on T1-weighted images, with a moderate increase in signal intensity if fluid-sensitive sequences such as T2-weighted (**Fig. 118F**) or STIR images are employed.
- Extensive fibrosis may accompany this, precluding significant increased signal with T2.
- Administration of intravenous (IV) gadolinium will almost invariably demonstrate extensive enhancement and also allows differentiation of the amyloid deposition within the soft tissues from surrounding joint effusions.
- In the spine, marrow and disk space replacement may mimic an infectious spondylodiskitis on MRI, particularly in patients who are symptomatic. The extent of changes demonstrated on MRI almost invariably correlates with the length of time the patient has undergone hemodialysis, with changes being more frequent with long-term treatment.

Treatment

- Low-dose prednisolone
- Symptomatic relief tends to follow rapidly after renal transplantation, although it is thought that this is due to the concomitant steroids.
- Changing to a biocompatible hemodialysis membrane can lead to an improvement in symptoms.

Prognosis

With increasingly refined techniques for biochemical monitoring of patients undergoing hemodialysis and the use of high-flux synthetic membranes, the prevalence of amyloid arthropathy secondary to dialysis has been declining.

PEARLS

- The lack of osteophytes helps to differentiate amyloid spondyloarthropathy from simple degenerative disk disease.
- Amyloid arthropathy typically affects multiple levels in the spine, unlike infection, which is usually confined to one disk space.
- Similarly, no paravertebral abscess will be present in amyloid arthropathy, aiding in the differentiation between it and infection.

PITFALLS

- Extensive fibrosis may accompany amyloid deposition, precluding the demonstration of significant increased signal on T2-weighted images.
- In one third of patients, the progression of the changes may be so rapid as to simulate infection.
- The administration of IV gadolinium may not help to distinguish infection from amyloid arthropathy, because in the absence of fibrotic change in the latter, both conditions will exhibit enhancement.

Suggested Readings

Floege J, Ketteler M. Beta$_2$-microglobulin-derived amyloidosis: an update. Kidney Int Suppl 2001;78:S164–S171

Kessler M, Netter P, Azoulay E, Mayeux D, Pere P, Gaucher A. Dialysis-associated arthropathy: a multicentre survey of 171 patients receiving haemodialysis for over 10 years. Br J Rheumatol 1992;31:157–162

Leone A, Sundaram M, Cerase A, Magnavita N, Tazza L, Marano P. Destructive spondyloarthropathy of the cervical spine in long-term hemodialyzed patients: a five-year clinical radiological prospective study. Skeletal Radiol 2001;30:431–441

PART VIII Other Conditions

CASE 119

Anthony G. Ryan, Nizar Al-Nakshabandi, and Peter L. Munk

Clinical Presentation

A 37-year-old man presented with discomfort and swelling of the right knee that had gradually progressed over a 2- to 3-year period. This was aggravated by activity, which often produced a marked increase in swelling.

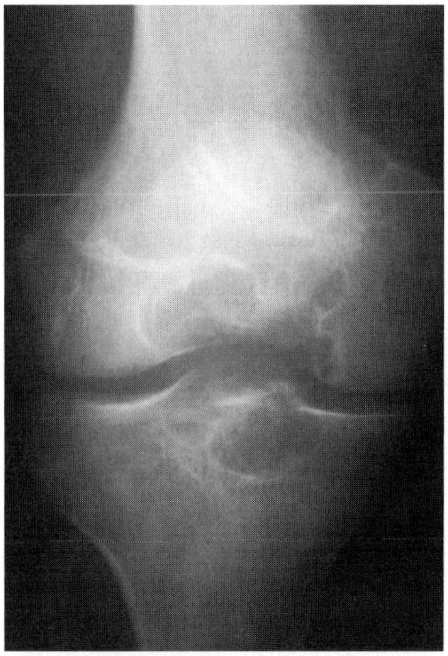

Figure 119A

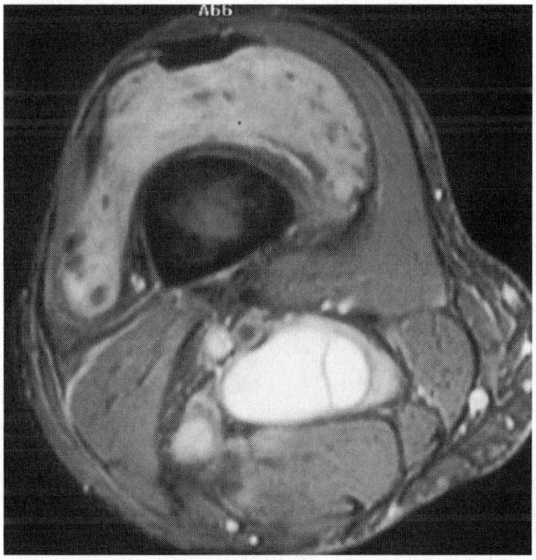

Figures 119B

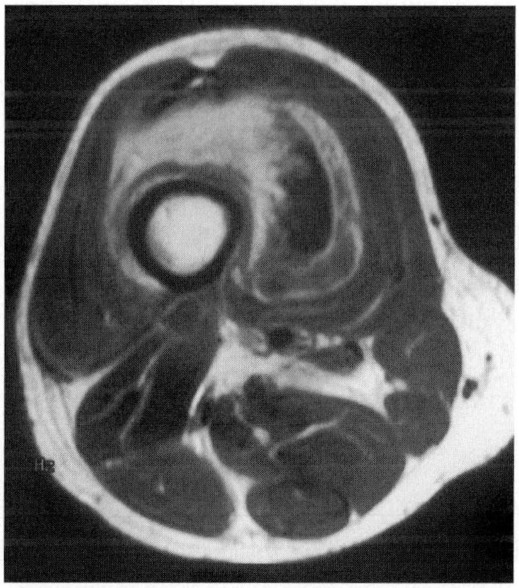

Figures 119C

Radiologic Findings

The anteroposterior view of the knee (**Fig. 119A**) shows erosions involving both the femur and the tibia centered in the region of the intercondylar notch. The erosions are well defined with slightly sclerotic borders, consistent with a slowly enlarging soft-tissue mass.

An MRI examination shows a large effusion distending the suprapatellar bursa (**Figs. 119B,119C**). On the gradient echo image (**Fig. 119B**), multiple punctate foci of low signal intensity are present, consistent with areas of hemosiderin deposition. Following administration of intravenous (IV) gadolinium contrast, extensive masslike enhancement is noted (**Fig. 119C**).

Diagnosis

Pigmented villonodular synovitis (PVNS).

Differential Diagnosis

- Rheumatoid arthritis
- Indolent infection
- Synovial sarcoma
- Hemophilia
- Lipoma arborescens

Other hemosiderin-containing lesions include

- Hematoma
- Hemangioma

Discussion

Background

PVNS is a rare benign proliferative diffuse intra-articular growth of the synovium of obscure etiology, first described in 1941 and representing part of a disease spectrum that includes a localized form (giant cell tumor of the tendon sheath [GCTTS]). The more common (75 to 85%) of the two entities, GCTTS differs from PVNS in location, as it is classically extra-articular, located around the tendon sheaths of the hand, and usually measures < 2 cm in size.

Etiology

Although some debate persists regarding the etiology of the condition, in its diffuse form, it is widely held to be neoplastic, as evinced by the presence of mononuclear clonality and rare reported cases of metastases. Alternative etiologies suggested include an inflammatory process of unknown cause and an abnormality of local lipid metabolism. The localized form is held by some to be a local granulomatous reaction; however, a causative agent has not been identified.

Pathophysiology

Repetitive trauma to the friable villi causes bleeding, resulting in synovitis, effusion, pain, and limited joint motion. Bone erosions contribute to the pain and limited range of motion.

Clinical Findings

The annual incidence of PVNS in the United States is 1.8 to 2 per million persons, with no significant gender predisposition. It is most frequently encountered in the third and fourth decades of life. The joint most commonly affected is the knee, followed by the hip, ankle, shoulder, and elbow joints, although almost all joints have been reported to be affected.

Symptoms are usually nonspecific (e.g., pain, warmth, and swelling), and on examination, tenderness and an effusion are present. Joint mobility commonly becomes restricted as the lesion expands.

Joint aspiration yields blood 75% of the time and yellow fluid 25% of the time. Laboratory investigations are usually unrewarding, as they are almost invariably normal.

Complications

- Effusion
- Joint pain
- Limited motion
- Local recurrence after excision

Pathology

GROSS

PVNS demonstrates thickening of the synovium with villous or nodular proliferation and diffuse hemosiderin staining secondary to intra-articular hemorrhage, the latter leading to intra- and extracellular hemosiderin deposition.

MICROSCOPIC

Histology characteristically reveals cellular lobularity beneath an intact synovial layer with brown granular deposits of hemosiderin. The cellular lobules are seen to be composed of macrophages laden with hemosiderin and lipid, plump mononuclear cells, and multinucleated osteoclast-like giant cells. Accompanying fibrotic changes are typical. Other conditions causing recurrent hemarthroses, such as hemophilia, hemochromatosis, and hemosiderosis, also demonstrate hemosiderin on histological section; however, the pigment is largely confined to the synovial cells and macrophages, whereas the distribution in PVNS is more diffuse. Multinucleated giant cells and histiocytes, seen in PVNS, are not features of these conditions.

Imaging Findings

RADIOGRAPHY

The features of PVNS on plain films are nonspecific; yet, together with the clinical findings, they are likely to suggest the diagnosis.

- Well-defined erosions are noted early in the disease, with relative preservation of the joint space.
- With progression, joint space loss may become severe and concentric, particularly when involving joints with a limited volume capacity, such as the hip (**Fig. 119D**).
- Extrinsic erosion may give rise to a geographic lytic lesion.

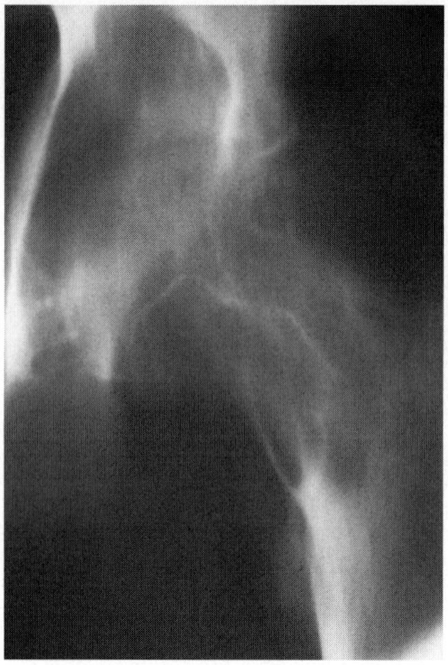

Figure 119D A single slice from a tomogram of the left hip. The hip joint itself is markedly narrowed. Large erosions involve both the neck of the femur and the acetabulum.

- A dense joint effusion is often visualized, representing the soft-tissue mass mixed with large amounts of hemosiderin.
- Normal bony mineralization is the rule, and soft-tissue calcification is rare.

ARTHROGRAPHY

- Typically, arthrography demonstrates multinodular filling defects. Dark brown fluid consistent with altered blood may be aspirated.

COMPUTED TOMOGRAPHY

- Due to the high hemosiderin content, PVNS appears as a soft-tissue mass of high density in relation to surrounding muscle.
- Underlying well-defined bone erosions or cysts with sclerotic margins can be especially well appreciated.
- Soft tissue may take the form of multiloculated nodular soft tissue.
- CT air arthrography can at times advantageously delineate the nodular nature and distribution of the intra-articular portions of the tumor, although similar information can usually be obtained from IV contrast-enhanced CT.
- PVNS shows variable enhancement, which can be striking.

MAGNETIC RESONANCE IMAGING

- The signal characteristics reflect the histological composition of the tissue, particularly hemosiderin, lipids, and inflammatory fibrosis.
- Hemosiderin is the most striking of these due to its magnetic susceptibility properties. This is manifested as low-signal "blooming" artifact, best appreciated on gradient/echo sequences (**Fig. 119B**).
- The mass is usually heterogeneous and low in signal intensity, which is best appreciated on T1 sequences.
- Areas of high signal seen on T1 sequences represent either lipid-laden macrophages or hemorrhage. The edges of the lesion are well demarcated by a low signal intensity capsule due to either fibrosis or hemosiderin.

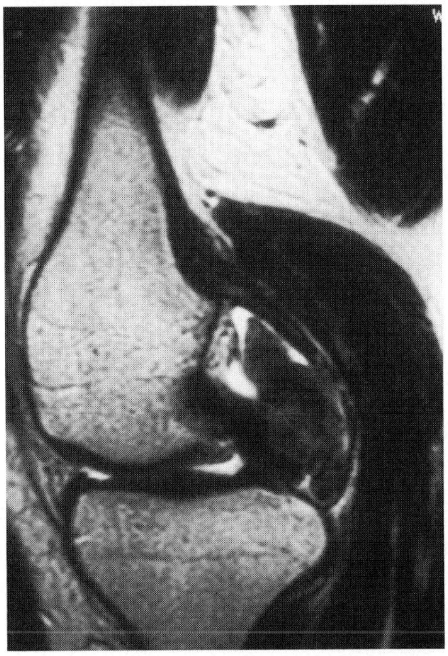

E

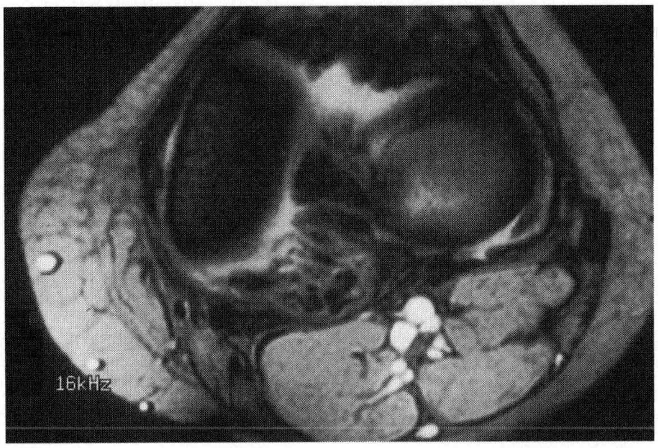

F

Figures 119E,119F 119E An oblique sagittal image shows a low signal area posterior to the posterior cruciate ligament. This mass is outlined by high-signal joint effusion. On excision, it was found to represent focal PVNS. **119F** An axial gradient-echo image shows multiple foci of low signal within the lesion consistent with "blooming" due to the presence of hemosiderin.

- The pattern of distribution, crucial for surgical planning, varies as the abnormal tissue can be focal or diffuse (**Figs. 119E,119F**).
- Marked enhancement is typical with administration of IV gadolinium (**Fig. 119C**).

Treatment

- If a prearthroscopic diagnosis is required, image-guided biopsy by ultrasound or CT may be undertaken and is likely to yield positive histology.
- The treatment of choice is surgical synovectomy, although radiation-induced synovial ablation is performed using injected yttrium 90 as the source.

Prognosis

- There is a high recurrence rate after surgical resection of up to 40 to 50%.

PEARLS

- GCTTS differs from PVNS in location, as it is classically extra-articular, located around the tendon sheaths of the hand, and usually measures < 2 cm in size.
- A dense joint effusion is often seen, representing the soft-tissue mass mixed with large amounts of hemosiderin.
- Hemosiderin is the most striking tissue characteristic on MRI due to its magnetic susceptibility properties. This is manifested as a low-signal "blooming" artifact, best appreciated on gradient-echo sequences.

PITFALLS

- Extrinsic erosion may give rise to a geographic lytic lesion, mimicking an aggressive bone malignancy.
- Well-defined erosions noted early in the disease, with relative preservation of the joint space, may mimic indolent infection, although the erosions of the latter are less well defined and rarely have sclerotic margins in the early phase of infection.
- Although intense enhancement after IV gadolinium is common, the pattern varies considerably, depending on the degree of fibrosis and the amount of hemosiderin present.

Suggested Readings

Al-Nakshabandi NA, Ryan AG, Choudur H, et al. Pigmented villonodular synovitis. Clin Radiol 2004;59:414–420

Cotten A, Flipo RM, Chastanet P, Desvigne-Noulet MC, Duquesnoy B, Delcambre B. Pigmented villonodular synovitis of the hip: review of radiographic features in 58 patients. Skeletal Radiol 1995;24:1–6

Hughes TH, Sartoris DJ, Schweitzer ME, Resnick DL. Pigmented villonodular synovitis: MRI characteristics. Skeletal Radiol 1995;24:7–12

Llauger J, Palmer J, Roson N, Cremades R, Bague S. Pigmented villonodular synovitis and giant cell tumors of the tendon sheath: radiologic and pathologic features. Am J Roentgenol 1999; 172:1087–1091

Wong K, Sallomi D, Janzen DL, Munk PL, O'Connell JX, Lee MJ. Monoarticular synovial lesions: radiologic pictorial essay with pathologic illustration. Clin Radiol 1999;54:273–284

CASE 120

Anthony G. Ryan and Peter L. Munk

Clinical Presentation

A 26-year-old woman presented with vague hip pain.

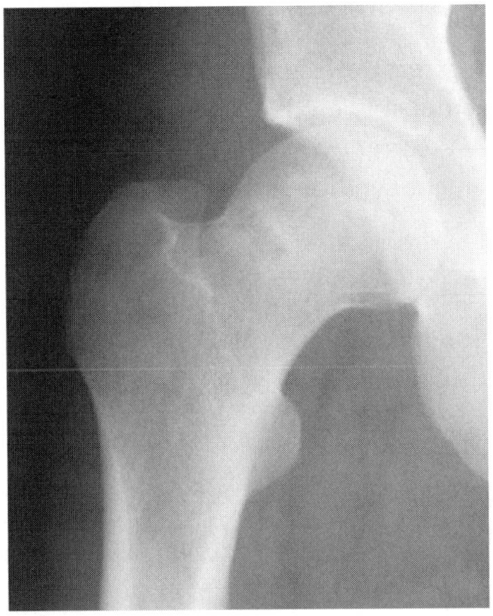

Figure 120A

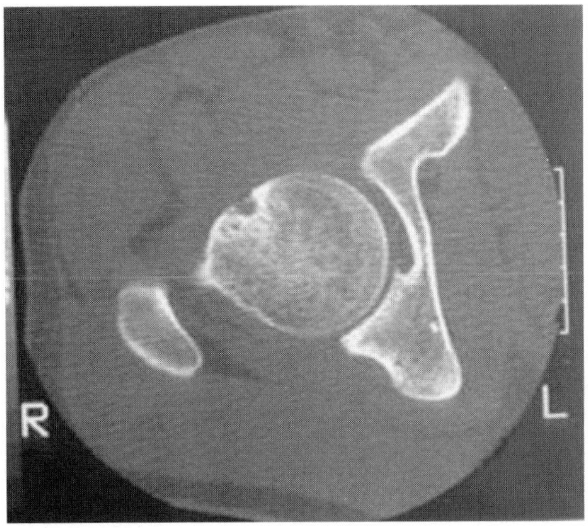

Figure 120B

Radiologic Findings

An anteroposterior radiograph of the hip (**Fig. 120A**) shows an apparent ill-defined lucency with a surrounding rim of sclerosis projected through the superior aspect of the femoral neck.

A transaxial CT at the level of the lesion (**Fig. 120B**) on the radiograph confirms the presence of a lucent defect surrounded by a moderate sclerotic margin at the junction of the femoral head and neck.

Diagnosis

Synovial herniation pit (Pitt's pit)

Differential Diagnosis

- Osteoid osteoma
- Geode

Discussion

Background

Patients very commonly present with hip pain that often is nonspecific in character. Virtually all of these patients will go on to have radiography. A frequently encountered finding is that of a synovial herniation pit.

Etiology

Although unclear, mechanical stress is thought to be responsible. The level of the herniation appears to be related to the thickest portion of the capsule and the ligaments in the hip joint, where the fibers of the zona orbicularis cross and intermingle with the iliofemoral ligament. This area becomes tightest in extension and internal rotation.

Pathophysiology

It is thought that, secondary to an adherent joint capsule, long-term erosion is produced due to mechanical stress and cortical remodeling. The cortex can be completely eroded in some cases, and the soft tissues can migrate into the medullary bone. Controversy currently exists, as some of these "herniation pits" may be causally related to acetabular impingement syndrome.

Clinical Findings

Most patients who have synovial herniation pits have them found as an incidental observation, as the pits are typically entirely asymptomatic, particularly when small.

Complications

Occasionally, very large synovial herniation pits can be seen, which gradually increase over time and even predispose to insufficiency fractures, although these are quite rare.

Pathology

GROSS

The joint capsule is found to be adherent to the underlying cortex, which is eroded centrally with a sclerotic margin secondary to cortical remodeling.

MICROSCOPIC

The cortex is completely eroded, occasionally with migration of the synovial soft tissues into the medullary bone.

Imaging Findings

RADIOGRAPHY

Round or oval radiolucencies are seen, typically with thin, sclerotic margins, most of which will be < 1 cm in diameter. These are typically found in the superior quadrant of the femoral neck and occasionally are bilateral.

The radiographic appearance of a lucent defect surrounded by a moderate sclerotic reaction can mimic an osteoid osteoma; however, the symptomatology is usually markedly different; that is, nocturnal pain may be relieved by aspirin in osteoid osteoma, whereas the herniation pit is typically painless and is discovered incidentally.

COMPUTED TOMOGRAPHY

On CT, a defect is noted in the cortex, and reactive sclerosis is commonly encountered around the lesion (**Fig. 120B**).

MAGNETIC RESONANCE IMAGING

The MRI appearance is quite variable, depending on the degree of sclerosis, which results in low signal on all sequences, and how much soft tissue has herniated into the bone. Typically, the soft tissue will be of intermediate to higher signal on T2-weighted sequences.

Treatment

Unless the pit has increased to a size where pathologic fracture may occur, no treatment is necessary.

Prognosis

- Usually self-limiting

PEARLS

- Occasionally, very large synovial herniation pits can be seen, which gradually increase over time and even predispose to insufficiency fractures, although the latter are quite rare.
- Although some cortically based lesions may demonstrate enhancement after gadolinium, neither the central fluid-containing portion of the pit nor the sclerotic margins of a herniation pit should enhance.
- The absence of other stigmata of osteoarthritis reduces the likelihood that such a lesion is a geode.

PITFALLS

- Herniation pits are typically entirely asymptomatic, particularly when small. Therefore, in the patient presenting with hip pain, a further cause for the pain should be sought rather than ascribing it to the pit.
- The radiographic appearance of a lucent defect surrounded by a moderate sclerotic reaction can mimic an osteoid osteoma; however, the symptomatology is usually markedly different; that is, nocturnal pain may be relieved by aspirin in osteoid osteomas, whereas the herniation pit is typically painless and is discovered incidentally in an older age group.

Suggested Readings

Daenen B, Preidler KW, Padmanabhan S, Brossmann J, et al. Symptomatic herniation pits of the femoral neck: anatomic and clinical study. Am J Roentgenol 1997;168:149–153

Lee A, Manolios N, De Costa R, Howe G, Spencer D. Herniation pit of the femoral neck. J Rheumatol 2000;27:2278–2280

Pitt MJ, Graham AR, Shipman JH, Birkby W. Herniation pit of the femoral neck. Am J Roentgenol 1982;138:1115–1121

CASE 121

George Nomikos, Anthony G. Ryan, Mark Murphey, and Peter L. Munk

Clinical Presentation

A 57-year-old man presented with a short history of increasing posterior right knee pain.

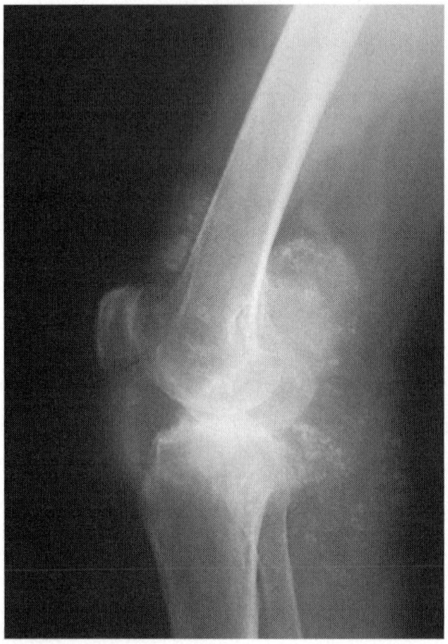

Figure 121A

Radiologic Findings

A lateral radiograph of the knee (**Fig. 121A**) shows erosions involving the tibia and patella, as well as a soft-tissue mass in the popliteal fossa. Multiple small calcifications are also visible in the mass. Axial CT images at the level of the femoral condyle and tibial plateau (**Figs. 121B,121C**) demonstrate multiple similarly sized calcified bodies in a popliteal cyst. Multiple erosions are identified in the tibia.

Diagnosis

Primary (idiopathic) synovial chondromatosis.

Differential Diagnosis

- Pigmented villonodular synovitis (PVNS)
- Osteoarthritis with secondary (osteo)chondromatosis
- Rheumatoid arthritis
- Septic arthritis
- Amyloid arthropathy
- Lipoma arborescens with osteochondral metaplasia

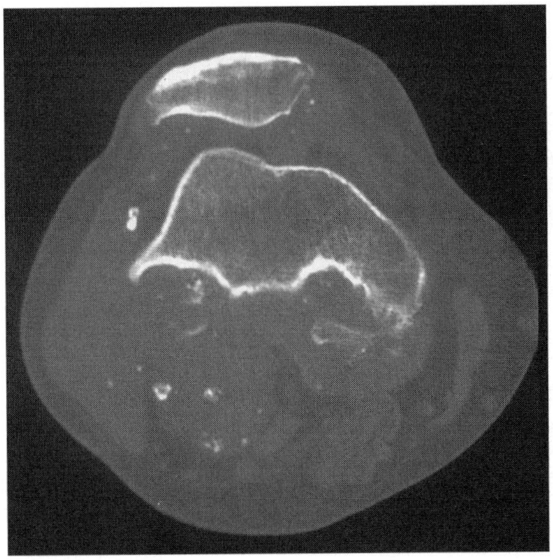

Figure 121B

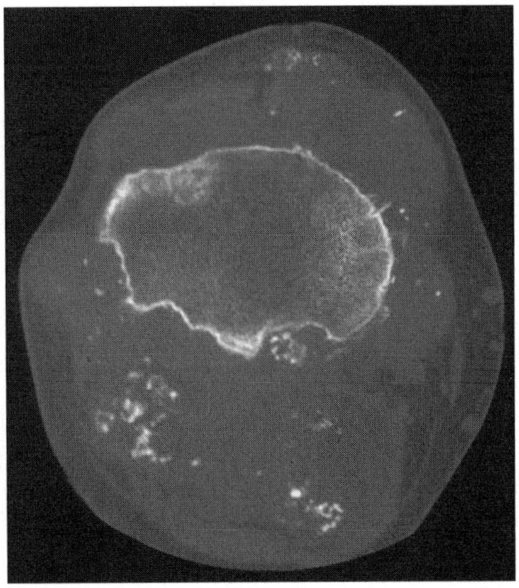

Figure 121C

Discussion

Background

Primary synovial chondromatosis (PSC) is a rare condition characterized by formation of multiple cartilaginous or osteocartilaginous bodies, usually of similar size, in a synovial joint. It must be distinguished from secondary (osteo)chondromatosis, in which multiple intra-articular bodies (IABs) are a result of another primary joint abnormality, such as osteoarthritis, osteonecrosis, neuropathic disease, trauma, osteochondritis dissecans, or rheumatoid arthritis. The IABs may be mineralized or nonmineralized.

Etiology

Synovial osteochondromatosis is a condition of unknown etiology in which synovial tissue undergoes benign reactive cartilaginous metaplasia to form multiple (osteo)cartilaginous nodules ranging from 1 mm to 3 cm in size. These osteochondral fragments in primary synovial chondromatosis tend to be similar in size and innumerable, unlike secondary osteochondromatosis, in which the fragments are usually of varying size and few in number. These chondral fragments may be free in the joint or may become reattached to synovium.

Clinical Findings

Patients are usually between 20 and 40 years old, and there is a 2:1 male:female predominance. Although usually monoarticular, multiple joints are rarely involved in the same patient. The most common presentation is with arthritic symptoms, including a painful swollen joint with limited range of motion. Palpable nodules are sometimes found on physical examination. Large joints, particularly the knee (> 50% of cases), are most commonly affected; however, smaller joints, such as the acromioclavicular joint, temporomandibular joint, vertebral facet joints, and distal radioulnar joint, among others, are occasionally involved. Although the process is most commonly seen in synovial joints, it may rarely occur in tendon sheaths (particularly the flexor side—tenosynovial chondromatosis) or bursae (bursal chondromatosis).

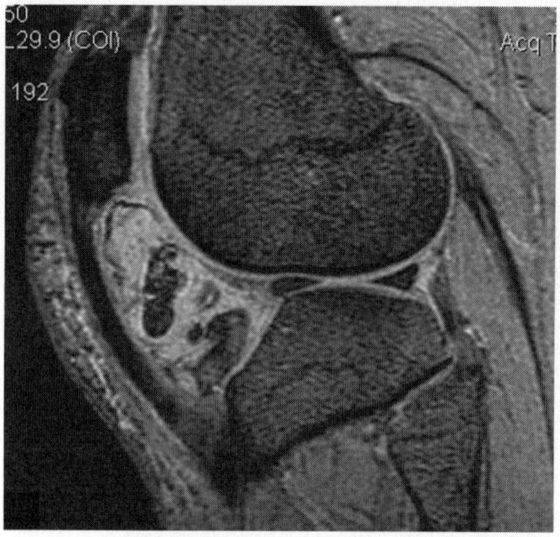

D

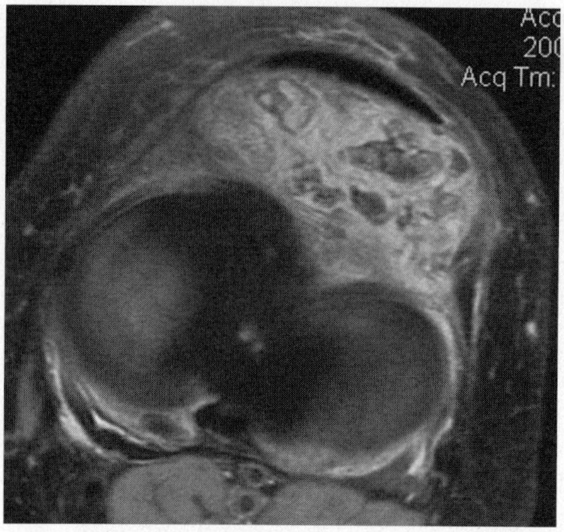

E

Figures 121D,121E Sagittal gradient (**121D**) and axial proton density fat-saturated (**121E**) images show a large, partially calcified synchondroma arising from the anterolateral tibia that fills Hoffa's fat pad and bows the patellar tendon. Note the cartilaginous signal on the gradient sequence (**121D**) with foci of low signal intensity calcifications.

Complications

If untreated, PSC may cause progressive joint destruction and secondary degenerative joint disease. Although extremely rare, malignant degeneration to chondrosarcoma has been reported. This possibility should be considered when there is evidence of spread outside the joint capsule (or known bursal recesses) or medullary invasion.

Pathology

There may be either focal or diffuse involvement of the synovium by multiple cartilaginous nodules. The nodules are most commonly identified in the connective tissue just below the synovium and may contain areas of bone formation and marrow elements. Giant solitary synovial chondromatosis is a rare variant in which a single large, solitary nodule is present (**Figs. 121D,121E**). Despite microscopic features of hypercellularity, enlarged chondrocytes, and nuclear pleomorphism, the process almost invariably demonstrates benign behavior.

Imaging Findings

RADIOGRAPHY

- Multiple mineralized (ring and arc appearance typical of a cartilage lesion) intra-articular bodies of similar size and shape are seen throughout the joint.
- The areas of mineralization range from small areas of calcification to larger areas of mature-appearing bone.
- Calcification is absent in 5 to 30% of cases, particularly in areas of complex anatomy, such as the hip.
- There may appear to be a soft-tissue mass about the involved joint secondary to the presence of hyperplastic synovium and multiple nonossified IABs.
- A joint effusion may be seen.
- Osseous erosions and scalloping are not uncommon, particularly in less capacious joints, such as the hip and wrist.

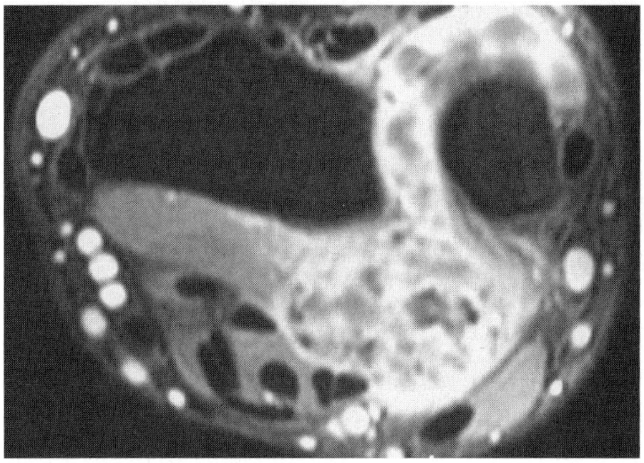

Figure 121F Transaxial T1-weighted fat-saturated image after intravenous gadolinium shows intense enhancement and excludes simple effusion as the cause of low signal intensity demonstrated on nonenhanced T1-weighted images.

COMPUTED TOMOGRAPHY

- Intra-articular low attenuation mass with or without calcifications
- Best modality to detect areas of calcification
- May demonstrate both mineralized and nonmineralized IABs
- Nonmineralized IABs are better demonstrated with CT arthrography.
- Calcifications and extrinsic erosions (usually with sclerotic margins) are better seen than with radiographs.

MAGNETIC RESONANCE IMAGING

- May appear as areas of low to intermediate signal intensity on T1-weighted images and high signal intensity on T2-weighted images with no areas of signal void (could be confused with a joint effusion)
- Low-signal septae corresponding to areas of fibrosis are often seen and may help distinguish PSC from a simple joint effusion, especially if no calcifications are present.
- Areas of calcification appear as regions of signal void with or without central areas of marrow signal intensity (**Fig. 121E**).
- Intravenous (IV) gadolinium may be useful to distinguish PSC from a joint effusion in cases that lack calcification (**Fig. 121F**).

Treatment and Prognosis

- Synovectomy and removal of intra-articular bodies
- 11% recurrence rate
- Malignant degeneration very rare

PEARLS

- The osteochondral fragments in primary synovial chondromatosis tend to be similar in size and innumerable, unlike secondary osteochondromatosis, in which the fragments are usually of varying size and few in number.
- Nonmineralized intra-articular bodies are better demonstrated with CT arthrography.
- The low-signal septae corresponding to areas of fibrosis may help distinguish PSC from a simple joint effusion, especially if no calcifications are present.

- Similarly, IV gadolinium may be useful to distinguish PSC from a joint effusion in cases that lack calcification.

PITFALLS

- The absence of calcification does not exclude the diagnosis, as it is absent in up to 30% of cases, particularly in areas of complex anatomy, such as the hip.
- It must be remembered that extra-articular synovium rarely gives rise to the condition.
- In the absence of IV gadolinium, synovial osteochondromatosis may appear as areas of low signal intensity on T1-weighted images and high signal intensity on T2-weighted images and thus may be mistaken for a joint effusion.

Suggested Readings

Crotty JM, Monu JU, Pope TL Jr. Synovial chondromatosis. Radiol Clin North Am 1996;34:327–342

Hermann G, Abdelwahab IF, Klein M, Kenan S, Lewis M. Synovial chondromatosis. Skeletal Radiol 1995;24:298–300

Kramer J, Recht M, Deely D, et al. MR appearance of idiopathic synovial chondromatosis. J Comput Assist Tomogr 1993;17:772–776

Wong K, Sallomi D, Janzen D, Munk P, O'Connell JX, Lee MJ. Monoarticular synovial lesions: radiologic pictorial essay with pathologic illustration. Clin Radiol 1999;54:273–284

CASE 122

George Nomikos, Hema N. Choudur, Anthony G. Ryan,
Peter L. Munk, and Mark Murphey

Clinical Presentation

A 74-year-old man presented with right leg pain.

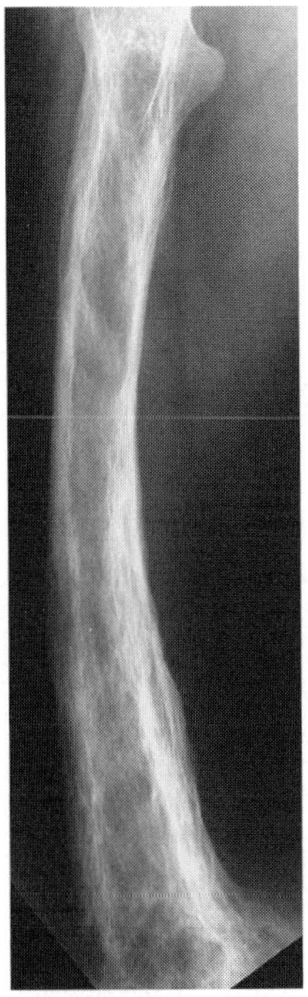

Figure 122A

Radiologic Findings

A plain radiograph of the right femur (**Fig. 122A**) shows gross deformity and diffuse expansion. Mixed sclerotic and lucent areas are interspersed in the deformed bone, with loss of the normal trabecular pattern.

Diagnosis

Paget's disease (mixed phase).

Differential Diagnosis

- Osseous metastases
- Chronic osteomyelitis

Discussion

Background

Paget's disease of bone (osteitis deformans) is a common nonhormonal metabolic bone disorder characterized by progressive skeletal deformation due to abnormal bone resorption and remodeling, resulting in osseous overgrowth and weakening. It occurs more frequently in the axial than in the appendicular skeleton. The relative frequency of involvement is, from most involved to least, pelvis, femur, skull, tibia, and vertebrae.

It is most common in Great Britain and in countries colonized by the British, such as the United States, New Zealand, and Australia. It is also common in continental Europe, but it is uncommon in Asia and Africa.

Paget's disease affects 3 to 4% of the population over 40 years old and 10 to 11% of the population over age 80; there is an overall mild male predominance (1.8:1 male:female ratio). It is uncommon in patients younger than 40 years old.

Etiology

Although the etiology is still uncertain, two entities have been implicated, one, a virus and the other, a genetic predisposition. The viral theory is favored by those authorities pointing to the presence of intranuclear inclusions in the osteoclasts of pagetic bone and the presence of giant osteoclasts. The genetic theory is prevalent, as the condition is known to occur in families.

Pathophysiology

At the outset, there is abnormal resorption of bone due to uncontrolled osteoclastic activity. This is followed by fibrous tissue formation, with disorderly trabeculae being laid down by the osteoblasts; however, the matrix is undermineralized and therefore structurally soft. As the disease progresses, more dense bone is laid down in a haphazard manner.

Clinical Findings

Symptoms of Paget's disease are variable, and many patients are initially asymptomatic. Common musculoskeletal symptoms include pain, tenderness, warmth (secondary to hypervascularity), osseous enlargement, bowing deformities, and kyphosis. Exacerbation of the pain at rest and at night is typical. Patients may present with a pathological fracture or an increasing bone or soft-tissue mass secondary to malignant transformation (osteosarcomas, chondrosarcomas, malignant fibrous histiocytoma, and giant cell tumors have all been reported in patients with Paget's disease).

Osseous expansion may lead to nerve compression syndromes, particularly involving the cranial nerves, producing deafness and visual disturbances. Skull deformity and enlargement can lead to increased intracranial pressure and hydrocephalus. Vertebral body enlargement can lead to narrowing of the spinal canal and consequent neurologic deficit, including weakness and incontinence or cranial nerve deficits.

High-output congestive heart failure has been associated with Paget's disease because of the hypervascularity of the abnormal bone. Aortic stenosis, heart block, and bundle branch block have also been associated with Paget's disease.

Laboratory values mirror the increased turnover of bone associated with this condition. During the lytic phase, serum and urine levels of hydroxyproline are increased and can be used to assess the degree of bone resorption. Serum alkaline phosphatase is elevated during the mixed and sclerotic phases due to increased bone formation during these phases. Serum calcium and phosphorus are normal.

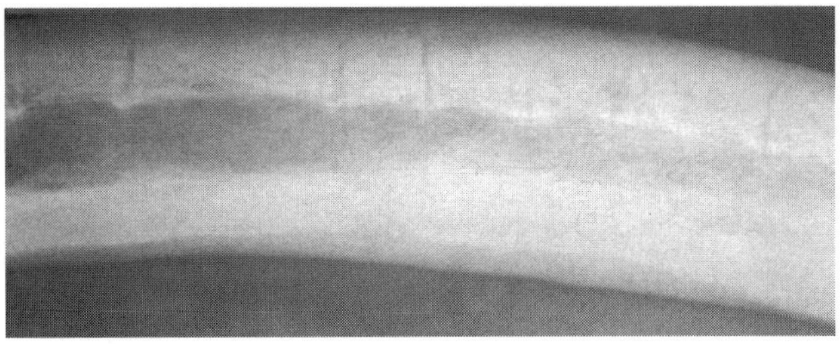

Figure 122B Multiple fractures are evident on the convex side of the bone, which is bowed with gross cortical thickening.

Stages of Disease

- *Lytic phase* Characterized by bone resorption due to excessive osteoclastic activity
- *Mixed phase* A phase of simultaneous resorption and bone formation
- *Blastic phase* Characterized by erratic bone formation

Complications

- Deformity and bowing secondary to osseous weakening
- Scoliosis
- Anterior bowing of the femur or tibia
- Acetabuli protrusio
- Fractures, which usually develop on the convex side of the involved bone and may progress to become complete (**Fig. 122B**)
- Secondary osteoarthritis owing to abnormal mechanics, most commonly involving the hip and knee
- Gout, calcium pyrophosphate dehydrate deposition disease, and rheumatoid arthritis have also been associated with Paget's disease.
- Neurologic complications secondary to osseous expansion causing nerve compression, including spinal stenosis and compression of cranial nerves. Paget's occurs in the skull in about 30% of cases.
- In the spine, cord compression may occur due to the enlargement of the vertebral bodies, intraspinal soft-tissue overgrowth, ossification of epidural fat, platybasia, bleeding, sarcomatous degeneration, vertebral fracture, or subluxation.
- Spinal ischemia can occur when blood is diverted due to a steal phenomenon.
- Recrudescence of the lytic phase, which may be associated with trauma to pagetic bone or after restriction of weight bearing, may simulate a malignant process.
- Sarcomatous transformation ($<$ 1% with long duration of disease, but up to 5 to 10% in those with extensive polyostotic disease), most commonly in the proximal femur, pelvis (**Fig. 122C**), and shoulder

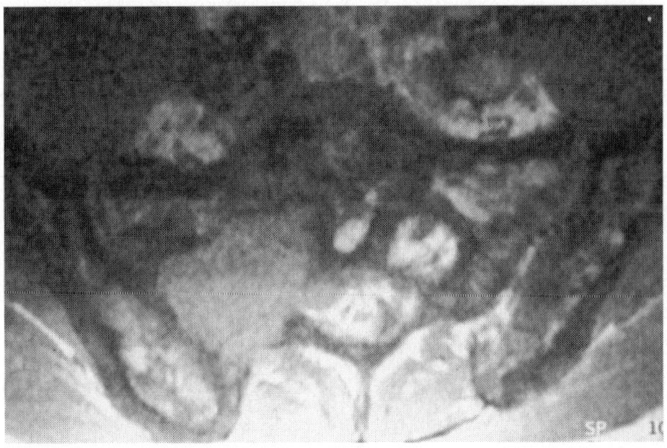

Figure 122C Transaxial T2-weighted image at the level of the sacral ala shows low signal intensity cortical thickening and a large right-sided multilobular mass, subsequently demonstrated to be sarcomatous transformation within pagetic bone.

- Sarcomatous transformation is most commonly to osteosarcoma, followed by malignant fibrous histiocytoma/fibrosarcoma, and chondrosarcoma.
- There is an association between giant cell tumors (both solitary and multiple) and Paget's disease.
- Giant cell tumors of the skull and facial bones are almost always associated with Paget's disease.
- Metastatic disease, myeloma, and lymphoma may all occur in pagetic bone, although whether or not there is an increased or decreased incidence of metastatic disease in pagetic bone remains controversial.

Pathology

Three phases have been classically described, as above: the incipient-active (lytic) phase, the active (mixed) phase, and the late-inactive (blastic) phase.

Initially (lytic phase), there is prominent bone resorption by osteoclasts without attempted repair. Over time, osteoblastic activity increases, in an attempt at repair (mixed phase), and eventually overtakes osteoclastic activity. During the blastic phase, osteoblastic activity gradually diminishes.

Different stages of the disease often coexist in the same patient.

The end-stage pathologic changes are a "mosaic" or "jigsaw" pattern of disordered trabecular bone. Cement lines, due to osseous resorption and inadequate repair, are seen along the enlarged trabeculae. Both the cortical and trabecular bone demonstrate thickening. This thickened trabecular bone is architecturally abnormal, and thus, although it appears thick, it is actually weaker (pumice bone) than normal bone. Pagetic bone is also hypervascular and demonstrates prominent vascular channels.

During the lytic phase of disease, the normal fatty marrow is replaced with fibrovascular tissue. This in turn is replaced by fat as the disease progresses, eventually leading to an increase in the overall amount of marrow fat (atrophic marrow) compared with normal yellow marrow.

Imaging Findings

RADIOGRAPHY

- The most common sites of involvement include the pelvis (30 to 75%), spine (30 to 75%), skull (25 to 65%), and proximal long bones, such as the femur (25 to 35%) and humerus (31%).
- Polyostotic disease is encountered in the majority of cases (65 to 90%).
- The monostotic form typically involves the clavicle or the tibia.
- When the jaws are affected, this is sometimes referred to as a further "facial" subtype.
- Pelvic and appendicular involvement is often unilateral.
- In long bones, Paget's disease often begins as a subchondral lucency that extends from the epiphysis to the diaphysis at a rate of about 1 mm per month, producing a "blade of grass" or flame-shaped configuration (**Fig. 122D**). These sharply lytic lesions may cause cortical scalloping.
- Rarely, it may involve the diaphysis alone.
- The lytic phase is most commonly seen in the skull (osteoporosis or osteolysis circumscripta) (**Fig. 122E**).
- Skull involvement is usually more prominent in the inner table (as opposed to fibrous dysplasia, which tends to involve the outer table preferentially).
- The mixed lytic and sclerotic phase of the disease is the most commonly encountered form.
- Characteristic findings in the mixed phase include cortical thickening (ilioischial and iliopectineal lines commonly thickened in the pelvis), with interspersed lucencies and trabecular coarsening, usually along the lines of stress (**Fig. 122F**). In addition, at this stage, the bone may be grossly deformed.

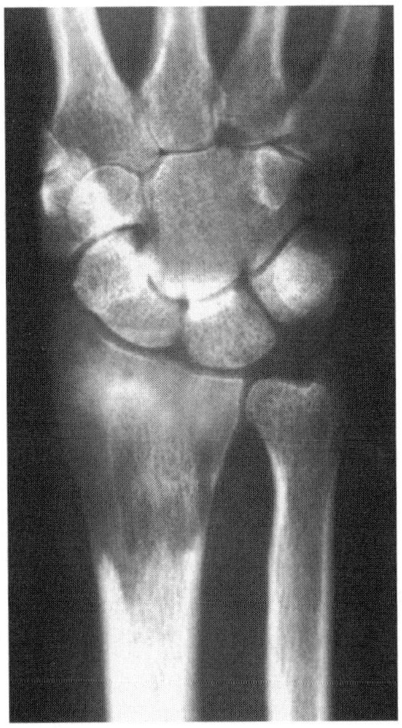

D

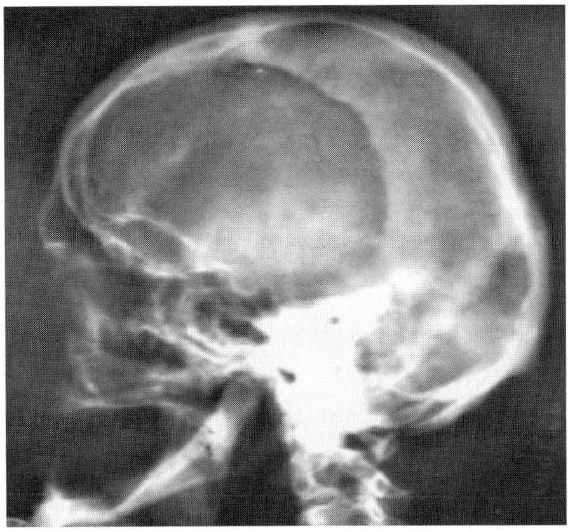

E

Figures 122D,122E 122D An anteroposterior (AP) radiograph of the distal radius and ulna show a sharply demarcated lucency in the distal radius extending from the epiphysis to the diaphysis: classic "blade of grass" appearance. **122E** A lateral radiograph of the skull shows a large sharply demarcated circular lucency in the frontal and parietal bones, typical of osteolysis circumscripta, found in the lytic phase of the disease.

- Pelvic changes are often asymmetric, with greater involvement of the right side.
- In the spine, a "picture frame" appearance is common in affected vertebral bodies due to thickening around all margins of the involved bone (**Fig. 122G**).
- Vertical trabecular thickening in the spine is common and appears more coarse than the corduroy appearance typically seen in spinal hemangiomas.
- Extensive sclerosis is the hallmark of the blastic phase (**Table 122–1**), producing dense, irregular trabeculae within thickened, deformed, and bowed bones (usually the tibia and femur).

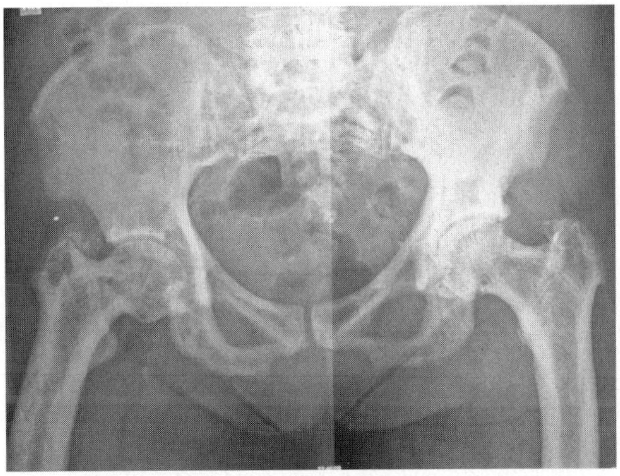

F

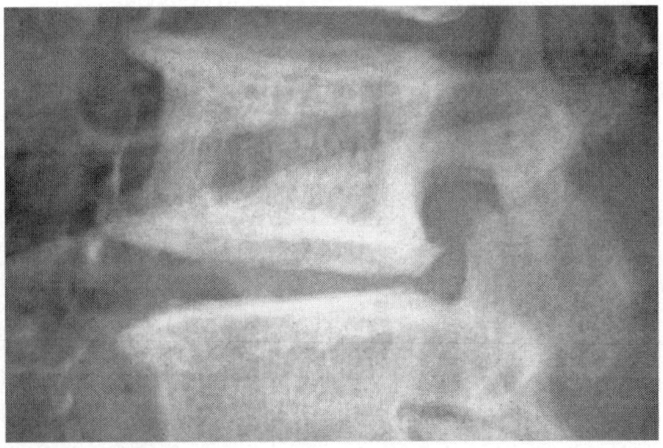

G

Figures 122F,122G 122F An AP radiograph of the pelvis shows trabecular coarsening and cortical thickening (including the ilioischial and iliopectineal lines). There is mixed lucency and patchy sclerosis throughout the pelvis, as well as mild expansion of the pubic rami and ischium. There is associated coxa vara deformity of the right hip. **122G** Image shows a typical "picture frame" appearance secondary to marginal thickening of the vertebral body.

Table 122–1 Diffuse Sclerosis: Differential Diagnosis

Metastatic disease (particularly breast and prostate)
Lymphoma
Myelofibrosis
Mastocytosis
Fluorosis
Renal osteodystrophy
Sickle cell disease
Gaucher's disease

- Osseous enlargement is most commonly associated with the blastic phase.
- Patchy, round areas of sclerosis that cross the sutures may produce a "cotton wool" appearance in the mixed phase (**Figs. 122H–122J**).
- Marked thickening of the inner table of the skull may be seen in the late phase ("tam-o'-shanter" skull) (**Fig. 122J**).
- Vertebral bodies often demonstrate diffuse sclerosis and enlargement during this phase, producing an "ivory vertebrae" appearance (**Fig. 122K**).

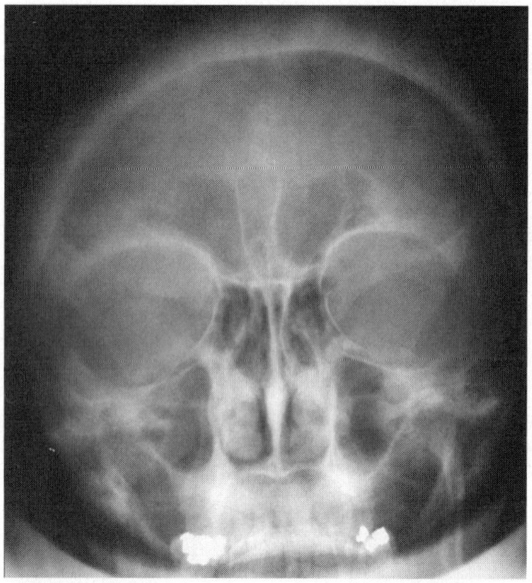

H

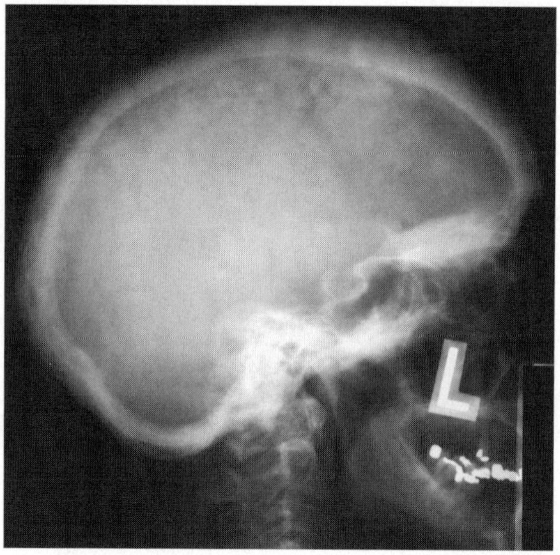

I

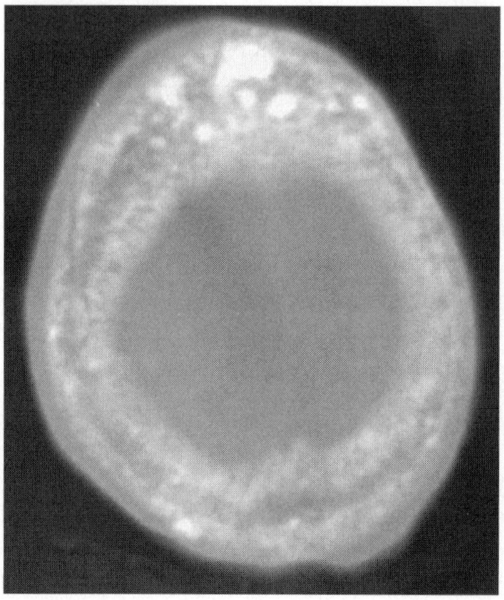

J

Figures 122H–122J AP (**122H**) and lateral (**122I**) radiographs of the skull and accompanying CT head on bone windows (**122J**) show innumerable patchy, round areas of sclerosis crossing sutural lines, producing a "cotton wool" appearance typical of the mixed phase. Note also the dramatic thickening of the inner table, which is likely to lead eventually to the so-called tam-o'-shanter skull of the late phase.

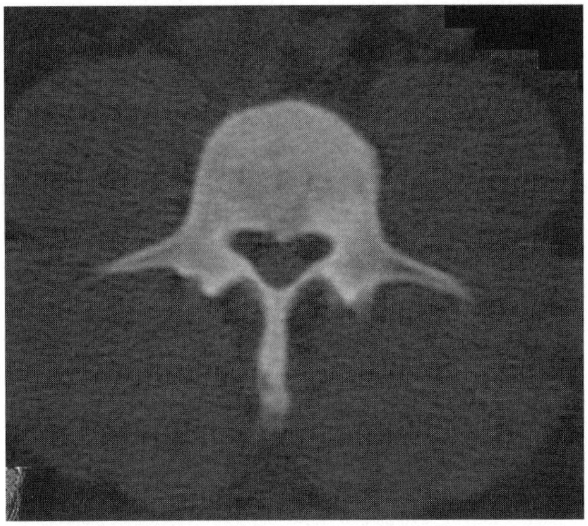

Figure 122K Transaxial CT through a vertebral body demonstrating the typical "ivory vertebra" appearance secondary to diffuse sclerosis and enlargement.

- The presence of bone enlargement (vertebral body with or without involvement of the posterior elements) is useful in distinguishing Paget's disease from other causes of an ivory vertebral body (**Table 122–2**).
- Pathological fractures are clearly depicted on plain radiographs.
- Sarcomatous transformation is seen as focal enlargement with overlying soft-tissue swelling with or without a pathological fracture.

SCINTIGRAPHY

- Intense increased activity in all three phases is typical (because of the hypervascularity of pagetic bone).
- Scintigraphy helps to identify the location and multiplicity of lesions in the polyostotic variety.
- In osteolysis circumscripta, only a rim of increased uptake is seen.
- Unlike metastatic disease, the region of increased activity is usually elongated in shape.
- Scintigraphic changes may be seen before radiographic changes.
- The radioisotope uptake varies in the three stages of the disease: in the late phase, increased activity may not be present.

COMPUTED TOMOGRAPHY

- Changes are similar to those seen on radiographs (lytic areas, disordered trabecular coarsening, cortical thickening, lytic/sclerotic medullary changes, osseous enlargement).
- Fatty marrow attenuation is most commonly seen.
- Trabecular disorganization is well seen.
- Cortical destruction should not be seen in uncomplicated Paget's disease.
- CT is often used to delineate spinal canal and nerve root involvement and to confirm the presence of sarcomatous changes.

Table 122–2 Ivory Vertebral Body: Differential Diagnosis

Paget's disease
Metastatic disease (particularly breast and prostate cancer)
Lymphoma
Chordoma
Unusual infection (tuberculosis)

MAGNETIC RESONANCE IMAGING

- Variable appearances, depending on the stage of disease
- Cortical thickening and trabecular coarsening are more difficult to appreciate on MRI than on radiographs or CT.
- Heterogeneously low signal on T1-weighted images and heterogeneously high signal on T2-weighted images in the active/lytic phase, likely related to fibrovascular marrow replacement
- Small islands of residual marrow should be identifiable in the active/lytic phase.
- In the mixed phase, marrow fat is largely preserved.
- There may even be increased fat in the marrow of pagetic bone relative to normal bone marrow during the mixed phase.
- When coarsened, the trabeculae appear hypointense on T1- and T2-weighted images intermixed within the marrow fat (**Figs. 122L–122N**).
- Focal fat collections ("fat cysts") may also be seen (**Figs. 122O–122P**).
- The size of the medullary cavity may be diminished secondary to cortical thickening.
- Diffuse low signal on T1- and T2-weighted images during the late/blastic phase

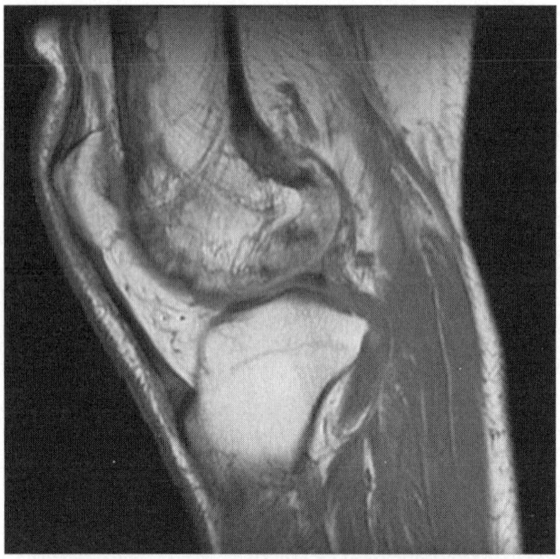
L

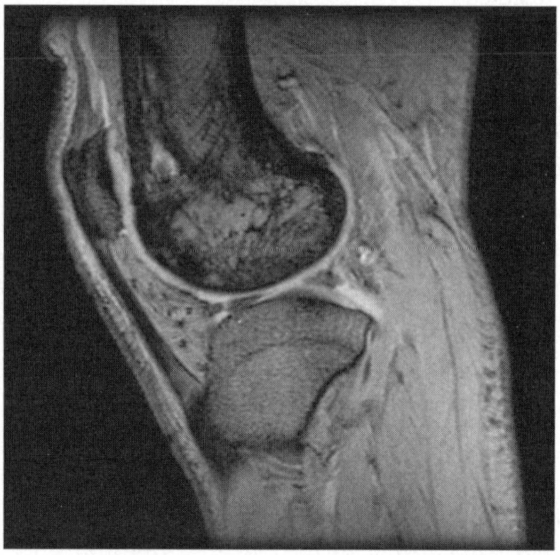
M

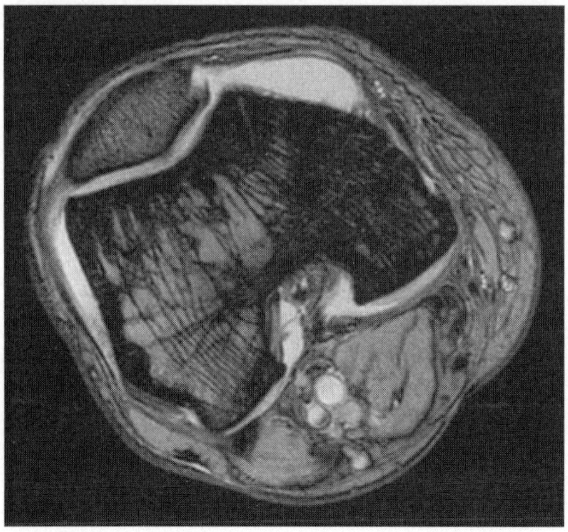
N

Figures 122L–122N Asymptomatic Paget's disease (mixed phase) of the femur discovered incidentally on imaging the knee joint. Sagittal T1-weighted (**122L**), sagittal T2-weighted (**122M**), and transaxial gradient-echo (**122N**) images show coarsened trabeculae as hypointense striations intermixed within the marrow fat. The cortex is grossly thickened and of predominantly low signal. There is a subtle reduction in marrow fat signal intensity when compared with that of the tibia, consistent with a degree of fibrous change.

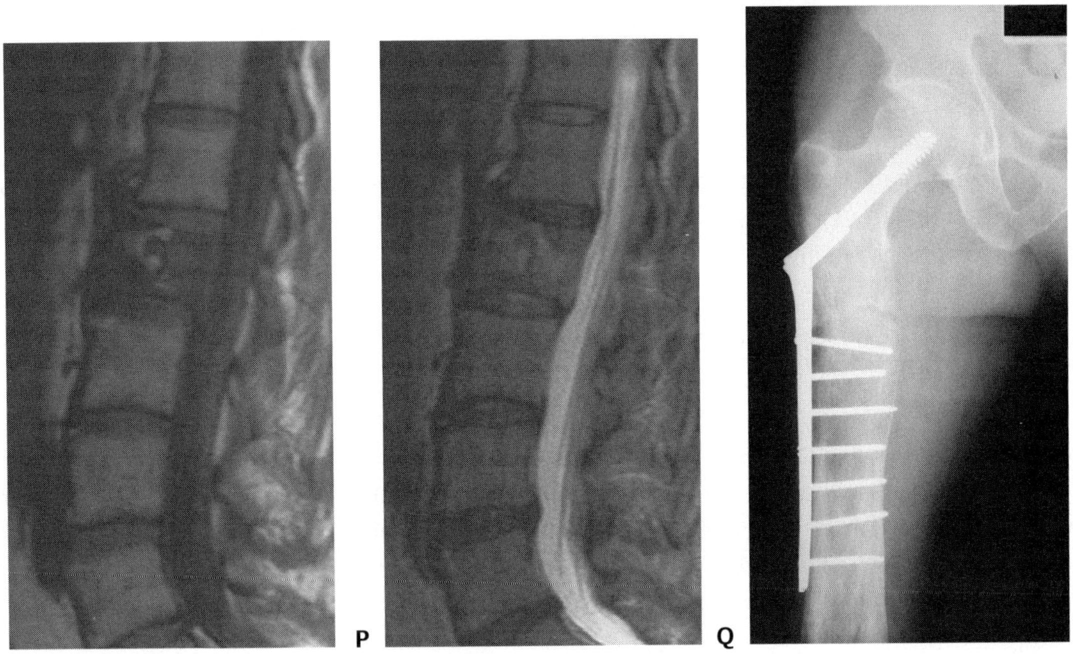

Figures 122O–122Q Sagittal T1-weighted (**122O**) and T2-weighted (**122P**) images of the lumbar spine show a focal fat collection ("fat cyst") (high signal intensity on both sequences) in an expanded vertebral body. **122Q** The image shows an open reduction and fixation with a dynamic hip screw of a pathological fracture through a severely affected proximal femoral shaft.

- A "pseudomass," due to elevation of the periosteal membrane in active Paget's disease, may rarely be seen and may simulate a tumor, but this should not be associated with bone destruction or marrow replacement.
- Cortical enhancement may be prominent during the active phase of disease.
- Medullary enhancement is usually in a speckled pattern.

Treatment

- Treatment is generally symptomatic with oral bisphosphonates, which reduce pain by decreasing bone resorption and formation.
- Calcitonin is also used to inhibit osteoclast activity.
- Pharmacologic treatment for pagetic spinal stenosis is very effective; therefore, surgical decompression is instituted only when secondary neural compression occurs due to pathologic fractures, or if dislocations, syringomyelia, platybasia, spontaneous epidural hematoma, or sarcomatous transformation has occurred.
- Long-bone deformities can be treated with corrective osteotomy.
- Pathologic fractures are reduced and fixed as necessary, often combined with osteotomy to correct the characteristic deformity (**Fig. 122Q**).
- Malignant transformation requires histologically appropriate surgery.

Prognosis

- Usually good unless there is malignant transformation
- Pagetic sarcoma has a poor prognosis, with a $<$ 90% 3-year survival rate.
- Fixation of pathological fractures may be complicated by delayed union or nonunion.

PEARLS

- Plain radiographic findings are very characteristic, and the only other modality needed is a bone scan to rule out the polyostotic variety. However, the risk of sarcomatous transformation (1%) warrants close follow-up with cross-sectional imaging.
- The pathological fractures of long bones occur on the convex aspect compared with the concave aspect in osteomalacia (Looser's zones).
- Skull involvement is usually more prominent in the inner table (as opposed to fibrous dysplasia, which tends to involve the outer table preferentially).

PITFALLS

- Involved vertebral bodies are dense and enlarged in size (picture frame appearance), as seen in lymphoma and metastasis. The presence of bone enlargement (vertebral body with or without involvement of the posterior elements) is useful in distinguishing Paget's disease from other causes of an ivory vertebral body.
- Unlike metastatic disease, the region of increased activity on radionuclide bone scanning is usually elongated in shape.
- Scintigraphic changes may be seen before radiographic changes.
- The radioisotope uptake varies in the three stages of the disease: in the late phase, increased activity may not be present.

Suggested Readings

Paget J. On a form of chronic inflammation of bones (osteitis deformans). Med Chir Tr 1877;60:37

Roberts MC, Kressel HY, Fallon MD, Zlatkin MB, Dalinka MK. Paget disease: MR imaging findings. Radiology 1989;173:341–345

Smith J, Botet JF, Yeh SD. Bone sarcomas in Paget disease: a study of 85 patients. Radiology 1984;152:583–590

Smith SE, Murphey MD, Motamedi K, Mulligan ME, Resnik CS, Gannon FH. From the Archives of the AFIP. Radiologic spectrum of Paget disease of bone and its complications with pathologic correlation. Radiographics 2002;22:1191–1216

CASE 123

George Nomikos, Anthony G. Ryan, Peter L. Munk, and Mark Murphey

Clinical Presentation

A 34-year-old man presented to the emergency department with leg pain. He had no history of trauma.

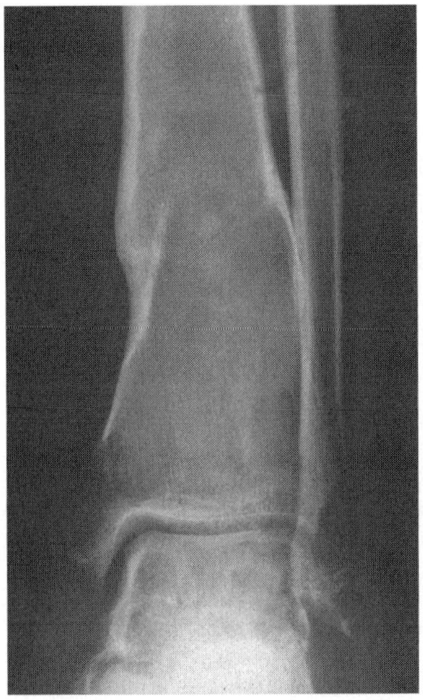

Figure 123A

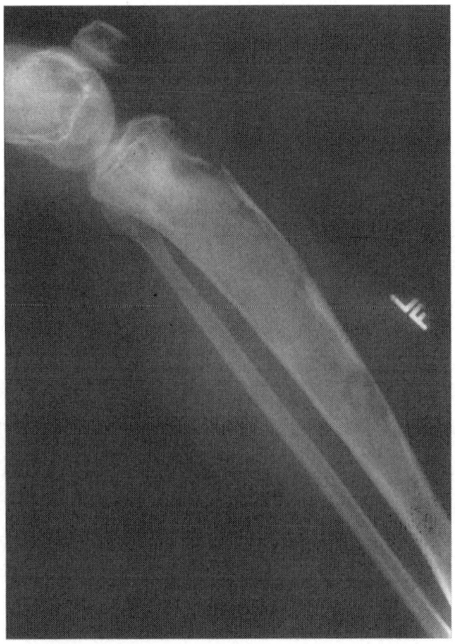

Figure 123B

Radiologic Findings

An anteroporsterior (AP) radiograph of the ankle and a lateral radiograph of the lower leg are provided (**Figs. 123A,123B**). These images show two lesions in the tibia, both of which demonstrate mild expansile remodeling of the bone and an internal ground glass appearance. There is associated cortical thinning and endosteal scalloping without evidence of cortical penetration. There is evidence of an old healed pathologic fracture through the more distal lesion.

Diagnosis

Polyostotic fibrous dysplasia.

Differential Diagnosis

None.

Discussion

Background

This process may affect a single bone or be polyostotic. The vast majority of cases affect a single bone, with approximately a quarter of patients having multiple bones affected. When a single bone is affected, the rib, femur, tibia, or mandible is most frequently involved, although virtually all osseous structures may be affected. In patients with polyostotic dysplasia, a single limb may be affected, or a single side of the body. The entire skeleton is never affected.

Etiology

Fibrous dysplasia (a separate and distinct entity from osteofibrous dysplasia) is not a true neoplasm, but rather a noninherited developmental marrow-packing abnormality caused by a mutation that alters the gene controlling osteoblastic cell growth and differentiation.

Pathophysiology

The normal contents of the medullary canal are replaced by immature fibro-osseous tissue due to abnormal differentiation of osteoblasts. The affected osteoblasts do not undergo normal development and maturation, resulting in immature woven bone being present in the afflicted structures. Bowing of affected bones occurs because the bones are weakened by expansion of the lesion in the intramedullary aspect of the bone. Microfractures result in progressive deformity, and these patients are also prone to pathologic fractures and stress fractures. Typically, these bowing deformities are unilateral.

Clinical Findings

Patients may also present with leg length discrepancies and cosmetic deformities, particularly when the disease affects the facial bones and mandible. Patients with monostotic disease may have the disease noted incidentally when radiography is performed for some other indication.

Although the onset is usually in childhood, patients are most commonly adolescents or young adults at the time of diagnosis, with 75% presenting before age 30. There is a relatively equal sex predilection.

The monostotic form accounts for the majority (~80%) of cases. Patients with the polyostotic form of the disease tend to present earlier. Small lesions are often asymptomatic. Although the lesions are often painless, common presenting symptoms may include pain and swelling, which may, on occasion, be caused by pathologic fracture. Alternatively, bowing deformity may bring the patient to clinical attention. Vaginal bleeding has been reported as the presenting complaint in up to 25% of female patients with polyostotic fibrous dysplasia due to associated hormone abnormalities (see below). Involvement in the polyostotic form of the disease may be diffuse. Lesions may become more active during pregnancy, leading to increased pain, pathologic fracture, and secondary aneurysmal bone cyst (ABC) formation.

Extensive involvement of frontal and facial bones may produce a lionlike facies (leontiasis ossea).

Up to 30% of patients with polyostotic fibrous dysplasia may demonstrate café-au-lait spots. The combination of polyostotic fibrous dysplasia (usually unilateral), café-au-lait spots (usually ipsilateral), and endocrine abnormalities (e.g., precocious puberty in females) is called McCune-Albright syndrome. Mazabraud's syndrome is a noninherited, nonfamilial association of soft-tissue myxomas of muscle in association with fibrous dysplasia.

Complications

- Pathologic fracture
- Deformity
- Neurologic and cranial nerve abnormalities may be associated with skull and facial lesions.
- Malignant transformation (usually to osteosarcoma) is rare (< 1% of cases).
- Malignant transformation is more common in the polyostotic form of the disease but also occurs in monostotic disease.

Pathology

GROSS

Areas of hemorrhage, cyst formation, and secondary ABC formation may occur.

MICROSCOPIC

Histologically, fibrous dysplasia is composed of irregular spindles of woven bone trabeculae, which are irregular in morphology and have been described as resembling Chinese text characters. This woven bone is usually nonmineralized and is surrounded by a fibrocellular matrix. Areas of cartilage may be present. Lesions containing more woven bone tend to appear denser radiographically than those containing more fibrous tissue.

Imaging Findings

RADIOGRAPHY

Normal trabecular and cortical bone on radiography is noted to be replaced with bone that has a rather hazy appearance that has classically been described as ground glass. Patients who have a significant fibrous or cystic component to the bone may appear frankly radiolucent.

In children, there is progressive growth of lesions. As the skeleton matures, growth typically slows down appreciably and may cease entirely. Although true cystic change can typically be seen in fibrous dysplasia of the ribs, this is encountered less frequently elsewhere in the skeleton.

- Common sites of disease in the monostotic form include the ribs, proximal femur, and craniofacial bones.
- Commonly affected areas in the polyostotic form include the craniofacial bones, femur, tibia, pelvis, feet, shoulder, and spine (**Figs. 123C,123D**).
- Lesions may be central or eccentric and usually involve the diametaphysis when they occur in long bones.
- Epiphyseal involvement before closure of the physis is rare.
- Lesions do not arise from the cortex.
- Polyostotic fibrous dysplasia may be unilateral or bilateral (although usually predominant on one side of the body) and is more commonly associated with deformities than the monostotic form of the disease.
- Endosteal scalloping, cortical thinning, and expansile remodeling are common.
- A thick sclerotic rim may be present.
- Lesions without a sclerotic margin usually have a narrow zone of transition.
- May demonstrate a loculated appearance due to subperiosteal bone reinforcement (**Figs. 123E,123F**)
- Periosteal reaction indicates pathologic fracture or malignant transformation (rare).
- Characteristic "ground glass" appearance due to the spicules of woven bone in the fibrous tissue (**Fig. 123G**)

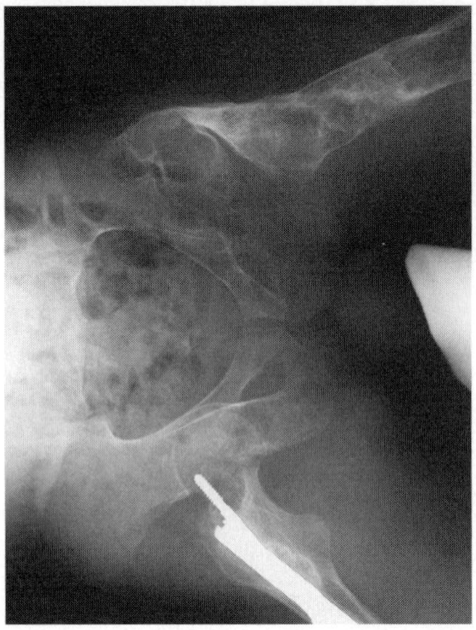

C

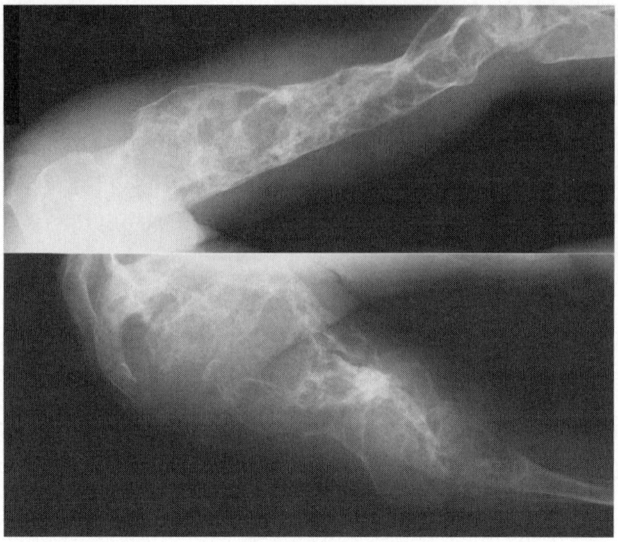

D

Figures 123C,123D Multiple examples of polyostotic fibrous dysplasia. **123C** Radiograph demonstrates bilateral involvement; affecting the right hip (previously fractured and repaired), right ischium, and left hip, where a prominent "shepherd's crook" type deformity is present. **123D** Radiograph demonstrates bilateral upper limb involvement resulting in severe deformity of both humeri, particularly the right, where marked shortening is evident. In addition, lesions are evident in both ulnae.

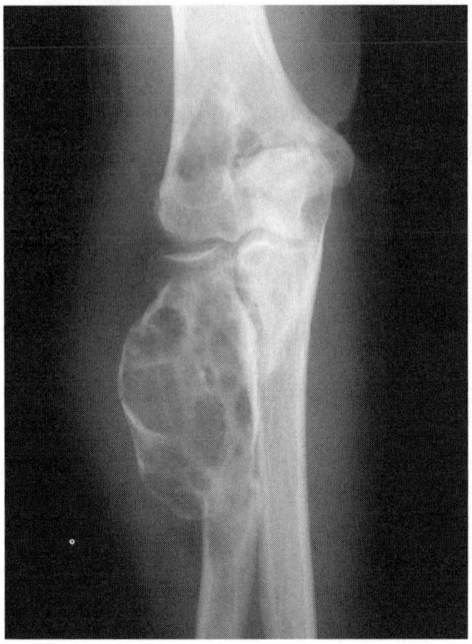

E

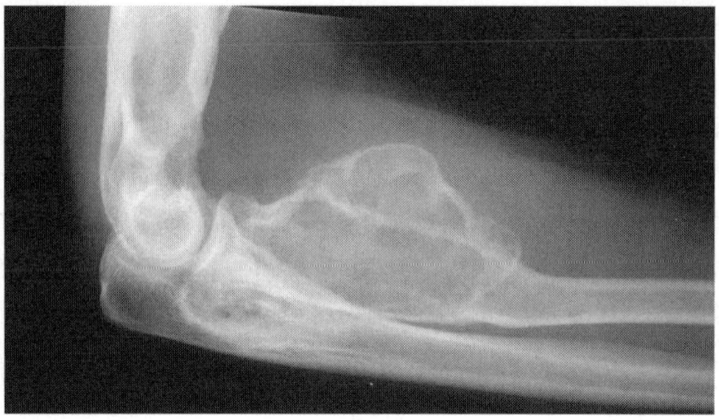

F

Figures 123E,123F AP (**123E**) and lateral (**123F**) radiographs of the elbow show a loculated appearance of the proximal radial diametaphysis due to subperiosteal bone reinforcement.

- Punctate or flocculent calcification possible (in areas of cartilage)
- Skull lesions often cause expansion of the diploic space and predominant remodeling of the outer table (**Figs. 123H,123I**).
- Shepherd's crook deformity (varus bowing) of the proximal femur is common in proximal lesions (**Figs. 123C,123J**).
- Pre-CT, conventional tomography was used to demonstrate rib lesions elegantly (**Fig. 123K**).

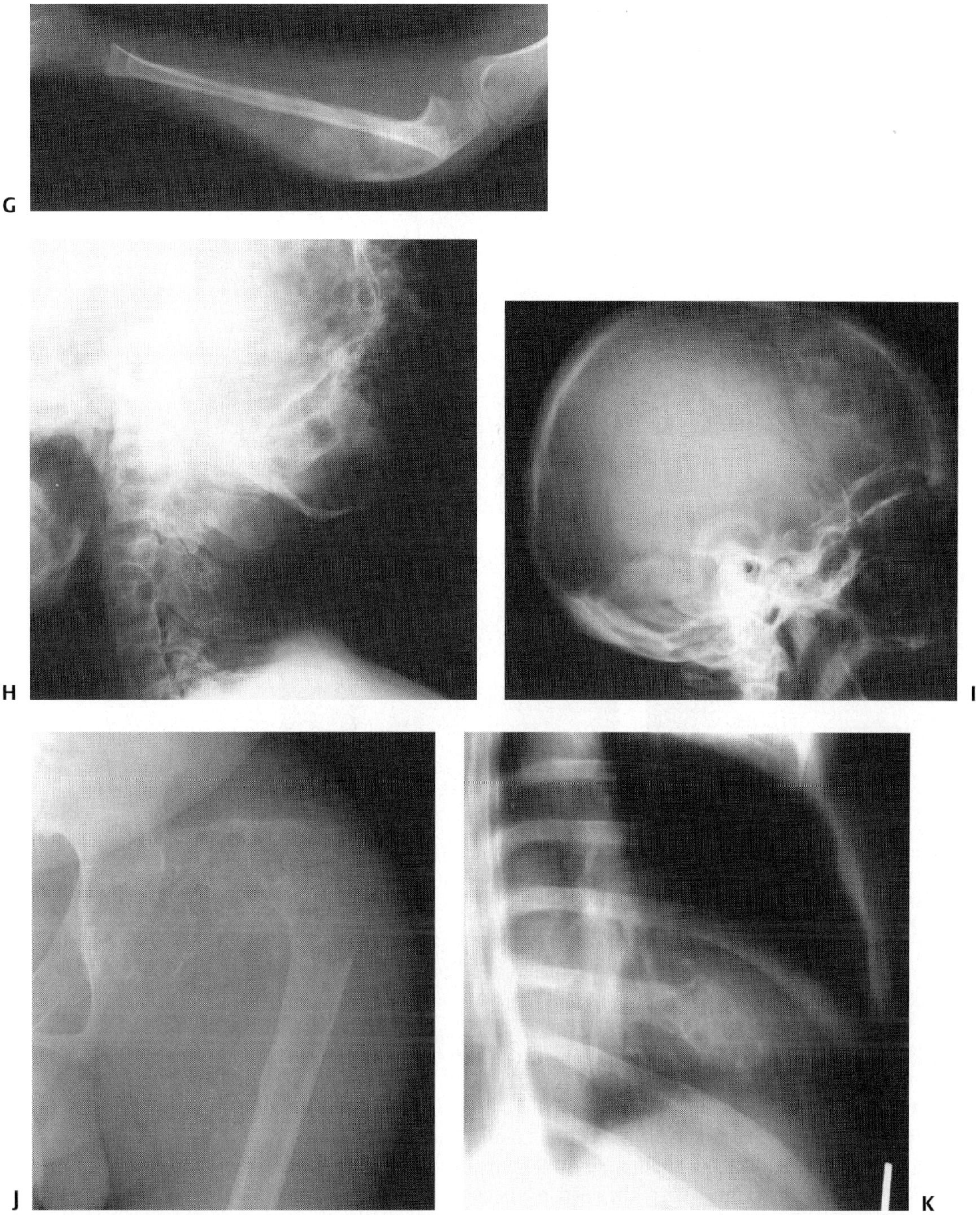

Figures 123G–123K **123G** Lateral radiograph of the forearm in a child with fibrous dysplasia affecting almost the entirety of the ulna demonstrates the characteristic "ground glass" appearance. **123H,123I** Radiographs of the skull in two patients with polyostotic fibrous dysplasia, affecting the occipital bone in **123E** and the frontal bone in **123H**. **123J** Radiograph of the left hip shows a classic shepherd's crook deformity (varus bowing) of the proximal femur. **123K** Conventional tomography of the posterior ribs clearly shows an expansile loculated lesion of the left 10th rib.

SCINTIGRAPHY

- Best method to determine extent of disease
- Activity often only mildly increased in first two phases but usually markedly increased on images of the third phase

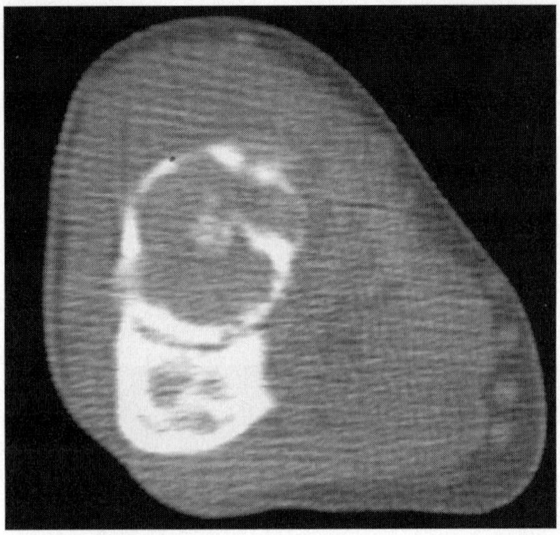
L

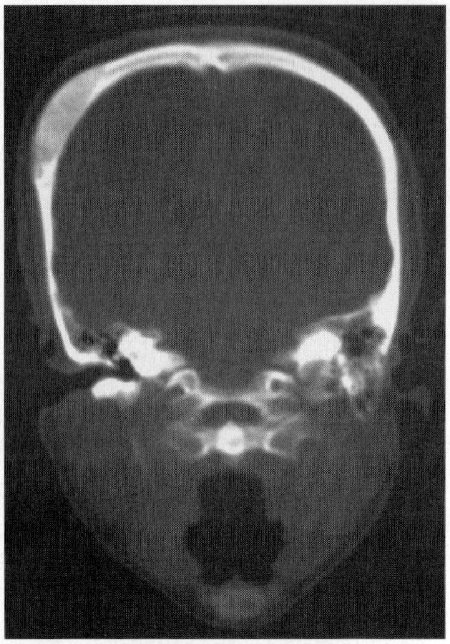
M

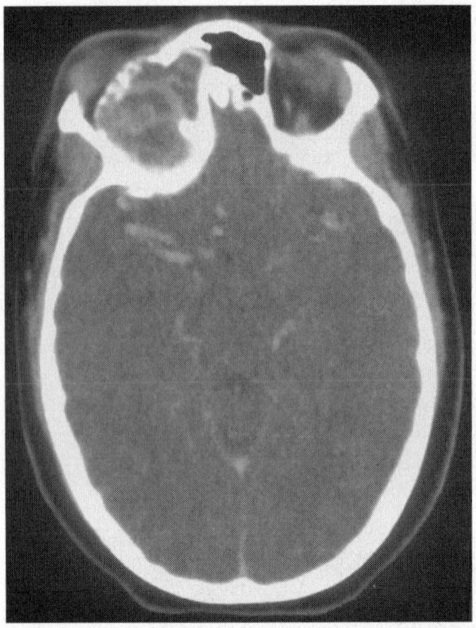
N

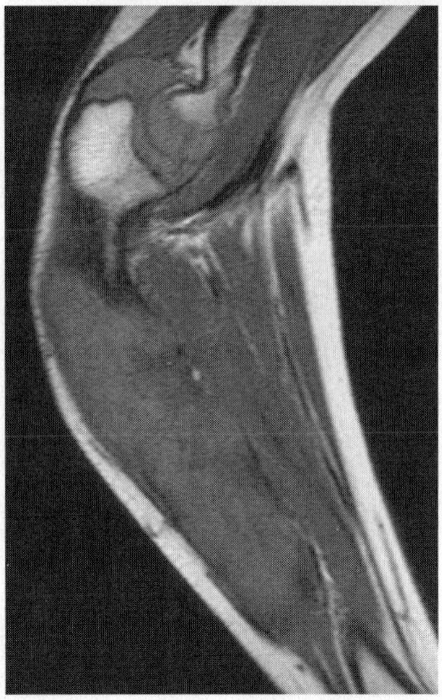
O

Figures 123L–123O **123L** Transaxial image from CT of the radial lesion in **Figs. 123E** and **123F** shows expansion, loculation, and marked cortical thinning. **123M** Coronal image from CT of the head shows an expansile lesion of the right parietal bone with a "smoky" internal attenuation affecting primarily the outer table. **123N** Transaxial image from CT of the head in a patient with a right orbital lesion shows sclerosis and modeling deformity of the superior orbit and heterogeneous internal architecture. (See **123P** and **123V** for corresponding MRI.) **123O** Sagittal T1-weighted MRI of the ulnar lesion shown in **123G**, showing signal intensity slightly hyperintense to skeletal muscle.

COMPUTED TOMOGRAPHY

- Useful for the further characterization of lesions demonstrated on conventional radiography (**Fig. 123L**), evaluation of craniofacial lesions (**Figs. 123M,123N**), impingement on adjacent structures, or suspected malignant transformation
- Variable appearance depending on amount of mineralization, hemorrhage, cyst formation
- Fluid levels may be visible in secondary ABC component.

MAGNETIC RESONANCE IMAGING

- Excellent for determining extent of involvement
- Usually similar to muscle on T1-weighted images (**Fig. 123O**), although areas of hemorrhage (secondary ABC formation) may be high signal on T1-weighted images
- Variable on T2-weighted images
- Lesions appear hyperintense to fat on T2-weighted images (60% of cases) (**Figs. 123P–123U**), intermediate on T2-weighting (20% of cases), or low signal intensity on T2-weighting (20% of cases).
- Low signal intensity in some lesions on T2-weighted images may be due to an increased number of osseous trabeculae.
- MRI demonstrates fluid levels in areas of secondary ABC formation well (**Fig. 123V**).
- Contrast enhancement is variable (**Fig. 123W**).

Treatment and Prognosis

- Dependent on the extent of disease and associated complications

PEARLS

- Although a thick sclerotic rim may be present, lesions without a sclerotic margin usually have a narrow zone of transition.
- The combination of polyostotic fibrous dysplasia (usually unilateral), café-au-lait spots (usually ipsilateral), and endocrine abnormalities (e.g., precocious puberty in females) is called McCune-Albright syndrome.
- The association of fibrous dysplasia and intramuscular myxomas is designated Mazabraud's syndrome.

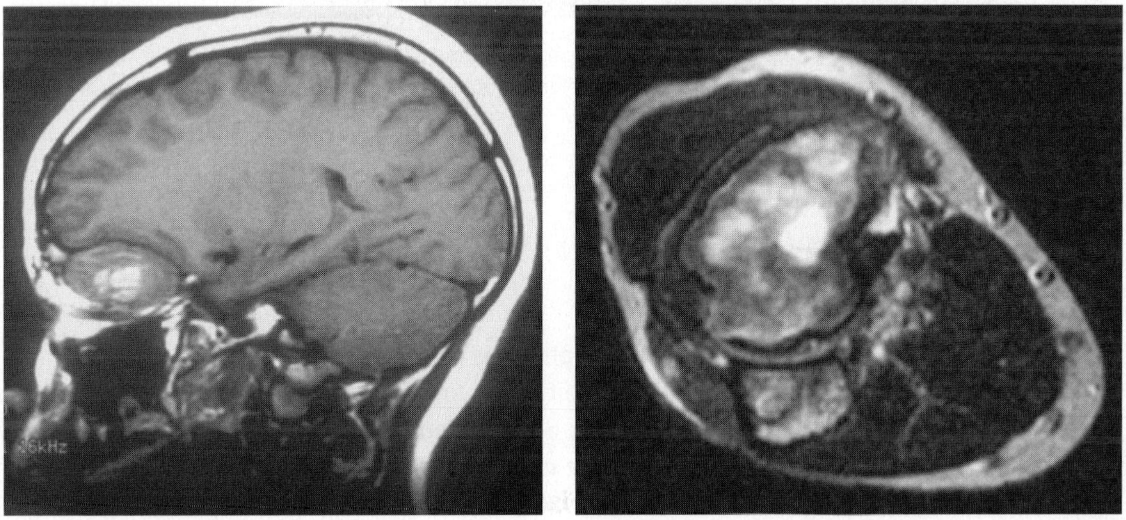

P Q

Figures 123P,123Q The sagittal T2-weighted head (**123P**) shows high signal intensity (hyperintense to fat) with the orbital lesion, and the transaxial (**123Q**) image of the ulnar lesion (in **123O**) shows internal high signal intensity throughout with areas of more focally increased intensity.

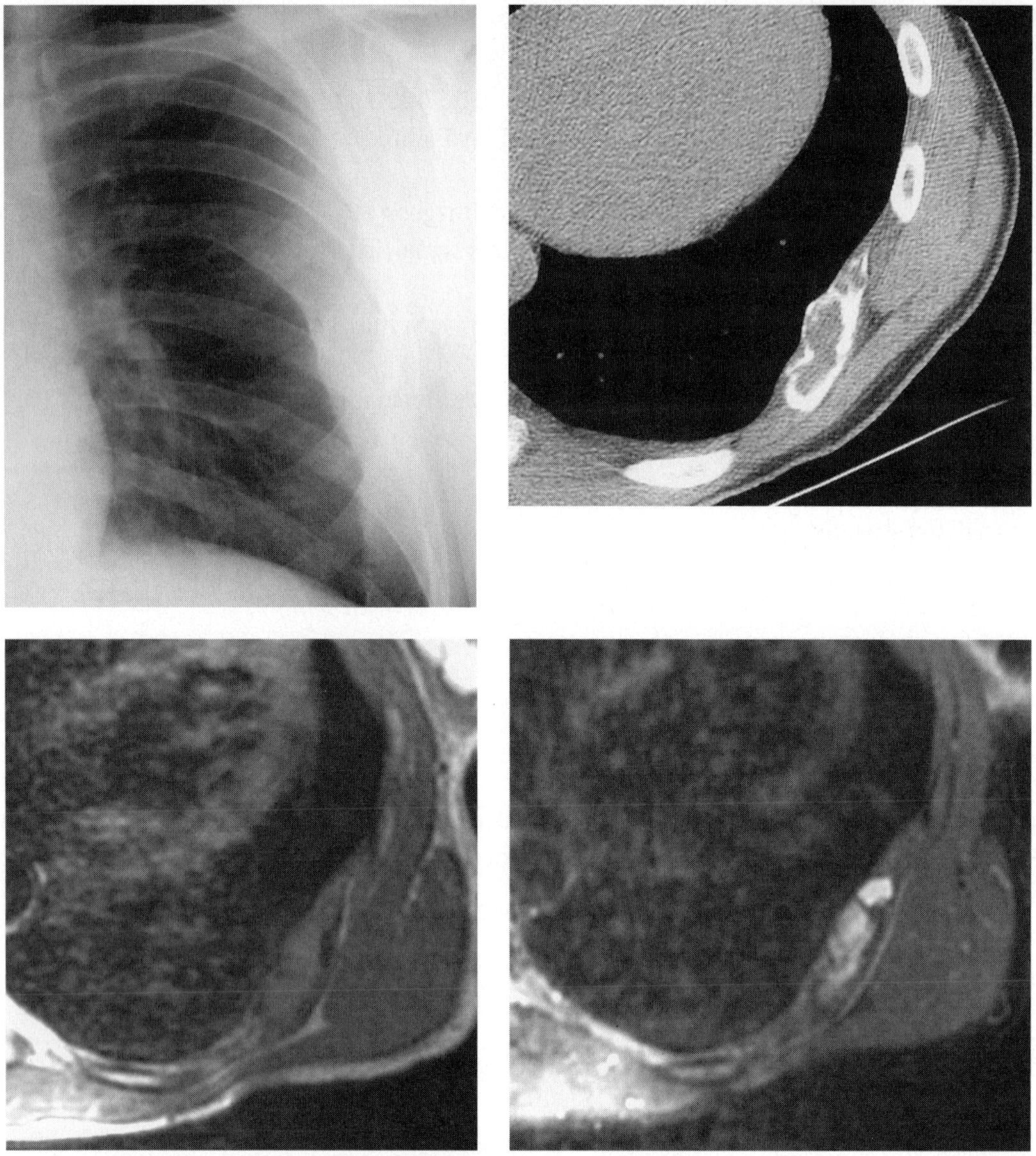

Figures 123R–123U Conventional radiograph (**123R**) and corresponding CT (**123S**) show an expansile monostotic rib lesion demonstrating relative hyperintensity to skeletal muscle on T1-weighted (**123T**) and hyperintensity on T2-weighted fat-saturated (**123U**) images.

PITFALLS

- Epiphyseal involvement before closure of the physis is rare.
- Skull lesions often cause expansion of the diploic space and predominant remodeling of the outer table as compared with Paget's disease, which affects predominantly the inner table.
- Of note, cherubism is a distinct disorder to the extensive involvement of frontal and facial bones seen in fibrous dysplasia (producing a lionlike facies: leontiasis ossea). The underlying pathologic process in cherubism is not fibrous dysplasia but rather a process pathologically indistinguishable from giant cell reparative granuloma. In cherubism, there is extensive involvement of the mandible and maxilla.

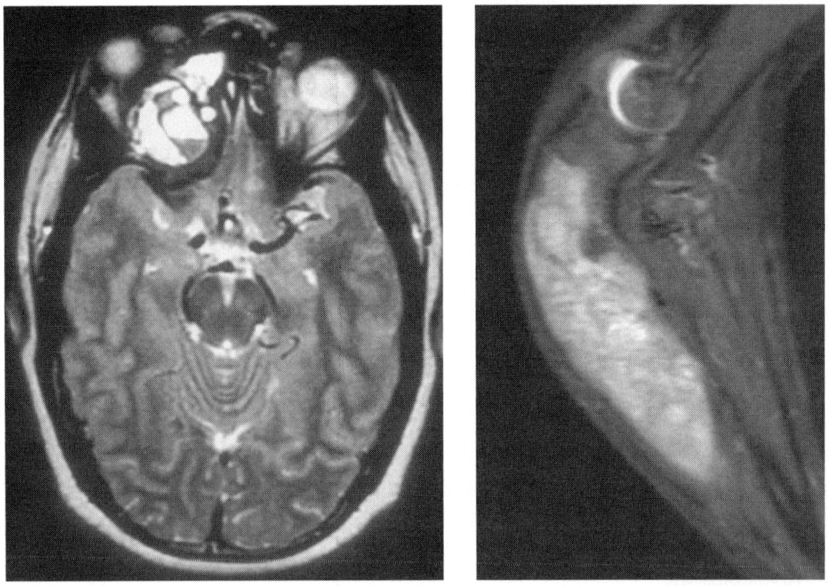

V W

Figures 123V,123W 123V Transaxial T2-weighted image of the orbital lesion shows fluid levels in areas of secondary aneurysmal bone cyst formation. **123W** T1-weighted fat-saturated image after intravenous gadolinium shows diffuse, but not intense, contrast enhancement.

Suggested Readings

Fitzpatrick KA, Taljanovic MS, Speer DP, et al. Imaging findings of fibrous dysplasia with histopathologic and intraoperative correlation. Am J Roentgenol 2004;182:1389–1398

Iwasko N, Steinbach LS, Disler D, et al. Imaging findings in Mazabraud's syndrome: seven new cases. Skeletal Radiol 2002;31:81–87

Jee WH, Choi KH, Choe BY, Park JM, Shinn KS. Fibrous dysplasia: MR imaging characteristics with radiographic correlation. Am J Roentgenol 1996;167:1523–1527

Kransdorf MJ, Moser RP Jr, Gilkey FW. Fibrous dysplasia. Radiographics 1990;10:519–537

Smith SE, Kransdorf MJ. Primary musculoskeletal tumors of fibrous origin. Semin Musculoskelet Radiol 2000;4:73–88

Struk DW, Munk PL, Lee MJ. Musculoskeletal case 8. Mazabraud's syndrome—intramuscular myxoma associated with fibrous dysplasia. Can J Surg 2000;43:15,62–63

CASE 124

Peter L. Munk and Anthony G. Ryan

Clinical Presentation

A 58-year-old man presented with pain in his leg, with erythema and swelling visible overlying his shin distally.

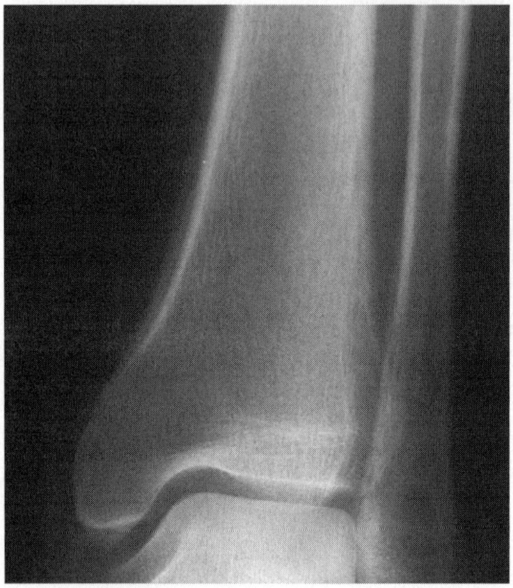

Figure 124A

Radiologic Findings

A coned view of the distal tibia (**Fig. 124A**) shows a subtle sclerotic line paralleling the medial aspect of the tibial cortex.

Diagnosis

Secondary hypertrophic pulmonary osteoarthropathy (HPOA) (Marie-Bamberger disease).

Differential Diagnosis

Differential of a periosteal reaction, including underlying osteomyelitis or neoplasm.

Discussion

Background

This condition is composed of a triad consisting of clubbing of the digits and painful joints (secondary to synovitis) with accompanying periosteal new bone formation.

Etiology

HPOA is most frequently associated with underlying intrathoracic causes. Other conditions producing chronic inflammation have also been reported to precipitate this condition. The vast majority of patients have bronchogenic carcinoma (particularly adenocarcinoma and squamous carcinoma), although other conditions, such as mesothelioma, pulmonary abscess, and bronchiectasis, as well as metastatic disease, have been reported as causes. It is estimated that at least 5% of patients with bronchogenic carcinoma will develop HPOA.

Nonthoracic causes have also been described, including chronic liver disease (e.g., biliary cirrhosis and Wilson's disease), Crohn's disease, gastrointestinal tract malignancies, and chronic infection of vascular grafts. More recently, HPOA has been described as a noninfectious musculoskeletal association of acquired immunodeficiency syndrome.

In the pediatric age group, a common underlying condition is cystic fibrosis.

Pathophysiology

Although the underlying cause is unclear, the condition appears to be neurogenically mediated, as a paraneoplastic syndrome, producing the release of vasodilators and leading to increased blood flow, particularly noted in the distribution of the vagus nerve. Other theories suggest a hormonal origin, with estrogen, prostaglandin, and various growth factors implicated; 10% of bronchogenic carcinomas have a hormonal output.

Clinical Findings

The majority of patients are middle-aged men, frequently presenting initially with clubbing of the digits, which, in the case of bronchogenic carcinoma, may be of relatively rapid onset and quite painful. This is secondary to soft-tissue hypertrophy and is not associated typically with changes in the underlying phalangeal tufts.

Associated symptoms in the joints may be present at this time or develop later. Synovitis is said to develop in as many as 40% of patients with bronchogenic carcinoma. Patients usually present with one or several burning, painful, tender joints. Most commonly affected are the ankles (88%), wrists (83%), and knees (75%). Synovial effusions are common.

Symptoms tend to be aggravated by movement and are worse at night.

The skin overlying the affected joints may be warm and reddened, or pale and cyanosed, and may be associated with paresthesias and sweating. The symptomatology may resemble that of rheumatoid arthritis, and the two conditions are often mistaken in the acute phase.

Associated gynecomastia is relatively common.

Pathology

GROSS

- Thick periosteal new bone formation

MICROSCOPIC

- Synovitis and periostitis, the latter representing a reaction to round cell infiltration of the outer fibrous layer followed by new bone proliferation

Imaging Findings

RADIOGRAPHY

- Radiography of the hands may demonstrate the soft-tissue swelling underlying the patient's clubbing, and joint effusions may be detectable.

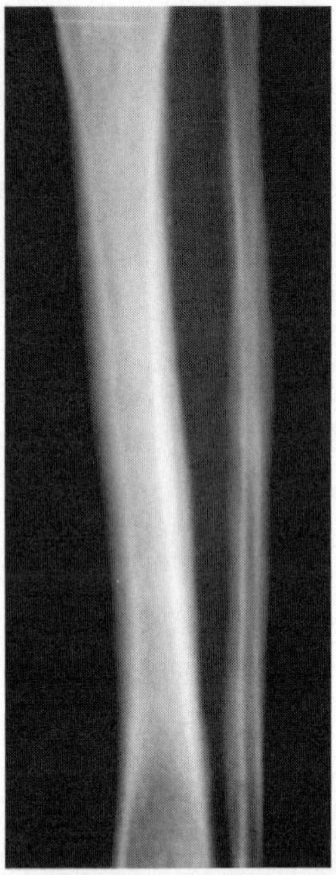
B

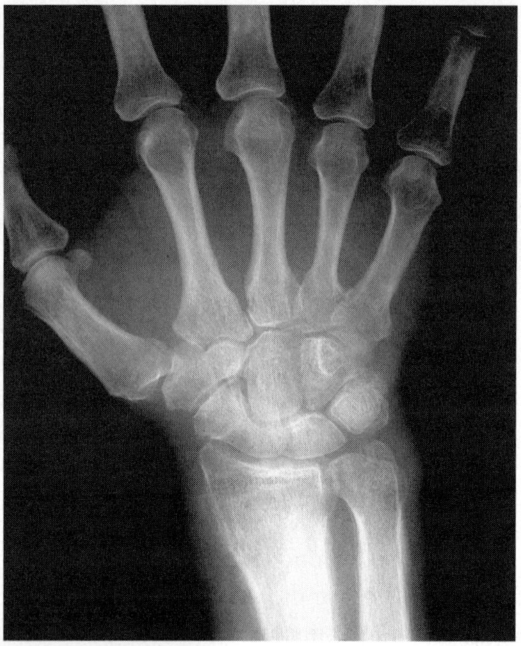
C

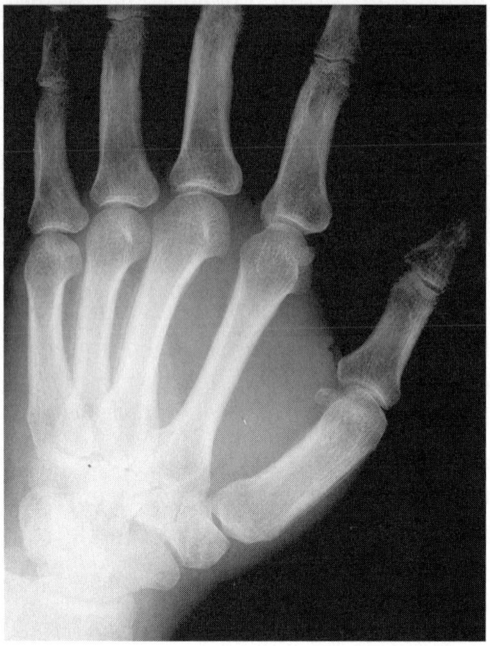
D

Figures 124B–124D 124B An anteroposterior (AP) radiograph of the tibia and fibula shows a thick periosteal reaction along the length of the fibula. A more subtle reaction is evident on the fibular aspect of the tibia. **124C** An AP radiograph of the wrist shows a subtle periosteal reaction affecting the distal extent of both the radius and the ulna. **124D** Oblique view of the hand shows a thin periosteal reaction affecting the lengths of the first, third, and fourth metacarpals.

- Periostitis is the principal finding, giving rise to the most striking change seen in this disorder: a marked periosteal reaction that may be thick and undulating (**Fig. 124B**) or smooth and thin, especially early in the process.
- The diaphyses are usually affected initially, although, as the disease progresses, metaphyseal involvement is noted.
- The tibia and fibula are typically affected, as are the radius and ulna (**Fig. 124C**), although other long bones, including phalanges (**Fig. 124D**), may be affected.
- Spiculated and hair-on-end periosteal reaction has also been reported. Even with correction of the underlying disease process, radiographic changes are slow to resolve.

RADIONUCLIDE IMAGING

- Unsurprisingly, changes are evident earlier than on radiography, as increased cortical uptake along the shafts of the affected bones produce a "double stripe" or "parallel track" sign.
- Increased periarticular uptake is evident in those with an associated synovitis.
- Scapular (66%) and mandibular (40%) involvement is common.

MAGNETIC RESONANCE IMAGING

- Periosteal reaction is evident as a thin, wavy, hypointense line outside a rim of hyperintensity on T2-weighted images.
- Edema may be present in the adjacent muscles.
- Well-defined soft-tissue swelling overlying the femoral cortex, high on T2-weighted and STIR images, is thought to represent inflammatory change, including round cell infiltration of the outer fibrous layer.
- Adjacent joint effusion may be evident.

Treatment

- Nonsteroidal anti-inflammatory drugs (NSAIDs) and intercostal nerve blocks are given to relieve pain initially.
- Vagal interruption, either by percutaneous ablation or at thoracotomy, may cause regression.
- Interestingly, thoracotomy is reported to frequently relieve symptoms in these patients even if resection of the underlying precipitating cause is not possible.

Prognosis

Although radiographic changes are slow to resolve with correction of the underlying disease process, relief of symptoms secondary to the arthropathy is usually rapid.

In cases where it is not possible to treat the underlying cause, the associated pain may be controlled with NSAIDs, steroids, and bisphosphonates.

PEARLS

- The demonstration of HPOA on a radiograph should initiate further investigation, starting with a chest radiograph.
- Metaphyseal involvement is usually a late feature, and if it appears dominant in relation to the diaphyseal involvement, the adjacent epiphysis and joint should be carefully examined for evidence of septic arthritis. Obviously, this does not apply when the osseous involvement is bilaterally symmetric.
- The periosteal new bone formation is most marked on the concavity of the tubular bones affected.
- HPOA may be differentiated from metastatic disease on radionuclide imaging by its distribution throughout the appendicular skeleton in a symmetric diffuse fashion, compared with metastatic disease, which is characteristically manifested by focal, irregular, asymmetric distribution throughout the axial skeleton.

PITFALLS

- The symptomatology may resemble that of rheumatoid arthritis, and the two conditions are often mistaken in the acute phase.

- The clubbing associated with HPOA is secondary to soft-tissue hypertrophy and is not associated typically with changes in the underlying phalangeal tufts.
- In cases where no underlying cause is evident, the differential for bilaterally symmetrical periosteal reaction in adults applies:
  - Vascular insufficiency (venous or arterial; in the former, the presence of phleboliths suggests the diagnosis)
  - Thyroid acropachy (the clinical setting should be self-explanatory)
  - Fluorosis (diffuse osteosclerosis is usually evident; ligamentous calcification is a prominent feature)
- Pachydermoperiostosis is described as a primary form of HPOA, and is responsible for a bilaterally symmetrical periosteal reaction, but this typically affects adolescent males of African descent as a primary phenomenon rather than as a manifestation of underlying malignancy or chronic suppuration.

Suggested Readings

Capelastegui A, Astigarraga E, Garcia-Iturraspe C. MR findings in pulmonary hypertrophic osteoarthropathy. Clin Radiol 2000;55(1):72–75

Davies RA, Darby M, Richards MA. Hypertrophic pulmonary osteoarthropathy in pulmonary metastatic disease: a case report and review of the literature. Clin Radiol 1991;43(4):268–271

Morgan B, Coakley F, Finlay DB, Belton I. Hypertrophic osteoarthropathy in staging skeletal scintigraphy for lung cancer. Clin Radiol 1996;51(10):694–697

CASE 125

Peter L. Munk and Anthony G. Ryan

Clinical Presentation

A 37-year-old man presented with a complaint of lower back pain.

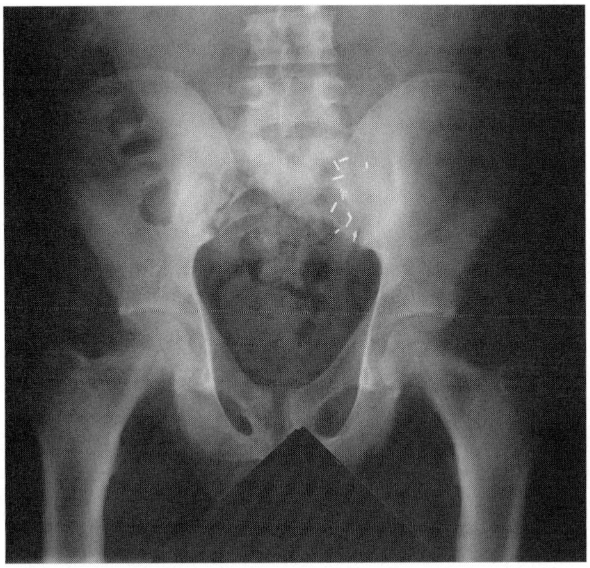

Figure 125A

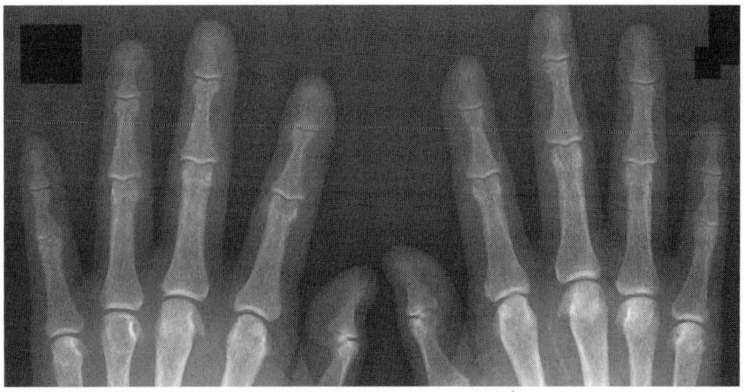

Figure 125B

Radiologic Findings

An anteroposterior radiograph of the pelvis (**Fig. 125A**) shows multiple surgical clips in the left lower quadrant, marked osteoporosis of both femoral heads, and apparent healing fractures of the pubic rami bilaterally.

A coned view of the distal hands (**Fig. 125B**) shows osteoporosis with cortical irregularity and subperiosteal lucency on the radial aspects of the phalanges and subtle lucency of the distal phalangeal tufts.

Diagnosis

Renal osteodystrophy (secondary hyperparathyroidism).

The pubic abnormalities are Looser's zones: pseudofractures secondary to osteomalacia. The surgical clips are in relation to a renal transplant (failed).

Differential Diagnosis

None.

Discussion

Background

Renal osteodystrophy is a constellation of clinical, pathologic, and radiologic manifestations seen in patients with chronic renal disease.

The radiological manifestations are diverse and fall into several categories. With the increasing utilization of hemodialysis and aggressive management of patients with renal disease, patients with imaging manifestations of renal osteodystrophy are increasingly encountered. These changes are in many cases reversible following renal transplantation, although they may take years to regress.

These changes can be broadly categorized under several headings.

Etiology

The osseous changes due to renal osteodystrophy are for the most part due to secondary hyperparathyroidism.

Pathophysiology

Patients with renal failure often undergo hypertrophy of the hyperparathyroid glands induced by hyperphosphatasemia due to decreased renal excretion. Increased circulating levels of parathyroid hormone (PTH) then alters bone metabolism, leading to a protean constellation of changes. In particular, PTH promotes the development of osteoclasts, osteoblasts, and osteocytes, giving rise to bone resorption, periosteal reactions, and brown tumors. Osteosclerosis, osteoporosis, and osteomalacia may all occur; hence the sobriquet "active bones disease."

Osteoclastic bone resorption is probably the most consistent feature and may affect any portion of the bone, that is, subperiosteal, cortical, subchondral, trabecular, endosteal, or at entheses.

Patients with renal failure due to chronic disease affecting the glomeruli also develop alterations in vitamin D metabolism, frequently showing decreased sensitivity to the vitamin. This in turn also alters bone metabolism, with osteomalacia or rickets developing. Metabolic interactions become very complex, and often several manifestations of disease are present simultaneously.

Clinical Findings

- Secondary hyperparathyroidism may occur in patients with renal failure of any etiology.
- Resorption of adjacent ligaments and tendons may lead to "spontaneous" tendon rupture.
- Rickets may actually be the initial feature for the presence of chronic renal disease in children.
- Bone may soften and lead to bowing, particularly of the lower limbs. Hip pain secondary to slipping of the femoral epiphyses due to weakening of the bone may occur. Frank fractures may occur secondary to the weakened bone. Bowing of bone and pathologic fractures may also occur in the mature skeleton. Insufficiency fractures also occur with increased frequency in these patients.

Complications

- Secondary hyperparathyroidism
- Osteopenia secondary to intracortical resorption
- Endosteal bone resorption
- Resorption of adjacent ligaments and tendons
- Resorption of bone subjacent to the insertion of ligaments and tendons

- Brown tumors: osteoclastomas
- Osteosclerosis
- Rickets and osteomalacia (rickets seen in the growing bone and osteomalacia in the mature skeleton), leading to bone softening and bowing in children and occasionally epiphyseal slipping or frank fractures. Bowing of bone and pathologic fractures may also occur in the mature skeleton.
- Insufficiency fractures
- Metastatic calcification in cartilage and periarticular soft tissues

Pathology

GROSS

- Involved bones may be softened and bowed or fractured.
- Brown tumors may be evident.
- Resorption of bone adjacent ligaments and tendons may lead to "spontaneous" tendon rupture.
- Patients may show juxta-articular erosions, particularly likely to be manifested in the hands and feet, as well as resorption of the lamina dura around the teeth.

MICROSCOPIC

- Subperiosteal resorption of bone is seen. Patients may also show changes of osteoporosis with intracortical resorption and an appearance of tunneling and endosteal bone resorption. Subchondral resorption of bone demonstrates collapse of cortical bone and overlying cartilage. Subligamentous and subtendinous bone resorption is also seen.
- Also seen is trabecular coarsening due to resorption of secondary trabeculae as a result of the underlying osteoporosis that may or may not occur in combination with osteosclerosis.
- Brown tumors, also referred to as osteoclastomas, represent accumulations of giant cells and vascularized fibromatous material that replace bone and appear as destructive, often expansile lesions in bone. They may necrose and liquefy, producing cysts (osteitis fibrosa cystica).
- Patients with rickets may demonstrate abnormal physes, with physeal widening and demineralization.
- Metastatic calcification may be evident in cartilage and periarticular soft tissues.

Imaging Findings

RADIOGRAPHY

Hyperparathyroidism

- Subperiosteal resorption of bone produces a lacelike irregularity of the cortical margin that progresses to scalloping and spiculation. It is frequently seen in the tufts of the distal phalanges of the fingers, although resorption is also seen at many other sites, including the diametaphyses of the middle phalanges, particularly on their radial aspects (**Figs. 125B–125D**), the inferior surface of the ribs and calcaneus, the medial aspects of the proximal tibia, humerus, and femur, and the inferior aspect of the clavicles, particularly distally.
- Patients may show juxta-articular erosions, likely to be manifested in the hands and feet, as well as resorption of the lamina dura around the teeth.
- Patients may also show changes of osteoporosis with intracortical resorption and an appearance of tunneling (**Figs. 125C,125D**) secondary to intrahaversian osteoclasis.
- Endosteal bone resorption is typically seen in the upper extremities, particularly the hands, as scalloped areas along the cortex. When CT head is performed for other reasons, endosteal scalloping

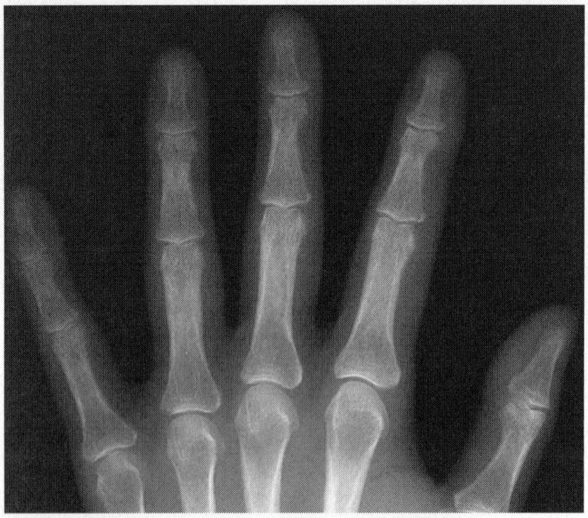
C

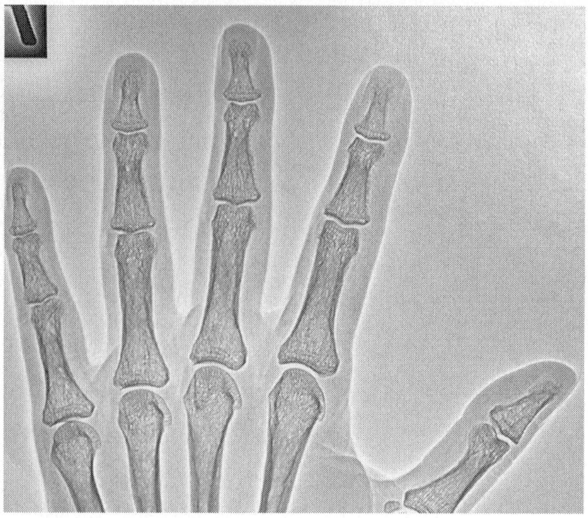
D

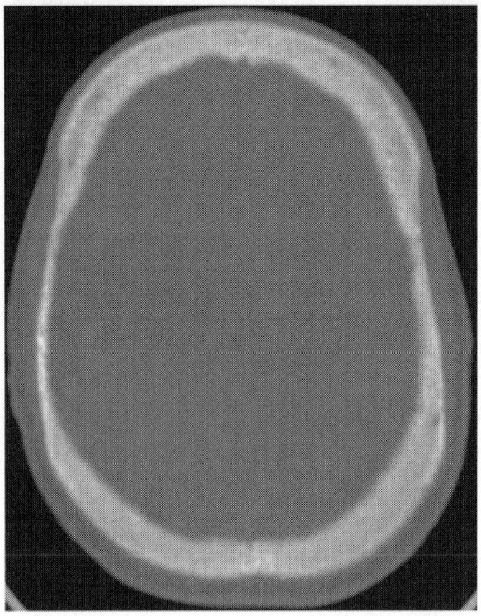
E

Figures 125C–125E Radiograph (**125C**) and xeroradiograph (**125D**) show subperiosteal resorption and consequent "tunneling" on the radial aspects of the phalanges and rendered more conspicuous on the xeroradiograph, the latter of only historical interest now. Subtle acrolysis of the distal tufts is also evident, especially in the second digit. **125E** A transaxial image from a CT head displayed on bony windows shows loss of distinction of the inner table with focal scalloped areas most evident in the left parietal bone.

may be evident as small focal scalloped areas on the inner table (**Fig. 125E**). When many areas are present, they are evident on plain films, giving rise to the classic "salt and pepper" appearance.

- Resorption of bone subchondrally can occur in any joint, especially the small joints of the hands and including the discovertebral junction of the spine and the sacroiliac joints. This resorption can simulate erosions and give rise to pain in as many as 50% of affected patients.
- Subtendinous and subligamentous resorption is evinced by surface scalloping at entheses, which may be either smooth or irregular. This is most frequently seen on the inferior calcaneus, the greater and lesser trochanters, and the anterior inferior iliac spine. Resorption of adjacent ligaments and tendons has also been reported.

Brown tumors

- Brown tumors, also referred to as osteoclastomas, represent accumulations of giant cells and fibromatous material that produce destructive, often expansile lesions in bone. These are particularly frequent with primary hyperparathyroidism. However, most brown tumors are seen in relation to secondary hyperparathyroidism, as this is a far more common condition. Almost always, other radiographic manifestations of hyperparathyroidism are seen in association with a brown tumor, although not invariably so.

F 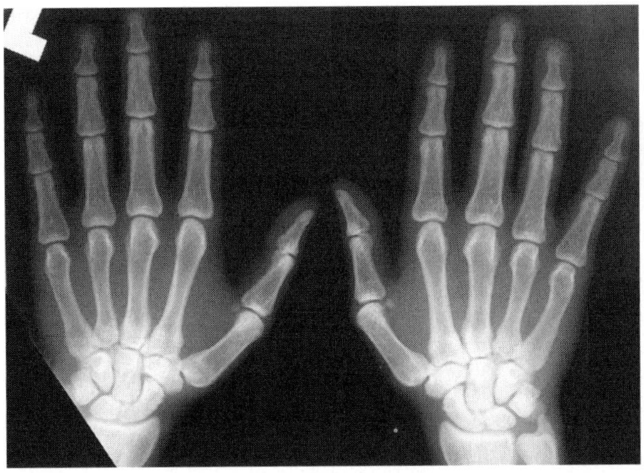 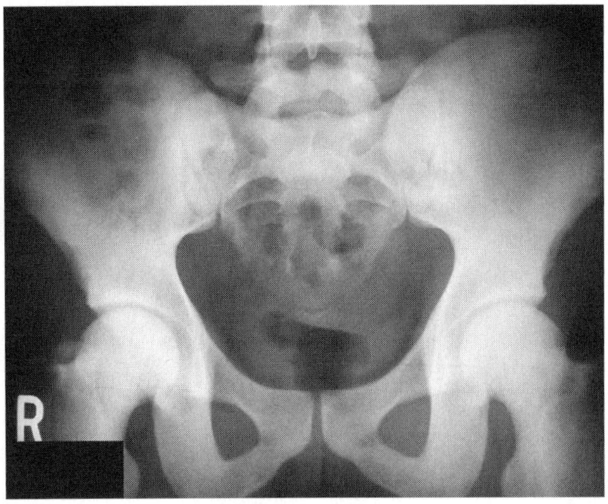 G

Figures 125F,125G Hands (**125F**) and pelvis (**125G**) show diffuse marked osteosclerosis secondary to chronic renal failure.

- Brown tumors are often solitary but may be multiple. They are frequently eccentric or cortical in the long bones. They may give rise to endosteal scalloping and occasional expansion. Brown tumors are most frequently seen in the ribs, pelvis, facial bones, and femora. They may heal following correction of the underlying condition, demonstrating calcification, sclerosis, and eventual disappearance.

Osteosclerosis

- Trabeculae often appear coarsened in patients with renal osteodystrophy (**Figs. 125F,125G**). This appearance may be due to resorption of secondary trabeculae as a result of the underlying osteoporosis, which may or may not occur in combination with osteosclerosis. The condition can often be diffuse, affecting the entire skeleton, although in its initial stages, osteosclerosis is manifested as increased density along the vertebral end plates, producing a so-called rugger-jersey spine appearance (**Fig. 125H**), after the horizontal stripes seen on many rugby jerseys. The underlying physiologic mechanism for producing these changes has not been clearly elucidated. Although treatment of the underlying failure by transplantation may "heal" the increased sclerosis, it is more common in fact for the sclerosis to increase.

Rickets and osteomalacia

- This is a manifestation of altered vitamin D metabolism in patients with chronic renal disease secondary to parenchymal renal loss and consequent reduction in activation of inactive vitamin D. Rickets and osteomalacia form a continuity of the disease process, with rickets seen in the growing bone and osteomalacia in the mature skeleton.
- Rickets is more confidently diagnosed in patients with renal osteodystrophy, as the findings are more striking in this setting.
- In the mature skeleton, rickets at times can only be diagnosed through biopsy, as imaging manifestations are often subtle. Rickets may actually be the initial feature for the presence of chronic renal disease in children.
- Patients may demonstrate abnormal physes with widening and demineralization, along with disorganization and poor definition of the metaphyses. The metaphyses also acquire a cupped configuration and become widened. The bone may soften and become bowed.
- Children may demonstrate slipping of the epiphyses due to the weakening of the bone, or frank fractures may occur.

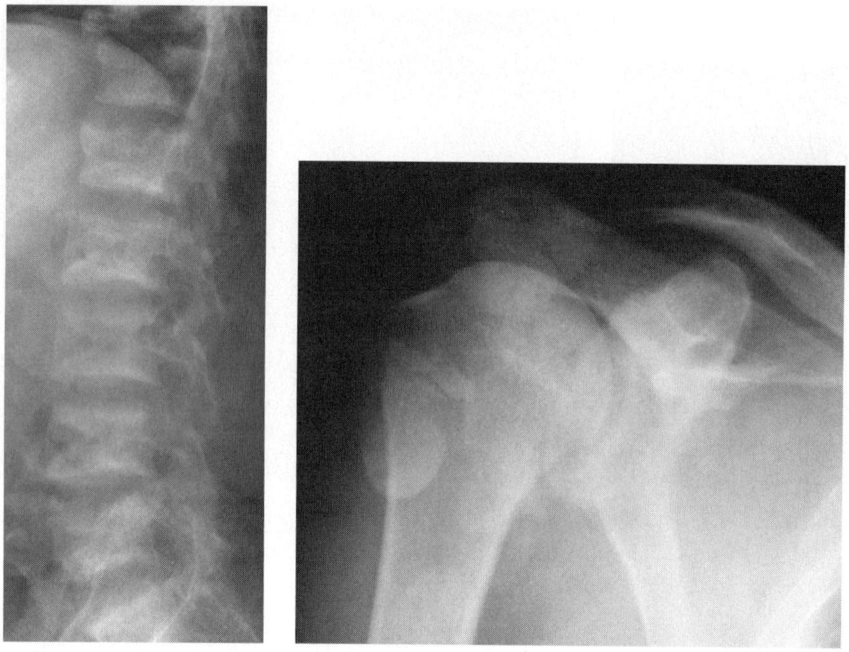

H I

Figures 125H,125I 125H A lateral radiograph of the lumbar spine shows the prominent vertebral body osteopenia and increased end plate sclerosis producing multiple horizontal "stripes"; thus the sobriquet "rugger-jersey" spine. Note also the marked Schmorl's nodule with indentation and deformity of the superior end plate of L1. **125I** An AP radiograph of the shoulder shows dense, cloudlike periarticular metastatic calcifications.

- Bowing of bone and pathologic fractures may occur in the mature skeleton.
- Insufficiency fractures also occur with increased frequency in these patients.
- Patients may also develop metastatic calcification, which is particularly common in cartilage and periarticular soft tissues (**Fig. 125I**), occurring in over half the patients receiving more than 4 years of hemodialysis. The calcifications, which may or may not be symptomatic, consist of chalky, paste-like hydroxyapatite.

Treatment

Correction of renal failure helps to correct some of the osseous changes, particularly if transplantation is successful.

Prognosis

Prognosis is entirely dependent on the degree of success of treating the underlying failure; however, some features are likely to progress or become more conspicuous after treatment, such as tendon rupture, crystal deposition, infection, and avascular necrosis.

PEARLS

- Subperiosteal resorption of bone is frequently seen in the tufts of the distal phalanges of the fingers and classically on the radial aspect of the diametaphyses of the phalanges.
- Rickets may actually be the initial feature for the presence of chronic renal disease in children.
- Almost always, other radiographic manifestations of hyperparathyroidism are seen in association with a brown tumor, although not invariably so.

PITFALLS

- Brown tumors are particularly frequent with primary hyperparathyroidism; however, radiologists encounter brown tumors most frequently in relation to secondary hyperparathyroidism, as this is a far more common condition.
- In the mature skeleton, rickets at times can only be diagnosed through biopsy, as imaging manifestations are often subtle.
- Patients may show juxta-articular erosions, likely to be manifested in the hands and feet, resulting in possible confusion with gout.

Suggested Readings

Adams JE. Dialysis bone disease. Semin Dial 2002;15:277–289

Jevtic V. Imaging of renal osteodystrophy. Eur J Radiol 2003;46:85–95

Murphey MD, Sartoris DJ, Quale JL, Pathria MN, Martin NL. Musculoskeletal manifestations of chronic renal insufficiency. Radiographics 1993;13:357–379

Tigges S, Nance EP, Carpenter WA, Erb R. Renal osteodystrophy: imaging findings that mimic those of other diseases. Am J Roentgenol 1995;165:143–148

CASE 126

Brian Edward Reeves, Anthony G. Ryan, Peter L. Munk, and Thomas Pope

Clinical Presentation

A 26-year-old woman presented with painless stiffness and swelling in her right elbow.

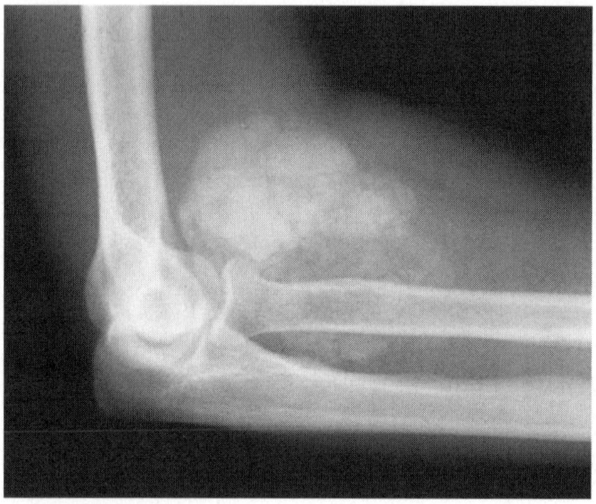

Figure 126A

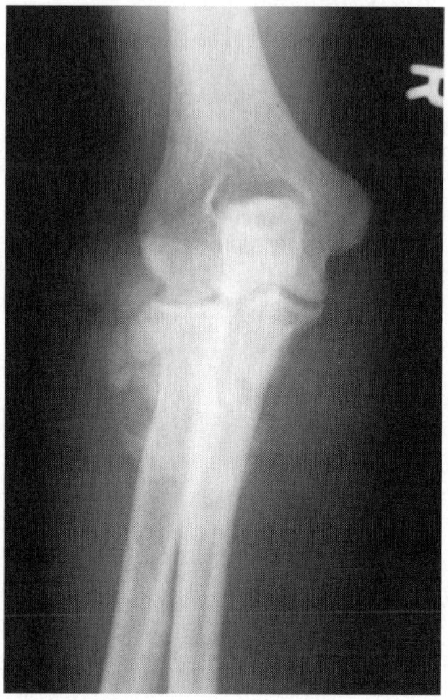

Figure 126B

Radiologic Findings

Lateral (**126A**) and anteroposterior (**126B**) radiographs of the right elbow show a lobulated homogeneous, calcific mass within the antecubital fossa. The articular space is normal, and there is no erosion of bone.

Diagnosis

Tumoral calcinosis.

Differential Diagnosis

- Renal osteodystrophy
- Calcinosis universalis
- Calcinosis circumscripta
- Milk-alkali syndrome
- Hypervitaminosis D
- Metastatic calcification
- Heterotopic calcification

- Scleroderma
- Dermatomyositis
- Tumoral calcinosis secondary to chronic renal failure

Discussion

Background

Idiopathic tumoral calcinosis is a rare and poorly understood entity consisting of calcium salt deposition in the extracapsular soft tissues adjacent to joints. It occurs most commonly in the first or second decade, predominantly affects African Americans, and is seen more frequently in men.

Etiology

One third of the cases are thought to be familial, and the inheritance is likely autosomal dominant with variable expression. There is some evidence suggesting that tumoral calcinosis may be caused

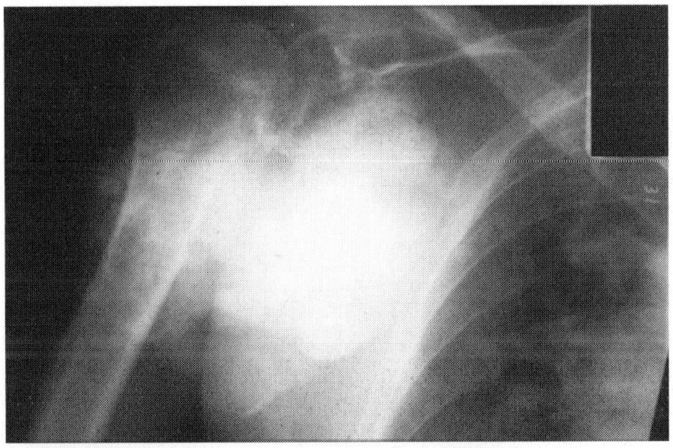
C

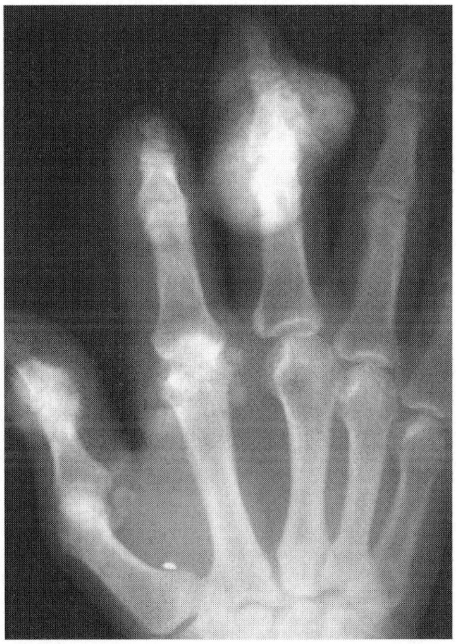
D

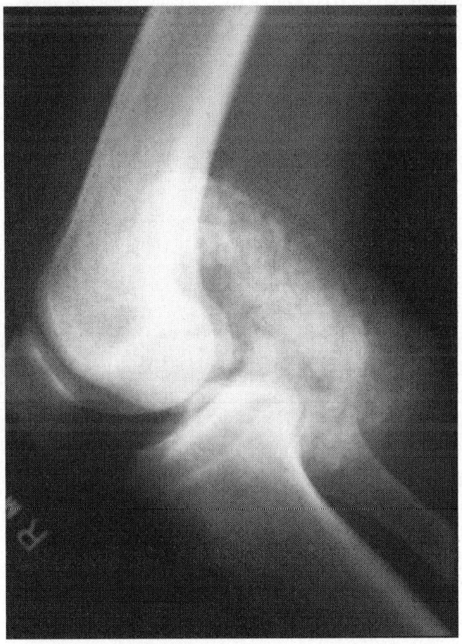
E

Figures 126C–126E The images show tumoral calcinosis affecting the shoulder (**126C**), hand (**126D**), and knee (**126E**).

by an inborn abnormality of phosphorus metabolism; other metabolic defects, collagen vascular disorders, and trauma have also been suggested as pathogenic mechanisms.

Clinical Findings

Patients usually present with painless swelling around one or more joints. Joints involved in the order of the frequency of involvement are hips, elbows, shoulders, and feet (**Figs. 126C–126E**).

The masses range from 1 to 20 cm in diameter and may grow large enough to cause symptoms by compression of adjacent nerves. Softened calcium-containing material may discharge through skin sinuses. Renal and parathyroid function are usually normal. Serum calcium, phosphorus, uric acid, and alkaline phosphatase may be normal or slightly elevated.

Complications

- Compression of peripheral nerves
- Erosion through the skin with chalky drainage
- Osseous erosions
- Amyloidosis

Pathology

Pathologic analysis reveals lobulated soft-tissue masses with well-defined capsules and thick septae, which are filled with calcareous material (calcium phosphate, calcium carbonate, and calcium hydroxyapatite) and fluid.

Imaging Findings

RADIOGRAPHY

- The radiographic findings are characteristic.
- The calcific material is homogeneous radiographically, and the masses are most common on the extensor surfaces of the joints.
- Initially, there are small calcified nodules, which progress to large, multilobular calcific deposits in the periarticular tissues.
- A cobblestone appearance may also be seen and is created by fibrous septae.
- Fluid-fluid levels may be seen if there is milk of calcium in the lesion.

COMPUTED TOMOGRAPHY

- The calcified deposits appear smoothly marginated and hyperdense on CT.
- The lesions may be small and solid or large and cystic.
- Usually, there is a clear tissue plane between the lesion and the underlying bone.
- Edema may also be present in the surrounding tissues.

MAGNETIC RESONANCE IMAGING

- The masses replace rather than invade adjacent tissues and are hypointense on T1- and T2-weighted sequences.
- Areas of high signal intensity on T2-weighted sequences may be seen in the lesion or adjacent soft tissues and correspond to edema and/or granulomatous reaction.

NUCLEAR MEDICINE

- Radioisotope bone scans will show increased tracer accumulation within the lesions.

Treatment

The masses of calcification can be removed surgically, but recurrence is common if the masses are incompletely excised. Dietary phosphorus restriction and phosphate-binding antacids may be effective; however, steroids, radiation therapy, and parathyroidectomy are ineffective modes of treatment.

PEARLS

- The calcium salt deposition in tumoral calcinosis occurs in the extracapsular soft tissues adjacent to joints, whereas the calcification associated with tuberculous arthritis is clearly intracapsular.
- Patients with tumoral calcinosis usually present with painless swelling around one or more joints, and myositis ossificans is usually associated with one region only; there is usually a history of trauma, and the lesion is painful initially.
- The masses replace rather than invade adjacent tissues and are hypointense on both T1- and T2-weighted sequences.

PITFALLS

- Softened calcium-containing material may discharge through skin sinuses, which may be confused with the caseous granulomatous material that may discharge secondary to intra-articular tuberculosis.
- Although osseous erosions in association with calcific juxta-articular material may occur and raise the differential of tophaceous gout, the erosions in tumoral calcinosis will be clearly deep to the calcific mass, whereas the erosions in gout will be in the typical juxta-articular location.
- Radioisotope bone scans will show increased tracer accumulation within the lesions, in common with other calcific or ossific lesions, and are thus not discriminatory.

Suggested Readings

Martinez S. Tumoral calcinosis: 12 years later. Semin Musculoskelet Radiol 2002;6:331–339

Senol U, Karaal K, Cevikol C, Dincer A. MR imaging findings of recurrent tumoral calcinosis. Clin Imaging 2000;24:154–156

Steinbach LS, Johnston JO, Tepper EF, Honda GD, Martel W. Tumoral calcinosis: radiologic-pathologic correlation. Skeletal Radiol 1995;24:573–578

CASE 127

Peter L. Munk and Anthony G. Ryan

Clinical Presentation

A 47-year-old woman presented with swelling and discomfort in the fingers.

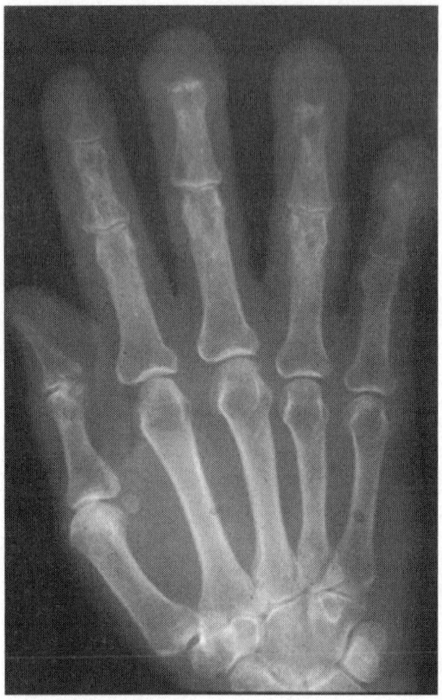

Figure 127A

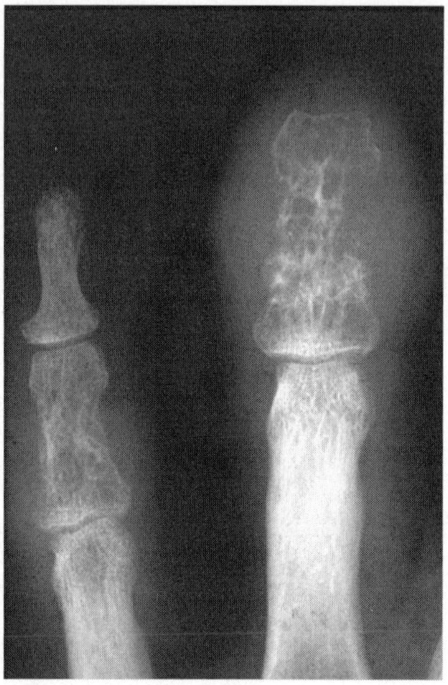

Figure 127B

Radiologic Findings

Radiographs of the hand were obtained (**Fig. 127A**) with coned views of the distal phalanges of the contralateral hand (**Fig. 127B**). Mild soft-tissue swelling is present over the distal aspect of the fingers bilaterally. The underlying bone of the fingertips shows irregular destruction, with almost complete destruction of the tufts and distal phalanges of the third through fifth digits of the hand (**Fig. 127A**). Irregular radiolucency affects the distal metaphyses of the proximal and middle phalanges of several fingers. The coned view shows a lacelike pattern of destruction in the distal phalanx (**Fig. 127B**).

Diagnosis

Osseous sarcoidosis.

Differential Diagnosis

The osseous findings are typically very characteristic, and in the face of other manifestations, such as lymphadenopathy (especially pulmonary hilar), a confident diagnosis can be made.

Occasionally, other conditions should be considered, such as

- Tuberous sclerosis
- Enchondromatosis
- Fibrous dysplasia

Discussion

Background

Sarcoidosis is a disease that, in most cases, involves soft tissues, especially lymph nodes, skin, lungs, and other organs. Only about 10% of patients have bone involvement, with the hands and feet being the most common sites. Recognition of musculoskeletal involvement has increased considerably with the advent of MRI, which permits soft-tissue and marrow lesions to be more readily seen.

Etiology

Unknown.

Clinical Findings

Patients typically present between age 20 and 40. People of African descent are more commonly afflicted than Caucasians. Patients may have very mild symptoms but may also present with lymphadenopathy, fever, anemia, weight loss, hepatosplenomegaly, skin or ocular lesions, or pulmonary fibrosis/infiltrates. Most patients have a favorable clinical outcome and may have resolution of their condition without treatment, although steroids are frequently used. Lung parenchymal or multiorgan involvement indicates a poorer prognosis.

Pathology

- Noncaseating granulomas, increased lymphocytes (helper T cells), giant cells of the Langerhans' type, and plasma cells
- Elevated angiotensin-converting enzyme

Imaging Findings

RADIOGRAPHY

- Bone sarcoid is typically bilateral, and its epicenter of involvement is cortical, with preservation of the periosteum.
- The hands and feet are frequently afflicted, with the ends of the bones being the most common site of lesions.
- The lesions themselves are typically radiolucent with surrounding sclerosis and have a "punched out" cystic or lacelike character, with relatively little disturbance of the surrounding soft tissues until the lesions become advanced.
- If the articular surface of the bone is affected, soft-tissue swelling and effusions can be expected. In fact, arthritis occurs in as many as 10 to 35% of cases, more commonly than focal osseous lesions.
- Generalized osteopenia is common, and coarsening of trabeculae, leading to the typical lacy pattern, can be expected.
- When these lesions are in weight-bearing bones, collapse or fracture may occur.
- Rarely, an osteosclerotic pattern may be encountered, particularly in the spine, pelvis, and skull. Involvement of the long tubular bones, extremities, and ribs is unusual.

COMPUTED TOMOGRAPHY/MAGNETIC RESONANCE IMAGING

- Cross-sectional imaging may demonstrate lesions within bone, especially in the marrow space, that may not be evident on radiography (**Figs. 127C–127E**).

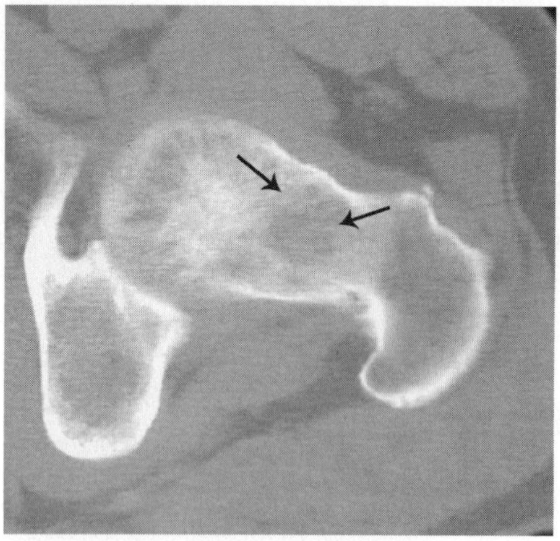

C

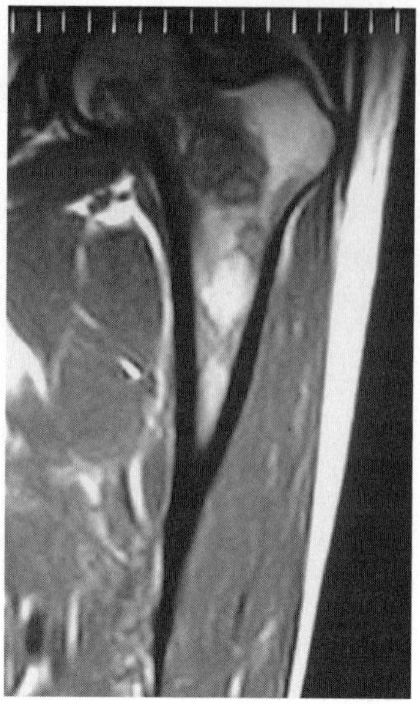

D

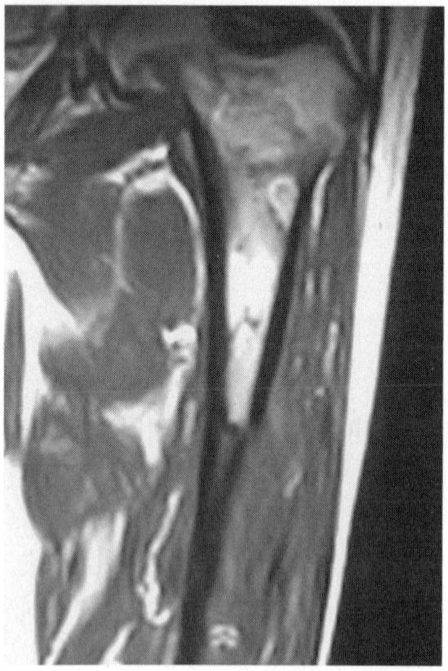

E

Figures 127C–127E 127C Axial CT images through the proximal femur show an area of radiolucency (arrows) representing destruction of trabeculae by a granuloma. **127D** and **127E** Coronal T1-weighted (**127D**) and T2-weighted (**127E**) MRIs from the same patient show geographic areas of abnormal signal intensity within the marrow, corresponding to sarcoid granulomas.

- It should be remembered that radiographic osseous involvement with sarcoid is rarely encountered without the presence of skin lesions. The osseous manifestations, however, may be significantly more prominent.
- Involvement of the subcutaneous compartment has also been reported, and lesions often present as masses (T1-weighted in **Fig. 127F**; T2-weighted in **Fig. 127G**). These nodules tend to be encountered in a slightly older population, and osseous lesions may be absent. The lesions are typically painless and highly vascular. Muscle involvement is also well described and will be detected in the majority of patients on biopsy.
- Patients may have a myopathy, with significant accompanying weaknesses in some instances. Discrete lesions in muscle can be seen in up to 1.4% of patients although positive findings of sarcoidois on biopsy are much higher (50 to 80%).
- Multifocal areas of high signal intensity are seen on T2-weighted fat-suppressed sequences or contrast-enhanced T1-weighted sequences (**Fig. 127G**). Typically, lesions will be bilateral and are more commonly seen in the lower extremities.

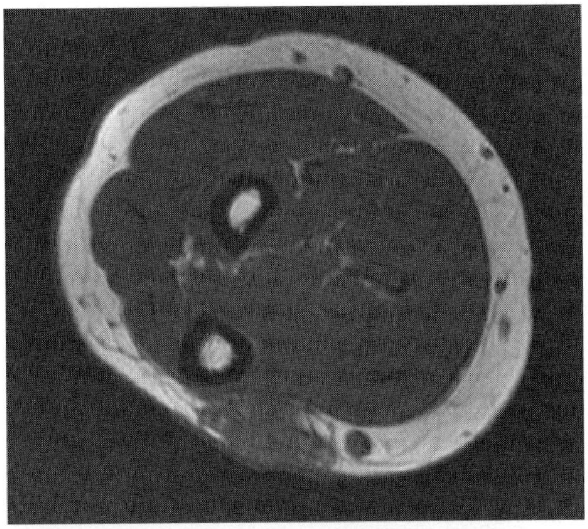
F

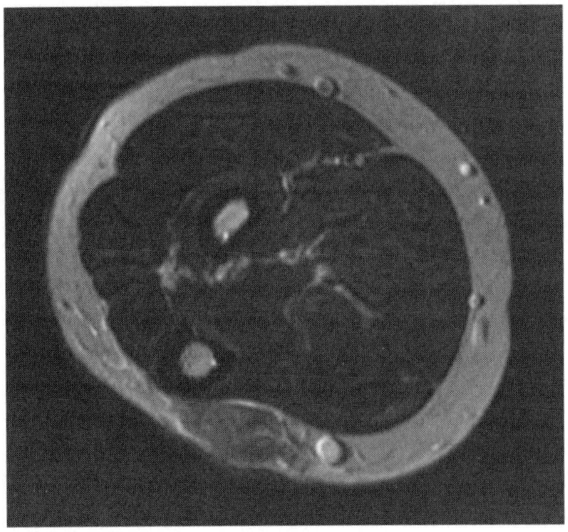
G

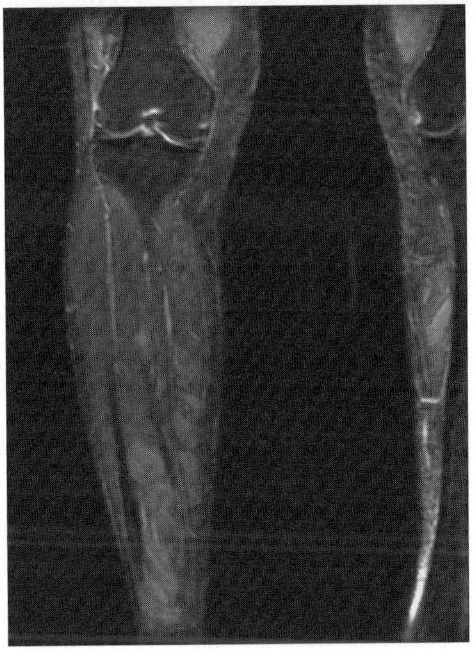
H

Figures 127F–127H Axial T1-weighted (**127F**) and axial T2-weighted (**127G**) images show a reasonably well-defined subcutaneous nodule with nonspecific characteristics: low/intermediate signal intensity, hypointense relative to fat, and slightly hyperintense to muscle on both sequences. **127H** Coronal fat-suppressed inversion recovery (STIR) image of the legs shows numerous areas of moderately increased signal within muscle in a patient with clinical moderately severe sarcoid myopathy.

- With long-standing disease, a marked myopathy can evolve with atrophy and fatty replacement.
- Other diseases and conditions that produce a similar pattern of lesions are gout, rheumatoid arthritis, tubular sclerosis, fibrous dysplasia, and infection with a granulomatous organism, such as tuberculosis or fungus.

PEARLS

- The lacelike involvement of the phalanges is almost pathognomonic of osseous sarcoidosis.
- Radiographic osseous involvement with sarcoidosis is rarely encountered in the absence of skin lesions, and the majority of patients will also have the typical pattern of hilar lymphadenopathy.
- Subcutaneous involvement often presents as painless and highly vascular nodules, which tend to be encountered in a slightly older population and in the absence of osseous lesions.

PITFALLS

- Although the subcutaneous nodules of sarcoidosis are typically well defined, this cannot be taken as pathognomonic. Biopsy is frequently required to exclude more aggressive lesions, such as metastases and fibromatosis.
- Tuft resorption is seen in scleroderma; however, calcifications are invariably present within the tissues of the pulp.
- Rarely, an osteosclerotic pattern can be encountered, particularly in the spine, pelvis, and skull. Involvement of the long tubular bones, as well as the extremities and ribs, is unusual.

Suggested Readings

Beasley EW III, Peterman SB, Hertzler GL. An unusual form of tibial sarcoidosis. Am J Roentgenol 1987;149:754–756

Moore SL, Teirstein AE. Musculoskeletal sarcoidosis: spectrum of appearances at MR imaging. Radiographics 2003;23:1389–1399

Otake S. Sarcoidosis involving skeletal muscle: imaging findings and relative value of imaging procedures. Am J Roentgenol 1994;162:369–375

CASE 128

Anthony G. Ryan and Peter L. Munk

Clinical Presentation

A 60-year-old man presented with bilateral painful hands.

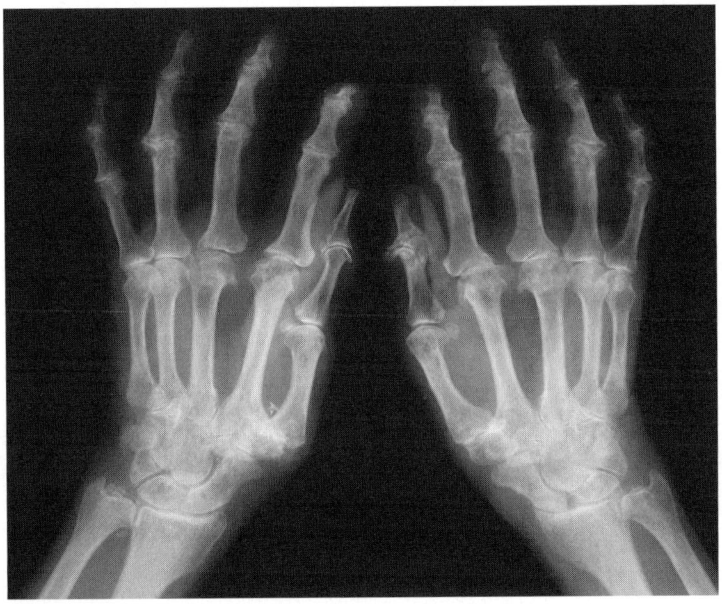

Figure 128A

Radiologic Findings

An anteroposterior radiograph of both hands (**Fig. 128A**) shows joint space reduction affecting the metacarpophalangeal, radiocarpal, and interphalangeal joints; diffuse osteopenia; and prominent hooked osteophytes on the radial aspect of the second and third metacarpals, the heads of which are enlarged by the presence of the osteophytes. Variable lucencies, marginated by thin, sharply defined rims of sclerosis, are evident within the metacarpal heads. Chondrocalcinosis is evident in the triangular fibrocartilage bilaterally. The scapholunate interval is of normal size.

Diagnosis

Hemochromatosis arthropathy.

Differential Diagnosis

- Pseudogout (should demonstrate no evidence of arthropathy)
- Psoriatic arthritis (should have the typical skin and nail changes with this degree of cartilaginous and bony change)
- Osteoarthritis (affects predominantly the distal joints of the hands)
- Rheumatoid arthritis
- Gout (in which chondrocalcinosis may also be seen)

Discussion

Etiology

Hemochromatosis may occur as a primary or secondary (acquired) condition.

The primary, idiopathic form is transmitted as an autosomal recessive trait, with only homozygotes demonstrating the clinical condition, or via indeterminate inheritance (e.g., there is an abnormal iron-loading gene present in thalassemia and sideroblastic anemia, resulting in increased iron absorption with a normal dietary load).

Acquired hemochromatosis occurs secondary to

- Excessive iron absorption in anemias, myelofibrosis, and portacaval shunt
- Exogenous administration of iron, multiple blood transfusions, porphyria cutanea tarda, and drinking beer brewed in iron vessels

Both primary and secondary causes result in deposition of excessive iron in the liver, pancreas, spleen, gastrointestinal tract, kidney, gonads, heart, and endocrine glands, resulting in fibrosis, which leads to eventual organ failure.

Pathophysiology

Iron deposition in the synovium leads to an arthropathy in 30 to 50% of cases. Synovitis is also caused and/or exacerbated by secondary calcium pyrophosphate deposition (CPPD), leading to chondrocalcinosis, most frequently found in the triangular fibrocartilage of the wrist, the menisci, the anulus fibrosus, the ligamentum flavum, the symphysis pubis, the Achilles' tendon, and the plantar fascia.

The calcification is due to deposition of calcium pyrophosphate crystals, perhaps resulting from iron inhibition of pyrophosphatase.

Clinical Findings

- Hemochromatosis typically affects persons of middle age (older than 40 years), with a significant (10:1) male predominance.
- "Bronze"/slate gray skin pigmentation secondary to deposition of melanin, hepatomegaly, and diabetes mellitus are the classic triad of findings in the presence of gross iron deposition.
- Cirrhosis, congestive heart failure, arrythmias, and hypogonadism
- Arthritic symptoms are present in 30% of patients.
- Blood tests reveal an overall increase in serum iron and ferritin.

Complications

- Hemochromatosis arthropathy occurs in 30 to 50% of patients affected with the disease, secondary to iron deposition with or without concomitant CPPD deposition (in up to 50%).
- Congestive heart failure occurs in 30% of cases.
- Cirrhosis is seen in 30% of cases, leading to hepatic failure.
- Hepatoma is seen in up to 30% of cases, although this rarely occurs in patients in whom cirrhosis has not yet developed, and is thus preventable if excess iron is removed.

Pathology

GROSS

- Osteoarthritic-like changes

MICROSCOPIC

- Synovitis secondary to both iron and CPPD deposition

Imaging Findings

RADIOGRAPHY

The arthropathy resembles degenerative/osteoarthritic arthropathy demonstrating subchondral cyst formation (small subchondral cystic lesions with a fine rim of sclerosis is a typical feature in the metacarpal heads), subchondral sclerosis, joint space narrowing, which tends to be uniform, and osteophyte formation. Despite these similarities, hemochromatosis has a characteristic distribution affecting unusual locations rarely affected by osteoarthrosis, for example, the radiocarpal and metacarpophalangeal joints.

Prominent osteophytes affecting the metacarpal heads, described variably as hooked, beaked, or drooping, are a characteristic finding. The pronounced osteophyte formation makes the metacarpal heads appear enlarged and blocklike or "squared."

Unlike osteoarthrosis, generalized osteoporosis is a frequent finding.

The joints affected by the arthropathy are, in decreasing frequency,

- Hands
- Carpus (where pericapitate narrowing is common)
- Proximal interphalangeal joints (although the interphalangeal joints of the thumb are usually spared)
- Knees
- Hips

Chondrocalcinosis, involving both fibrous and hyaline cartilage and evident in 20 to 60% of patients, is usually secondary to CPPD and may occur in the triangular fibrocartilage of the wrist, the menisci, the anulus fibrosus, the ligamentum flavum, the symphysis pubis, the Achilles' tendon, and the plantar fascia.

The arthropathy follows the same distribution and hypertrophic changes as in CPPD; however, in distinguishing hemochromatosis arthropathy from that due to CPPD, the following findings favor a diagnosis of hemochromatosis:

- More prevalent narrowing of the metacarpophalangeal joint spaces, including those in the fourth and fifth digits
- Hooklike osteophytes on the radial aspect of the metacarpal head
- There is less prevalent scapholunate separation in hemochromatosis than is seen in CPPD disease.

MAGNETIC RESONANCE IMAGING

In hemochromatosis arthropathy, MRI demonstrates the bony degenerative changes with similar sensitivity to plain films, but also enables additional visualization of both cartilaginous and meniscal deformity.

Despite the sensitivity of gradient sequences to iron, MRI does not confirm reliably the presence of intra-articular iron, nor is any correlation observed between synovial fluid MR signal intensity and the severity of the observed degenerative changes.

Treatment

PLEBOTOMY

Excess iron needs to be removed as a matter of urgency (500 mL twice weekly initially), and must be continued for up to 2 years, after which three or four venesections a year are usually adequate to prevent recurrent overload.

CHELATION THERAPY

Deferoxamine has a role in the treatment of patients who do not tolerate venesection (e.g., patients with severe heart failure or anemia).

SCREENING OF RELATIVES

First-degree relatives should all be offered screening by testing serum ferritin levels.

Prognosis

Although life-prolonging, venesection has no effect on established chondrocalcinosis, diabetes, or testicular atrophy.

Overall, the prognosis is poor, with death from congestive heart failure occurring in 30% and hepatic failure in 25% of cases.

PEARLS

- The arthropathy of hemochromatosis looks like osteoarthritis out of place, that is, affecting the metacarpal and radiocarpal joints.
- In differentiating CPPD from hemochromatosis, the following features are more specific to hemochromatosis:
  - More prevalent narrowing of the metacarpophalangeal joint spaces, including those in the fourth and fifth digits
  - Hooklike osteophytes on the radial aspect of the metacarpal heads
  - Less frequent separation of the scaphoid and the lunate

PITFALLS

- Despite the sensitivity of gradient sequences to iron, MRI does not confirm reliably the presence of intra-articular iron, nor is any correlation observed between synovial fluid MR signal intensity and the severity of the observed degenerative changes.
- Because the arthropathy may precede the other findings, the radiologist must keep this diagnosis in mind when an arthropathy is encountered, as its discovery may be potentially life-saving.

Suggested Readings

Adamson TC III, Resnik CS, Guerra J Jr, Vint VC, Weisman MH, Resnick D. Hand and wrist arthropathies of hemochromatosis and calcium pyrophosphate deposition disease: distinct radiographic features. Radiology 1983;147:377–381

Eustace S, Buff B, McCarthy C, MacMathuana P, Gilligan P, Ennis JT. Magnetic resonance imaging of hemochromatosis arthropathy. Skeletal Radiol 1994;23:547–549

Hirsch JH, Killien FC, Troupin RH. The arthropathy of hemochromatosis. Radiology 1976;118:591–596

CASE 129

Anthony G. Ryan and Peter L. Munk

Clinical Presentation

A 25-year-old man presented with a chronically painful knee, having experienced spontaneous dramatic knee swelling.

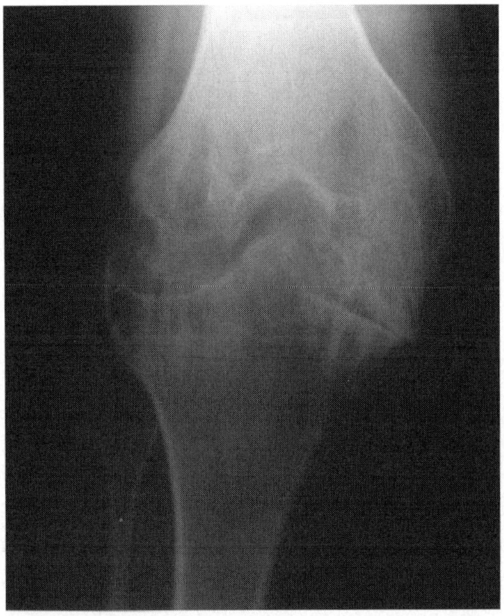

Figure 129A

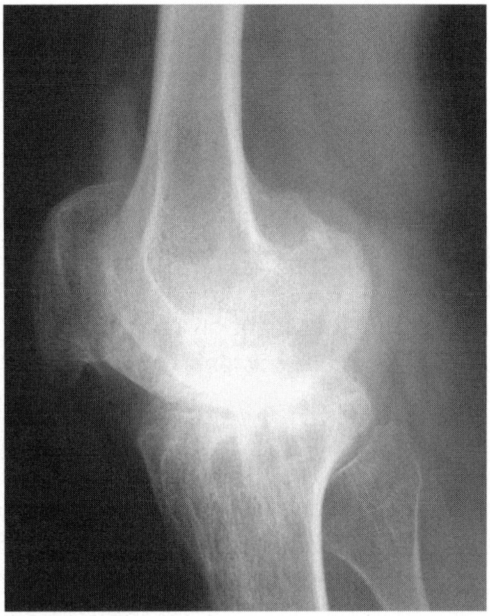

Figure 129B

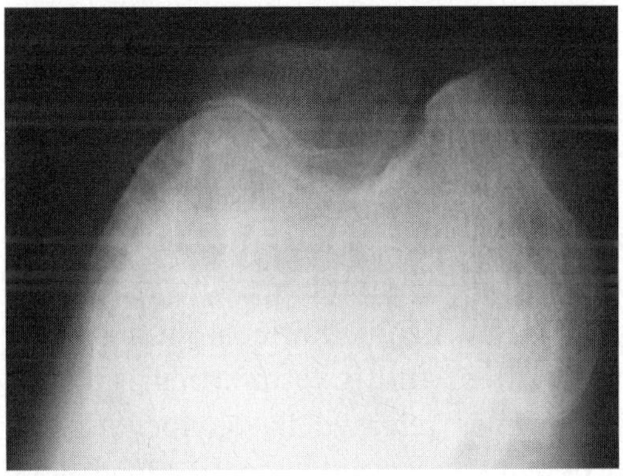

Figure 129C

Radiologic Findings

Anteroposterior (AP), lateral, and skyline views (**Figs. 129A–129C**) of the right knee show a dense joint effusion and osseous changes consistent with advanced degeneration, that is, large subchondral cysts, irregularity, and sclerosis of the osseous articular surface with marginal osteophytosis. There is overgrowth of the medial epiphysis in particular. Valgus deformity is evident. The intercondylar notch is widened. The joint space is narrowed; however, it is relatively preserved, given the severity of the other changes present. The inferomedial aspect of the patellofemoral joint demonstrates the most marked joint space narrowing.

Diagnosis

Hemophilic arthropathy.

Differential Diagnosis

- Advanced degenerative osteoarthritis
- Chronic juvenile rheumatoid arthritis (JRA)
- Chronic tuberculous arthritis
- Synovial hemangioma

Discussion

Background

In patients with severe hemophilia (< 1% of factor VII:C), 85 to 90% of all bleeding events involve the joints, frequently occurring spontaneously. The frequency and severity of bleeds decrease with increasing levels of the factor. Musculoskeletal bleeds account for most of the morbidity associated with the condition, although transfusion-related human immunodeficiency virus (HIV) remains the most frequent cause of death (intracranial hemorrhage was more common in the pre-HIV era).

Etiology

This is an X-linked recessive condition occurring in 1 in 500 to 1 in 10,000 males, causing deficiency of coagulation factor VIII:C (hemophilia A), and in the case of Christmas disease, factor IX (hemophilia B). Although transmissible, it should be remembered that as many as one third of hemophilias are secondary to sporadic genetic mutations or deletions.

Pathophysiology

The initial bleed occurs in the synovium and extends into the joint space. Repeated hemorrhages cause ongoing irritation of the synovial lining, resulting in chronic synovitis. The hypertrophied synovium is hyperemic and more prone to injury, leading to a cycle of bleeding, synovitis, and further bleeding.

The hypertrophied synovial membrane causes progressive degeneration of the articular cartilage, commencing as fissuring and extending to erode the cortical and subchondral bone. The characteristic large subchondral cysts are thought to be secondary to the pannus and additional intraosseous hemorrhage rather than the invariable superimposed secondary osteoarthritis. Intra-articular blood, elevated intra-articular capsular pressure, and proteolytic enzymes released by leukocytes and inflamed synovium contribute further to cartilaginous and osseous erosion. Increased blood flow secondary to chronic synovitis causes periarticular osteoporosis (exacerbated by the immobility induced by the pain), epiphyseal overgrowth, and premature physeal closure.

The synovium becomes infiltrated by plasma cells and monocytes, followed by hemosiderin deposits and adhesions, leading to subsynovial fibrosis. The subsynovial fibrosis develops early and is later accompanied by intra-articular and capsular fibrosis, leading to joint contractures. Fibrosis within and around the joint further impairs cartilage nutrition.

In acute hemorrhages, the joint capsule may become distended with blood and diminish the range of motion.

In addition to spontaneous hemarthroses, 15 to 30% of hemophiliac bleeds are extra-articular, occurring along fascial planes, within muscle, and within bone. Intramuscular bleeds are most common in the quadriceps and iliopsoas muscles.

Clinical Findings

Repeated hemorrhage occurs more frequently into the joints than into the gastrointestinal or genitourinary tracts in patients with hemophilia. Most patients have their first hemarthrosis between 1 and 5 years of age. After the age of 10, bleeds occur less often. Typically, the same joint suffers the repeated hemorrhages.

With acute hemarthrosis, the patient complains of pain in the joint, which, on examination, is tense, red, and warm with a markedly decreased range of motion secondary to intra-articular blood and accompanying muscle spasm. There is usually a fever and elevated white cell count, raising the differential diagnosis of a septic arthritis. Joint aspiration, urgent Gram's stain, and culture and sensitivity are performed in this instance. The knee is most commonly affected, followed by the elbow, ankle, hip, and shoulder, in order of decreasing frequency.

In the setting of recurrent bleeds, flexion contractures are likely to develop, especially in the knees and elbows.

Not surprisingly, studies have repeatedly shown a poor correlation between physical examination and the extent of cartilaginous destruction demonstrated on MRI.

Stages of Disease

Hemarthroses usually begin in the first two decades of life. Each bleeding episode usually involves a single joint (70% of episodes are monoarticular). Over the course of the patient's lifetime, however, a few or several joints may be involved. The number of joints affected tends to stabilize by age 20.

Complications

ARTHROPATHY AND OSTEOARTHRITIS

- In the hip, osteonecrosis may occur, usually due to compromise of the blood supply secondary to increased intracapsular pressure. Protrusio acetabuli and secondary degeneration may occur secondary to the bone softening induced by hyperemia. Slipped epiphysis may occur secondary to hemorrhage into the growth plate. Coxa valga may result from delayed weight bearing.
- In the shoulder, hemarthroses may cause pseudosubluxation. Rotator cuff tears are common when there is accompanying glenohumeral joint degeneration.

PSEUDOTUMOR

A hemophiliac pseudotumor occurs in 1 to 2% of hemophiliacs. This is a chronic posthemorrhagic cystic collection of encapsulated hemorrhagic fluid within muscle and bone characterized by pressure, necrosis, and destruction. Pseudotumors arise secondary to intraosseous or subperiosteal hemorrhage or less often within the medullary cavity, giving the appearance of an expansile lytic process.

There are two distinct subtypes of pseudotumor, juvenile and adult forms. The juvenile form usually consists of multiple intramedullary expansile lesions without soft-tissue mass in the small bones of the hands or feet, occurring before epiphyseal closure.

The adult form is usually a single intramedullary expansile lesion with a large soft-tissue mass in the ilium or femur. Soft-tissue involvement of the retroperitoneum, psoas muscle, bowel wall, or renal collecting system may be seen.

These lesions are typically painless, expanding masses that may cause pressure on adjacent organs. Pseudotumors destroy soft tissue, erode bone, and cause neurovascular compromise and are most commonly found in the femur, pelvis, and tibia. They are usually asymptomatic until there is a pathologic fracture.

Hemorrhage into the growth plate may give rise to a limb length discrepancy. There may or may not be calcification associated. Osteonecrosis secondary to intraosseous hemorrhage may occur.

Pathology

GROSS

- Hypertrophic synovium
- Articular cartilage degeneration
- Erosion of cortical and subchondral bone
- Subchondral cysts
- Periarticular osteoporosis
- Epiphyseal overgrowth and premature physeal closure
- Subsynovial fibrosis develops early and is later accompanied by intra-articular and capsular fibrosis leading to joint contractures.
- Pathologically, pseudotumors are hematomas with thick, fibrous capsules caused by intraosseous, subperiosteal, or soft-tissue hemorrhage.

MICROSCOPIC

- Chronic hemosiderotic hypertrophic synovitis
- Pannus formation
- Synovial loss and replacement by fibrous bands stained with iron
- Marked iron staining of the eburnated bone

Imaging Findings

RADIOGRAPHY

Radiographic findings vary according to the stage of the disease. Arnold and Hilgartner have proposed a five-stage classification, which has proven useful in the assessment of the bony changes:

- *Stage 1* Soft-tissue swelling, joint effusion (dense and cloudy secondary to hemorrhage and, later, iron deposition), but bone and joint surfaces normal
- *Stage 2* Soft-tissue swelling accompanied by periarticular osteoporosis; epiphyseal overgrowth ± premature ossification of epiphyseal centers in the immature skeleton; joint integrity maintained
- *Stage 3* Persistent soft-tissue swelling, osseous erosion, sclerosis, hypertrophic osteophytes, and subchondral cysts; joint width space preserved
- *Stage 4* The osseous abnormalities of stage 3 are more marked and are accompanied by cartilaginous destruction with focal or diffuse joint space narrowing.
- *Stage 5* The joint is stiff and contracted, with advanced degenerative changes. There is severe joint space narrowing with bony erosion, multiple subchondral cysts, partial collapse of the articular surface, eburnation, and sclerosis of subchondral bone and osteophytosis.

In clinical studies, the Arnold-Hilgartner scoring has been shown to be a useful predictor of synovial hypertrophy, with sensitivity, specificity, positive predictive value, and negative predictive value of 100%, 100%, 100%, and 100%, respectively, for knees and 82%, 100%, 100%, and 82%, respectively, for ankles (this compares favorably with clinical symptomatology, which has sensitivity, specificity, and positive and negative predictive values for the knee of 100%, 78%, 78%, and 100%, respectively, and for the ankle 83%, 75%, 83%, and 75%, respectively).

Table 129–1 Pettersson Score (Radiograph: 0 to 13 Points)

Osteoporosis	Yes	1
Epiphyseal widening	Yes	1
Irregular subchondral bone surface	Incomplete: 1	Complete: 2
Joint gap	Gap > 1 mm: 1	Gap < 1 mm 2
Subchondral cysts	1 cyst: 1	More than 1 cyst: 2
Erosions of the joint's edges	Yes	1
Incongruence of the joint's edges	Slight: 1	Increased: 2
Joint deformity (i.e., dislocated)	Slight: 1	Increased: 2

The Pettersson scoring system (**Table 129–1**) was developed to provide a reproducible means by which arthropathy could be placed on a scale of severity. It can be used to assess the results of treatment in the individual and to allow standardization of reporting for research purposes.

Within the knee, there are distinct findings, such as widened intracondylar notch secondary to hemorrhage into the cruciate ligament attachment. Squaring of the inferior pole of the patella is thought to occur secondary to premature cessation of growth. Overgrowth of the patella may cause it to be elongated and thin.

Enlargement of epiphyses (36.1%) and an irregular subchondral surface (32.9%) are the most frequently seen findings, whereas osteoporosis (5.4%) is rarely seen. Varus or valgus deformities are common.

It is often said that JRA and hemophilia are radiographically indistinguishable. The classic findings of overgrowth of the ends of the bones (epiphyseal enlargement) and gracile diaphyses are common to both, although the latter are more common in JRA. As outlined above, joint destruction may or may not be present. Widening of the intercondylar notch is said to be classic for both JRA and hemophilia, but this has a further differential, including tuberculous arthritis.

A disused joint secondary to paralysis may mimic JRA and hemophilia. Some authors propose that the disuse common to JRA, hemophilia, and paralysis is the reason for epiphyseal overgrowth.

An uncommon intra-articular vascular tumor that may mimic a hemophilic joint is synovial hemangioma. This is seen in adolescent and young women, causing pain, swelling, and a diminished range of motion. The diffuse synovial proliferative form can present with intermittent pain, hemarthrosis, and increased limb length. The radiographic features are very similar to those of hemophilia, demonstrating joint space narrowing secondary to cartilage destruction, epiphyseal overgrowth, and synovial proliferation.

In the elbow, growth disturbances are common, with accelerated appearance of ossification centers and overgrowth at the radial head producing an enlarged trochlear notch. There may be pressure erosions of the radial notch of the ulna. Large osteolytic areas are common in the proximal ulna.

In the shoulder, cyst formation predominates on the humeral aspect of the joint (**Fig. 129D**).

At the ankle (where hemophilic arthropathy tends to be most severe), asymmetric growth of the distal tibia epiphysis causes it to slope downward medially, resulting in tibiotalar slant. The dome of the talus may be flattened. The posterior talocalcaneal joints are most often involved. There may be flattening and irregularity of the joint surface and widening or narrowing of the joint space. Widening of the sinus tarsi has been reported.

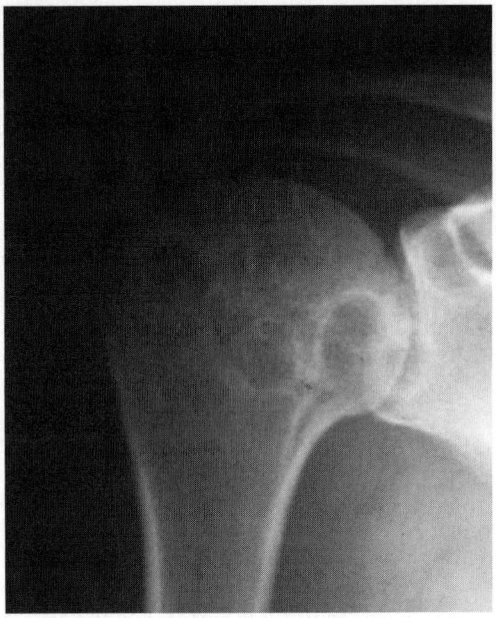

Figure 129D An AP shoulder radiograph shows marked subchondral cyst formation on the humeral aspect of the joint. A solitary cyst with a well-demarcated sclerotic margin is present on the glenoid aspect in its inferior half.

In the hip, concentric joint space narrowing has been described in association with chronic hemosiderotic synovitis, such as occurs in hemophilia; however, this is not a specific sign, as it occurs in rheumatoid arthritis, infective arthritis, and pigmented villonodular synovitis.

In the hands and feet, the metacarpophalangeal (MCP) and metatarsophalangeal (MTP) are most frequently affected.

Radiographically, a hemophilic pseudotumor is represented by a mixed cystic expansile lesion eroding adjacent bone with a variable soft-tissue mass. Pathologic fracture may be evident. Unresorbed hematoma may increase in size over time. Periosteal elevation with new bone formation at the edge of the lesion is common, as are internal calcifications.

ULTRASOUND

Ultrasound may be useful in the diagnosis of the acute hemarthrosis and to guide aspiration, particularly if synovial hypertrophy is marked. Sonography may also be useful in following the progression of soft-tissue hematomas.

COMPUTED TOMOGRAPHY

CT is rarely employed in the assessment of a hemophilic joint, although it may be useful in evaluating subtle bony erosion. CT is particularly useful, however, in the assessment of pseudotumor.

The central component of the lesion demonstrates low attenuation due to the presence of fluid or coagulant. There may be relatively higher attenuation at the periphery due to the variable fibrous capsule. Areas of calcification may be evident (**Fig. 129E**).

Secondary infection is a rare complication. Gas may be present secondary to infection or communication with a perforated intestine.

MAGNETIC RESONANCE IMAGING

The facility of MRI to demonstrate and stage the earliest (nonosseous) signs of arthropathy undetectable by physical examination or radiographs makes it the investigation of choice early in the presentation, when treatment is likely to be most beneficial.

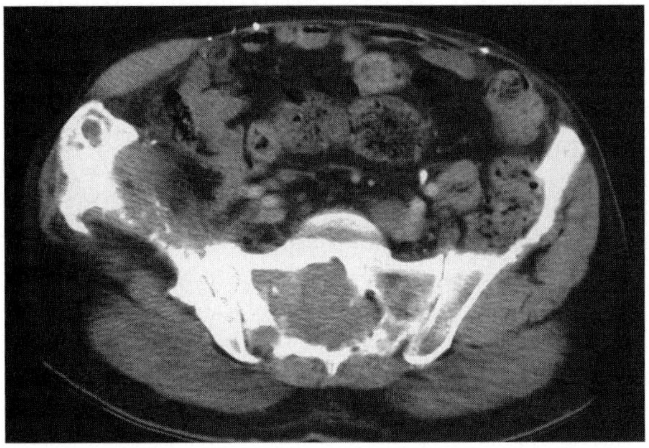

Figure 129E A transaxial CT image of the pelvis at the level of the iliac crests and first sacral vertebra shows three pseudotumors. The first occupies the midportion of the right iliac wing, which is eroded centrally and associated with a soft-tissue component anteriorly that contains scattered calcifications. Lateral to this is a second central intraosseous pseudotumor. Both of these lesions are associated with reactive sclerosis and osseous hypertrophy in the adjacent ilium. A third large pseudotumor has eroded a large quantity of bone in the right sacral ala, the S1 vertebral body, and extends as far as the left sacral foramen, which it partially occupies. Relative hyperdensity is visible within the right side of this sacral pseudotumor, consistent with hemorrhage occurring at a different time than in the rest of this lesion. Reactive sclerosis is present throughout the right sacrum.

MRI should also establish whether ongoing pain is secondary to recurrent hemorrhage or degenerate joint disease and, in postsynovectomy patients, will confirm or refute the recurrence of synovial hemorrhage and proliferation.

Similar to the Pettersson score for radiographs, numerous MRI scoring systems are in use. The NUSS variant is shown in **Table 129–2**. Studies comparing the various MRI scoring systems with the Pettersson scoring system, not surprisingly, show that increasing severity of hemophilic arthropathy is demonstrated at an earlier stage by MRI.

- Intra-articular hemorrhage usually has a nonspecific appearance of a large joint effusion. Although the effusion may be frankly hemorrhagic, most cases are in fact simple effusions.
- Fluid-fluid levels may be seen (secondary to hemorrhage of differing ages) and are most conspicuous on T2-weighted images.
- Intra-articular clot may be evident by the presence of areas of very low signal intensity within a joint effusion.
- Gradient-echo sequences may demonstrate subtle intrasynovial hemorrhage and hemosiderin deposition by the presence of magnetic susceptibility artifact (so-called blooming), in addition to synovial hypertrophy and cartilaginous destruction.

Table 129–2 Nuss Score (MRI: 0 to 13 Points)

Hemorrhage	
Slight	1
Moderate	2
Large	3
Hemosiderin	
Present	1
Synovial hypertrophy	
Slight	1
Moderate	2
Large	3
Subchondral cysts/erosion	
One cyst and partial surface erosion	1
> One cyst and partial surface erosion	2
> One cyst and complete surface erosion	3
Cartilage defects	
< 50%	1
≥ 50%	2
Complete	3

- It is thought that gadolinium-enhanced examinations may increase the sensitivity for the detection of early synovial hypertrophy before hemosiderin deposition occurs.
- Chronically thickened synovium returns intermediate to low signal intensity on T1-weighted and proton density images, and very low signal intensity on T2-weighted images.
- Subchondral cysts and chondral and osteochondral defects are all visible on MRI prior to radiography.

The subchondral cysts of hemophilia have been categorized using four progressive stages:

- *Stage1* Hemorrhagic cyst containing methemoglobin (high signal on both T1 and T2)
- *Stage 2* Nonhemorrhagic fluid (low on T1, high on T2)
- *Stage 3* Complex cyst with variable heterogeneous signal due to fluid, synovium, fibrous tissue, hemosiderin, and recurrent hemorrhage. Expansion of this cyst, leading to destruction of subchondral bone, may be due to increased marrow pressure, osmotic pressure, and intraosseous hemorrhage.
- *Stage 4* Fibrous tissue and hemosiderin predominate, producing low signal intensity throughout. Subchondral cysts of different stages may occur in the same bone.

A peripheral rim of low signal intensity on both T1- and T2-weighted images is more frequently seen in pseudotumors affecting solely soft tissues than in osseous pseudotumors, reflecting fibrous tissue and hemosiderin deposition. Although the center of the lesion is usually hyperintense, blood products of varying age and fluid-blood levels may be present, resulting in a more heterogeneous signal pattern. Peripheral nodules of heterogeneous signal intensity may be present, likely representing small hematomas from the most recent hemorrhage.

Treatment

Staging of the arthropathy, ideally by MRI, is important, because the appropriate therapy depends on the degree of synovial hypertrophy and cartilaginous destruction present.

Prophylactic replacement factor is the treatment of choice (now proven to be superior to on-demand therapy) and should be started when the number of hemarthroses is three or more. Plasma factor levels should be maintained at least above 1%. It has been shown that if prophylaxis is started in children between the ages of 1 and 3, hemophilic joint destruction does not occur. This treatment also greatly reduces the development of pseudotumors.

If untreated, or if undertreated, more than three bleeds per year invariably result in hemophilic arthropathy.

In the acute event, intravenous replacement of clotting factor (to 20 to 30% of normal or to > 50% if severe) is used to treat bleeding episodes. The use of recombinant clotting factors virtually eliminates the risk of transfusion-related disease, such as HIV.

Subsequently, physical therapy is used to prevent intra-articular fibrosis, maintain a functional range of motion, and prevent muscle atrophy.

In recurrent cases, the goal of treatment is to prevent hemarthrosis, consequently preventing progression of synovitis and its sequelae.

TREATMENT FOR CHRONIC SYNOVITIS

Corticosteroids

A 3- to 4-week course has been used to decrease synovial hypertrophy, resulting in temporary remission; however, synovial regrowth is quite likely when the steroids are withdrawn.

Nonsteroidal anti-inflammatory drugs

Used for acute pain and to reduce inflammation. Ibuprofen and Motrin are not recommended, as they are occasionally associated with increased bleeding.

Surgery, sclerotherapy, radiosynovectomy, and arthroplasty

Surgical synovectomy is indicated in cases of refractory synovitis and is effective in preventing hemarthrosis; however, rehabilitation is prolonged, and the functional outcome, in terms of range of motion, may be suboptimal. The latter problems are considerably reduced by the use of the arthroscopic approach, in addition to the lesser volumes of replacement factor required for the actual surgery itself.

An alternative to surgical synovectomy is percutaneous intra-articular sclerotherapy, using either chemical corrosives or radiotherapeutic agents.

Radiosynovectomy (P-32 colloid synoviorthesis) involves ^{32}P chromic phosphate injection into the joint (1.0 mCi [37.0 MBq] in adult knees and 0.5 mCi [18.5 MBq] in adult elbows). In a study with over 2 years of follow-up, 67% of patients were associated with improvement in range of motion, 80% with improvement in frequency of hemorrhage, and 80% with improvement in quality-of-life activities. Follow-up is required (at least 2 months) to exclude leakage from the joint. The liver also requires surveillance to detect systemic absorption.

Arthroplasty to replace end-stage joints must be undertaken by a surgeon with hemophilia experience, as the difficulties in exposure of the joint, diminished bone stock, joint deformities, quadriceps contracture, and adhesions make the procedure more complicated than in the nonhemophiliac population.

TREATMENT OF HEMOPHILIC PSEUDOTUMOR

In an acute bleed, procoagulation factor concentrate transfusion should be administered. Radiation therapy may be successful in destroying the friable vessels that bleed within the lesion. Embolization may occasionally be helpful in the treatment of symptomatic pseudotumors.

Prognosis

The number and degree of complications are directly related to the number and frequency of hemarthroses, and, consequently, to the severity of the underlying hemophilia. In the absence of treatment, most hemophilic joints will develop severe secondary osteoarthrosis, joint contractures, and severe disability.

Improved outcomes have been demonstrated in those patients receiving a larger amount of replacement factor than those regularly receiving smaller amounts on demand; in these patients starting regular replacement therapy at 2 to 3 years of age, hemophilic arthropathy did not occur.

Although slowed by synovectomy, joint degeneration invariably occurs over time. Hip arthroplasty typically results in good pain relief, but the complication rate is high. Aseptic loosening of cemented components is common secondary to microhemorrhages at the bone–cement interface. Arthroplasty failure or infection is treated with arthrodesis.

PEARLS

- When a joint appears to have advanced degenerative disease but has a relatively preserved joint space, hemophilic arthropathy should be considered (the clinical history may not be available or may not have been provided by the referring physician).
- On plain films, the effusion appears more radiodense than a nonhemorrhagic effusion.
- Gradient-echo sequences may demonstrate subtle intrasynovial hemorrhage and hemosiderin deposition by the presence of magnetic susceptibility artifact (so-called blooming), in addition to synovial hypertrophy and cartilaginous destruction.

PITFALLS

- Using plain film scoring systems such as the Pettersson system will underestimate the degree of synovial hypertrophy present, a crucial point in deciding the most appropriate treatment.
- All requests to biopsy or aspirate pseudotumors should be resisted strongly, as these procedures may lead to the formation of fistulous tracts, infection of the pseudotumor, and uncontrolled bleeding.
- MRI may not confidently differentiate between pseudotumor, abscess, or neoplasm, and the possibility of the latter entities must always be considered, even in the classic setting.

Suggested Readings

Abrahams TG, Pavlov H, Bansal M, Bullough P. Concentric joint space narrowing of the hip associated with hemosiderotic synovitis (HS), including pigmented villonodular synovitis (PVNS). Skeletal Radiol 1988;17:37–45

Arnold WD, Hilgartner MW. Hemophilic arthropathy. Current concepts of pathogenesis and management. J Bone Joint Surg Am 1977;59:287–305

Goldner BD. Osteolytic gluteal hematoma in hemophilia. Am J Roentgenol 1988;151:833

Hamel J, Pohlmann H, Schramm W. Radiological evaluation of chronic hemophilic arthropathy by the Pettersson score: problems in correlation in adult patients. Skeletal Radiol 1988;17:32–36

Hermann G, Gilbert MS, Abdelwahab IF. Hemophilia: evaluation of musculoskeletal involvement with CT, sonography, and MR imaging. Am J Roentgenol 1992;158:119–123

Hilgartner MW. Current treatment of hemophilic arthropathy. Curr Opin Pediatr 2002;14:46–49

Kulkarni MV, Drolshagen LF, Kaye JJ, et al. MR imaging of hemophilic arthropathy. J Comput Assist Tomogr 1986;10:445–449

Ng WH, Chu WC, Shing HK, et al. Role of imaging in management of hemophilic patients. Am J Roentgenol 2005;184:1619–1623

Nuss R, Kilcoyne RF, Geraghty S, et al. MRI findings in haemophilic joints treated with radiosynoviorthesis with development of an MRI scale of joint damage. Haemophilia 2000;6:162–169

Pettersson H, Ahlberg A, Nilsson IM. A radiologic classification of hemophilic arthropathy. Clin Orthop Relat Res 1980 in June;153–159

Siegel HJ, Luck JV, Jr, Siegel ME, Quines C, Anderson E. Hemarthrosis and synovitis associated with hemophilia: clinical use of P-32 chromic phosphate synoviorthesis for treatment. Radiology 1994;190:257–261

PART IX Protheses

CASE 130

Peter L. Munk, Anthony G. Ryan, and Laurel O. Marchinkow

Clinical Presentation

A 73-year-old woman presents with persistent pain in her left hip 18 months after total hip arthroplasty.

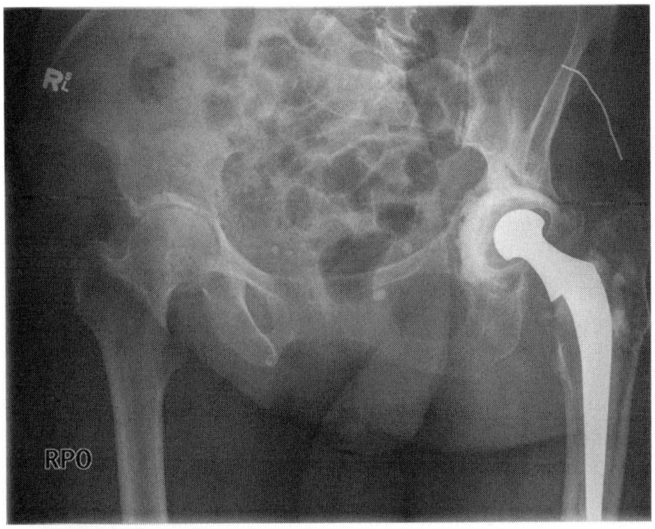

Figure 130A

Radiologic Findings

Left anterior oblique (LAO) radiograph (**Fig. 130A**) of the pelvis shows a lucent rim around the acetabular component at the cement–bone interface.

Diagnosis

Loosened acetabular component secondary to infection with an indolent organism.

Differential Diagnosis

- Sterile loosening
- Histiocytic response

Discussion

Etiology

The vast majority of arthroplasties are performed on the hip for chronic degenerative joint disease. Arthroplasty for smaller joints is more commonly performed to treat inflammatory arthropathies unresponsive to the best medical management and when function is severely limited.

Imaging Findings

RADIOGRAPHY

Hip

The most common arthroplasties are of the hip, and it is with these that the greatest experience has been accrued. A wide variety of different types of hip arthroplasty devices have been developed over the past several decades, and these are in constant evolution, with new types being introduced every year.

Metal, plastic, and ceramic are used in varying combinations and designs. The exact appearance and orientation of the arthroplasties varies from one design to the next; therefore, only certain broad generalizations can be made.

The acetabular component is normally anteverted, although some varieties are held in neutral position. The degree of anteversion requires measurement from a true lateral film. The femoral component is normally seated centrally within the medullary cavity of the proximal femur, although slight valgus orientation is frequently noted and considered acceptable.

Both acetabular and femoral components may be cemented or uncemented. Occasionally, one component may be cemented and the other uncemented. Uncemented components normally have a slightly corrugated surface due to the presence of numerous tiny beads adherent to the surface to promote bone ingrowth for long-term fixation.

A small amount of radiolucency between the bone and cement is a common finding, typically measuring 1 to 2 mm in width. In the long term, a thin radiodense line or neocortex between the cement and inner cortex may form, which should not be misinterpreted as loosening.

A small amount of resorption of bone at the medial calcar region, where the femoral stem rests against the medial cortex, is also common. This is due to a relatively reduced stress load on the cortex at this site, referred to as stress shielding (**Figs. 130B–130E**).

Knee

Knee arthroplasty is also frequently performed. The most common type of arthroplasty is a total knee arthroplasty, where both medial and lateral compartments of the knee are resurfaced. This may or may not include resurfacing of the patellar surface. Occasionally, a single compartment (medial or lateral) may be resurfaced if little disease is present in the opposite compartment.

Typically, both the femoral and tibial components have a peg projecting into the medullary space of the respective bone. Arthroplasties that have undergone revision, that is, second or third arthroplasties, typically have much longer stems to provide stability.

In most instances, a plastic tray is present on the tibial component that is of variable thickness, depending on the amount of bone that must be resected (**Fig. 130F**). A thicker plastic component helps maintain leg length, especially where there has been bone loss.

Shoulder

In the upper extremity, the most common type of arthroplasty is shoulder arthroplasty. This may consist of simply a humeral component, particularly in the case of complex proximal humeral fractures, or a total joint arthroplasty, where a resurfacing button is placed in the glenoid fossa of the scapula (more commonly used in patients with arthritis).

Because stability of the shoulder joint is provided largely by ligaments and tendons, the structures must be carefully assessed prior to performing an arthroplasty. The principal indication for shoulder arthroplasty is improvement of patient pain rather than improvement of joint function.

Commonly after arthroplasty, slight cranial displacement of the humeral component in relation to the scapula is noted, partly as a result of loss of bone in the upper scapula due to arthritic change. Marked cranial displacement usually reflects the presence of rotator cuff rupture.

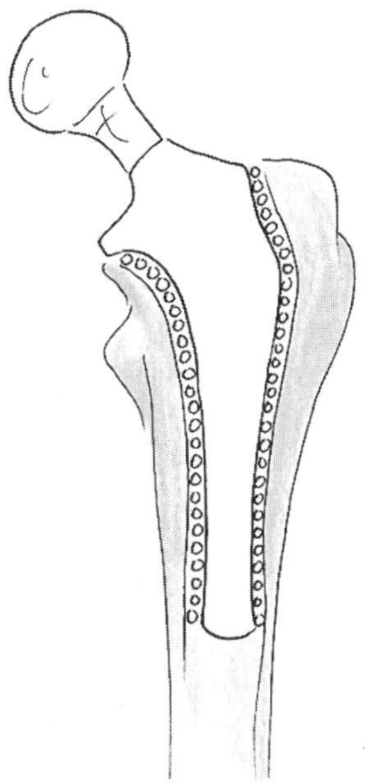

B

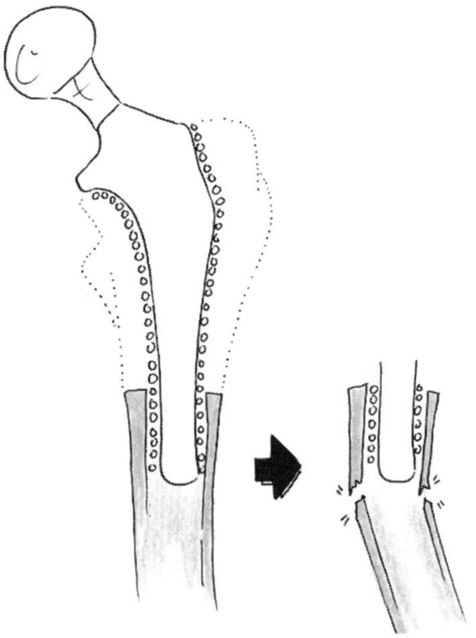

C

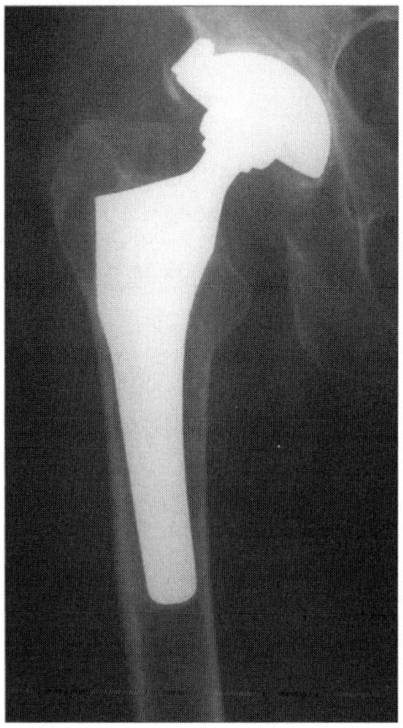

D

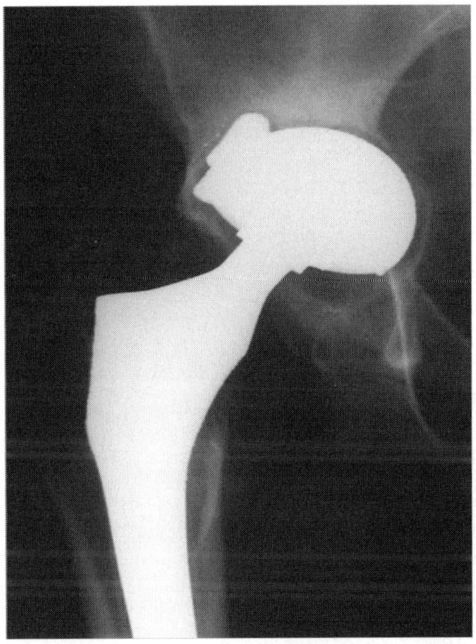

E

Figures 130B–130E 130B Stress shielding diagram shows the femoral component in place. **130C** Stress shielding diagram shows relative thinning of the femoral cortex, yielding a periprosthetic fracture at the level of the tip. **130D** Stress shielding. Relative osteoporosis of the medial femoral cortex is evident. **130E** Stress shielding. Relative osteoporosis and periprosthetic lucency around the acetabular component are consistent with stress shielding. (See also **Figures 130B** and **130C** in color insert.)

Other joints

Less common arthroplasties are noted elsewhere in the upper extremity, such as the elbow (**Figs. 130G,130H**), distal ulna, wrist, and carpal bones (**Figs. 130I–130M**), as well as the metacarpophalangeal joints (**Fig. 130N**).

The most common indication for this type of arthroplasty is arthritis, particularly rheumatoid arthritis or, in the case of carpal bones, trauma or avascular necrosis. In the case of many smaller bones or joints, the arthroplasty may employ a plastic or metal spacer or hinge rather than a complex joint device (**Figs. 130J–130L**).

Arthroplasties in the lower extremity below the knee are infrequently performed, although a few centers do perform ankle joint replacement (**Figs. 130O,130P**). These are technically challenging procedures with an unpredictable clinical outcome.

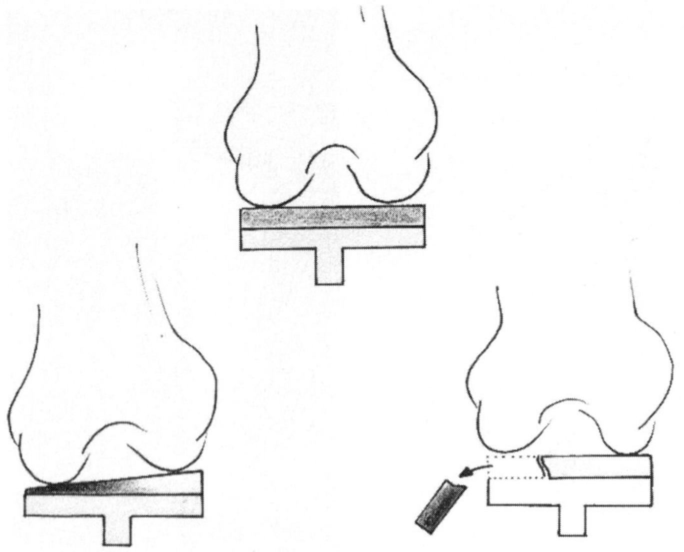

Figure 130F A line diagram shows various tibial liner morphologies (i.e., straight and beveled) and a diagrammatic example of fracture and displacement of one component of a liner.

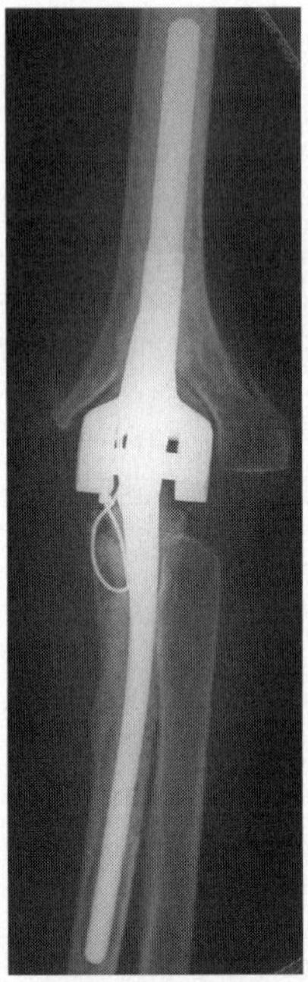

G

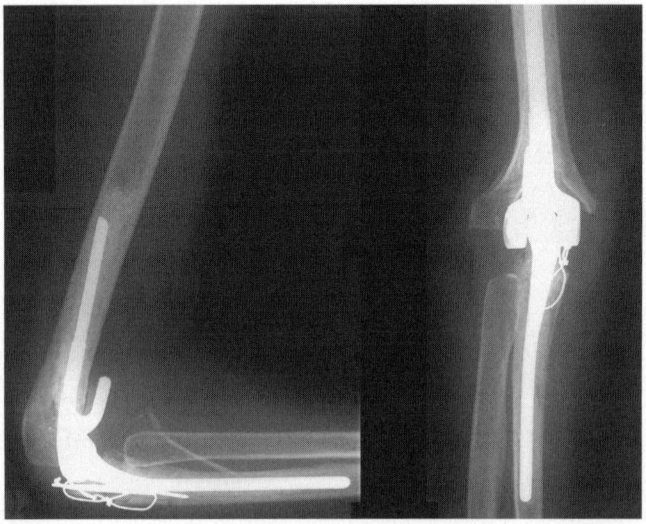

H

Figures 130G,130H **130G** An anteroposterior (AP) radiograph of the elbow shows a loosened ulnar component of a total elbow arthroplasty, as evinced by periprosthetic lucency. **130H** AP and lateral radiographs of the elbow show a loosened ulnar component of a total elbow arthroplasty, with an accompanying fracture of the proximal ulna (seen best on the lateral view).

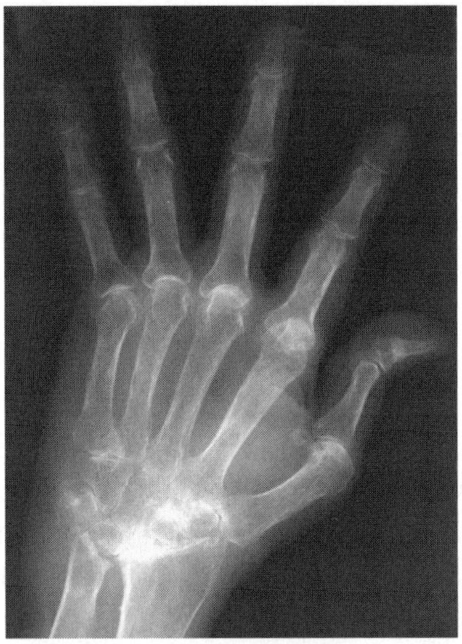
I

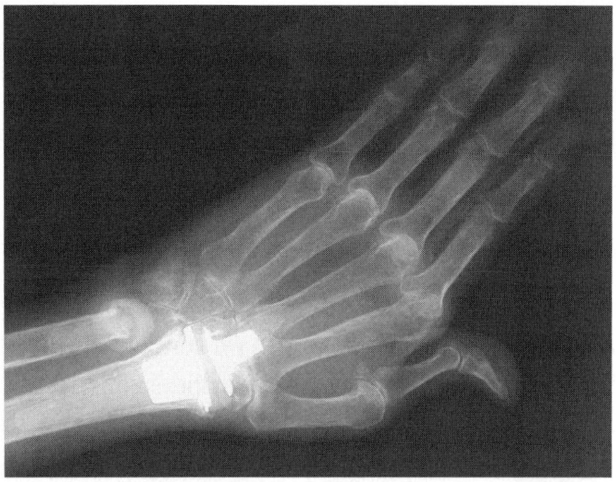
J

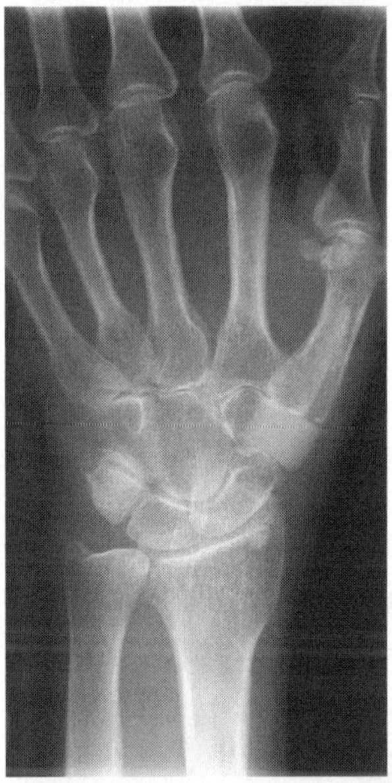
K

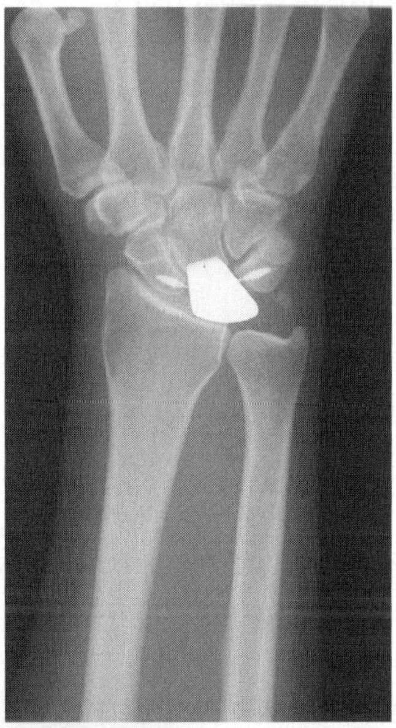
L

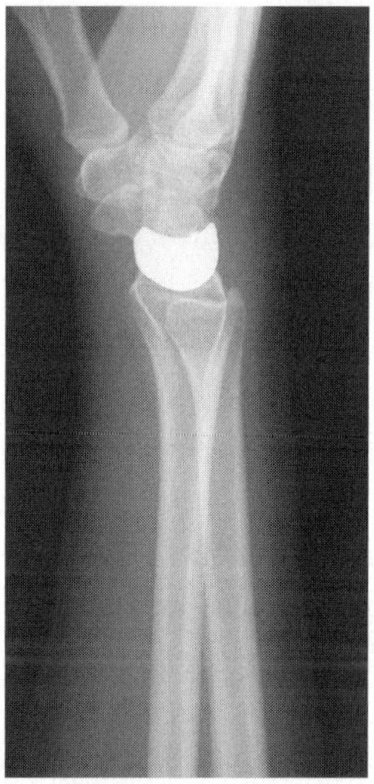
M

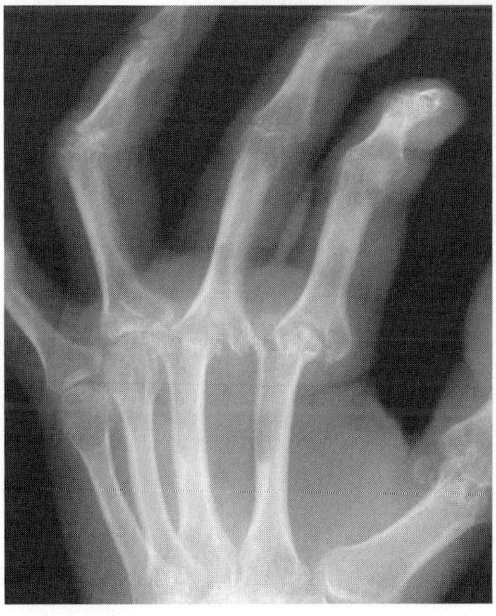
N

Figures 130I–130N **130I** Scapholunate advanced collapse (SLAC) wrist is seen on a preoperative AP radiograph. **130J** Postoperative AP wrist image shows a Silastic dome on the distal ulna and arthroplasty of the radiocarpal joint. **130K** An AP radiograph of the wrist shows a Silastic replacement trapezium. **130L** and **130M** AP (**130L**) and lateral (**130M**) radiographs of the wrist show a screw-fixated metallic replacement lunate. **130N** A dorsal oblique radiograph of the hand shows total Swanson arthroplasties of the second and third metacarpophalangeal joints in a patient with rheumatoid arthritis. Note the subtle components projecting into the shafts of the metacarpals and phalanges. The arthroplasties are subluxated.

Complications

TYPES OF ARTHROPLASTY FAILURE

A wide variety of different causes of arthroplasty failure exist, regardless of the joint involved. Most of the current experience in the management of these complications has been obtained through arthroplasty failure of hip and knee joints.

Mechanical loosening

This is the most common indication for arthroplasty revision. It is said to occur in 4 to 13% of hip arthroplasties and in 7 to 10% of knee arthroplasties. Despite marked patient symptomatology, imaging will at times demonstrate minimal, if any, findings.

Radiolucency at the bone–cement or cement–prosthesis interface of > 2 mm is a worrisome finding, particularly if this is increasing in width on serial examinations (**Figs. 130G,130H** and **130Q–130U**). It should also be noted that patients who have undergone revision arthroplasty will frequently demonstrate a radiolucent zone that is wider than this. Evidence of shifting in position or movement of the arthroplasty is a reliable indicator of mechanical loosening.

With noncemented arthroplasty, shedding of beads from the surface of the arthroplasty is also a reliable finding.

Nuclear medicine bone scanning is a helpful adjunct in assessment of failure on the basis of loosening.

Arthrography is a very insensitive method, although tracking of contrast between interfaces if demonstrated is diagnostic. The debris within the joint will often prevent tracking of contrast into these lucent interfaces.

Infection

Infection occurs in 1 to 4% of arthroplasties. One third of cases occur in the first 3 months following surgery, one third occur between 3 and 12 months, and one third occur more than 12 months after. Many patients with infected arthroplasties may be markedly symptomatic but demonstrate only minimal findings on imaging. This is because many patients with infections have a relatively indolent organism, which may not produce extensive destructive change (**Figs. 130V,130W**).

Rapidly progressive destruction of bone with formation of a sinus track occasionally occurs.

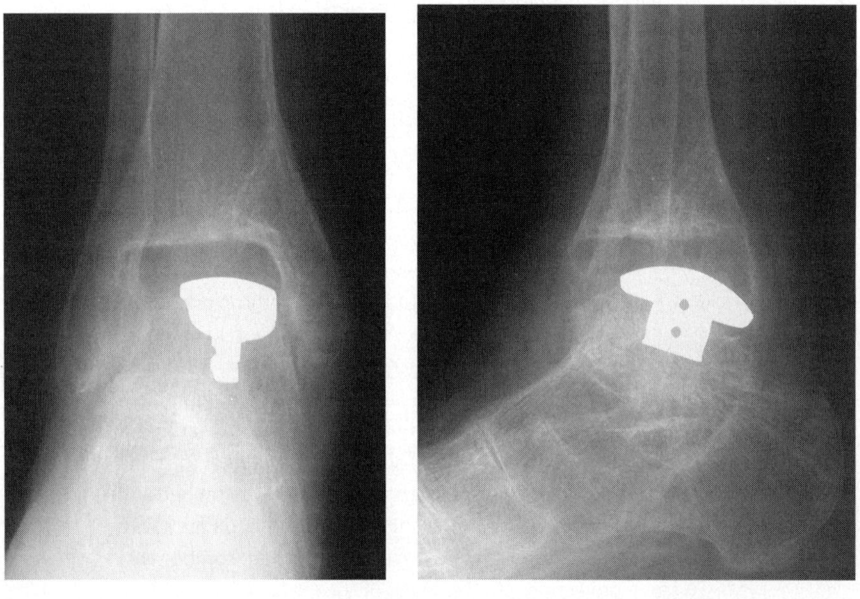

O P

Figures 130O,130P AP (**130O**) and lateral (**130P**) radiographs of the ankle show a total ankle arthroplasty consisting of a metallic talar stud and a plastic tibial plafond prosthesis.

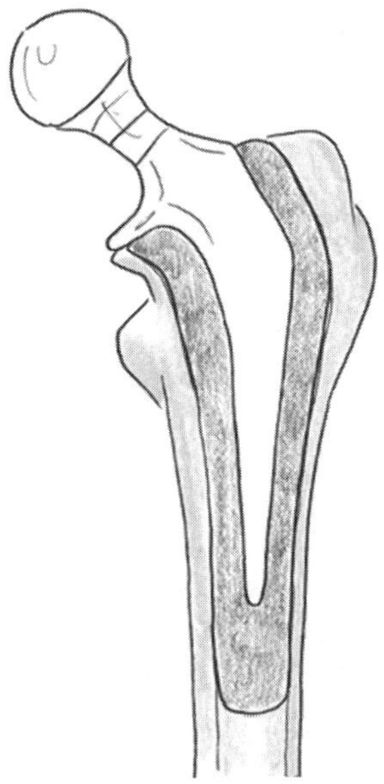
Q

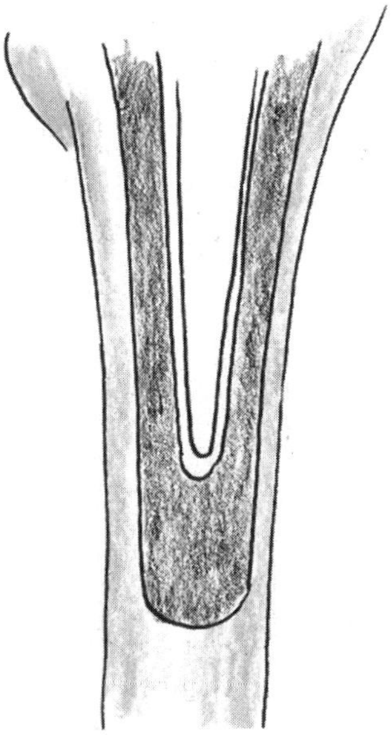
R

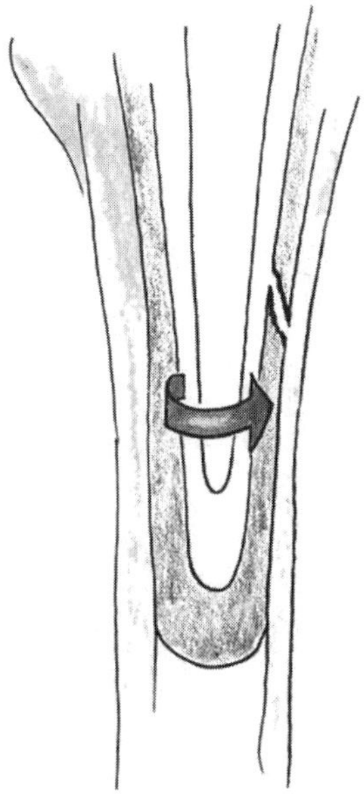
S

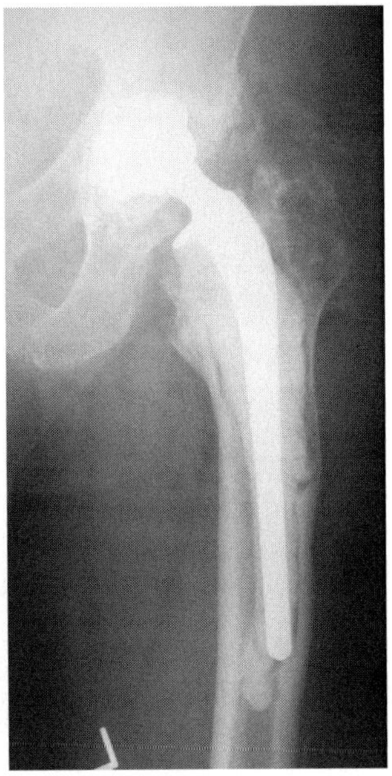
T

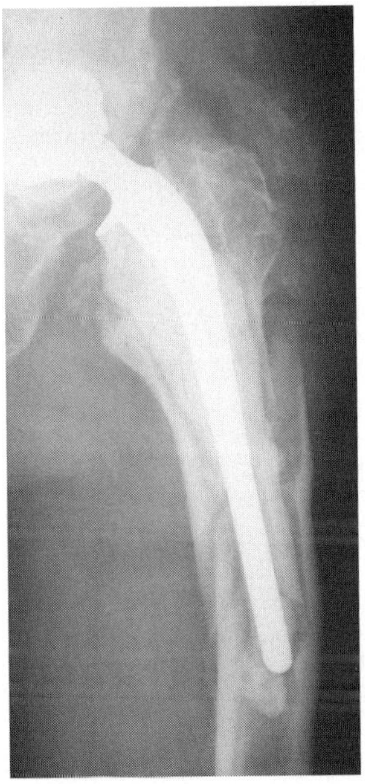
U

Figures 130Q–130U **130Q** Line diagram showing the expected immediate postoperative appearances of a cemented prosthesis, that is, close apposition of bone–cement and cement–prosthesis. **130R** Line diagram showing the interval development of lucency between the prosthesis and the cement. **130S** Line diagram showing how the increased periprosthetic space permits a degree of prosthetic movement, building considerable torque forces that can give rise to cement fractures, as shown. **130T** An AP radiograph of a total hip prosthesis shows loosening as in the diagrams above; however, in the radiograph, the lucency is evident at the bone–cement interface. Fractures of the cement at its caudal tip and at its lateral midpoint are present. **130U** The same hip as in **130T**, showing progression of the findings with fracture through the obviously thinned lateral cortex, extending obliquely from below the greater trochanter inferiorly to exit at the level of the tip of the femoral component. (See also **Figures 130Q**, **130R**, and **130S** in color insert.)

Nuclear medicine studies can be invaluable in establishing the presence of an infectious process in selected cases.

Often the only reliable way of determining whether infection exists is aspiration and culture of the joint. In many centers, this is routinely performed in the assessment of symptomatic arthroplasties prior to revision to exclude indolent infection.

Histiocytic response

Also known as cement disease, histiocytic response is the result of macrophage reaction to some component of the arthroplasty. It would appear that several different components may elicit this response, including components of the cement as well as the debris from plastic liners or metal.

Typically, lesions form scalloped radiolucencies around the components (**Fig. 130X**) and most frequently occur between 1 and 5 years after installment of the arthroplasty. At times, the appearance is indistinguishable from that of an infectious process. These lesions may loosen the device or significantly weaken bone, resulting in fracture.

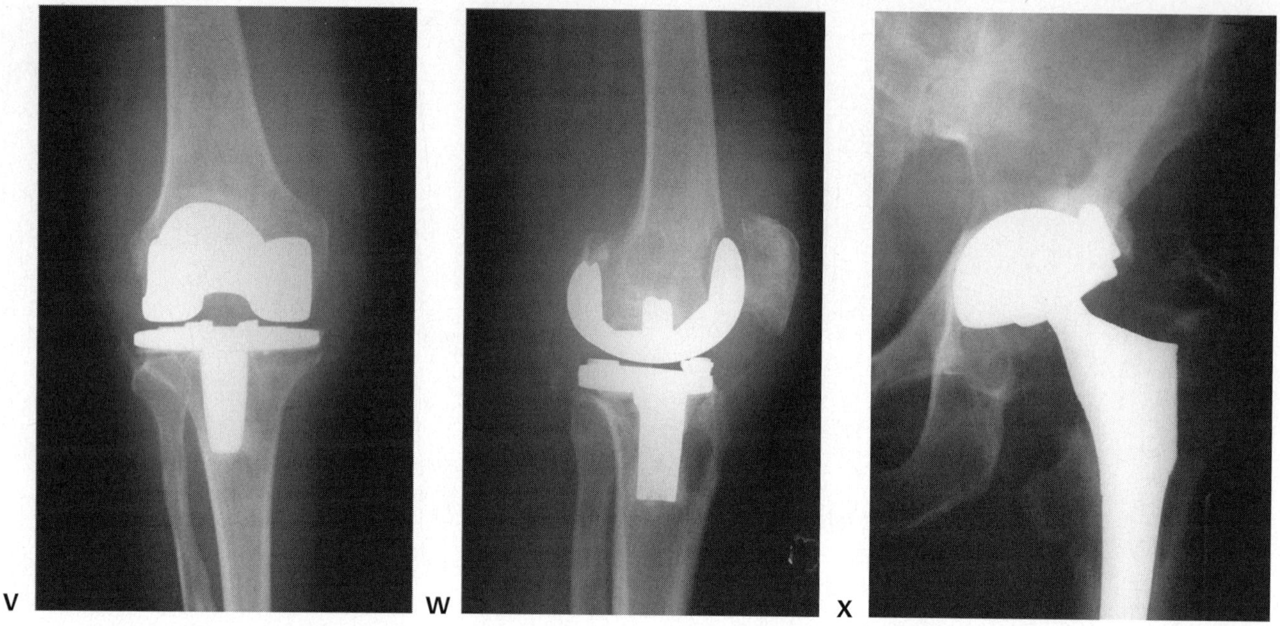

Figures 130V–130X AP (**130V**) and lateral (**130W**) radiographs of the knee (4 months after arthroplasty) in a patient with an infected total knee arthroplasty show multiple periprosthetic lucent foci (cephalad to the central stud of the femoral component, posterior to the anterior portion of the femoral component, anterior to the stem of the tibial component, and caudad to each of the horizontal portions of the tibial component). **130X** An AP radiograph of the left hip after total hip replacement shows a large lucency projected superior to the acetabular component, consistent with histiocytic granuloma.

Stress shielding

Placement of an arthroplasty alters the way in which stress is transmitted through bone, thereby altering the balance of absorption versus synthesis of bone. In areas where stress is unloaded, focal osteoporosis and resorption of bone can occur; this is frequently seen in the femoral component around hip arthroplasties (**Fig. 130B–130E**). Stress shielding can also lead to significant weakening and fracture of bone around the arthroplasty.

PSEUDOBURSAE

Pseudobursae form frequently around hip and knee arthroplasties and consist of irregular synovial recesses that communicate with the joint (**Figs. 130Y—130Z2**). Bursae in relation to the greater trochanter occur most frequently (50%), with supra-acetabular and iliopsoas bursae seen in 33% and 17%, respectively.

These can become inflamed and markedly symptomatic, and may contain large amounts of hemorrhage and other debris, preventing ready demonstration of their continuity with the joint on arthrography. Should these become infected, they may also communicate with the skin surface to produce a sinus track.

At times, a selective injection of the pseudobursa with steroids and Marcaine may significantly improve patient symptoms.

FRACTURES

Fractures can occur in the bone adjacent to arthroplasties, particularly in osteoporotic patients or patients who have stress shielding or infection. Patients may develop stress or insufficiency structures

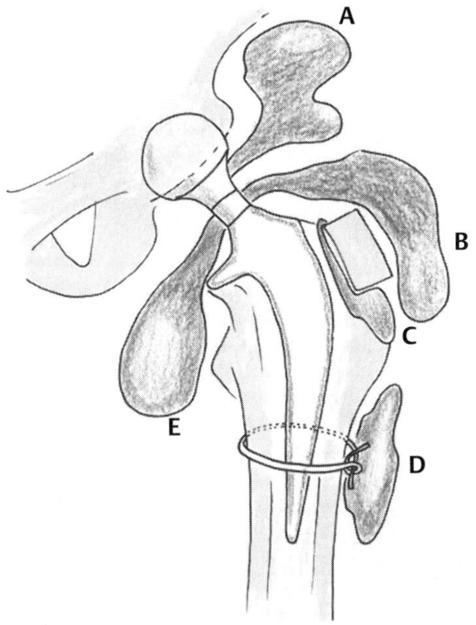

Y

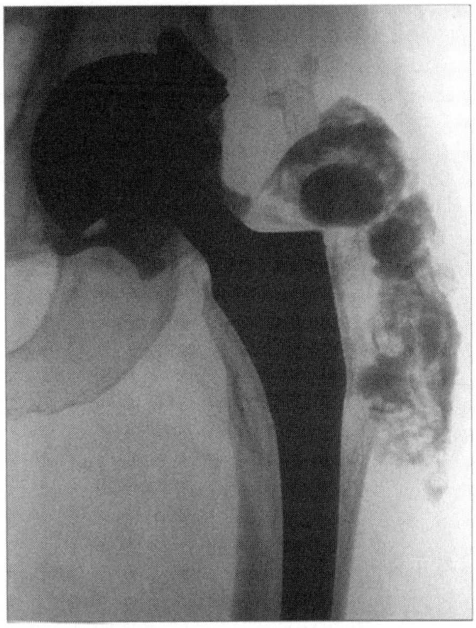

Z1

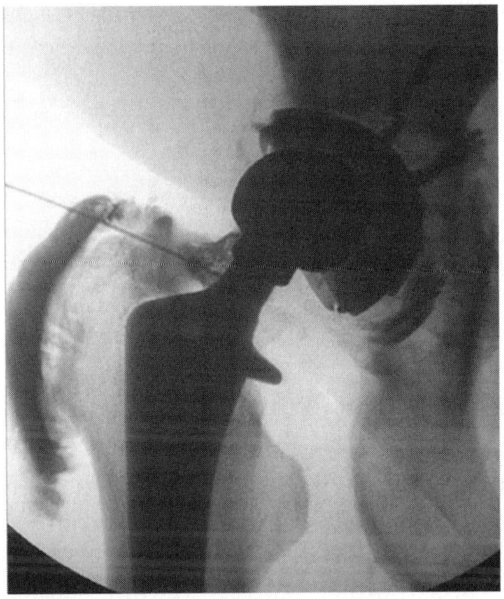

Z2

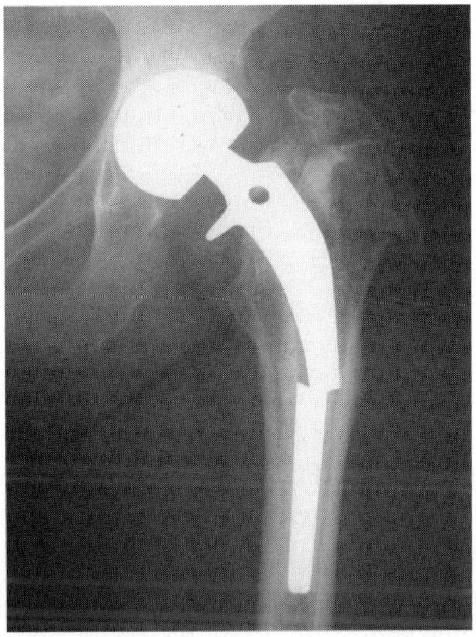

Z3

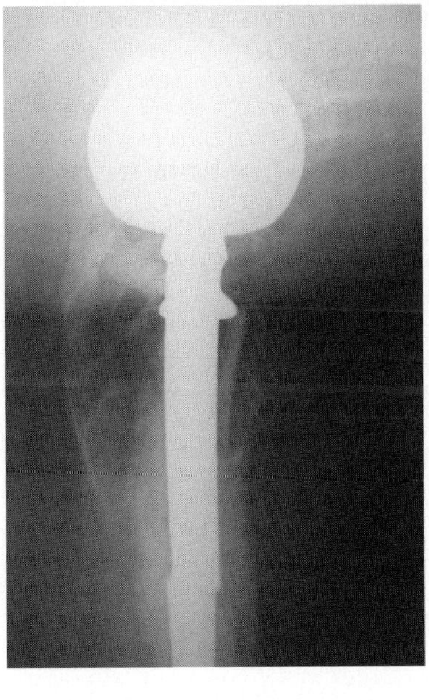

Z4

Figures 130Y–130Z4 130Y Line diagram showing the bursae and pseudobursae that may be seen on arthrography of a total hip arthroplasty. A, supra-acetabular; B, trochanteric; C, subtrochanteric; D, sutural; E, iliopsoas bursa. **130Z1** Exposure from arthrographic examination of painful arthroplasty shows a large lateral pseudobursa. **130Z2** Exposure from arthrographic examination of painful arthroplasty shows a large trochanteric bursa in communication with the joint. **130Z3** and **130Z4** AP (**130Z3**) and lateral (**130Z4**) radiographs show a fractured stem of a Thompson hemiarthroplasty prosthesis. (See also **Figure 130Y** in color insert.)

Z5
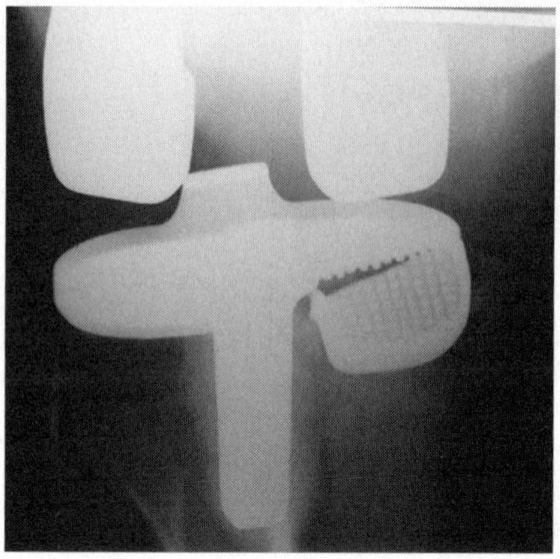
Z6
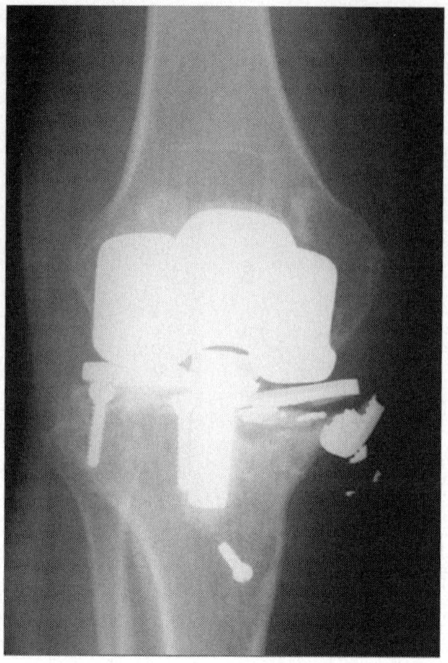
Z7
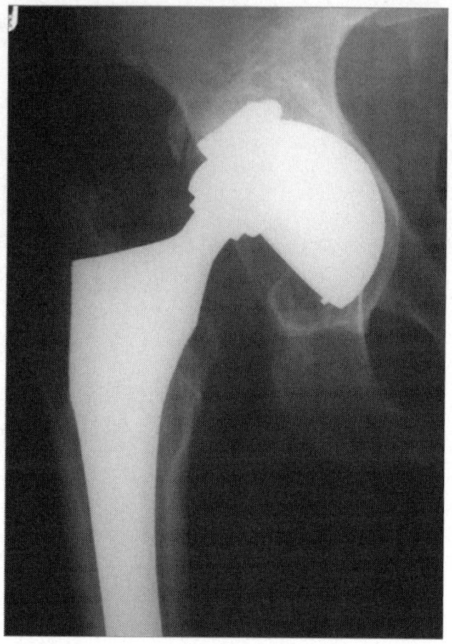

Figures 130Z5–130Z7 130Z7 An AP radiograph shows a simple fracture of the medial portion of a tibial component. **130Z6** An AP radiograph shows a shattered tibial component. **130Z7** Although the femoral head equivalent remains within the confines of the acetabular component, it is clearly internally displaced: this image shows a case of erosion of the acetabular liner with consequent subluxation.

in adjacent bone after placement of an arthroplasty, in part as a result of increased activity after treatment of a painful joint (**Figs. 130Z3–130Z6**).

Fractures of the components themselves can occur, at times related to severe or low-grade repetitive trauma or metal fatigue. Dissociation of components such as plastic liners from metal backing is also encountered. Displacement of a radiolucent component can at times be difficult to visualize on radiography and may be facilitated by injection of contrast within the joint. Malalignment of the metal components may suggest the diagnosis of a failed (**Fig. 130Z5**) or displaced plastic liner.

DISLOCATION OR SUBLUXATION

This may occur in any joint due to poor muscle tone and ligamentous laxity. Trauma or technical factors, such as malalignment of components, also may cause this.

Dislocation or subluxation may at times be subtle, and more than one projection is often required to confirm malalignment (**Figs. 130Z7—130Z11**).

METALLOSIS

Occasionally, plastic liners may displace, and chronic articulation of metal on metal may occur. Some arthroplasties are designed to articulate directly metal to metal. This may result in shedding of small amounts of metal into the joint on a chronic basis. Synovium inside the joint reacts to this and produces significant hypertrophy.

On radiography or cross-sectional imaging, increased density indicating the presence of metal within the contents of the joint may be apparent (**Figs. 130Z12,130Z13**).

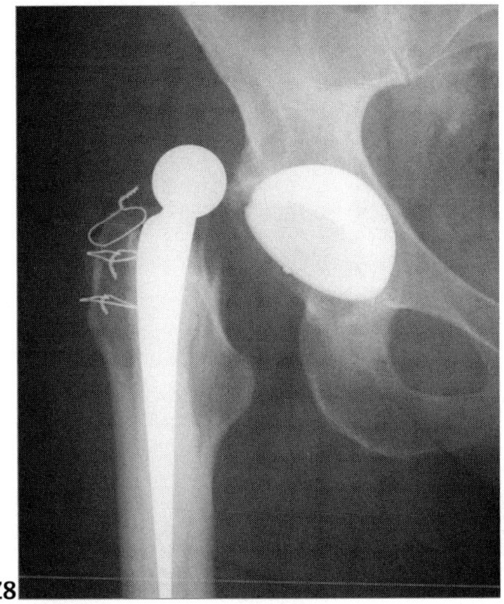

Z8

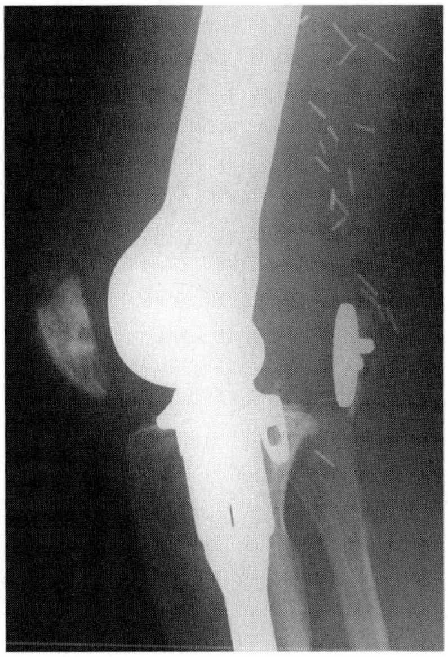

Z9

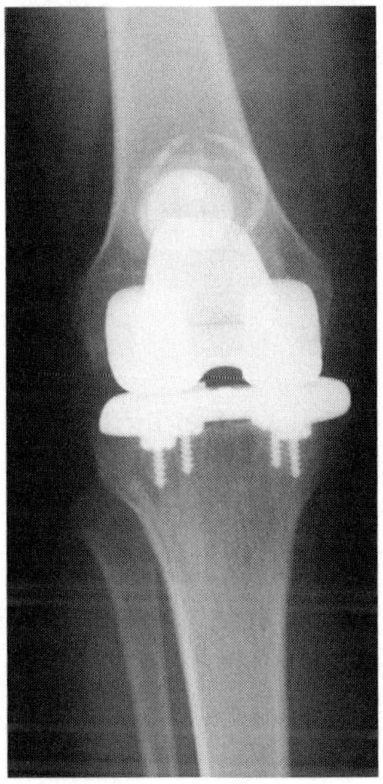

Z10

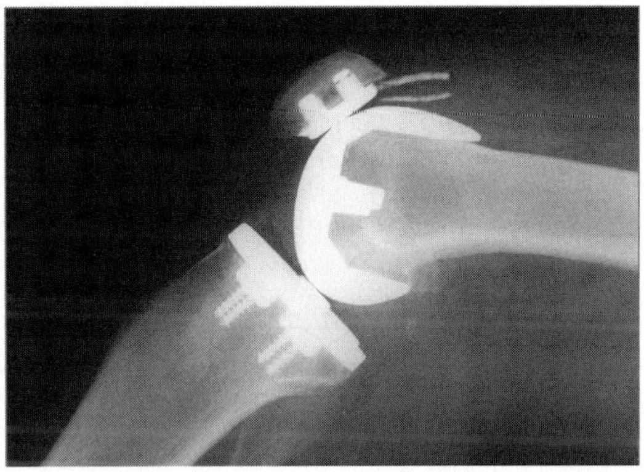

Z11

Figures 130Z8–130Z11 130Z8 An AP radiograph suggests subluxation. **130Z9** A lateral radiograph shows frank dislocation of the patellar component in a revised tricompartmental arthroplasty. The patellar disk is seen projected through the posterior capsular space, but it should obviously be apposed against the shaved posterior patellar surface. **130Z10** and **130Z11** AP (**130Z10**) and lateral (**130Z11**) radiographs of a tricompartmental arthroplasty show a displaced patellar liner as a circular density that assumes an almost tramline configuration on the lateral projection.

PEARLS

- Radiolucency at the bone–cement or cement–prosthesis interface $>$ 2 mm is a worrisome finding, particularly if this is increasing in width on serial examinations. Although this distance may increase in the initial 6 to 9 months after surgery, any increase after this should be viewed with suspicion.

Z12
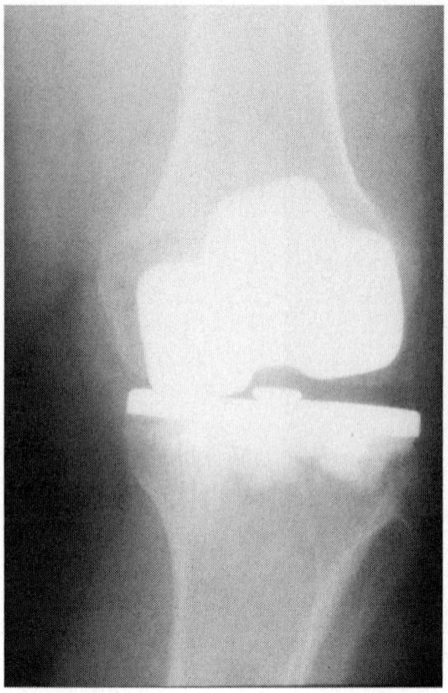
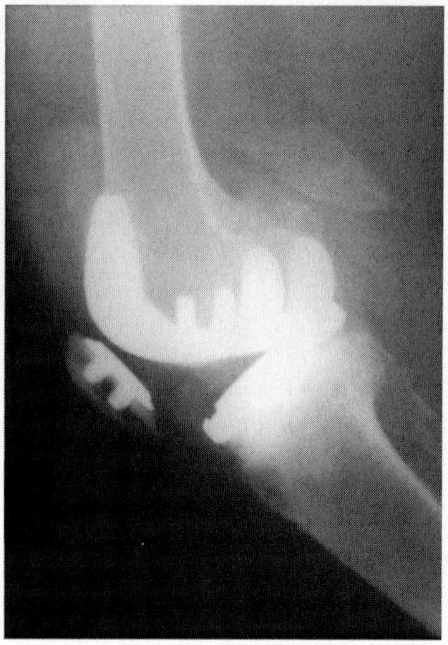
Z13

Figures 130Z12,130Z13 AP (**130Z12**) and lateral (**130Z13**) radiographs show a knee with a tricompartmental arthroplasty. The medial portion of the tibial liner has become displaced (as in **130Z6**), allowing metal-on-metal articulation, resulting in metallosis. Diffuse increased density and linear increased density in the capsular recesses are evident within the joint space, indicating the presence of articular metal particles.

- Commonly after arthroplasty, slight cranial displacement of the humeral component in relation to the scapula is noted, partly as a result of loss of bone in the upper scapula due to arthritic change. Marked cranial displacement usually reflects the presence of rotator cuff rupture.
- Prevention of metallosis is possible if the prosthetic joint is surveyed routinely and liner displacement is recognized soon after the event.

PITFALLS

- It should be noted that patients who have undergone revision arthroplasty will frequently demonstrate a radiolucent zone at the bone–cement or cement–prosthesis interface that is wider than 2 mm. Progression after 9 months postsurgery remains suspicious.
- Increased activity on a standard radionuclide bone scan is expected around the prosthesis for up to 9 months after surgery; activity after this is suspicious for loosening/infection.
- Gallium 67 radionuclide scanning is less accurate than the combination of a bone scintigram and indium 111 labeled white blood cell scanning. The latter has a sensitivity of between 50 and 100% and specificity of between 45 and 100%.

Suggested Readings

Gelman MI, Dunn HK. Radiology of knee joint replacement. Am J Roentgenol 1976;127:447–455

Goergen TG, Dalinka MK, Alazraki N, et al. Evaluation of the patient with painful hip or knee arthroplasty: American College of Radiology. Radiology 2000; 215(S):295–298

Keogh CF, Munk PL, Gee R, Chan LP, Marchinkow LO. Imaging of the painful hip arthroplasty. Am J Roentgenol 2003;180:115–120

Pritchard RW. Total elbow joint arthroplasty in patients with rheumatoid arthritis. Semin Arthritis Rheum 1991;21:24–29

Slawson SH, Everson LI, Craig EV. The radiology of total shoulder replacement. Radiol Clin North Am 1995;33:305–318

Wiseman BN. Imaging of the total hip replacement. Radiology 1997;202:611–623

INDEX

Page numbers followed by *f* or *t* indicate materials in figures or tables, respectively.

O